QUANTITATIVE ANALYSIS

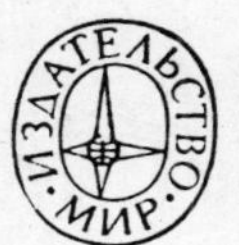

В. АЛЕКСЕЕВ

КОЛИЧЕСТВЕННЫЙ АНАЛИЗ

ИЗДАТЕЛЬСТВО
«ХИМИЯ»
МОСКВА

V. ALEXEYEV

QUANTITATIVE ANALYSIS

Translated from the Russian
by
E. UVAROV

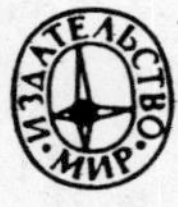

Mir Publishers Moscow

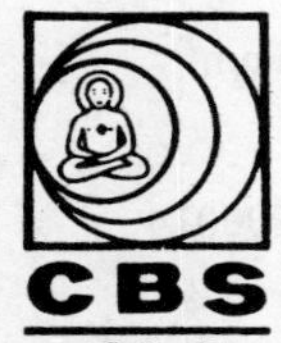

CBS Publishers & Distributors Pvt. Ltd.

New Delhi • Bengaluru • Chennai • Kochi • Kolkata • Mumbai
Hyderabad • Nagpur • Patna • Pune • Vijayawada

ISBN: 81-239-0293-X

First Indian Edition: 1994
Reprint: 1998, 2004, 2005

This edition has been published in India by arrangement with
Mir Publishers, Moscow

Published by **Satish Kumar Jain** and produced by **Varun Jain** for
CBS Publishers & Distributors Pvt. Ltd.,
4819/XI Prahlad Street, 24 Ansari Road, Daryaganj, New Delhi - 110002
delhi@cbspd.com, cbspubs@airtelmail.in • www.cbspd.com
Ph.: 23289259, 23266861, 23266867 • Fax: 011-23243014

Corporate Office: 204 FIE, Industrial Area, Patparganj, Delhi - 110 092
Ph: 49344934 • Fax: 011-49344935
E-mail: publishing@cbspd.com • publicity@cbspd.com

Branches:
- ***Bengaluru:*** 2975, 17th Cross, K.R. Road, Bansankari 2nd Stage, Bengaluru - 70 • Ph: +91-80-26771678/79 • Fax: +91-80-26771680 E-mail: cbsbng@gmail.com, bangalore@cbspd.com
- ***Chennai:*** No. 7, Subbaraya Street, Shenoy Nagar, Chennai - 600030 Ph: +91-44-26681266, 26680620 • Fax: +91-44-42032115 E-mail: chennai@cbspd.com
- ***Kochi:*** Ashana House, 39/1904, A.M. Thomas Road, Valanjambalam, Ernakulum, Kochi • Ph: +91-484-4059061-65 Fax: +91-484-4059065 • E-mail: cochin@cbspd.com
- ***Kolkata:*** 6-B, Ground Floor, Rameshwar Shaw Road, Kolkata - 700014 Ph: +91-33-22891126/7/8 • E-mail: kolkata@cbspd.com
- ***Mumbai:*** 83-C, Dr. E. Moses Road, Worli, Mumbai - 400018 Ph: +91-9833017933, 022-24902340/41 • E-mail: mumbai@cbspd.com

Printed at:
J.S. Offset Printers, Delhi (India)

CONTENTS

EDITORIAL NOTE

The author of this book, Vladimir Nikolayevich Alexeyev, was born in 1888 and died in 1958.

He started his practical and teaching work in the field of analytical chemistry in 1915. During the many years of his teaching activity he wrote a number of textbooks on analytical chemistry for universities and technical colleges. Besides his *Quantitative Analysis*, the books *Qualitative Analysis*, *Course of Qualitative Chemical Semimicroanalysis* and *Course of Analytical Chemistry* are well known.

In each of these books Alexeyev strove to give new facts discovered by science and to give new analytical methods, experimentally verified (in most cases by himself).

Alexeyev's books have won deserved recognition among students and teachers of analytical chemistry. He was always distinguished by his ability to present in simple language, logically and lucidly the fundamentals of theory and practice of analytical chemistry. Alexeyev's books have been and are being used by thousands of students, and many analytical chemists use them in their practical work.

The present book is a sequel to the author's *Qualitative Analysis* and *Course of Qualitative Chemical Semimicroanalysis.* Therefore it does not deal with many theoretical questions, which are fully discussed in these books, at equal length in a course of quantitative analysis. In all such instances merely a brief mention is made of the relevant principles and results, with a reference to the appropriate sections in the textbooks of qualitative analysis.

Exceptions are made in discussion of the theoretical principles of activity, the salt effect (Sec. 20) and oxidation potentials (Sec. 78). These subjects are the most difficult for students and, moreover, they are often considered only in courses of quantitative analysis.

The author's aim was to correlate theory with the practice of analysis and, as in the textbooks of qualitative analysis, to make the theory easily understood by students.

The question of physico-chemical methods of analysis and their place in a course of quantitative analysis is a very serious problem. Only two such methods are considered in detail in the book: colorimetry (visual) and electrogravimetric analysis. Conductometry, potentiometry, polarography, and photocolorimetry are considered only in outline, without descriptions of the methods or examples of determinations.

CHAPTER I

INTRODUCTION

1. The Subject of Quantitative Analysis

Analytical chemistry is divided into two parts, qualitative analysis and quantitative analysis. Qualitative analysis shows what elements (or ions) a given substance contains. The aim of quantitative analysis is determination of the quantitative contents of individual elements or compounds present in a substance.

Analytical results are usually expressed in percentages. For example, in analysis of calcium carbonate it is found what percentages of calcium, carbon and oxygen it contains. In view of the fact that $CaCO_3$ may be regarded as a compound of calcium oxide CaO with carbonic anhydride CO_2, the composition of this salt is also often expressed in percentages of the oxides CaO and CO_2.

Sometimes the determination of the total contents of individual elements (or their oxides) in a sample is insufficient and it is also necessary to know in the form of what compounds these elements are present and what the relative proportions of these compounds are. For example, carbon may be present in ferrous alloys both in the free state, as graphite, and in the combined state, in the form of carbides. The properties of an alloy greatly depend on the form in which carbon is present. Therefore, in addition to the total carbon content the amounts of free and bound carbon in an alloy are also sometimes determined. In the same way, in analysis of clays or bauxites in addition to the total contents of SiO_2, Al_2O_3, Fe_2O_3, chemically bound water, etc., it is also necessary to find how much SiO_2 is present as quartz and how much in the form of various silicates. Determination of individual compounds present in a given substance is known as *phase analysis*. In phase analysis the compound to be determined is first separated (for example, by making use of different behaviour towards solvents or differences of various physical properties) from other compounds of the same element present in the substance, and the compound is then analysed.

Analytical chemistry, including quantitative analysis, is of enormous importance in science and industry. For example, the chemical formula of an unknown substance is found from the percentage contents of its constituents, found by analysis. Chemical analysis is a most important method of investigation and is widely used in all branches of science which are related to chemistry. For example, it is of great importance in mineralogy, geology, physiology, microbiology, and medical, agricultural and technical sciences. Chemical analysis is no less important in industry. The technologist must know at every stage of the production process both the qualitative and the quantitative composition of the materials undergoing conversion. For example, a furnace charge in the production of cast iron or glass can be made correctly only if the composition of the charge materials is known; for most efficient leather tanning the contents of tanning materials in the extracts must be known, etc.

At the present time no material is taken into production or released without analytical data which characterize its quality and suitability for various purposes. These results not only form the basis of all the processing calculations but they also determine the costs of the materials, which form the basis of financial estimates.

Analysis of intermediate products (for example, smelting control in metallurgy, etc.) is of enormous importance. The technologist uses the results of such analysis for the most efficient utilization of the raw material, for prevention of troubles in the course of the process and therefore for prevention of spoilage.

The great importance of proper chemical control of production is obvious. Therefore, in nearly every factory one of the most important sections is the analytical laboratory for chemical control of production.

When quantitative analysis is undertaken, the qualitative composition of the given substance must be accurately known; qualitative analysis must be used even if the presence of a particular element in the substance is definitely known, because the correct method for quantitative determination of the element in question can be chosen only if the qualitative composition of the substance is known.

In practice, however, the analyst's problem is usually simplified considerably, because the qualitative composition of most of the investigated substances (ores, alloys, fertilisers, etc.) is well known. Approximate contents of individual elements are also quite often known.

Obviously, in such cases not only is preliminary qualitative analysis unnecessary, but the choice of the most suitable method of quantitative analysis becomes very much easier.

2. Methods of Quantitative Analysis

The same ionic reactions as are used in qualitative analysis are generally utilized in quantitative analysis. For example, chlorine (or, more correctly, chloride ion) is determined quantitatively by precipitation by silver ions:

$$Cl^- + Ag^+ = AgCl$$

Chlorine content may be determined by various methods on the basis of this reaction. For example, the precipitated AgCl can be filtered off, washed thoroughly, carefully heated (or dried) and accurately weighed. From the weight of the AgCl precipitate and its formula it is easy to calculate its chlorine content.

Thus, in the analysis of 0.0536 g NaCl the precipitate weighed 0.1290 g; since one gram-molecule (i.e., 143.3 g) AgCl contains one gram-atom (i.e., 35.45 g) Cl, we can write:

143.3 g AgCl contains 35.45 g Cl
0.1290 g AgCl contains x g Cl

$$x = \frac{0.1290 \times 35.45}{143.3} = 0.03192 \text{ g Cl}$$

Since all the chlorine was originally present in the weighed samples of common salt (NaCl) the percentage chlorine content of the latter is easily found:

0.0536 g NaCl contains 0.03192 g Cl
100 g NaCl contains y g Cl

$$y = \frac{0.03192 \times 100}{0.0536} = 59.6\%$$

This method is known as *gravimetric analysis*, because the weight of the reaction product is used for finding the amount of an element present.

The amount of chlorine in common salt can also be found in another way, by means of *titration*, i.e., measurement of the volume of a reagent solution ($AgNO_3$) of accurately known concentration, required to precipitate the Cl^- ions. These two quantities—the volume and the concentration of the reagent solution—are quite sufficient to calculate the chlorine content of the substance. For example, if 18.00 ml of $AgNO_3$ solution 1 ml of which contains 0.0085 g of this salt was required to precipitate all the chlorine in a solution of a weighed sample in water, then obviously the amount of $AgNO_3$ taken for the whole reaction is 18.00 × 0.0085, i.e., 0.1530 g. The equation for the reaction

$$NaCl + AgNO_3 = \downarrow AgCl + NaNO_3$$

shows that to precipitate one gram-ion (i.e., 35.45 g) of Cl one gram-molecule (i.e., 169.9 g) of $AgNO_3$ is required. Therefore we can write:

Precipitation of 35.45 g Cl takes 169.9 g $AgNO_3$
Precipitation of x g Cl takes 0.1530 g $AgNO_3$

$$x = \frac{0.1530 \times 35.45}{169.9} = 0.03192 \text{ g Cl*}$$

* Other and more convenient calculation methods will be considered later. They are discussed in Sec. 56.

Then, as before, it only remains to calculate the percentage of chlorine in the samples.

The method based on accurate measurement of the volume of a reagent solution of accurately known concentration, taken for a reaction, is known as *volumetric analysis.*

In volumetric determinations it is evidently necessary to establish exactly the end point of the reaction; this is not always possible. Moreover, the reaction itself must satisfy a number of conditions, and therefore the applicability of volumetric analysis is more restricted than that of the gravimetric method. An important advantage of the volumetric method is its greater speed, which is very important in practice, as for example in chemical control of production.

Reactions accompanied by colour changes are often used in qualitative analysis. For example, when the Fe^{+++} ions are detected by means of NH_4CNS or KCNS, soluble iron thiocyanate $Fe(CNS)_3$ of a deep red colour is formed:

$$FeCl_3 + 3NH_4CNS = Fe(CNS)_3 + 3NH_4Cl$$

This reaction can also be used in quantitative analysis. By this method the unknown solution and a "standard solution", i.e., a solution of a ferric salt of accurately known concentration, are treated with NH_4CNS or KCNS under the same conditions. If both solutions give the same colour, then the content of Fe^{+++} must also be the same. If the colour of the unknown solution is deeper (or less deep) than that of the standard, then the concentration of Fe^{+++} ions in it must be higher (or lower) than that of the standard.* The analytical method based on comparison of colour intensities is known as *colorimetric analysis.*

Instead of reactions involving colour changes, reactions accompanied by formation of sparingly soluble substances are sometimes used. The amount of a given element in solution is estimated from the degree of turbidity of the solution produced by some reagent or other, compared with the turbidity of a corresponding standard solution. Methods based on this principle are known as *nephelometric.*

Colorimetric (and nephelometric) determinations are possible only if the colours (or turbidities) of the solutions are not too intense. Extremely dilute solutions are used for such determinations. In practice the colorimetric and nephelometric methods are most commonly used when the content of the unknown element in the material is very low and therefore the gravimetric and volumetric methods are unsuitable. Colorimetric methods are also used widely because of their high speed.

---

* This is only true for fairly dilute solutions. The eye cannot distinguish differences between intensely coloured concentrated solutions.

Several other methods are used in quantitative analysis. For example, we must mention *gas analysis*, which generally consists in determining the volumes of individual components in a gas mixture, for example, by absorption in various reagents. The decrease of the gas volume is a measure of the absorbed component. There are also volumetric methods of gas analysis, in which the amount of an element is found by measurement of the volume of gas formed in a reaction. For example, carbon in iron or steel is usually determined from the value of CO_2 formed in combustion of a weighed sample in a current of oxygen at 1000-1250°C in a special electric furnace.*

Electrogravimetric analysis is widely used (especially for analysis of non-ferrous metals and alloys). In this method the element (in the free state) is isolated by electrolysis on a previously weighed electrode (certain elements are liberated in electrolysis in the form of oxides, such as MnO_2 or PbO_2). The increase in the weight of the electrode shows the amount of the element liberated.

There are also methods of *electrovolumetric analysis*, which are based on the usual principle of volumetric determinations (see above) but the end point of the reaction is established either by measuring the electrical conductivity of the solution (*conductometric method*), or by measuring the potential of an electrode immersed in the solution (*potentiometric method*). The electrochemical methods also include the so-called *polarographic method*. In this method the amount of an element (or ion) in a solution is estimated from the character of the volt-ampere curve (or "polarogram"), obtained in electrolysis of the solution carried out in a special apparatus known as a polarograph.

Mention must also be made of analytical methods based on the use of *labelled atoms*, i.e., radioactive isotopes of the elements to be determined. The fact that these isotopes are radioactive, while their properties are identical with the properties of the corresponding stable isotopes, makes it possible to use counters which measure various radiation intensities. It is then very easy to solve problems which are very difficult and sometimes impossible to solve by the usual analytical methods. The following example illustrates this. In order to find how phosphorus is distributed between metal and slag in the smelting of steel, calcium phosphate containing the radioactive phosphorus isotope with a half-life of 14.3 days is introduced into the smelting furnace. Samples of metal and slag are taken

* To measure the volume of CO_2 formed, the gas mixture $CO_2 + O_2$ leaving the furnace is passed through a concentrated KOH solution which absorbs CO_2; the reaction proceeds according to the equation:

$$2KOH + CO_2 = K_2CO_3 + H_2O$$

The decrease in the volume of the gas mixture shows the amount of CO_2.

during the smelting and their radioactivity is determined by means of a counter. This gives a rapid and easy answer to the problem of the distribution of phosphorus between steel and slag, and the factors on which this distribution depends. The labelled atom method is extremely sensitive which is another of its valuable characteristics.

Another method used in analytical practice is the *chromatographic method*. This is based on selective adsorption of dissolved substances or ions by various solids (adsorbents), such as aluminium oxide, permutite, various synthetic resins, etc. Chromatography is particularly valuable for separation of various substances or ions. Experience shows that even slight differences in the composition or structure of substances are usually enough to cause considerable differences in their adsorption. Because of this the chromatographic method can be used for separating substances which are so similar in properties that they cannot be separated by other methods or are only separated with great difficulty.

All the above methods of quantitative analysis can be divided into *chemical* and *physico-chemical methods*. The former group includes gravimetric, volumetric and gas analyses and the second group includes colorimetric, nephelometric, electrochemical and chromatographic analyses.

In addition there are *physical methods* of quantitative determination, such as quantitative spectroscopic analysis, luminescence analysis, etc.

Both in quantitative and in qualitative analysis a distinction is made between macro-, micro-, and semimicromethods.

In *macroanalysis* relatively large samples (about 0.1 g or more) of solids or large volumes (tens of millilitres or more) of solutions are taken.

The essential instrument for this method is the analytical balance, which can be used for weighing to an accuracy of 0.0002 g (or 0.2 mg).

In addition to the macromethod, micro- and semimicromethods of quantitative analysis are coming into increased use. In these methods samples weighing between 1 mg and 50 mg and solution volumes between tenths of a millilitre and several millilitres are used.

In such cases, to obtain the necessary accuracy it is necessary to use a more sensitive balance, such as a microbalance (accurate to 0.001 mg) and more accurate apparatus for measurement of solution or gas volumes. The main advantages of the micro- and semimicromethods are their high speed and the need for only very small amounts of material. Despite these advantages the classical macromethod, which is the oldest and the most convenient method of quantitative analysis is the one most widely used at the present time.

Only the methods of quantitative macroanalysis are considered in this book.

3. The Analytical Balance

The balance is the principal instrument used in quantitative analysis. The analytical results obtained by any method must be referred to a definite quantity of the given substance; for example, as a percentage of its weight. Therefore, the first stage in analysis is usually to weigh out a definite portion (sample) of the substance for investigation.

Weighing is also used in other operations of quantitative analysis; for example, to find the weight of a precipitate, to prepare solutions of accurately known concentration, etc.

One of the most important requirements in quantitative analysis is a sufficiently high degree of precision. The required degree of precision depends on the purpose of the analysis and may differ in different cases. In analytical work of moderate precision the error usually does not exceed a few tenths of one per cent of the quantity measured. This degree of precision must be reached with relatively small samples, as work with large amounts of substance is inconvenient and very time-consuming. On the other hand, with small samples the required degree of precision can only be obtained if the accuracy of weighing is high enough.

The analytical balance used in quantitative macroanalysis can be used for weighing objects not heavier than 100-200 g to a precision of 0.0002 g, i.e., 0.2 mg.

The most usual design of a balance of this type is shown in Figs. 1 and 2.

The most important part, the beam, has three knife edges made of agate or very hard steel (*1* and *2*, Fig. 2*a*). The central knife edge rests on a special very smooth agate plate on top of the balance column. The balance pans are suspended from the terminal knife edges by means of ***stirrups*** (Fig. 2*b*).

A pointer *3* (Fig. 1) is fixed to the centre of the beam; as the balance swings the lower end of the pointer moves along the scale *9*, at the bottom of the column. All three knife edges must be strictly parallel and in the same plane for correct operation of the balance; furthermore, the precision of weighing on an analytical balance depends to a considerable extent on the sharpness of the three knife edges and the smoothness of the plates on which they rest.

The knife edges and plates gradually wear out and the balance becomes less precise. To reduce wear as much as possible the balance is provided with an *arrest device* whereby the balance beam can be raised and the balance "arrested". When the balance is arrested the knife edges do not touch their plates. The arrest knob *2* (Fig. 1) is attached to the underside of a glass or marble slab on which the balance column and case are mounted. The balance must be arrested when not in use.

Sharp jerks and movements cause particularly serious wear of the balance. Therefore, *great care is necessary when using an analytical balance: in particular, the balance must never be touched when it is*

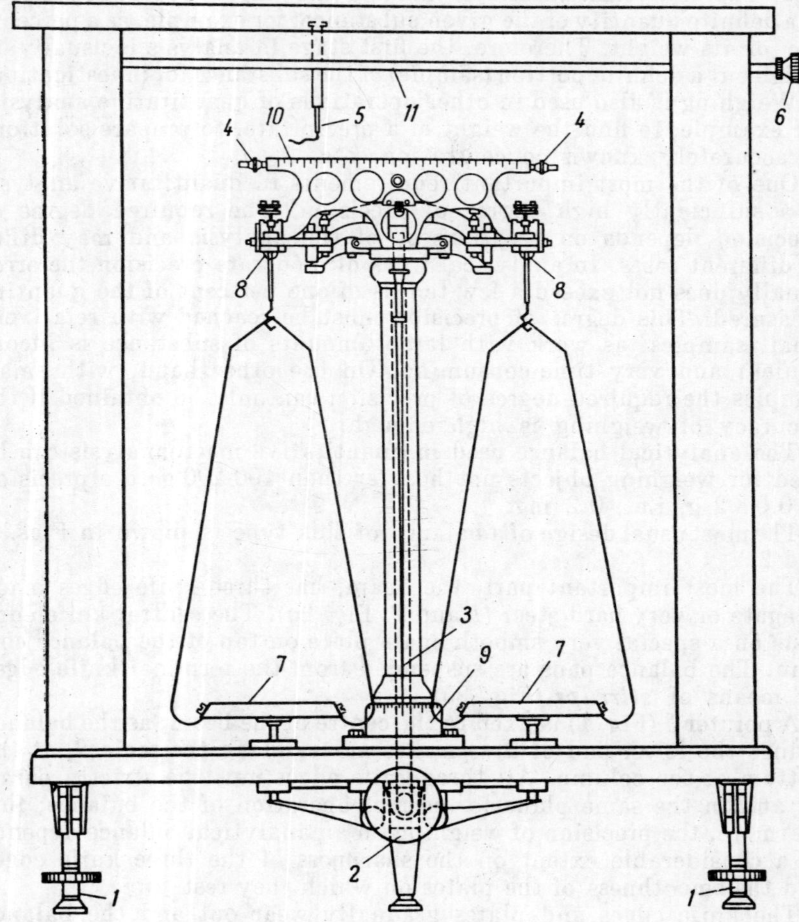

Fig. 1. Analytical balance

1—adjusting screws; *2*—arrest knob; *3*—pointer; *4*—screws for zero point adjustment; *5*—rider hook; *6*—knob of rider carrier; *7*—balance pans; *8*—stirrups; *9*—scale; *10*—graduated beam; *11*—rider carrier

free to swing. The balance must always be arrested before the weighed object or weights are put on or taken off the pans. Sharp jerks must also be avoided during the actual arresting. The arrest knob is turned carefully and smoothly, and this movement is made when the pointer approaches the centre of the scale.

The balance is enclosed in a glass case which protects it from dust, air movements, the operator's breath, etc.

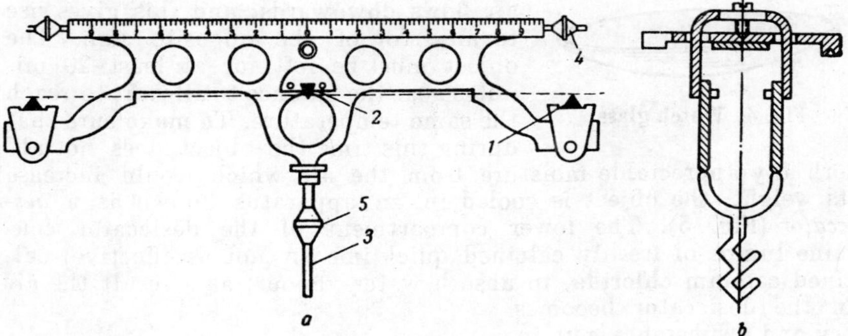

Fig. 2. Parts of analytical balance:
a—beam; *b*—stirrup. *1*—terminal knife edge; *2*—central knife edge; *3*—pointer; *4*—screw for zero point adjustment; *5*—weight for sensitivity adjustment

The base of the balance rests on screws *1* (Fig. 1), whereby the knife edges and agate plates on which they rest are brought into horizontal position by means of a plumb bob attached to the balance column (at the back). These knife edges and plates must be strictly horizontal for proper operation of the balance.

The balance pans *7* are made of some light metal which is nickel-plated or coated with gold or platinum to prevent oxidation. Obviously substances should never be put directly on the balance pans because this spoils the balance. Neither is it permissible to put substances on pieces of paper, as is usually done in weighing on less accurate technical balances. The reasons are, first, paper is hygroscopic and, second, it is impossible to transfer all the substance from it without loss into the vessel where it is to be dissolved (some of the substance always remains on the paper). Therefore, substances are weighed either in special weighing bottles with ground-glass lids (Fig. 3), or on watch glasses (Fig. 4), or in crucibles, test tubes, etc.

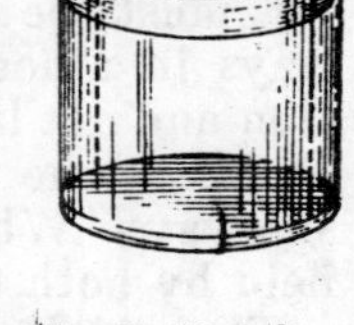

Fig. 3. Weighing bottle

For the results of weighing to be accurate the weighed object must be of the same temperature as the balance. If a hotter (or colder) object is placed on a balance pan, this has the effect of lengthening (or shortening) the corresponding arm of the beam resulting in incorrect readings. Moreover, a hot object warms the air in contact with it and makes it rise. The moving air pushes the corresponding balance pan upwards, and therefore the error is increased further. Conversely, if a cold object is weighed a current of air flows downwards, and this gives rise to an error of the opposite sign. The object must be left for at least 20 minutes near the balance to allow it to reach the same temperature. To make sure that during this time the object does not absorb any appreciable moisture from the air which would increase its weight, the object is cooled in an apparatus known as a *desiccator* (Fig. 5). The lower compartment of the desiccator contains lumps of freshly calcined quicklime or (not as effective) calcined calcium chloride, to absorb water vapour; as a result the air in the desiccator becomes dry and a substance put in the upper compartment (on the porcelain plate shown on the right of the diagram) does not absorb water vapour as it cools.

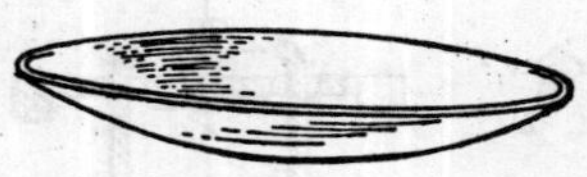

Fig. 4. Watch glass

The ground-glass rim of the desiccator lid must be thoroughly greased with a thin layer of petroleum jelly melted together with beeswax or paraffin wax. To open the desiccator the lid must be moved sideways in a horizontal direction and not lifted upwards. In the same way to close the desiccator the lid is gradually slid on sideways. When the desiccator is carried about the lid must be held by both thumbs, as otherwise it may fall and break.

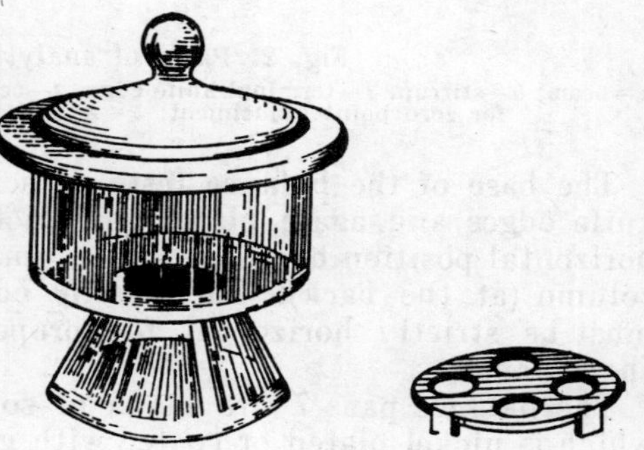

Fig. 5. Desiccator and porcelain plate

The weights used with analytical balances are contained in a special box (Fig. 6) which also contains a pair of forceps for lifting the weights and putting them on and off the balance pans. The forceps should be ivory-tipped. *The weights must never be touched by hand.*

The weights are coated with gold or platinum to prevent corrosion and consequent changes of weight. The small weights (fractions of a gram) are made of some metal which is not corroded in air, for example, aluminium or platinum.

The weights are arranged in the box in definite order. There are two usual systems corresponding to the numbers 5 : 2 : 2 : 1 or 5 : 2 : 1 : 1 : 1. In accordance with the first system the box would contain weights of 50, 20, 20, 10, 5, 2, 2, 1 g, and in accordance with the second, weights of 50, 20, 10, 10, 10, 5, 2, 1, 1, 1 g. Fractions of a gram follow the same systems and are made of different shapes so that small weights are easier to distinguish. For example, fractional weights with the figure 5 (i.e., 0.5 and 0.05 g) are made in the shape

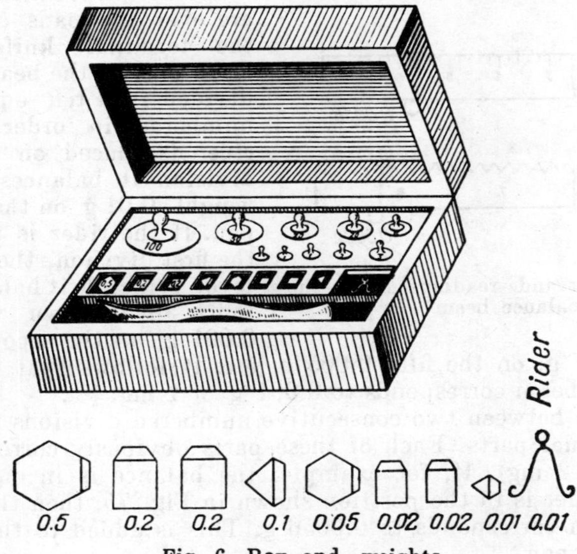

Fig. 6. Box and weights

of regular hexagons, weights with the figure 2 (i.e., 0.2 and 0.02 g) are squares, and weights with the figure 1 (i.e., 0.1 and 0.01 g) are triangles. Each fractional weight has an edge bent at right angle by which it is lifted with the forceps.

When a weighing is finished each weight must be put in its proper place in the box. If this rule is strictly obeyed it is possible to check the weights first by the empty spaces in the box, and then as each weight is removed from the balance and is put back into the box. This checking is absolutely essential as any error made in counting the weights spoils the entire analysis which may take several days.

By means of the weights an object can be weighed to an accuracy of 0.01 g. Thousandth and ten-thousandth fractions of a gram are weighed by means of the so-called *rider*.

The rider (Fig. 7*a*) is a thin bent wire (usually aluminium) weighing 0.01 g or 0.005 g; it is attached with the aid of the forceps by its loop on the hook *5* (Fig. 1). This hook is fixed to the horizontal rod *11* with the knob *6* outside the balance case. This rod is rotated or moved to place the rider at any desired point on the beam.

The beam has a scale *10* the graduations of which differ in different balances.

In the most usual type of balance the zero division is exactly over the fulcrum (i.e., over the central knife edge), and the tenth divisions are over the pans (i.e., over the terminal knife edges). Each arm of the beam is thus divided into ten equal parts numbered in order. If the rider is placed on the tenth division it balances its own weight, 0.01 g on the opposite pan. If the rider is placed on the first division, then, by the lever principle it balances one-tenth of its own weight or 0.001 g, on the second it balances 0.002 g, on the fifth 0.005 g, etc. It follows that each division on the beam corresponds to 0.001 g or 1 mg.

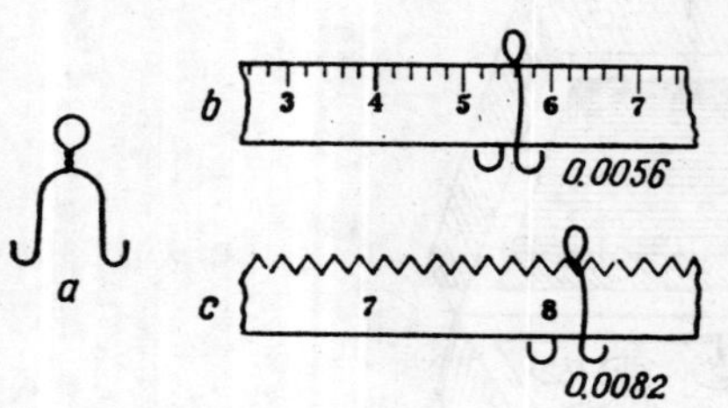

Fig. 7. Rider and readings along the balance beam

The space between two consecutive numbered divisions is divided into five equal parts. Each of these parts obviously corresponds to 0.0002 g (0.2 mg). If, for example, the balance is in equilibrium when the rider is in the position shown in Fig. 7*b*, then the reading on the beam corresponds to 0.0056 g. This is added to the weights on the scale pan.

In another type of balance the zero of the scale is not in the centre of the beam but over the left-hand knife edge. The tenth division is over the right-hand knife edge, and the fifth division is above the balance pivot. Here the distance between the divisions is twice as much as in balances with a central zero. It is therefore possible to divide each division into ten parts and not five, so that the precision of the beam readings is doubled.

For convenience the beam in this type of balance is notched, so that each notch corresponds to a small scale division. The rider in a balance of this type weighs 0.005 g (5 mg) and not 0.01 g. The balance is so adjusted as to be in equilibrium in the unloaded state when the rider is on the zero division of the scale.

Obviously, if the rider is moved from the zero division to the fifth (i.e., exactly over the central knife edge), this is equivalent to removal of 0.005 g from the left-hand pan or a similar increase of the load on the right-hand pan. In the same way, if the rider is moved to the tenth division this is equivalent to a further increase of 0.005 g on the right-hand pan, which makes a total of 0.01 g. Therefore in a balance of this type each large scale division (numbered) corresponds to 0.001 g (1 mg). The small divisions (of which there are twice as many as in balances with central zero) obviously correspond to 0.0001 g and not 0.0002 g.

Therefore, if the balance is in equilibrium with the rider in the position shown in Fig. 7*c*, then the beam reading is 0.0082 g.

4. Sensitivity, Stability, Accuracy and Precision of the Balance

The scale division at which the pointer comes to rest is known as the *zero point* when the pans are empty, and the *rest point* with a load on the balance.* In weighing these points must coincide; this shows that the loads on the two pans are equal.

The weighing procedure will be described fully later. Here we consider the question of the sensitivity of the balance.

If the balance is at rest and a small additional weight is put on one of the pans, then the rest point shifts along the scale. The greater this shift, the more sensitive is the balance. Therefore, the number of divisions by which the rest point is shifted under an additional load of 1 mg can be used as an indication of the sensitivity.

The sensitivity of a balance is more accurately represented by the ratio:

$$\frac{\tan\alpha}{p}$$

Here α is the angle through which the pointer is deflected as the rest point is shifted from one position to another by the additional load p (Fig. 8).**

The above ratio can be written:

$$\frac{\tan\alpha}{p} = \frac{l}{qd} \qquad (1)$$

It follows from formula (1) that the sensitivity $\frac{\tan\alpha}{p}$ increases with: increase of the length of the beam arm (l); decrease of the mass (q) of the beam (together with the pans and loads); decrease of the

---

* In practice it is not necessary to wait until the pointer stops. The position of the zero point or rest point is found from the swings as described in Sec. 6.

** Since the angle α is small, its tangent is very nearly equal to the corresponding arc, and the above practical definition of sensitivity is fairly close to the theoretical.

distance (d) between the fulcrum and the centre of gravity of the moving parts of the balance.

For the balance to be *stable*, so that when the beam has left the rest point it returns to it, and does not remain in any position in which it is left (neutral equilibrium), or does not turn over (unstable equilibrium), the centre of gravity must be below the fulcrum. The greater the distance (d) between the centre of gravity and the fulcrum, the more stable the balance.

It might seem that, by formula (1), to increase the sensitivity the length of the arm (l) must be as large as possible. In practice, however, lengthening of the arms is disadvantageous, because the weight (q) increases in greater proportion since a longer beam must be considerably more massive to keep it rigid.

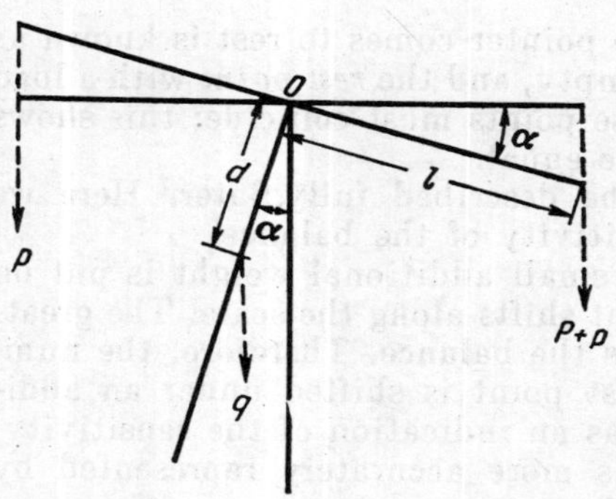

Fig. 8. Determination of the sensitivity of the balance

Therefore, in practice the sensitivity of the balance is regulated by variation of the distance between the centre of gravity of the moving parts of the balance and the fulcrum. This is done by means of the weight 5 (Fig. 2) on the pointer, which can be raised or lowered by means of a screw thread.

When we raise the weight we raise the centre of gravity and bring it nearer the fulcrum; this increases the sensitivity of the balance. We must remember, however, that the stability of the balance is thereby reduced, and the rest point is easily displaced by external forces, so that the accuracy can even become less rather than greater.

Moreover, the time of swing increases with decrease of the distance d, which slows down weighing considerably.

It follows that the sensitivity can be raised only up to a certain limit by variation of the centre of gravity of the beam. This operation may be carried out only by the instructor and *never by the student himself*.

It must be remembered that the sensitivity of the balance is represented by formula (1) only under the condition that all three knife edges are in the same horizontal plane. In reality this condition is hardly ever satisfied, because even if it was observed exactly when the balance was assembled, the beam gradually sags slightly under the influence of the weighed loads. The magnitude of this sag is represented by the angle β between the horizontal plane passing through the central knife edge and the lines joining the central and terminal knife edges. If the beam is bent the relationship between sensitivity and the other quantities is represented by the more complex formula:

$$\tan \alpha = \frac{pl \cos \beta}{qd + (2P - p)\, l \sin \beta} \tag{2}$$

Here P is the load on the balance pans; p is the excess load on one of the pans.

It follows from Equation (2) that the sensitivity of the balance also depends on the load P and on the angle β, decreasing as they increase. It is clear from this that the balance must not be overloaded above the permissible limit, as this would cause considerable bending of the beam and would spoil the balance.

In addition to sensitivity, attention should also be paid to the accuracy and precision of the balance. The *accuracy* of a balance is characterized by the difference between the true weight of an object and the weight as given by the balance. The following conditions must be satisfied for accurate weighing: (a) the arms (i.e., the distances between the central knife edge and the two terminal knife edges) must be equal; (b) all three knife edges must be parallel; (c) the two arms with their pans must be equal in weight.

The *precision* of a balance is indicated by the differences between the results of repeated weighings of the same object. The less these results differ, the more precise is the balance. For example, when we say that the precision of an ordinary analytical balance is 0.0002 g this means that with proper use the results of repeated weighings would not differ from each other by more than 0.0002 g.

A balance may be precise, i.e., it may give very similar results in repeated weighings, and yet these results may be incorrect if, for example, the balance arms are of unequal length. In Sec. 8 it is explained how correct results may be obtained by weighing with such a balance.

The state of the knife edges and of the plates on which they rest has a very great influence on the precision. For example, if a knife edge becomes blunt it makes contact with the plate not along a line but by a flat plane. In consequence, as the balance swings the beam rests sometimes on one and sometimes on the other edge of this plane, so that the position of the rest point changes and the precision diminishes. Accurate readings of the position of the pointer are of great importance too. Therefore, in the most modern balances the pointer swings are observed by means of a lens or a microscope.

5. Rules for Handling the Analytical Balance

In weighing it must be remembered that the analytical balance is a precise physical instrument which must be handled with very great care.

To avoid damage to the balance and to ensure accurate weighing the following rules must be strictly observed:

1. Check the state of the balance before each weighing (or series of consecutive weighings). Remove dust from the pans with a soft brush and find the zero point of the balance (see Sec. 6).
2. Whatever faults you may find in checking the balance, and whatever may happen to the balance during use, never attempt to mend the balance yourself, but always ask the instructor.
3. The unarrested balance must not be touched. The balance must be arrested before the object and weights are put on the pans or taken off them. The balance must be arrested before the rider is moved along the beam. The arrest knob must be turned slowly and carefully.
4. Do not move the balance from its place.
5. Never overload the balance above the permitted load (usually 100 g) as this causes damage. In case of doubt, the object must first be weighed on a rough balance and only when it is certain that it is not too heavy may the analytical balance be used.
6. Do not place wet or dirty objects on the balance. Do not spill anything inside the balance case.
7. Do not put the object to be weighed directly on the balance pan. Do not use pieces of paper; put the substance on a watch glass, or in a weighing bottle, crucible, test tube, etc.
8. Hygroscopic substances and liquids (especially if they give off corrosive vapours) must be weighed in hermetically closed vessels (weighing bottles).
9. Do not weigh hot (or very cold) objects. The object to be weighed must reach the temperature of the balance; it must therefore be left for at least 20 minutes in a desiccator near the balance.
10. Always use only the side doors of the balance case when weighing. The front door, which protects the balance and the weighed object from heat given off by the operator and from water vapour and carbon dioxide breathed out, must be shut all the time.
11. Do not touch the balance, weights or rider with the fingers. The weights must be handled by special forceps, with ivory tips. The same forceps are used for hanging the rider on the hook or taking it off.
12. Do not muddle the weights. Each weight must be put in its proper place in the box.
13. To reduce the effect of weighing errors on the analytical results all weighings must be done on the same balance and with the same set of weights.

14. Do not lean on the bench on which the balance stands, to avoid displacing the balance and disturbing its horizontal position.

15. Remain in the balance room only while weighing. Do not talk to your neighbours, as this may lead to errors.

6. Weighing

Determination of the Zero Point. As already stated, the zero point is the point on the scale at which the pointer of the unloaded balance comes to rest. Before weighing is started the zero point is first determined, because it often changes through a number of accidental causes.

In practice, of course, it is not necessary to wait until the pointer stops, as this would greatly delay weighing, but the zero point is found from the positions of the pointer during its swings in each direction. Obviously, the deviations on each side of the zero point are equal and so the position of the zero point on the scale can be easily found.

The zero point is found as follows. With the balance case closed, the arrest knob is carefully turned fully to the left and the pointer swings are observed. The swings on each side of the central division must not be more than ten divisions, or preferably not more than four. If the pointer does not reach the desired amplitude at once, the balance is carefully arrested and then released again.

When the desired amplitude has been reached, the first two swings of the pointer are disregarded. Starting with the third swing, the extreme positions of the pointer on the scale are read off to the nearest tenth of a division (estimated by eye).

In these readings either the central division or one of the end divisions of the scale is taken as zero. In the former case both extreme divisions of the scale are denoted by the same number 10. Therefore, to show the direction of the pointer, swings to the right of the zero are taken as positive and to the left as negative.

If one of the end divisions is taken as the scale zero, the other end division is indicated by the number 20 and the central division by 10. Negative numbers are then unnecessary.

It is particularly convenient to take the extreme right-hand division as zero, because with increasing mass of the weights put on the right-hand pan the rest point shifts in the direction of increasing scale divisions.

The pointer swings gradually die down because of air resistance and friction. To allow for the damping an *odd* number of readings, usually three (or five), is taken when the zero point is determined.

Suppose, for example that the scale zero is on the right and that the following readings were obtained with the empty balance:

Left	Right
$l_1=16.4$	$l_2=4.7$
$l_3=16.2$	
Average 16.3	

Consequently, the zero point is:

$$l_0=\frac{16.3+4.7}{2}=10.5$$

It is easy to show that this value (10.5) is the true zero point by calculating the deflections of the pointer on each side of it:

Right $10.5-4.7=5.8$ divisions
Left $16.3-10.5=5.8$ divisions

The zero point can also be calculated from the formula:

$$l_0=\frac{l_1+2l_2+l_3}{4}=\frac{16.4+2\times4.7+16.2}{4}=\frac{42}{4}=10.5$$

The following example shows how the zero point is found when the centre of the scale is taken as zero and five readings are taken:

Left	Right
-5.0	$+6.2$
-4.6	$+5.9$
-4.4	
Average -4.7	Average $+6.1$

$$l_0=\frac{-4.7+6.1}{2}=+0.7$$

This result shows that the zero point is 0.7 of a division to the right of the middle of the scale.

Such a small discrepancy between the zero point and the middle of the scale is of no significance. If it is too large (for example, more than two divisions) the balance must be adjusted by means of the screws *4*. (See Fig. 1.) Of course, the students should not do this themselves; the balance should always be adjusted by the instructor.

It should be remembered that, if the zero on the beam scale of a balance is on the left and not in the centre, to find the zero point the rider (0.005 g) must first be put at the zero division. A balance of this type should be at equilibrium with the rider in this position.

It should be noted that in ordinary analytical work determination of the zero point (and also the rest point) can be much simplified by the *method of short swings*. The principle of this method is that if the pointer does not swing by more than 4 divisions on each side of the central division, then the decrease of amplitude is so small that it may be neglected. Therefore, the zero point can be found with sufficient accuracy from two swings (one to the left and the other to the right).

Weighing. When the zero point has been found, the weighing is performed. The balance is arrested and the side doors are carefully opened. The object to be weighed (crucible, weighing bottle, watch glass, etc.), which has reached the temperature of the balance, is put in the middle of the left-hand pan and the left door is closed. Weights are placed on the right-hand pan by means of the forceps. For quicker weighing the weights must be put on the pan in the same order as they are in the box, and not at random.

Let us consider the following example of a weighing operation. Suppose that a weighing bottle has to be weighed. First, take a weight which is obviously too heavy, for example 20 g. Put this on the scale pan and turn the arrest knob slightly to see in which direction the needle swings. In this case it swings to the left. Therefore this weight is too heavy. Arrest the balance, take off this weight and put on the next one in sequence (10 g). Suppose that this is too light. Arrest the balance and put on the 5 g weight. This is too heavy. Take this off and put on 2 g (too light) and again 2 g (still too light). Since 5 g was too heavy there is no point in adding 1 g. Instead, use exactly the same procedure with the fractional weights.

When the pan with the weights begins to swing over on addition of one-hundredth of a gram (for example, if 14.78 g is too light and 14.79 g is too heavy) thousandth and ten-thousandth fractions of a gram are found by means of the rider. This is done with the doors of the balance case shut. There are several methods for finding these fractions.

The Coincidence Method. Put the rider on the hook *5* of the horizontal rod (see Fig. 1) and shut the doors of the case. Make sure that the balance is arrested and by means of the horizontal rod *11* put the rider on the middle (fifth) division of the right-hand arm. Raise the hook by a turn of the knob *6*, release the arrest and note the swings. Find in which direction the swing is greater, and move the rider by means of the same rod to the right or left, *making sure that the balance is arrested each time.* Finally, find the position of the rider at which the rest point, found in the same way as the zero point (p. 29), coincides with sufficient precision with the latter.*

* The precision to which the two should coincide can be easily found if the sensitivity of the balance is known. If the rest point and the zero point do not coincide, the resultant error can be neglected if it does not exceed the precision limits of the balance, i. e., 0.2 mg. If the sensitivity of the balance is, say,

When this has been done, check the weights against the empty spaces in the box and write them down. Confirm this by removing the weights from the pan and putting them back in the box. Then read off the position of the rider on the beam. This gives the third and fourth decimal points. For example, if the weights on the pan added up to 14.78 g, and the scale reading is 44, the weight of the object is 14.7844 g.

Method of Swings. Find two positions of the rider, differing by one large scale division (1 mg), such that one is too light and the other is too heavy. For example, suppose that 14.784 g was too light whereas 14.785 g is heavier than the object; then the true weight of the object is somewhere between the two. To find the thousandth and ten-thousandth fractions of a gram, the rest point of the balance is found in the usual way for both positions of the rider. Suppose that the following results are obtained:

	Too light (14.784 g) Left	Right		Too heavy (14.785 g) Left	Right
	13.7	—		15.8	—
	13.5	3.8		15.6	7.7
Average	13.6		Average	15.7	

Rest point

$$l_1 = \frac{13.6 + 3.8}{2} = 8.7 \qquad l_2 = \frac{15.7 + 7.7}{2} = 11.7$$

Therefore, the sensitivity of the balance is 11.7 — 8.7 = 3.0 divisions. Evidently, each division corresponds to 1/3 mg. If the zero point (l_0) is 10.5, then to reach equilibrium the rest point must be displaced by 10.5 — 8.7 = 1.8 divisions from its position when the weights are too light. Since each scale division corresponds to 1/3 mg the required additional weight is $1.8 \times 1/3 = 0.6$ mg = 0.0006 g. Therefore, the weight of the object is 14.7846 g.

Denoting the value of a scale division by S and noting that $S = \frac{1}{l_2 - l_1}$, the calculations can in general be represented by the following formulas:

$$x = S\,(l_0 - l_1)\ \text{mg} \tag{1}$$

$$x = \frac{l_0 - l_1}{l_2 - l_1}\ \text{mg} \tag{2}$$

where x is the required additional weight (in mg) which must be added to find the weight of the object.

3.0 divisions/mg then the maximum permissible discrepancy is found by proportion:

1 mg corresponds to 3.0 divisions

0.2 mg corresponds to x divisions

$$x = 3 \times 0.2 = 0.6 \text{ division}$$

Therefore the difference between the rest and zero points may be disregarded if it does not exceed 1/5 of the sensitivity at the given load. Determination of the sensitivity is described below.

Formula (2) shows that the sensitivity of a balance is not constant but falls slightly with increasing load. Therefore, the sensitivity must either be found each time by experiment, as described above, or found in advance for different loads (0; 10; 20; 30; 40; 50 g, etc.). These results are then used to plot a sensitivity curve (Fig. 9) which is used to find the sensitivity of the balance at a given load.

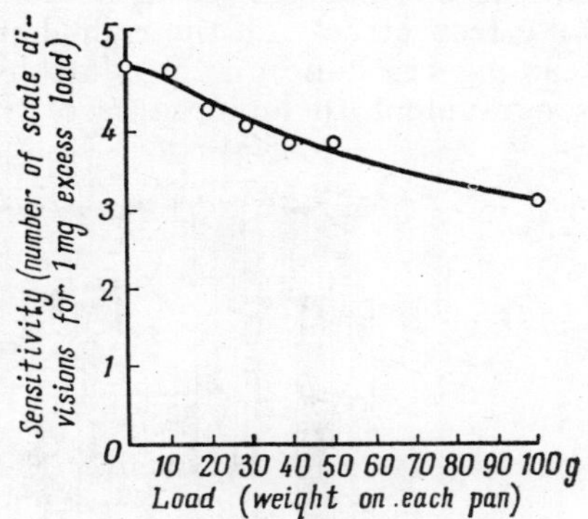

Fig. 9. Sensitivity curve

The method of swings is more convenient when an object is being weighed for the first time. On the other hand, the coincidence method is more convenient for a repeated weighing of the same object (for example, a crucible which is being heated to constant weight).

7. The Damped Balance and Its Use

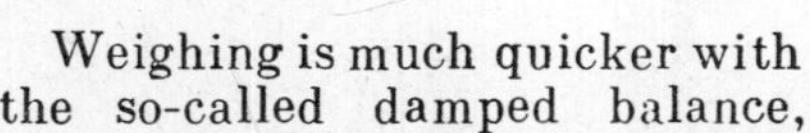

Weighing is much quicker with the so-called damped balance, such as the АДВ-200 balance made by the "Gosmetr" factory (Fig. 10)*.

The main feature of the design of this balance is that it is equipped with an air damping device which causes the beam to cease swinging very quickly. This balance also has an automatic device for putting on small weights and a special mechanism for taking the pointer readings.

The damping devices are hollow aluminium cylinders closed at the top and open below. They are suspended by hooks from the stirrups, one over each balance pan (in other types of damped balances they may be underneath the balance pans). Each cylinder is within another aluminium cylinder of slightly larger diameter open at the top and closed below. The latter cylinders are fixed on the balance column. When the arrest is released the inner cylinders begin to swing together with the beam and pans, and move up or down inside the outer cylinders. The resultant air friction stops the swinging almost at once. The pointer stops in a definite position corresponding to the zero point (or the rest point if the balance is loaded).

On the right-hand stirrup and at right angles to the beam is a horizontal plate on which fractional weights totalling from 10 to 990 mg are suspended. These weights are in the form of rings which hang above this plate. They are hung on the plate by means of a system of levers operated by a hand knob fitted on the outside, on the right-hand side of the balance case. This knob consists of two graduated

* The code mark АДВ-200 represents the Russian term for an analytical damped balance of 200 g maximum load.

discs which can be rotated in either direction. Weights of 100, 200, 300... 900 mg may be put on the plate by rotation of the outer disc. This is obviously equivalent to putting weights of 0.1, 0.2, 0.3... 0.9 g respectively on the right-hand pan. In the same way 10, 20, 30 ...90 mg are hung on the plate by rotation of the inner disc, which is equivalent to hundredths of a gram on the right-hand pan.

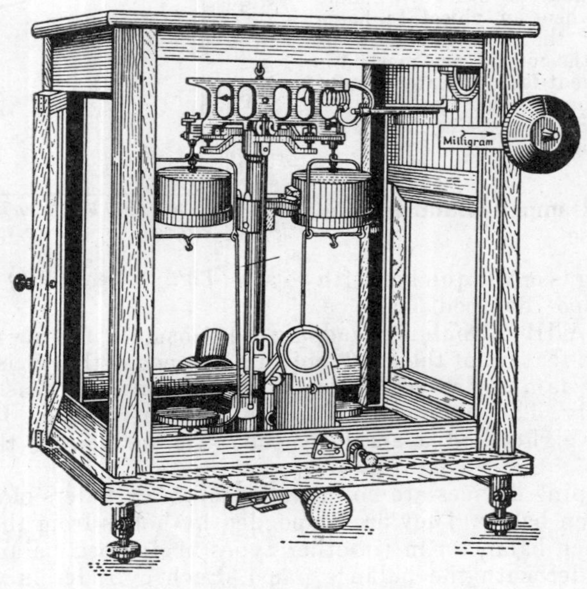

Fig. 10. АДВ-200 damped balance

The total weight of all these weights is found by means of a fixed pointer (in the form of an arrow) near the disc. If, for example, the figure 8 on the outer disc and the figure 3 on the inner disc are opposite this arrow, this means that 830 mg or 0.83 g has been put on the plate or (which is the same) on the right-hand pan.

Milligrams and tenths of milligrams are found from the deviation of the pointer. This deviation is read off by means of an optical device with an illuminated screen which shows an enlarged image of a micro-scale fixed on the pointer. This screen is illuminated by a lamp fixed in the back of the case, which is automatically switched on (through a transformer) when the arrest knob is turned.

The sensitivity of the balance is so adjusted that when one of the pans is overloaded by 10 mg the pointer with the micro-scale deviates by exactly ten divisions from the zero point. In other words, if the balance is so adjusted that in absence of load the image of the zero division of the micro-scale coincides with a vertical line (used for taking the readings) on the screen, then if 10 mg is put on the right-hand pan, when the pointer stops this line exactly coincides with the tenth division of the scale.* Each numbered scale division therefore corresponds to 1 mg. Since the space between two adjacent positions is divided into ten equal parts each of which corresponds to 0.1 mg, the scale reading on the illuminated screen gives milligrams and tenths of milligrams, i.e., the third and fourth decimal places.

It is clear from this that weighing is much quicker and simpler with a damped balance. There is no need to record the pointer swings and calculate the zero and rest points; the rather lengthy operations with the rider for finding milligrams and tenths of milligrams are also unnecessary. They are replaced by a single scale reading on the illuminated screen. Moreover, automatic operation makes it quicker and simpler to determine the first two decimal places. The accuracy of a damped balance is of the same order as that of an ordinary analytical balance.

The speedier weighing with a damped balance is especially important in factory laboratories for production control, where speed of analysis is often decisive.

Weighing on a Damped Balance

1. First plug in the lamp into the lighting circuit.

2. Check the position of the zero point. To do this, carefully turn the arrest knob all the way without opening the balance case. This automatically lights the lamp and a magnified image of the micro-scale attached to the pointer appears on the screen. While the pointer is moving the image of the micro-scale also moves along the screen. However, the damping devices stop the pointer almost at once and the image also stops. With no load on the balance the zero on the scale must coincide exactly with the vertical line on the screen. If it does not, the head of the regulating screw which is outside the balance case above the arrest knob must be turned until the zero and the line coincide.

3. Put the object on the left-hand pan and weights from the box on the right-hand pan, and thus find in the usual way the number of whole grams in the total weight, i.e., weight to the nearest 1 g.

4. Close the balance case and proceed to find the tenths and hundredths of a gram. To do this turn the outer disc of the automatic

* The sensitivity of the balance may alter with time. It can be readjusted by turning a nut on a vertical rod fixed in the middle of the beam. Of course, *the students themselves must never make this adjustment.*

device which places fractional weights on the pan, and bring different numbers on the disc against the fixed arrow, checking each time in which direction the pointer swings. As always, whenever any weights are put on or taken off, i.e., *with every turn of the disc, the balance must be arrested.*

When the tenths of a gram have been found, proceed to find hundredths by means of the inner disc in exactly the same way.

5. Having found the weight to the nearest 0.01 g as described above, turn the arrest knob to the end, and when the swinging has stopped read off the position of the vertical line along the scale on the screen. The large divisions on this scale, corresponding to whole milligrams, are marked with numbers with plus or minus signs. A plus sign means that the value of the reading must be added to the sum of the weights on the balance. Conversely, if the scale reading has a minus sign, it must be subtracted from the weights.

For example, if the weights on the balance total 11.83 g and the screen reading is 2.7 mg (0.0027 g) then if this reading is positive the weight of the object is 11.83 + 0.0027 = 11.8327 g. Conversely, if the reading is negative it would be 11.83 — 0.0027 = 11.8273 g.*

When the weighing is finished, remove the object and weights from the balance. To remove the fractional weights, bring the zero divisions of both discs against the fixed pointer.

8. Elimination of the Effect of Unequal Arm Length. Reduction of the Weight of an Object to Its True Value in a Vacuum

Direct weighing does not give the true weight (or more correctly the mass) of an object, because of errors due to inequality of the balance arm lengths and to losses of weight because the weighing is performed in air.

In most usual analytical work these errors may be disregarded because they have the same (or nearly the same) effects both on the weight of substance (q), and on the amount of the component (a) being determined. Therefore, they do not affect the final results, i.e., the percentage content of the component. The percentage content is found from the formula:

$$p = \frac{a}{q} \times 100\%$$

If the arm lengths are unequal and as a result the weights found (a and q) are, for example, 1% below the true values, the result is

* If the reading is greater than 5 mg, for greater accuracy the load on the right-hand pan should be increased by 10 mg if the reading is positive, or decreased by 10 mg if it is negative. A new reading is then taken and used for finding the weight of the object.

the same whether we take this into account or not. This is shown by the following equation:

$$p = \frac{a+0.01a}{q+0.01q} \times 100 = \frac{1.01a}{1.01q} \times 100 = \frac{a}{q} \times 100\%$$

However, sometimes it is necessary to know the true weight of a substance or object, and then the errors caused by inequality of arm length or weighing in air cannot be disregarded. For example, this applies to calibration of weights, to determination of the capacities of measuring vessels for liquids or gases (from the weight of water contained in them), to determination of atomic weights of elements, etc.

Sometimes the true weight must be known even in analysis. For example, the nitrogen content of saltpetre is found by measurement of the volume of gaseous NO, formed by the reaction:

$$NaNO_3 + 3FeCl_2 + 4HCl = 3FeCl_3 + NaCl + 2H_2O + NO\uparrow$$

The weight of NO is found by calculation from its measured volume. In this case the weighing errors are not compensated and therefore the true weight of the saltpetre taken for analysis must be known.

We now consider how all these weighing errors can be eliminated.

Correction for Inequality of the Length of the Balance Arms. We know from physics that the balance is a lever of the first order with equal arms, and the balance can be correct only if the arms are exactly equal in length. In practice, however, this can never be achieved exactly. Therefore, the arms of every balance must be regarded as more or less unequal. Special weighing methods are used to eliminate the effect of this inequality on the weighing results.

Double Weighing. In this method the object is first put on the left-hand pan and the weights on the right-hand pan. The object is weighed and in this case the weight is P_1.

The weighing is then repeated with the object on the right-hand pan and the weights on the left. If the balance arms were exactly equal in length this weight would coincide with the first. However, in reality because of the unequal arm lengths we have a slightly different weight P_2.

Denoting the true weight of the object by P and the lengths of the right- and left-hand arms by l_1 and l_2, we can write in accordance with the lever principle:

$$l_2P = l_1P_1 \text{ (1st weighing)}$$

$$l_1P = l_2P_2 \text{ (2nd weighing)}$$

Multiplying these equations term by term, we have:

$$l_1 \cdot l_2 \cdot P^2 = l_1 \cdot l_2 \cdot P_1 \cdot P_2$$

and hence

$$P = \sqrt{P_1P_2}$$

Thus, the true weight of the object in air is the geometric mean of the two weighings. Since the values of P_1 and P_2 are similar, the geometric mean is almost identical with the arithmetic mean which is much easier to find;

it is then assumed that

$$P = \frac{P_1 + P_2}{2}$$

Method of Substitution. By this method the object is placed on either pan and counterbalanced with any suitable material on the other pan.

The object is then taken off and replaced with the necessary weights to obtain the same rest point.

Since the object and the weights are put on the same pan and therefore act on the same arm, the inequality of arm length has no effect and the true weight of the object is found directly.

The Method of D. Mendeleyev. The third method, proposed by D. Mendeleyev, is as follows. A load close to the limiting load of the balance is put on one of the pans and counterpoised by weights in the other pan. The object is then placed on the pan with the weights, and weights are then removed to obtain the same rest point as before.

The total of the weights taken off is clearly equal to the weight of the object.

Reduction of the Weight of an Object to Its True Value in a Vacuum. By Archimedes' principle a weighed object and the weights have an apparent loss of weight equal to the weight of the air displaced by them. Since the object and the weights differ in volume their losses in weight should also be different. This fact, like inequality of arm lengths, gives rise to errors in weighing.

To find the true weight of an object a correction must be applied for weighing in air (buoyancy).

It is easy to see that this correction is equal to the difference between the volumes of the objects and the weights, multiplied by the density of air (d_a). If the weight of the object (and therefore of the weights) in air is found to be P, and the densities of the object and the weights are d_{ob} and d_w, as the volume of an object is equal to its weight divided by the density, we can write:

$$P_0 = P + d_a\left(\frac{P}{d_{ob}} - \frac{P}{d_w}\right) \tag{1}$$

where P_0 is the weight of the object in vacuum.

The density of air d_a depends on the pressure, temperature and humidity of the air and can be calculated from a special formula. However, such calculations are unnecessary for ordinary analytical work. The value $d_a = 0.0012$ is sufficiently precise for practical purposes. The density of the weights can be taken as 8.4 for brass and 2.7 for aluminium.

Let us consider two numerical examples of the reduction of a weight to its weight in a vacuum.

Example 1. The weight of an AgCl precipitate (density 5.6) in air is 0.5000 g. Find its weight *in vacuo*.

Solution. Since aluminium weights were used we find from formula (1):

$$P = 0.5000 + 0.0012\left(\frac{0.5}{5.6} - \frac{0.5}{2.6}\right) = 0.5000 - 0.00012 = 0.49988 \text{ g}$$

This example shows that the correction for buoyancy in air (0.00012 g in this case) may be disregarded because it is smaller than the precision limits of weighing.

When large masses are weighed, as in calibration of measuring vessels, the error is much larger and must be taken into account.

Example 2. The weight of water contained in a measuring flask was found to be 250.80 g at 20°C when weighed on a technical balance. Find the weight of the water *in vacuo*.

Solution. **Since brass weights were used and the density of water at 20°C is 0.9982, we have:**

$$P=250.80+0.0012\left(\frac{250.80}{0.9982}-\frac{250.80}{8.4}\right)=250.80+0.27=251.07 \text{ g}$$

Thus, the true weight of the water differs by 0.27 g from its apparent weight in air. This difference is too large to be neglected, despite the fact that the weighing was carried out on a technical balance to an accuracy of 0.01 g.

9. Calibration of Weights

Although analytical weights are made to a high degree of precision, their weight may alter with time. Therefore weights must be checked or calibrated from time to time.

It should be noted that as a rule the relative rather than the absolute precision of the weights is important. In other words, *all the weights of a given set must be consistent between themselves*, i.e., the 1 g weight must be exactly twice as heavy as the 0.5 g weight, five times as heavy as the 0.2 g weight, etc.

As the set contains pieces of the same nominal weight (for example, pairs of weights with the number 2, or three weights with the number 1) they are distinguished by one or two dots near the corresponding number while the others are left unmarked.

When weights are being calibrated the effect of unequal arm lengths must be eliminated, for example, by double weighing.

The calibration itself can be conveniently carried out as follows: The weight of the rider is provisionally assumed to be exactly 0.01 g and all the other weights are compared with it (Table I).

First the 10 mg (0.01 g) weight is checked. It is first put on the left-hand pan, with the rider on the 10th division of the right-hand arm. The swings are observed and the rest point calculated. Suppose that it is 9.8 divisions (l_1). To compensate for unequal arm length, the weight is moved to the right-hand pan and the rider to the 10th division of the left-hand arm, and the rest point is again found.

Suppose that it is 10.3 divisions (l_2). It can be shown that the difference in weight between the tested weight (P_1) and the rider (P_2) in milligrams is:

$$P_1-P_2=1/2\,(l_2-l_1)\,S$$

where S is the value of a scale division. For example, if the sensitivity of the balance is 4 divisions per mg then $S=1/4=0.25$ mg per division and

$$P_1-P_2=1/2\,(10.3-9.8)\,0.25=+0.06 \text{ mg}$$

Thus, the 10 mg weight is heavier than the rider by 0.06 mg, $P_1 = 10.06$ mg = 0.01006 g.

One of the 20 mg weights (without mark) is next tested. It is put on the left-hand pan, with the 10 mg weight which has just been tested on the right-hand pan and the rider on the 10th division of the right-hand arm.

Suppose that the rest point l_1 was 10.5 divisions. The weights (and rider) are now changed over, and the new rest point is found: l_2 = 9.5 divisions. Therefore, the difference between the 20 mg weight (P_1) and the sum (P_2) of the 10 mg weight and the rider is:

$$P_1-P_2=1/2\,(9.5-10.5)\,0.25=-0.12 \text{ mg}$$

and since the 10 mg weight actually weighs 10.06 mg, the true weight of the 20 mg piece is:

$$P_1=10+10.06-0.12=19.94 \text{ mg}=0.01994 \text{ g}$$

The weight of the second 20 mg piece, marked with a dot (20˙) is next found. It is compared with the weight of the first 20 mg piece (without dot) and its weight ($P = 0.02000$ g) is found by the procedure described above.

The 50 mg weight is compared with the sum of the three weights: 20 mg + + 20 mg + 10 mg, etc. Thus, the weights P of all the pieces in the set are found (see the second column from the right in Table I), on the assumption that the rider weighs exactly 10 mg.

However, in practice it is more convenient to take as correct one of the larger weights, used relatively seldom, such as 10 g or 50 g, rather than the

Table I

Example of Weight Calibration *

P_1	P_2	l_1 div.	l_2 div.	S mg/div.	P_1-P_2 mg	P g	Δ mg
Rider	(10 mg)	—	—	—	—	**0.01000**	0.00
10 mg	Rider	9.8	10.3	0.25	+0.06	0.01006	+0.06
20 mg	10 mg + rider	10.5	9.5	0.25	—0.12	0.01994	—0.07
20˙ mg	20 mg	9.8	10.3	0.25	+0.06	0.02000	—0.01
50 mg	10 mg 20 mg 20˙ mg	10.1	9.9	0.25	—0.03	0.04997	—0.05
100 mg	10+20+20˙+50 mg	9.6	9.8	0.25	+0.03	0.10000	—0.04
200 mg	100+50+20+20˙+ +10 mg	9.2	10.0	0.25	+0.10	0.20007	—0.01
200˙ mg	200 mg	10.3	9.4	0.25	—0.11	0.19996	—0.12
500 mg	100+200+200˙ mg	9.5	10.3	0.25	+0.10	0.50013	—0.07
1 g	100+200+200˙+ +500 mg	9.2	10.7	0.25	+1.19	1.00035	—0.04
1˙ g	1 g	10.0	10.0	0.25	0.00	1.00035	—0.04
1˙˙ g	1 g	10.0	10.0	0.25	0.00	1.00035	—0.04
2 g	1+1˙ g	10.1	10.0	0.25	—0.01	2.00069	—0.09
5 g	1+1˙+1˙˙+2 g	10.2	10.4	0.25	+0.03	5.00177	—0.19
10 g	1+1˙+1˙˙+2+5 g	9.0	12.2	0.26	+0.41	**10.00392**	0.00
10˙ g	10 g	10.3	11.0	0.26	+0.09	10.00401	+0.09
20 g	10+10˙ g	9.9	12.4	0.29	+0.36	20.00829	+0.45
50 g	1+1˙+1˙˙+2+5+ +10+10˙+20 g	9.6	11.6	0.37	+0.37	50.02010	+0.50

* E. Alexeyevsky, R. Golts and A. Musakin, *Quantitative Analysis*, Goskhimizdat, 1957.

rider, which is in constant use and therefore is subjected to fairly rapid wear. For example, if the 10 g weight (which was found to weigh 10.00392 g) is taken as exactly 10 g, then all the other weights must be corrected in proportion, by multiplying them by the ratio 10 : 10.00392. The corrections are then found (see the last column in Table I) which must be added (with their signs taken into account) to the nominal weights. For example, if the 5 g + 2 g + 1· g + + 1·· g + 0.2 g + 0.02 g + 0.02· g weights were used, the total correction is: $\Sigma\Delta = (-0.19 - 0.09 - 0.04 - 0.04 - 0.01 - 0.07 - 0.01) = - 0.45$ mg = = −0.00045 g. Therefore the total weight of the weights used was 9.24 − − 0.00045 = 9.23955 g = 9.2395 g.

The table of corrections is kept in the box of weights or on the wall near the balance to which the set of weights belongs.

10. General Comments on Work in a Laboratory for Quantitative Analysis

When starting practical work on quantitative analysis the student must remember that he is working in a precision laboratory, where the slightest inaccuracy may distort the analytical results which may have taken a great deal of work and time to obtain.

It is therefore specially important to keep strictly to the usual rules concerning orderly and clean work. Care must be taken always to keep the work place clean and dry. It must not be cluttered up by unnecessary objects. Only what is necessary for the work in hand should be on the bench. Everything else must be put away.

The vessels required for a given determination must be prepared beforehand and washed thoroughly.* Everything needed for the analysis must be arranged on the bench so that nothing can be knocked over by the student or his neighbour.

All sharp movements must be avoided during work in the laboratory. Analyses are often spoiled because, before the very last operation—weighing of the precipitate—the crucible containing the precipitate is knocked over because of a clumsy movement or accidental collision with a neighbour. The whole analysis, which may have taken several hours of work, must then be repeated.

The established procedure must be followed carefully in individual quantitative determinations. It must be remembered that analytical results can be reliable only if all the conditions for which the particular method was developed and verified are strictly obeyed. Any deviation from these conditions leads to error and greatly diminishes the accuracy of the method.

Equal care must be taken to obey the rules concerning techniques for performing individual operations, such as filtration, washing, drying and ignition of precipitates, etc. Although some of these rules may seem very trivial, it must be remembered that they are all based on the vast experience of many generations of chemists and that only if they are obeyed most strictly can the required accuracy of the analytical results be obtained.

---

* See Sec. 12.

Faultlessly correct execution of all working techniques must become an unconscious habit. In order to attain this, it is necessary at first to pay the greatest attention to correct performance of every individual operation, and of every working movement. Only then can we acquire the skills of accurate experimentation, which is one of the principal aims of a course of quantitative analysis.

However, these skills are not enough in themselves. Even a person without any suitable chemical training can be taught to carry out analytical techniques correctly. However, such a person would be quite helpless when faced with the slightest deviation from the usual routine. For example, he would not be able to choose the most suitable methods for investigating a particular substance, to work out new methods of analysis, to interpret his results correctly, etc. All this requires a thorough knowledge of the theory of analysis, which must also be studied with very serious attention.

In conclusion we must consider the keeping of laboratory notes, which are very important in quantitative analysis.

Such notes must never be made on separate sheets or scraps of paper; a special laboratory log-book must be kept. Separate sheets or scraps of paper with the necessary numerical data are easily lost, and this wastes all the labour and time spent on the analysis itself. In analytical work for industrial purposes laboratory log-books are important for another reason. The laboratory log-book is then the main document for checking the results obtained by the analyst (sometimes even after a long time has elapsed) whenever they are doubtful for any reason.

The method of making notes will be demonstrated by concrete examples in the descriptions of different analyses. We will merely note here that such records must contain all the necessary data (results of weighings and volume measurements, calcutations, etc.) and should be kept so that they can be easily followed when the analyst's results are being checked.

As far as possible all the necessary data should be entered directly into the log-book, without copying from other notes, as this may give rise to errors.

Each determination should have a separate page, or better two, allotted to it. If two pages are used, the results of direct determinations and other information (time when the analysis was performed, method used, etc.) are written on one page, and all the necessary calculations on the other.

The numerical quantities with which an analyst deals may be exact or approximate. Exact quantities include:

1. Quantities taken as constant, for example, valences of elements, the atomic weight of oxygen which is taken as 16, etc;
2. Relationship between units; for example, 1 kg contains 1,000 g;

3. The results of counting numbers of objects or operations; for example, the number of known elements and their atomic numbers, the number of determinations carried out, etc.

Approximate quantities include all results of measurements, covering the results of weighing. No matter how accurately we try to weigh, the last figure of the weight found must be unreliable. For example, if we weigh a crucible on a technical balance and find its weight to be 7.12 g, this means that the weight lies between 7.11 and 7.13 g. If we weigh more accurately, we again find only the approximate weight of the crucible. For example, if the same crucible is weighed on an analytical balance and a weight of 7.1244 g is found, in view of what was said earlier about the accuracy of weighing on the analytical balance, we must conclude that the weight of the crucible must be between 7.1242 and 7.1246 g. These examples show that the last figure in the result of weighing is always unreliable. The same is true for any other measurement, for example, the measurements of liquid or gas volumes, determinations of atomic or molecular weights, etc.

Since this is so, *all measurement results should be recorded in such a way that only the last figure is unreliable.* For example, if the weight of a crucible was found to be exactly 7.12 g on the analytical balance, it would be quite wrong to record the weight in that form. In accordance with the above rule this weight must be recorded as 7.1200 g. When we use the analytical balance we can guarantee the correctness of the first three decimal places in the quantity 7.1200. Only the last figure in this number is unreliable, in agreement with the rule. On the other hand, if the same result is obtained when the crucible is weighed on a technical balance to an accuracy not greater than 0.01 g its weight should be written as 7.12 and not 7.120 or 7.1200 g.

By obeying this rule the analyst reflects the precision of his data in the very way they are recorded.

11. Preparation of Substances for Analysis

Before an analysis can be started, the substance must be prepared. Two cases may occur:

(a) the composition of some pure substance is to be determined;

(b) it is required to find the average composition of a large mass of substance, which is a more or less heterogeneous natural mixture or industrial product, such as ores, slags, cements, alloys, soils, fertilizers, etc.

In the first case the preparation of the substance for analysis must consist in removal of all possible impurities, i.e., in obtaining the substance in the chemically pure state. Solid crystalline substances which are often met in analysis are usually purified by *recrystallization.*

In the second case the aim is to obtain a correct idea of the composition of large masses of the substance (for example, of a whole production batch) by analysis of a small sample; therefore in preparing the substance for analysis the important thing is to obtain an *average sample*, which is a sample truly representing the average composition of the whole batch.

Purification. In recrystallization the substance to be purified is dissolved in the smallest possible amount of hot water, the solution is filtered to remove insoluble impurities, and the filtrate is cooled rapidly.

The solubility of a substance usually decreases on cooling, so that some of it is precipitated in the form of crystals. On the other hand, the water-soluble impurities, present in much smaller amounts, generally do not crystallize out on cooling but remain in the mother liquor. The crystals are separated by filtration and pressed out between sheets of filter paper, and the substance is obtained in a purer form.

Sometimes a single recrystallization is not enough, and it is then repeated two or three times. In some cases even repeated recrystallization does not give the desired results because the impurity enters the crystal lattice of the substance, forming *mixed crystals**.

Sometimes instead of recrystallization solid substances are purified by *sublimation.* In this process the substance to be purified (for example, iodine) is heated and converted into vapour on heating, without melting. When the vapour cools crystals free from non-volatile impurities are again formed.

To remove dissolved substances in liquids they are purified by *distillation*; the well-known process of distillation of water is an example.

Mixtures of liquids are separated by *fractional distillation.* This is described in detail in practical textbooks on organic chemistry.

Sampling. This is a very important operation, as on it depends the extent to which the analytical results correspond to the true composition of the material. If the average sample is taken incorrectly even the most careful and accurate analysis loses its value.

Sampling techniques may be quite different in different cases. Each type of material has its own special sampling instructions, which take into account the specific characteristics of the material, the quantity taken, its purpose, etc. These instructions are given in manuals on technical analysis. Here we shall only refer to the general principle on which sampling is based.

---

* Mixed crystals are considered in detail on p. 109.

This principle is that *the average sample must be composed of the largest possible number of portions of the substance taken quite automatically from different parts of the batch.*

To understand this, it must be remembered that the material for analysis is not uniform in composition. Different parts, lumps and grains may differ greatly in composition within a single batch. Clearly, the more portions of the substance taken from different parts, lumps, etc., go to make the average sample, the more likely it is that all accidental deviations from the average cancel out, and the composition of the sample approaches the average composition of the material.

The *primary average sample* obtained in this way is still unsuitable for direct analysis, because it is too large and very heterogeneous. It is therefore ground down (which makes it more homogeneous) and treated as described below in order to reduce the amount. One method often used is known as *quartering.* This is performed as follows. Lumps of the primary average sample, taken as described above, are first broken down to pieces about the size of a walnut, mixed, and spread out in an even layer in the form of a square. The square is divided diagonally into four triangles; one pair of opposite triangles is discharged and the contents of the other pair are mixed and ground down further.

The resultant material, which is much more homogeneous is again quartered and ground, and the process is continued until about 25 g (or sometimes more) of the substance remains. It is then ground very thoroughly and put in a jar with a ground-glass stopper. This very homogeneous material is used for the subsequent analysis.

In some cases grinding may cause changes in the substance; it may become oxidized or lose part of its water of crystallization. To prevent this the grinding should be performed rapidly; sometimes the substance is ground under a layer of liquid which protects it from the air.

12. Laboratory Vessels and Their Preparation for Analysis

Vessels made of glass are the most important in chemical analysis. In addition to glassware, vessels and instruments are made of porcelain, quartz, platinum, silver and other materials.

Glass. Glass varies in composition. Not every kind of glass is suitable for chemical work. The best kind is heat-resisting glass (Pyrex) which has a relatively low coefficient of expansion, a high softening temperature and good chemical resistance. Although heat-resisting glass and other types of resistant glass withstand the action of different solutions better than ordinary glass, even these types of glass are attacked by water and solutions, especially if hot.

Alkaline solutions have the strongest effect on glass; acid solutions (except those containing HF) have even less effect on glass than pure water.

When any glassware is heated it is necessary to avoid sharp changes of temperature and uneven heating of different parts of the vessel.* Glass vessels must be heated on a gauze, and never over a naked flame.

Porcelain. Porcelain vessels, such as crucibles, evaporating basins, beakers, etc., withstand relatively high temperatures. Porcelain is resistant to alkalies and other chemical reagents. However, if substances are fused with alkalies or carbonates, porcelain crucibles (or basins) are partially attacked, and the products of this attack subsequently contaminate the solution being analysed. Porcelain crucibles which are generally used for ignition of precipitates, are the commonest in laboratory practice. They are quite satisfactory for analyses of moderate precision. Platinum crucibles must be used for analyses of higher precision.

Quartz. In many cases vessels made from fused quartz are used instead of glassware. Such vessels are very resistant to abrupt temperature changes; quartz melts at a high temperature (about 1700°C). Caustic alkalies and even alkali carbonates attack quartz glass, but acids have no effect on it (with the exception of HF and to some extent H_3PO_4). Vessels from pure quartz are of two kinds: transparent like glass, and translucent.

Platinum. Because it is chemically very inert and its melting point is high (1770°C), platinum is a most valuable material for a variety of chemical apparatus and vessels (crucibles, basins, electrodes for electrogravimetric determinations, etc.). However, although platinum is very resistant, it is attacked by chlorine, bromine, aqua regia (a mixture of concentrated HNO_3 and HCl) and caustic alkalies. Platinum forms alloys with lead, antimony, arsenic, tin, silver, bismuth, gold, etc. Compounds of these elements must not be heated in platinum vessels.

Platinum combines with carbon, silicon and phosphorus which make it brittle and fragile. Therefore *platinum vessels must not be heated over a luminous (smoky) gas flame*; the inner blue cone of the flame, containing hydrocarbons, must not touch the bottom of the vessel (crucible, basin, etc.). When platinum crucibles are used for ignition of precipitates they are picked up by tongs with nickel or platinum tips and placed in triangles consisting of metal wire

* The degree of sensitivity to sharp changes of temperature depends on the type of glass. For example, glasses of type Б-2 and No. 846, which are generally used for chemical glassware, withstand rapid cooling from 120-140°C to room temperature. Pyrex glass does not crack when cooled rapidly from 220-240°C to room temperature.

enclosed in porcelain tubes, which protect the platinum from contact with the metal wire.

The use of platinum vessels is greatly restricted by its very high cost.

Cleanliness of Vessels. Before starting work, find out from the textbook what vessels are needed for the given determination. Then wash the necessary vessels thoroughly.

Cleanliness of the vessels is of enormous importance in quantitative analysis. A vessel can be called clean if no contamination of any kind can be seen even by very careful examination, and if water runs down its walls smoothly without leaving any drops. Drops are formed if the glass surface is greasy; the presence of grease is most undesirable, as precipitates formed in chemical reactions usually adhere very closely to the grease layer and are very difficult to transfer to the filter. Contamination with grease of vessels and apparatus used for exact measurement of volumes is particularly harmful, because when the liquid is poured out part of it remains in the form of drops on the walls of the vessel and the volume measurement becomes inaccurate.

Glassware is washed as follows. First the vessel is filled with hot water and rubbed thoroughly inside and out with special brushes. This procedure is then repeated with soap or soda solution instead of water, and the vessel is then washed out thoroughly with tap water. If the vessel is not clean after this treatment and drops remain on its inner walls, it is washed out with "chromic mixture" which is a mixture of potassium dichromate $K_2Cr_2O_7$ and concentrated sulphuric acid.* The chromic mixture is poured into the vessel so that its inside walls are wetted thoroughly. The chromic mixture should then be returned to its container; it can be used repeatedly.

Great care must be taken when using chromic mixture, as it can cause burns and damage clothing. If any chromic mixture gets on the hands or face it must be immediately washed off with a large amount of water, followed by $NaHCO_3$ solution.

Instead of chromic mixture laboratory ware can also be washed with a mixture of equal volumes of approximately 0.1 *N* solution of $KMnO_4$ and concentrated H_2SO_4. Sometimes alkaline formula $KMnO_4$, alcoholic solutions of KOH or NaOH, etc., are used. Grease is best removed by alkaline solutions.

After the vessel has been treated with chromic mixture (or the other solutions named above) it should be thoroughly washed with

---

* To prepare chromic mixture, dissolve 5-6 g of potassium dichromate in 100 ml of water and *carefully* add 100 ml of concentrated H_2SO_4 to this solution (*but not the other way round*).

tap water and finally rinsed with a small amount (5-10 ml) of distilled water. It should not be wiped inside with a cloth, as this will inevitably contaminate it again. In general chemical vessels are wiped only on the outside; if they must be dried inside, they are put into a special drying cabinet heated by gas or electricity. However, in most cases this is unnecessary.

Sometimes *steaming* is also used, especially to clean measuring vessels. The vessel is put on the tube of the apparatus shown in Fig. 11 and a current of steam from the flask containing boiling water is passed through it. The water condensing on the walls of the vessel runs back into the flask. Steaming is continued until no more drops can be seen on the walls of the vessel. This not only cleans the vessel thoroughly but leaches out soluble components from the glass, which is sometimes necessary.

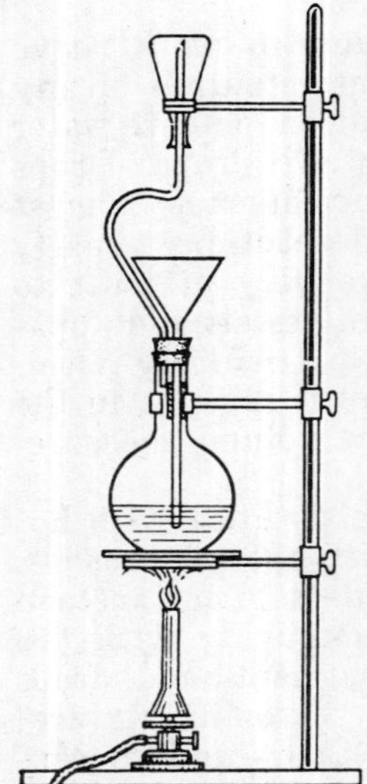

Fig. 11. Steaming of glassware

Porcelain crucibles in which precipitates are ignited are cleaned out with hot dilute (1 : 1) hydrochloric acid, then with chromic mixture and water. Often precipitates such as Fe_2O_3 or CuO which colour the crucible cannot be removed because they become fused into the glaze. Such crucibles are quite suitable for use.

13. Errors in Quantitative Analysis

No matter how carefully a quantitative determination is performed, the result always differs to some extent from the true content, i.e., it contains a certain error.

Analytical errors can be classified as follows: (a) systematic (determinate) errors; (b) random (indeterminate) errors; and (c) mistakes.

Systematic Errors. Systematic errors are errors which are constant in magnitude or vary in accordance with a definite law. Systematic errors can usually be foreseen and either avoided or suitably corrected. They may arise from various causes. The following types of systematic errors may be noted.

Errors of Method. These errors depend on specific characteristics of the analytical method used; for example, the reaction on which the determination depends may not be quite quantitative; the precipitate may be partially soluble, or various impurities may be precipitated with it; the precipitate may partially decompose or volatilize during ignition; the ignited precipitate may be hygroscopic; the main reaction may be accompanied by side reactions which distort the results of volumetric determinations; the indicator used in the titration may influence the results, etc. Errors of method are the most serious cause of incorrect results in quantitative determinations.

Errors Which Depend on the Apparatus and Reagents Used. These include errors caused by inequality of the balance arms or insufficient accuracy of the balance, the use of unchecked weights or uncalibrated measurement vessels, and errors which arise because extraneous substances enter the solution under investigation. The same category includes errors caused by contamination of the solution by decomposition products of the glass or porcelain of the vessels used for analysis; errors caused by the presence of the element being determined or of interfering substances in the reagents; errors caused by the use of incorrectly standardized solutions for titration,* etc.

Operative Errors. Operative errors are due to the faulty or careless execution of analytical operations. They include, for instance, underwashing of precipitates which gives consistently excessive results; sometimes (due to lack of experience) overwashing of precipitates, resulting in systematic losses. Systematic errors may also be due to undercalcining or overcalcining of precipitates, careless transfer of precipitates from beaker to crucible, incorrect draining of solutions from pipettes (p. 198), etc.

Operative errors are easy to detect and eliminate.

Individual Errors. These errors depend on the personal characteristics of the analyst himself; for example, his inability to detect exactly the end point in titration, etc. Individual errors also include the so-called *psychological errors*, due to a certain bias often met with in students. For example, in duplicate weighings or titrations, out of two adjacent scale divisions on the balance or burette,** the student often tends to choose the division which is closer to the previous determinations or even to those found by his fellow students rather than the one closer to the actual weight or volume. Obviously, this merely makes the results less accurate and sometimes may make them quite unacceptable. Therefore the student must make it a rule to be as objective as possible and not to allow any bias in estimating experimental results.

Random Errors. Random errors are indeterminate in magnitude and sign, and their appearance does not conform to any laws.

Random errors arise in every measurement, which includes any analytical determination, no matter how carefully it is performed.

* See Sec. 49.

** A burette (see Fig. 30) is a measuring vessel for liquids used in titration.

They are revealed by the fact that repeated determinations of a particular element in a sample, carried out by the same method generally give results which are not absolutely identical.

In contrast to systematic errors, random errors cannot be prevented or eliminated by corrections. However, they can be considerably reduced by increased care in work, and by increase of the number of replicate determinations (see below). The influence of random errors on analytical results can be estimated theoretically by statistical analysis (Sec. 14) of the results obtained in a series of repeated determinations.

Mistakes. Mistakes are crude errors which greatly distort the analytical results. They include errors caused by incorrect counting of weights or wrong readings on the scale in weighing, wrong burette readings in titration*, errors caused by spilling of the solution or precipitate during the determination, etc. A mistake makes the result of the given determination incorrect, and it is therefore rejected when the average of a series of replicate determinations is found.

Accuracy and Precision of Analytical Results. Systematic errors determine the degree of *accuracy* of the result; the smaller the systematic errors in the determination, the more accurate is the result considered to be. On the other hand, the magnitude of random errors determines the *precision* of the analytical result. It follows that the closer the results of replicate determinations are to each other, the more precise is the analysis considered to be.

It is easy to see that a high degree of precision does not prove that an analysis is accurate. This can be illustrated by the following example. Suppose that in a series of repeated titrations of equal volumes of a given alkaline solution very similar volumes of hydrochloric acid solution were taken; this shows that the precision was high. However, to find the final result it is necessary to calculate from the reaction equation the amount of alkali present from the volume and concentration of the HCl solution taken. If the concentration of the HCl solution had been inaccurately determined, the resultant systematic error will influence all the results of the separate determinations, and despite the good agreement the results would be quite incorrect.

Therefore, *the accuracy of an analytical result can be assessed from its precision only in the absence of systematic errors.* However, without overestimating the importance of precision, we must not forget that good precision shows the absence of any considerable random errors in the analysis. Even the most experienced and conscientious analyst may make such errors (and even mistakes); therefore, *every*

* The method of volumetric analysis known as titration is described in Sec. 49.

determination is performed at least twice, on two separate samples (*replicate determinations*). An analysis is regarded as satisfactory only if the results of the individual determinations are in good agreement; the average of these results is taken as the final result.

It can be proved by the mathematical theory of errors that the error of the average of n determinations is $\sqrt{n}$ smaller than the error of a single determination. However, this is true only if the errors are random and therefore fluctuate in magnitude on both sides of the quantity being measured, i.e., are smaller or larger than that quantity.

However, it may happen in analysis that the errors are all of the same sign. For example, the results of weighing of a hygroscopic substance are always greater and never less than the true weight. Obviously the average value must be further from the true weight than the lowest of the weights found. It is evident that the errors in this case are in fact systematic and not random.

Despite what was said above about the importance of replicate determinations, experiments on quantitative analysis are sometimes restricted (to save time) to single determinations with the use of recrystallized, chemically pure substances the composition of which can be easily calculated from their chemical formulas.

The errors in quantitative determinations, as in any other measurements, may be expressed in different ways. They may be classified into absolute and relative errors.

In most cases the relative rather than the absolute error is of the greater interest.

Absolute Error. The difference between the experimental result and the true (or most reliable) value, expressed in absolute units, is called the *absolute error*. Suppose, for example, that crystalline barium chloride was found to contain 14.70% of water of crystallization. The formula $BaCl_2 \cdot 2H_2O$ shows that in reality barium chloride should contain 14.75% of water of crystallization. Therefore, the absolute error (D) is:

$$D = 14.70 - 14.75 = -0.05\%$$

Relative Error. The absolute error expressed as a fraction of the value measured is known as the *relative error*. It is usually expressed as a percentage. For example, in the above example the relative error (D_0) is:

$$D_0 = \frac{-0.05}{14.75} \times 100 = -0.34\%$$

It is obvious that for a given magnitude of the absolute error the larger the value measured, the smaller the relative error. For example, if the same absolute error ($\pm 0.05\%$) occurs in the determination of barium in $BaCl_2 \cdot 2H_2O$, then, since the true content is 56.20%, the relative error is:

$$D_0 = \frac{\pm 0.05}{56.20} \times 100 = \pm 0.09\%$$

If the true value is unknown, the average (M) of the results is taken and each individual result (x) is compared with it. The resultant differences ($d = x - M$) are known as *deviations from the mean.* It will be shown more fully in Sec. 14 that these deviations can be used for estimating the precision of the results. Deviations from the mean can also be expressed either in absolute units or in relative units, with the mean taken as 100%.

Effect of Errors in Individual Measurements on the Result of Analysis. In quantitative determinations several separate measurements must be made; for example, weighing of the sample and of the precipitate obtained from it (or measurement of the volume of solution used in volumetric analysis), etc. When the analytical result is calculated the errors in the separate measurements may combine in various ways to introduce an error into the final result. How the individual errors combine depends on the type of mathematical operations carried out when the results are calculated. The formulas given below show how errors combine in different cases:

$$r = nxy \qquad \Delta r = \Delta x + \Delta y \qquad \text{(a)}$$

$$r = n\,(x : y) \qquad \Delta r = \Delta x - \Delta y \qquad \text{(b)}$$

$$r = n\,(x \pm y) \qquad \Delta r = n\left(\frac{x}{r}\,\Delta x \pm \frac{y}{r}\,\Delta y\right) \qquad \text{(c)}$$

$$r = nx^a y^b \qquad \Delta r = a\Delta x + b\Delta y \qquad \text{(d)}$$

Here Δx and Δy are the relative errors in the separate measurement of x and y;
Δr is the relative error of the calculated result (r);
n is a factor practically free from error (such factors include, for example, atomic and molecular weights, the errors in which are negligible in comparison with other errors).

Let us consider an example illustrating the use of the above formulas. Suppose that 0.5000 g of a certain substance is dissolved in water and the volume of the solution is made up to 250.0 ml. It is required to find the concentration (C) of the substance in solution. It is evidently

$$C = \frac{q}{V} = \frac{0.5}{250.0} = 0.002 \text{ g/ml}$$

where q is the weight taken in grams;
V is the volume of solution in ml.

We now calculate the precision to which this concentration was determined if the sample was weighed on an analytical balance to a precision of ± 0.0002 g, while measurement of the solution volume involves an error of $+0.5$ ml. The relative error in weighing is:

$$\Delta q = \frac{\pm 0.0002 \times 100}{0.5} = \pm 0.04\%$$

The relative error in the volume measurement is:

$$\Delta V = \frac{+0.5 \times 100}{250.0} = +0.2\%$$

Hence, from formula (b), we have:

$$\Delta C = \Delta q - \Delta V = \pm 0.04 - (+0.20)$$

Hence the relative error in preparation of a solution of the given concentration (0.002000 g/ml) lies between —0.16% and —0.24% (according to the sign of the error Δq when the sample was weighed).

Compensation of Errors. Formula (b) shows that if one measured value is divided by another for calculation of an analytical result *the errors in separate measurements may be partially or completely compensated.* This compensation of errors is very useful, and determinations should be carried out in such a way as to allow it to occur. That is why all weighings must be carried out on the same balance and with the same set of weights. This is because the weight of the element being determined, found from the weight of the precipitate, has to be divided by the weight of the sample taken. The more similar the weighing conditions, the greater the compensation of errors. It was also pointed out earlier that because of compensation of errors (use of the same balance) in many cases inequality of arm length may be disregarded and buoyancy corrections are unnecessary.

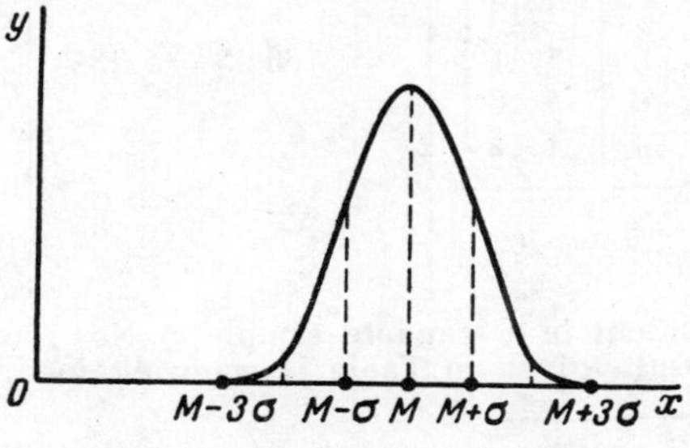

Fig. 12. Normal (Gaussian) distribution of random errors

14. Treatment of Analytical Results

As already stated (Sec. 13), to decrease the effect of random errors on the result of analysis usually not one, but two or more determinations are performed. As a rule, none of these determinations give the true value, because they all contain errors. Therefore, *the aim in analysis is to find the most probable value of the result and to assess its degree of precision.*

In absence of systematic errors, random errors conform to the so-called normal (Gaussian) distribution, represented graphically in Fig. 12. In this graph the values of the quantity being determined (x) are plotted against the corresponding probability of their occurrence in analysis.* It is clear from the curve in Fig. 12 that: (a) the most probable value is the arithmetic mean M of all the results; (b) positive and negative deviations from the arithmetic mean are equally probable; (c) small deviations are more probable than large.

The average deviation and the root mean square (standard) deviation of a single result are important in assessing the accuracy of a determination. The average deviation (d_{av}) is the average of individual deviations from the mean value, the signs of these deviations being disregarded. Therefore, if the absolute individual deviations are denoted by $[d_1]$, $[d_2]$, . . ., $[d_n]$, and the number of determinations by n, then the average deviation is:

$$d_{av}=\frac{[d_1]+[d_2]+\ldots+[d]_n}{n}=\frac{\Sigma [d]}{n} \tag{1}$$

The smaller the value of d_{av}, the more accurate the determination, i.e., the less the effect of *random* errors. However, the mathematical theory of errors shows that the magnitude of random errors is represented more correctly by the use of the *root mean square deviation* (standard deviation) σ, calculated from the formula**

$$\sigma=\sqrt{\frac{d_1^2+d_2^2+\ldots+d_n^2}{n-1}}=\sqrt{\frac{\Sigma d^2}{n-1}} \tag{2}$$

The probable random error of analysis can be calculated by using this value. This may be illustrated by the following example. In determining the chromium

Table II

Chromium Content of Standard No. 146 Steel Sample (determined by the persulphate method)

Detn. No.	Chromium content x, %	Mean M	Deviation from mean $d=x-M$	Square deviations d^2
1	1.12		$1.12-1.13=-0.01$	$0.01^2=0.0001$
2	1.15		$1.15-1.13=+0.02$	$0.02^2=0.0004$
3	1.11	$5.66:5=1.13\%$	$1.11-1.13=-0.02$	$0.02^2=0.0004$
4	1.16		$1.16-1.13=+0.03$	$0.03^2=0.0009$
5	1.12		$1.12-1.13=-0.01$	$0.01^2=0.0001$
$\Sigma x=5.66$			$d_{av}=0.018\%$	$\Sigma d^2=0.0019$

content in a standard sample of No. 146 steel by the persulphate method the results given in Table II were obtained.***

* The mathematical probability of any event is the ratio of the number of cases in which this event occurred to the total number of observed cases. For example, if in 20 determinations a particular result (for example, $x = 1.50\%$) was obtained in 4 cases, the probability of this result is $\alpha = 4:20 = 0.2$ (or 20%). Probability $\alpha=1$ represents complete certainty, and probability $\alpha = 0$ represents impossibility of the given event.

** With a large number of determinations $n-1$ is practically equal to n.

*** A. Dymov, *Technical Analysis of Ores and Metals* (in Russian), Metallurgizdat, 1949, p. 36.

For mathematical analysis of these results the arithmetic mean (M), deviations of the individual results from the mean, and the average deviation d_{av} are first found. The individual deviations are then squared and the sum of the squares (Σd^2) is found. Substituting this sum, and also the value of n into equation (2) we have:

$$\sigma = \sqrt{\frac{0.0019}{4}} = \pm 0.022\%$$

It should be noted that σ can be calculated with adequate precision for practical purposes trom the formula:

$$\sigma \approx \pm 1.25 \times d_{av} \tag{3}$$

Thus, in the present case

$$\sigma = \pm 1.25 \times 0.018 = \pm 0.022\%$$

According to the theory of errors, with a large number of measurements it can be asserted with *confidence* $\alpha = 0.997$ that the random error in the determination will not fall outside the limits of $\pm 3\sigma$ or $\pm 0.066\%$. In other words, in a very large number of measurements a result outside the limits of $1.13 - 0.066\%$ and $1.13 + 0.066\%$ (i.e., 1.064 and 1.196%) would be obtained in only three cases per thousand measurements.

If a smaller degree of confidence (α) is accepted, we have narrower limits for possible fluctuations of x, namely:

with $\alpha = 0.95$ $\quad x = M \pm 2\sigma$ $\quad$ (i.e., between 1.086% and 1.174%)

with $\alpha = 0.68$ $\quad x = M \pm \sigma$ $\quad$ (i.e., between 1.108% and 1.152%)

with $\alpha = 0.50$ $\quad x = M \pm \frac{2}{3}\sigma$ $\quad$ (i.e., between 1.115% and 1.145%)

Thus, virtually all random fluctuations of the measured value lie in the range $x = M \pm 3\sigma$. Therefore, errors exceeding 3σ should be rejected as mistakes.

The above results, based on the classical theory of errors, are valid only if the number of determinations is very large. In practice we always deal in analysis with relatively small numbers of determinations, so that the classical theory is inapplicable. Therefore, in estimating the influence of random errors on analytical results we must use modern methods of mathematical statistics which have been worked out for a small number of determinations. Here, as in the classical theory, the magnitude of the error is proportional to the root mean square deviation σ but the latter must be multiplied by a certain factor t_α which depends not only on α but also on the number of determinations n, and divided by $\sqrt{n}$. Therefore the probable analytical error in this case is:

$$\Sigma = \pm \frac{t_\alpha \cdot \sigma}{\sqrt{n}} \tag{4}$$

and the limits which contain the required value of x ("confidence limits") are given by the formula:

$$x = M \pm \Sigma = M \pm \frac{t_\alpha \cdot \sigma}{\sqrt{n}} \tag{5}$$

Values of t_α have been worked out for wide ranges of α and n, and are given in special tables.* An abbreviated table of this type is given in Appendix VIII. We use this table to find the probable random error and the confidence limits for the value determined (percentage of chromium in the standard steel sample). We first use Appendix VIII to find the value of t_α. When using this table we must remember that instead of the number of determinations it gives values of K, which are less than n by unity ($K = n - 1$). In the present case $K = 5 - 1 = 4$. We take the column for confidence $\alpha = 0.95$ (which is quite adequate for most cases) and in the horizontal row corresponding to $K = 4$ we find $t_\alpha = 2.78$. Substituting this into equation (4) we have

$$\Sigma = \pm \frac{2.78 \times 0.022}{\sqrt{5}} = \pm 0.027\%$$

This value of the probable error Σ is a measure of the precision of the analysis, i. e., the influence of random errors on the result. The confidence limits which contain the true value of x are:

$$x = 1.13 \pm 0.027\%$$

which is 1.103-1.157%.

If we took the confidence $\alpha = 0.99$ we would have

$$\Sigma = \pm \frac{4.60 \times 0.022}{\sqrt{5}} = \pm 0.045\%$$

and

$$x = 1.13 \pm 0.045$$

which corresponds to the range between 1.085% and 1.175%.

By the classical theory of errors these confidence values correspond to rather narrower confidence limits for x. They can be found from equation (5) by substitution of the value of t_α corresponding to $K = \infty$. Thus, with $\alpha = 0.99$ we have:

$$x = 1.13 \pm \frac{2.58 \times 0.022}{\sqrt{5}} = 1.13 \pm 0.025$$

which is between 1.105% and 1.155%.

The table shows that in every case t_α decreases rapidly with an increase in the number of determinations n. This decrease, like the increase of $\sqrt{n}$, must diminish the probable random error Σ and narrow the confidence limits for x. This effect must be most pronounced with small values of n, for example, as we pass from two to three, four or five determinations, as it is in such cases that t_α and $\sqrt{n}$ decrease especially rapidly with the increase of n. Subsequently this decrease slows down, and a point is very soon reached when the increase in precision is too small to justify the expenditure of labour, time, and reagents involved in the increased number of determinations.

We must remind once again that *the values of Σ calculated as described above characterize the influence only of random and not of systematic errors in analysis.* The analysis may prove quite wrong, despite a high degree of precision, i.e., a small value of Σ, if there were any systematic errors in the analysis. Absence of systematic errors may be established by comparison of the

* See V. Romanovsky, *Fundamentals of the Theory of Errors*, Gostekhizdat, 1947.

difference between the arithmetic mean analytical result (M) and the true content (A) of the element being determined ($\Delta = M - A$) with the probable random error Σ. If $\Delta < \Sigma$ there are no systematic errors. Conversely, if $\Delta \geqslant \Sigma$, there are systematic errors.

The true contents of elements in chemically pure substances can be calculated from their formulas. In the case of artificially prepared mixtures it is also usually possible to calculate A from the amounts and formulas of the components. On the other hand, the true contents of individual elements in various natural materials or industrial products are unknown and must be estimated from analytical results, which always contain errors of one kind or another. In such cases the true content of a particular element is taken to be the most reliable average value from a series of determinations carried out with the utmost care by several different methods in different laboratories. For example, standard steel No. 146, according to its accompanying certificate, has been analysed for chromium by five different methods in five leading laboratories of the USSR, the results being in the range of 1.12-1.16%. The arithmetic mean of all the results (1.14%) is known as the *established content* of the given element, and taken as the true content A. The established content is used whenever the standard is used in practice; for example, in verification of new analytical methods, in control of the work of laboratory assistants, in standardization of solutions of various reagents, etc.

The established content should also be used in deciding whether a particular analytical result (or method) is correct. For example, in the present instance we have: $A = 1.14\%$ and $M = 1.13\%$. Therefore, the accuracy of chromium determination by the persulphate method can be assessed by the magnitude of the error:

$$\Delta = M - A = 1.13 - 1.14 = -0.01\%$$

Comparing the value found for Δ with the value of Σ (for $\alpha = 0.95$) we see that $0.01 < 0.027$, so that the deviation of the analytical result from the true value is less than the probable random error of analysis. In other words, the actual error of the analytical result (—0.01%) is within the probable limits of random error, and therefore it may be concluded that the method is free from systematic errors.

To avoid systematic errors it is imperative to use well-verified analytical methods and reagents, which have been tested for purity. In such testing a so-called "*blank*" *experiment* is carried out; i.e., the element in question is determined with the reagents only, in absence of the actual material being analysed. A correction into the analytical results obtained with the given reagents can then be introduced from the results of the "blank" experiment.*

15. Calculations in Quantitative Analysis

The final result of an analysis is found by calculation from weight or volume data obtained during the analysis.

Calculation of the results is as much an integral part of analysis as any other operation. Calculation errors lead to the same consequences as errors in any other analytical operation.

---

* The subjects mentioned in this section are discussed in greater detail in V. Romanovsky's book: *Fundamentals of the Theory of Errors*, Gostekhizdat, 1947, and in the articles by: N. Komar, *Zhurnal Analit. Khim.*, 7, 325 (1952); E. Grachov, *Zhurnal Analit. Khim.*, 7, 42 (1952).

In industry the results of an analysis are often used to adjust a process immediately after they have been received from the laboratory. It is obvious that a calculation error is quite inadmissible in such cases. That is why a student must train himself to take the greatest care in calculations when he is studying quantitative analysis.

The numerical values used in such calculations are approximate (p. 43), therefore the calculation results must also be approximate. Since this is so, it is important to be clear about the degree of precision to which the result is to be presented. This is determined either by the precision of the analysis itself, or by the degree of precision required. Here we must consider two types of calculations which are met in quantitative analysis, namely, precise and approximate calculations.

Precise Calculations. These include calculations of the final result, which must be carried out *with the same precision as the analysis itself.* It would be obviously quite inadmissible as the result of an inaccurate calculation to lose the experimental precision which may have been obtained with great difficulty. However, it would be just as wrong to give a result to a greater number of decimal places than would correspond to the true precision of the determination.

The basic rule for deciding the degree of precision to which a calculation result should be presented was already indicated in Sec. 10. By this rule *the number of significant figures in a result should be such that only the last one is uncertain.*

Significant figures are all the figures in a number, apart from zeros, on the left, or of zeros on the right if these replace unknown figures or are written when the number is rounded off. For example, the number 0.0035 has two significant figures (3 and 5), as its three zeros are not significant but merely show the positions of the two significant figures. The zeros in the number 7.2500 are not significant if the number represents the weight of an object weighed on a technical balance, or is obtained by rounding off a weight determined more precisely. On the other hand, if the same number 7.2500 was obtained by weighing on an analytical balance to a precision of 0.0001-0.0002 g, both its zeros are significant figures. Zeros in the middle of a number, such as all the zeros in the number 10.0305 are also significant.

Significant figures must be distinguished from *decimal places.* For example, the number 0.0035 has four decimal places and two significant figures; the number 10.0305 also has four decimal places but six significant figures, etc.

The numerical quantities with which one deals in analysis may differ in their degree of precision. *The result of a calculation obviously cannot be any more precise than the least precise of the quantities used in the calculation*. Therefore, to perform a calculation most rationally, it is first necessary to find the least precise of the quantities used and decide accordingly how many decimal places or significant figures the result should contain.

If the calculation involves addition or subtraction of numerical quantities, the least precise is the one with the smallest number of decimal places. For example, if we have weights of 5.2727 g, 0.075 g, 3.7 g and 2.12 g, the least precise is 3.7 g, where the number of tenths of a gram is uncertain. The same number is obviously uncertain in the sum of all these weights.

It is therefore obvious that in the calculation there was no point in taking all the decimal places of the separate quantities, which should have been rounded off*. When this is done, it is usual to leave one additional figure, in this instance the second decimal place, which is then discarded from the final result. Therefore, this calculation should be performed as follows:

$$x = 5.27 + 0.08 + 3.7 + 2.12 = 11.17 \text{ g}$$

and finally

$$x = 11.2 \text{ g}$$

In multiplication and division the least precise number is the one with the fewest significant figures. The same number of significant figures should be left in the result. Here again it is advisable to keep one additional figure in each of the quantities; this is discarded in the final result. In illustration, let us calculate the percentage content of chlorine in common salt from the data on p. 15. This calculation is performed by the formula:

$$\%\text{Cl} = y = \frac{q \cdot A_{\text{Cl}} \cdot 100}{M_{\text{AgCl}} \cdot G}$$

where q is the weight of the AgCl precipitate (0.1290 g);
G is the weight of NaCl taken (0.0536 g);
A_{Cl} is the atomic weight of Cl (35.453);
M_{AgCl} is the molecular weight of AgCl (143.32).

Here the least precise number is 0.0536, which contains only three significant figures whereas the others have four of five.** Therefore, the analytical results should also have three significant figures. The other quantities in the calculation are rounded off to one addi-

* When a number is rounded off, the last figure retained is increased by 1 if the first rejected figure is 5 or more; this was done in this instance.

** The factor 100, used for conversion of the results into percentages is a precise number and therefore the number of its significant figures is not taken into account.

tional figure. This gives:

$$y = \frac{0.1290 \times 35.45 \times 100}{143.3 \times 0.0536} = 59.54\%$$

Finally, rounding off to three significant figures, we have $y = 59.5\%$. If the same calculation is performed without the additional figure, we have a somewhat different result, namely 59.6%. However, since the last figure of the result is uncertain, this difference is quite permissible. Hence it is clear that it is besirable but not essential to retain one additional figure in calculations. In certain cases (for example, in calculations with four-figure logarithms, when the additional figure would be a fifth significant figure) this cannot be done.

In the majority of cases the experimental data (weights and volumes) obtained in analysis are numbers of four significant figures. Therefore, the analytical results in such cases are also given to four significant figures. Calculations involving such numbers are most conveniently carried out by means of tables of four-figure logarithms and antilogarithms (see Appendix IX and X at the end of the book). These tables give just this degree of precision and at the same time make the calculations much easier. If the final result is to be given to three significant figures a slide rule may be used.

Approximate Calculations. As already stated, it is sometimes necessary during analysis to perform various approximate calculations which do not require a high degree of precision. Examples of these are calculations of the most suitable sample weights to be taken or of the amount of precipitant required for precipitation of a particular ion, etc. Quantities like these need not be known very precisely. For example, if the most suitable sample weight of a particular substance is 1 g, and we take 0.1-0.2 g more or less, this would not make any significant difference, as it is only important that the weight should roughly correspond to the optimum value. In just the same way there is no point in calculating the amount of precipitant precisely, as in practice considerably more than the calculated quantity is taken in order that the precipitation should be as complete as possible. It is therefore obvious that all such calculations should be carried out very approximately, the numbers used being rounded off very extensively. For example, let us consider the calculation of the amount of $AgNO_3$ required for complete precipitation of Cl^- from a solution containing 0.0536 g NaCl:

Precipitation of 58.443 g NaCl takes 169.88 g $AgNO_3$
Precipitation of 0.0536 g NaCl takes x g $AgNO_3$

Since we only want an approximate result, the original weight of NaCl, 0.0536 g, should be rounded off to 0.05 g. In that case, keeping one additional figure in all the other numbers, we have:

$$x = \frac{0.05 \times 170}{58} = 0.15 \approx 0.2 \text{ g}$$

The same calculation can be simplified still further if the additional figure is not retained, which is permissible in this case:

$$x = \frac{0.05 \times 200}{60} \approx 0.2 \text{ g}$$

It follows from this that quite often a calculation is greatly simplified if the required precision is taken into account.

QUESTIONS AND PROBLEMS
(on Secs. 1-15)

1. What are the essential principles of gravimetric and volumetric analyses?

2. To determine calcium in $CaCO_3$, 0.4116 g of the latter was dissolved in HCl, NH_4OH was added until alkaline, and Ca^{++} was precipitated by the action of ammonium oxalate $(NH_4)_2C_2O_4$ (write the equation for the reaction). The precipitated calcium oxalate $CaC_2O_4 \cdot H_2O$ was filtered off, washed, ignited and weighed. When the precipitate is ignited it is converted into CaO (write the reaction equation); the weight of CaO was 0.2302 g; calculate the percentage of calcium in $CaCO_3$.

Answer: 40.00%.

3. Neutralization of 20.00 ml of a solution of H_2SO_4 took 30.00 ml of caustic soda solution containing 0.004000 g NaOH per ml; calculate the number of grams of H_2SO_4 per litre of sulphuric acid solution.

Answer: 7.356 g.

4. What is the advantage of volumetric analysis over the gravimetric method?

5. What is the principle of colorimetric analysis? What is its most important field of application?

6. What is the percentage of carbon in a sample of cast iron if 1.0000 g of it, when burnt in an electric furnace (p. 17), gave 74.00 ml of CO_2?

Hint. The volume of CO_2 is reduced to standard conditions. The calculation is based on the fact that the volume of one gram-molecule of any gas under standard conditions (0° and 760 mm pressure) is 22.4 litres.

Answer: 3.97%.

7. What is the precision of weighing on an analytical balance?

8. What is the weight of a rider on a balance with the zero mark (a) in the centre of the beam scale; (b) at the left of the beam scale? What change of load on the right-hand balance pan corresponds to displacement of the rider by one (small) scale division?

9. What is the sensitivity of a balance? On what factors does it depend and how is it determined experimentally?

10. How is the sensitivity of a balance adjusted?

11. Why is it undesirable to decrease excessively the distance between the centre of gravity of the balance beam and the fulcrum?

12. Find the zero point of a balance from the following pointer readings:

left: 17.8; 17.6 divisions;
right: 4.0; 4.2; 4.4 divisions.

Answer: 10.9 divisions.

13. Find the sensitivity of a balance and the value of a scale division at the given load for the following pointer readings:

(a) with the rider on position marked 6:

left: 14.2; 14.0 divisions;
right: 2.4; 2.6; 2.8 divisions;

(b) with the rider on position marked 7:

left: 18.3; 18.1 divisions;
right: 4.3; 4.5; 4.7 divisions.

Answer: Sensitivity 3.0 divisions; value of a scale division 0.33 mg.

14. The zero point of a balance is 10.5 divisions. A crucible was weighed with 7.18 g on the right-hand pan. Determinations of the rest points for different positions of the rider gave the following results:

Rider position	Rest point
5th division	7.2 divisions
6th ditto	9.7 ditto
7th ditto	12.2 ditto
8th ditto	14.7 ditto

Find the weight of the crucible.

Answer: 7.1863 g.

15. The zero point of a balance is 9.5 divisions, and the sensitivity at a certain load is 3.0 divisions. Find: (a) the deviations of the rest point from the zero point which can be disregarded in weighing by the coincidence method; (b) the error which results if the weighing is terminated at a rest point of 9.1 divisions.

Answer: (a) 0.6 division or less; (b) 0.13 mg.

16. Explain why an object to be weighed must be at the same temperature as the balance.

17. A weighing bottle was found to weigh 12.7544 g on the left-hand pan, and 12.7538 g on the right-hand pan. Correct the weight of the bottle for inequality of the beam arms.

Answer: 12.7541 g.

18. The right and left arms of a balance beam are 79.90 and 80.00 mm long respectively. The weight of a crucible when weighed on the left-hand pan was found to be 7.1540 g. What is its true weight (in air)?

Answer: 7.1440 g.

19. A $BaSO_4$ precipitate (sp. gr. 4.5) weighed 0.6000 g in air. What is its weight in a vacuum? Aluminium weights (sp. gr. 2.6) were used; the density of air is taken as 0.0012 g/cu cm.

Answer: The correction for buoyancy in air is —0.000117 g; the weight of the precipitate in a vacuum is ~0.5999 g.

20. Explain why, in quantitative analysis, it is in most cases unnecessary to correct for inequality of balance arm length or for buoyancy in air. When are such corrections necessary?

21. How and why are substances recrystallized? Does recrystallization achieve its purpose in all cases?

22. Explain the principle and importance of average sampling.

23. A crucible weighs 8 g. How should this weight be written down if the crucible was weighed (a) on a technical balance; (b) on an analytical balance?

24. How many decimal places should be retained in a total obtained by addition of weights some of which were determined on a technical balance and some on an analytical balance?

25. How many significant figures are there in the following numbers: (a) 0.00012; (b) 2.7005; (c) 3.5700 (weight obtained on an analytical balance)?

Answer: (a) 2; (b) 5; (c) 5.

26. How many significant figures should be retained in values of atomic and molecular weights in calculation of the results of gravimetric or volumetric determinations? When should atomic and molecular weights be rounded off in calculations?

27. Explain the differences between systematic and random errors and mistakes. Point out the causes of systematic and random errors.

28. Explain the meaning of *accuracy* and *precision* of a determination or method. If the precision of a determination or method is high, can it be assumed accurate?

29. What is the average deviation of a single result? What is the root mean square deviation?

30. The following results were obtained in determinations of nickel in an alloy: 8.25%; 8.15%; 8.08%; 8.20%; 8.02%. Find the indeterminate error of analysis (assuming confidence $\alpha = 0.95$) and the confidence limits for the result.

Answer: $\Sigma = \pm 0.102\%$; $x = 8.14 \pm 0.102\%$ (i.e., from 8.038% to 8.242%).

CHAPTER II

GRAVIMETRIC ANALYSIS

16. The Principle of Gravimetric Analysis

The content of a given element (or ion) in a substance is usually found in gravimetric analysis from the weight of a precipitate formed when the element or ion is converted into an insoluble compound. In addition to *precipitation*, other methods are used. For example, volatile components (H_2O, CO_2, etc.) of a substance are often determined by *volatilization*; the substance is warmed or ignited and the amount of the component is found from the loss of weight. A volatile component (such as CO_2) can also be separated from the sample by a suitable method (for example, by the action of HCl) and determined by absorption in a suitable absorbent.* In this case the amount of CO_2 is found from the increase in the weight of the absorbent.

In each of these analytical methods the amount of a given component is found from the results of weighing. These methods can therefore be regarded as different varieties of gravimetric analysis.

The most important is the precipitation method, which is considered in detail below.

A weighed sample** of the substance to be analysed is brought into solution by a suitable method, and the element to be determined is then precipitated as an insoluble compound (or liberated in the free state). The precipitate is filtered off, washed thoroughly, ignited (or dried) and weighed accurately. The content of the element is calculated from the weight of the precipitate and its formula and expressed as a percentage of the sample taken.

The most important of the above operations is precipitation. The precision of analytical results depends to a considerable extent on the choice of precipitant, the amount of precipitant added, the conditions of precipitation, etc. Precipitation may be accompanied by complications (such as formation of a colloidal solution, coprecipi-

---

* In this case soda lime, which is a mixture of CaO with NaOH.

** See p. 19.

tation of impurities, etc.) which make the analytical results quite incorrect unless the analyst takes appropriate steps. Because of all this we must first consider the theory and practice of precipitation. Other operations in gravimetric analysis will be discussed later.

17. Requirements for Precipitates. Choice of Precipitant

If an insoluble compound of a particular element is to be used for gravimetric determination by the precipitation method, it must satisfy a number of requirements. Before considering these requirements, we should note that the precipitates formed during analysis are usually ignited. Many precipitates undergo chemical changes during ignition. Therefore, very often not the precipitated compound but some other compound is weighed. Accordingly, a distinction is made in gravimetric analysis between the precipitated form and the weighed form.

The precipitated form is the name given to the compound precipitated from solution by the action of the appropriate reagent, and the *weighed form* is the compound which is weighed for determination of the final result. For example, in determinations of Fe^{+++} and Al^{+++} the precipitated forms are usually the hydroxides $Fe(OH)_3$ and $Al(OH)_3$, formed by the action of NH_4OH on the solution. The weighed forms are the anhydrous oxides Fe_2O_3 and Al_2O_3, formed by ignition from the hydroxides, for example:

$$2Fe(OH)_3 = Fe_2O_3 + 3H_2O$$

In determination of Ca^{++} the precipitated form is calcium oxalate $CaC_2O_4 \cdot H_2O$, and the weighed form is calcium oxide CaO formed from it on ignition:

$$CaC_2O_4 \cdot H_2O = CaO + \uparrow CO_2 + \uparrow CO + \uparrow H_2O$$

In some cases the precipitated and weighed forms may both be the same compound. For example, Ba^{++} and SO_4^{--} ions are precipitated and weighed as barium sulphate which is not changed chemically when ignited. In just the same way in determination of Ag^+ ions (or Cl^- ions) the precipitated and weighed forms are both silver chloride AgCl, etc.

It is obvious that the precipitated and weighed forms must conform to different requirements. Let us consider them separately.

Requirements for the Precipitated Form. 1. The precipitated form should have *low solubility*, without which practically complete precipitation of the given ion or element is impossible. It is known that the solubility of a sparingly soluble electrolyte is character-zed by its solubility product (SP).* It is found in practice that in the case of binary electrolytes (compounds the molecules of which dissociate into pairs of ions, such as $BaSO_4$, AgCl, etc.) precipitation is practically complete only as long as SP of the precipitate does not exceed 1×10^{-8}. Therefore compounds with SP $> 10^{-8}$ are generally not used as precipitated forms in gravimetric analysis. Of course, the suitability of a particular compound for this purpose also depends on the degree of precision required in the analysis. In less precise determinations it is occasionally permissible to use as the precipitated forms compounds which cannot be used in more precise analysis.

2. It is also desirable that the structure of the precipitate should be such as to allow of rapid filtration and washing. Precipitates consisting of relatively large crystals are very convenient, because they hardly clog the filter pores, and, as their specific surface is not extensive they do not readily adsorb impurities from solution and are easily washed free from the latter.** Precipitates consisting of very small crystals, such as $BaSO_4$ or CaC_2O_4, are less convenient in this respect. Moreover, if the precipitation is not performed correctly such precipitates readily pass through the filter pores; of course, this is quite inadmissible in gravimetric analysis.

Amorphous precipitates, especially if gelatinous, such as $Al(OH)_3$, have extensive specific surfaces and therefore adsorb considerable amounts of impurities which are difficult to wash off. Moreover, filtration is very slow in such cases.

However, because of the lack of compounds of more convenient properties, it is often necessary to use such precipitates. In such cases the analyst tries to create conditions in which the disadvantages of amorphous precipitates are reduced to a minimum (Sec. 24).

3. Finally, the precipitated form must be converted fairly easily and completely into the weighed form.

Requirements for the Weighed Form. 1. The most important requirement is that its composition *should correspond exactly to its chemical formula*. Obviously, otherwise it would be impossible to calculate analytical results; for example, if the weighed precipitate was an indefinite mixture and not an individual chemical substance of a definite composition corresponding to its formula.

However, many precipitates obtained in analysis do not satisfy this requirement. For example, the ferric hydroxide precipitate

---

* See V. Alexeyev, *Qualitative Analysis*, Sec. 24, Goskhimizdat, 1960, V. Alexeyev, *Course of Qualitative Chemical Semimicroanalysis*, Sec. 28, Goskhimizdat, 1962.

** The entrainment of impurities from solution by precipitates as the result of adsorption and other causes is discussed more fully in Sec. 25.

formed in gravimetric determination of iron does not correspond exactly to the formula $Fe(OH)_3$, but contains variable amounts of water which depend on the precipitation conditions and which are not known exactly. Therefore, it would be more correct to write its formula as $Fe_2O_3 \cdot nH_2O$. When ferric hydroxide is ignited, all this water is removed and a compound of quite a definite composition is formed, exactly corresponding to the formula Fe_2O_3.

The compositions of precipitates originally formed often do not correspond to their formulas, and that is why they have to be ignited. Moreover, when a precipitate is ignited the water and any volatile impurities retained by it are completely removed, and the filter itself is converted into ash.

2. The weighed form *must have adequate chemical stability*. Analysis obviously becomes more difficult if the weighed form readily changes its composition, for example, by absorption of water vapour or CO_2 from the air, by oxidation or reduction, by decomposition at higher temperatures, and similar processes. If this happens the composition of the precipitate no longer corresponds to its formula. Such properties in a precipitate need not make the determination impossible, but would involve a number of measures for preventing changes of composition, which would complicate the analysis.

To avoid this, it is often preferred to convert a precipitate having such properties into a more convenient weighed form by treating it with suitable reagents. For example, CaO precipitates readily absorb H_2O and CO_2 from the air (which makes weighing difficult); therefore they are sometimes converted into $CaSO_4$ by treatment with sulphuric acid in the crucible, and excess acid is removed by evaporation.

The precipitate also has to be treated with reagents if it undergoes partial reduction during ignition by the action of carbon and of products of incomplete combustion of the filter. This occurs, for example, in determination of Cl^- in the form of AgCl (Sec. 40).

3. Finally, it is convenient if *the content of the element being determined in the precipitate should be as low as possible*,* because errors in the determination (for example, weighing errors, losses due to solubility of the precipitate or incomplete transfer to the filter, etc.) have less effect on the final result of the analysis.

For example, the same absolute error in weighing $BaCrO_4$ and Cr_2O_3 precipitates influences the content of chromium found 3.5 times as much in the second case as in the first.

---

* In other words, the conversion factor (Sec. 32) (i.e., the factor by which the weight of the precipitate is multiplied to find the content of the given element) must be as small as possible.

The loss of 1 mg of precipitate in analysis corresponds to the following errors in determination of the weight of chromium:

Weighed form Cr_2O_3	Weighed form $BaCrO_4$
152 mg Cr_2O_3 contains 104 mg Cr	253.3 mg $BaCrO_4$ contains 52 mg Cr
1 mg Cr_2O_3 contains x mg Cr	1 mg $BaCrO_4$ contains x mg Cr
$x=\frac{104}{152}\times 1=0.7$ mg Cr	$x=\frac{52}{253.3}\times 1=0.2$ mg Cr

The above requirements largely determine the choice of precipitant. In addition, the following considerations should be taken into account.

It is found in practice that precipitates formed during analysis always take various extraneous substances or ions from solution with them. These include ions of the precipitant which have to be removed from the precipitates by washing. Since such washing may prove incomplete, *it is convenient if the precipitant is volatile*, as in that case the part of it not removed by washing is volatilized during ignition. In view of this, Fe^{+++} is precipitated by NH_4OH rather than by KOH or NaOH; Ba^{++} by H_2SO_4 and not by Na_2SO_4 or K_2SO_4; Ag^+ by HCl and not by NaCl, etc.

Of course, it is not always possible to follow this rule. For example, when Cu^{++} is precipitated as $Cu(OH)_2$ it is not possible to use NH_4OH, because the precipitate is soluble in excess of this reagent, and NaOH or KOH must be used, etc.

Obviously, the precipitates must be washed with special thoroughness in such cases.

In practice, a particular ion usually has to be precipitated in presence of several other ions. Therefore, other sparingly soluble substances may be precipitated together with the one required. To avoid this it is very important to choose a precipitant which precipitates only the required ion but not the others present in solution; i.e., which is *specific* in its action.

This may be illustrated by the following example. The Al^{+++} ion is often determined by precipitation as $Al(OH)_3$ by the action of ammonia, followed by weighing of the Al_2O_3 formed by ignition of the precipitate. However, this method is inconvenient if the solution contains Fe^{+++} ions, also precipitated by ammonia as $Fe(OH)_3$. In that case it is better to use a more specific precipitant, namely, sodium thiosulphate $Na_2S_2O_3$, which reacts with Al^{+++} as follows:

$$2Al^{+++}+3S_2O_3^{--}+3H_2O=\downarrow 2Al(OH)_3+\downarrow 3S+\uparrow 3SO_2$$

The precipitate of $Al(OH)_3+S$ is filtered off, washed and ignited. The sulphur burns away, and $Al(OH)_3$ is converted into Al_2O_3.

Sodium thiosulphate does not precipitate Fe^{+++} ions but merely reduces them to Fe^{++}.

Of course, it is not always possible to find a specific precipitant. In such cases *masking* of the interfering ions is used; i.e., they are combined in fairly stable complexes which are not precipitated by the particular reagent; if masking is not possible, the ions are removed from solution by some suitable method. Such methods are descrided more fully later (Secs. 23 and 35).

18. Amount of Precipitant

We learn in qualitative analysis that a solution of a particular sparingly soluble electrolyte becomes saturated when the product of the concentrations (or, more correctly, the activities) of its ions reaches a certain value, constant for a given temperature, known as the solubility product (SP).

For lead sulphate solution saturated at 25°C we can write:

$$[Pb^{++}][SO_4^{--}] = SP_{PbSO_4} = 2.2 \times 10^{-8}$$

If

$$[Pb^{++}][SO_4^{--}] < 2.2 \times 10^{-8}$$

then the solution is not saturated, and some more lead sulphate can be dissolved in it.

If the solubility product is "exceeded", i.e.,

$$[Pb^{++}][SO_4^{--}] > 2.2 \times 10^{-8} \text{ (at 25° C)}$$

then the solution is supersaturated and a certain amount of $PdSO_4$ must be precipitated. Therefore, by the solubility product rule* *a precipitate is formed only when the product of the concentrations (or, more precisely, the activities)*** *of the corresponding ions exceeds the solubility product of the precipitated compound at a given temperature.*

Therefore, if equal volumes of 0.0001 M $Pb(NO_3)_2$ and Na_2SO_4 solutions are mixed $PbSO_4$ is not precipitated. When equal volumes of these solutions are mixed the concentration of each of the two substances is halved and becomes 0.00005 M or 5×10^{-5} M. Since salts are strong electrolytes and are therefore dissociated almost completely in aqueous solution, and each molecule of these salts dissociates to give one Pb^{++} ion or one SO_4^{--} ion, the concentrations of these ions after mixing are also equal:

$$[Pb^{++}] = [SO_4^{--}] = 5 \times 10^{-5} \text{ g-ion/litre}$$

---

* See V. Alexeyev, *Qualitative Analysis*, Sec. 26 Goskhimizdat, 1960, or V. Alexeyev, *Course of Qualitative Chemical Semimicroanalysis*, Sec. 28, Goskhimizdat, 1962.

** For fuller details, see p. 75.

Therefore, the ionic product (i.e., the product of the concentrations of the ions in solution) in this case is:

$$[Pb^{++}][SO_4^{--}] = 5 \times 10^{-5} \times 5 \times 10^{-5} = 25 \times 10^{-10} = 2.5 \times 10^{-9}$$

Since $2.5 \times 10^{-9} < 2.2 \times 10^{-8}$, i.e., is less than SP for $PbSO_4$ at this temperature, the solution is unsaturated with respect to $PbSO_4$ and this salt is not precipitated.

When the ionic product $[Pb^{++}][SO_4^{--}]$ exceeds 2.2×10^{-8}, the solution is supersaturated with respect to lead sulphate and the latter is precipitated. As this precipitation proceeds the concentrations of the respective ions in the solution gradually decrease, and when their product becomes equal to SP for the precipitate, dynamic equilibrium is established between the precipitate and solution and further precipitation ceases. The liquid phase is then a solution of $PbSO_4$ saturated at the given temperature.

Since no substance is absolutely insoluble in water, the solubility product can never be zero. It follows that *theoretically no precipitation can ever be quite complete*. Part of the ions being precipitated, corresponding to SP of the precipitate, always remains in solution. However, as in qualitative analysis, we are concerned with practical rather than theoretical completeness of precipitation. For qualitative analysis we can consider the precipitation of any given ion as practically complete when the amount remaining in solution is too small to interfere with any of the subsequent analytical operations. Similarly, *in gravimetric analysis precipitation is regarded as practically complete when the amount of the precipitated substance remaining in solution is beyond the precision limits of weighing, i.e., when it does not exceed 0.0002 g.*

For practically complete precipitation of a particular ion it is evidently necessary to take a sufficient amount of precipitant. The amount required can be approximately calculated from the reaction equation.

Suppose that it is required to determine the lead content of lead acetate $Pb(CH_3COO)_2 \cdot 3H_2O$ by precipitation of Pb^{++} ions with sulphuric acid:

$$Pb(CH_3COO)_2 \cdot 3H_2O + H_2SO_4 = \downarrow PbSO_4 + 2CH_3COOH + 3H_2O$$

If the weight of $Pb(CH_3COO)_2 \cdot 3H_2O$ taken for analysis was 0.6525 g, we can write:

1 mole of $Pb(CH_3COO)_2 \cdot 3H_2O$ takes 1 mole of H_2SO_4

0.6525 g of $Pb(CH_3COO)_2 \cdot 3H_2O$ takes x g of H_2SO_4

Since this calculation is only approximate and a high degree of precision is not required (p. 60) the quantities in the calculations should be rounded off. Thus, the weight 0.6525 g can be rounae off to 0.7 g, and the molecular weights of $Pb(CH_3COO)_2 \cdot 3H_2O$ and H_2SO_4 should be rounded off to 380 and 98 respectively. Then:

380 g of $Pb(CH_3COO)_2 \cdot 3H_2O$ takes 98 g of H_2SO_4
0.7 g of $Pb(CH_3COO)_2 \cdot 3H_2O$ takes x g of H_2SO_4

$$x = \frac{0.7 \times 98}{380} \approx 0.2 \text{ g}$$

Since the precipitant is generally used in the form of a solution of some known concentration, we must convert the weight of sulphuric acid to the volume of solution. Solution concentrations are expressed in percentages, moles (molar solutions) or gram-equivalents (normal solutions).

The percentage concentration of a solution represents the number of grams of substance in 100 g (weight percentage) or in 100 ml (volume percentage) of solution.

The molar concentration represents the number of moles (gram-molecules), and the normal concentration the number of gram-equivalents per litre of solution.

Suppose, for example, that a solution containing 10% (by volume) of H_2SO_4 is used for precipitating Pb^{++}. The required volume is found by proportion:

100 ml of solution contains 10 g H_2SO_4
x ml of solution contains 0.2 g H_2SO_4

$$x = \frac{0.2 \times 100}{10} = 2 \text{ ml}$$

The calculation becomes much simpler if the concentration of the precipitant is expressed in moles (or gram-equivalents) rather than in percentages. In such a case the volume of precipitant solution required can be found by simple proportion. For example, if the concentration of the sulphuric acid solution is 0.5 *M* (which is 1 *N*), since one gram-molecule of H_2SO_4 is contained in 2 litres of this solution, we can write:

380 g of $Pb(CH_3COO)_2 \cdot 3H_2O$ takes 2,000 ml 0.5 *M* H_2SO_4
0.7 g of $Pb(CH_3COO)_2 \cdot 3H_2O$ takes x ml 0.5 *M* H_2SO_4

$$x = \frac{0.7 \times 2{,}000}{380} \approx 4 \text{ ml}$$

Let us now consider how completely $PbSO_4$ is precipitated if the amount of precipitant calculated from the reaction equation is added. When this amount is added, one SO_4^{--} ion is introduced with each Pb^{++} ion, and therefore the concentrations of these ions must be equal at the end of precipitation. The product of these concentrations (at room temperature) is

$$[Pb^{++}][SO_4^{--}] = SP_{PbSO_4} = 2.2 \times 10^{-8}$$

and therefore the concentration of each is

$$[Pb^{++}] = [SO_4^{--}] = \sqrt{2.2 \times 10^{-8}} \approx 1.5 \times 10^{-4} \text{ g-ion/litre}$$

If all these Pb^{++} and SO_4^{--} ions remaining in solution were to combine and form a precipitate, 1.5×10^{-4} mole or $1.5 \times 10^{-4} \times$ $\times$ 303 g $PbSO_4$ would be obtained from each litre of solution. However, only about 100 ml of solution is used in the analysis here. Therefore, the loss due to solubility of the $PbSO_4$ precipitate in this case is approximately

$$\Delta = 1.5 \times 10^{-4} \times 303 \times 0.1 \approx 0.0045 \text{ g}$$

It is evident that the precipitation of Pb^{++} cannot be regarded as practically complete in this instance because the loss due to solubility of the precipitate is approximately 22 times the permissible value (0.0002 g).

19. Effect of Excess Precipitant on Completeness of Precipitation

It was shown in the preceding section that precipitation of a substance such as $PbSO_4$ (SP = 2.2×10^{-8}) is very incomplete if the equivalent amount of precipitant (i.e., the amount corresponding to the reaction equation) is used. Theory and practice both show that the precipitation can be much more complete if excess of precipitant is used.

According to the solubility product rule, *the product of the concentrations (more precisely, the activities) of the ions of any sparingly soluble electrolyte in a concentrated solution of that electrolyte is constant at a given temperature, and is equal to the* SP *of the electrolyte,** for example:

$$[Pb^{++}][SO_4^{--}] = SP_{PbSO_4} = 2.2 \times 10^{-8} \text{ (at 25° C)}$$

It follows from this equation that if it is required to precipitate Pb^{++} more completely, i.e., to reduce its concentration in the saturated $PbSO_4$ solution obtained at the end of the precipitation, the concentration of the precipitating SO_4^{--} ions must be correspondingly raised; i.e., excess of precipitant (H_2SO_4) must be added.

Suppose, for example, that instead of the 4 ml of 0.5 *M* H_2SO_4 solution, as required by calculation, we take 1.5 times as much, 6 ml. It is easy to calculate the loss due to solubility of the precipitate in this case.

---

* For the derivation of the solubility product rule, see: V. Alexeyev, *Qualitative Analysis*, Sec. 24, Goskhimizdat, 1960; and V. Alexeyev, *Course of Qualitative Chemical Semimicroanalysis*. Sec. 28, Goskhimizdat, 1962.

Of the 6 ml of H_2SO_4 taken, 4 ml is expended in precipitation of Pb^{++} and 2 ml remains in excess. Since the total volume of the solution is 100 ml, this excess amount of sulphuric acid becomes diluted 50-fold, from 2 to 100 ml, and the H_2SO_4 concentration in solution therefore becomes $0.5 : 50 = 0.01 = 10^{-2}$ *M*.

Since H_2SO_4 is a strong electrolyte, and each molecule gives one SO_4^{--} ion on dissociation, we can disregard the small amount of SO_4^{--} ions which form the $PbSO_4$ precipitate, and assume that $[SO_4^{--}] \approx 10^{-2}$ g-ion/litre. On the other hand, denoting the required solubility of $PbSO_4$ (in moles/litre) by x, we can write $[Pb^{++}] = x$.

Therefore,

$$[Pb^{++}][SO_4^{--}] = x \times 10^{-2} = 2.2 \times 10^{-8}$$

and hence

$$x = 2.2 \times 10^{-6}\ M$$

The loss due to solubility of $PbSO_4$ is

$$\Delta = 2.2 \times 10^{-6} \times 303 \times 0.1 = 0.00007\ g$$

which is beyond the precision limits of weighing. Thus, with the use of 50% excess of reagent the very incomplete precipitation of $PbSO_4$ becomes practically complete. The same is found for other cases of this kind if the solubility product of the precipitate is not too large (of the order of 1×10^{-8} or less). Therefore, *to diminish losses due to solubility of precipitate in gravimetric analysis the precipitant is usually added in 50% excess*, i.e., the amount added is 1.5 times the amount calculated from the reaction equation. However, when this method of lowering losses due to solubility of the precipitate is used, it should be remembered that *too great an excess of precipitant is not useful but harmful, as it raises and not lowers the solubility of the precipitate*. The increase in solubility is usually caused by formation of complex compounds or acid salts, or by the amphoteric character of the precipitated compound (hydroxide), etc.

For example, it often happens in qualitative analysis that a precipitate which is initially formed redissolves when excess precipitant is added. This is found, for instance, in the reaction between $HgCl_2$ and KI, when excess KI dissolves the HgI_2 precipitate owing to formation of the complex salt $K_2[HgI_4]$:

$$HgI_2 + 2KI = K_2[HgI_4]$$

In this reaction Hg^{++} and I^- ions which enter the solution from the precipitate combine with added excess I^- ions to form the very slightly dissociated complex ions $[HgI_4]^{--}$, the instability constant* of which is 5×10^{-31}.

* For fuller details see: V. Alexeyev, *Course of Qualitative Chemical Semimicroanalysis*, Goskhimizdat, 1962, p. 257.

It is known, however, that *if any of the ions of a precipitate are removed, the precipitate must dissolve completely or partially.* Because of this reaction the product of the precipitate ion concentrations in solution becomes less than the solubility product of the precipitate, and the previously saturated solution becomes unsaturated. Since this solution is in contact with the precipitate, it must dissolve the latter. In the same way, when Zn^{++} is precipitated by addition of NH_4OH, the $Zn(OH)_2$ precipitate dissolves in excess ammonia owing to formation of the complex ammine $[Zn(NH_3)_6](OH)_2$:

$$Zn(OH)_2 + 6NH_4OH = [Zn(NH_3)_6](OH)_2 + 6H_2O$$

Similarly, in precipitation of Ag^+ as AgCl the solubility of the latter rises owing to the formation of the complex compound $H[AgCl_2]$ or $Na[AgCl_2]$ if a large excess of precipitant (HCl or NaCl) is used. This is illustrated by the following data on the solubility of AgCl in NaCl solutions of various concentrations:

NaCl concentration, moles/litre	0	0.0039	0.0092	0.088	0.35	0.5	0.9	2.87
Solubility of AgCl, millimoles*/litre	0.013	0.00072	0.00091	0.0036	0.017	0.028	0.10	10.0

* One millimole = 0.001 mole (gram-molecule).

It follows from these data that at low NaCl concentrations the solubility of AgCl is lower than in pure water (the effect of introducing the common Cl^- ion). However, after reaching a minimum at about 0.004 *M* NaCl concentration, the solubility of AgCl rises again as the result of complex formation and at 2.87 *M* NaCl it is about 770 times as high as in pure water.

When ions are precipitated as sparingly soluble hydroxides, the precipitates may dissolve in presence of excess precipitant if the hydroxides are amphoteric, for example:

$$Al(OH)_3 + OH^- \rightleftarrows AlO_2^- + 2H_2O$$

Formation of aluminates in quantitative analysis must be taken into account even if NH_4OH is used as precipitant, because excess of it raises the solubility of $Al(OH)_3$ considerably and makes the precipitation incomplete.

When Pb^{++} is precipitated as sulphate, a large excess of precipitant raises the solubility of the precipitate because SO_4^{--} ions formed from it in solution combine with hydrogen ions to form HSO_4^- anions. The equation for this reaction is:

$$PbSO_4 + H_2SO_4 = Pb(HSO_4)_2$$

20. The Salt Effect

It was shown earlier that excess of precipitant is usually required for practically complete precipitation in gravimetric determinations. However, too great an excess is harmful, because the solubility of the precipitate may be raised rather than lowered, as the result of complex formation, formation of acid salts, or because of the amphoteric character of the precipitate (if it is a hydroxide). There is yet another reason why the use of too much precipitant should be avoided, namely: *various strong electrolytes present in solution usually increase the solubilities of precipitates in contact with them.* For example, I. Tananayev and I. Mizetskaya* found that the solubility of $PbSO_4$ is higher in the presence of such salts as KNO_3, $NaNO_3$, etc., and the increase is greater with higher total concentrations of such salts. This is known as the *salt effect*, and is explained as follows.

We know from qualitative analysis** that the solubility product is only approximately equal to the product of the ion concentrations in saturated solution. In reality, it is the product of the ion activities in saturated solution which is constant. *Activity*, it will be remembered, *is the effective or apparent concentration of an ion in accordance with which it takes part in chemical reactions.* For example, the true concentrations of H^+ and Cl^- ions in 0.1 *M* solution of HCl (which, in the modern view, is almost completely dissociated in aqueous solution) are also 0.1 g-ion/litre. However, these ions behave in various chemical reactions as if their true concentrations were only 0.0814 g-ion/litre. Therefore denoting activity by the symbol *a*, we can write***:

$$a_{H^+} = a_{Cl^-} = 0.0814 \text{ g-ion/litre}$$

The ratio of the activity (*a*) to the true concentration (*C*) of an ion is known as the *activity coefficient* and is denoted by f_a (or f with a subscript indicating the formula of the ion). Thus, in the present case:

$$f_{H^+} = f_{Cl^-} = \frac{0.0814}{0.1} = 0.814$$

In general, we may write:

$$f_a = \frac{a}{C} \quad (1)$$

---

* I. Tananayev and I. Mizetskaya, *Zhurnal Analit. Khim.*, 1, 94 (1946).

** V. Alexeyev, *Qualitative Analysis*, Sec. 24, Goskhimizdat, 1960, or V. Alexeyev, *Course of Qualitative Chemical Semimicroanalysis*, Sec. 28, Goskhimizdat, 1962.

*** This value of the activity (0.0814) is the mean activity of the ions. It is equal to $a = \sqrt{a_c a_a}$, where a_c and a_a are the activities of the cation and anion respectively.

From this equation it follows that

$$a = f_a C \tag{2}$$

Therefore, *the activity of an ion is the product of its concentration and the activity coefficient.*

As has already been stated, the concentration C for strong electrolytes is calculated on the assumption that they are almost completely dissociated in solution. By the modern theory of strong electrolytes,* the activity coefficient is a measure of the influence of electrostatic attraction and repulsion forces between the ions on the behaviour of an ion in chemical reactions. If $f_a < 1$, this means that the ion is restricted in its movements by interionic forces. In this case $a < C$, i.e., the ions present (C g-ions/litre) act as if there were fewer of them (a g-ions/litre). If $f_a = 1$, then $a = C$. This means that the ion acts in accordance with its concentration in solution. In the case of strong electrolytes this only occurs in very dilute solutions ($C = 0.0001\ M$ or less) where the interionic distances are so large that forces between the ions are of no practical significance.** In the same way, interionic forces may be disregarded for not very concentrated solutions of weak electrolytes, where only a small proportion of the molecules is dissociated into ions. For such solutions we may assume that $f_a = 1$ and $a = C$.

In accordance with the activity concept, ion activities and not concentrations must be used in all equilibrium equations, such as the equations for the dissociation constant and the solubility product. Activity coefficients were initially introduced in science as empirical factors for extending the law of mass action to cases where it is not applicable in its usual form. Their physical meaning was not clear. It was subsequently elucidated by means of the theory of strong electrolytes, whereby values of f_a could be calculated. In general, such calculations are rather involved, because the formula used contains three constants. It becomes fairly simple only for calculations relating to very dilute solutions (for values of μ not greater than 0.1)***:

$$\log f_a = -0.5z^2 \frac{\sqrt{\mu}}{1+\sqrt{\mu}} \tag{3}$$

---

* V. Alexeyev, *Qualitative Analysis*, Sec. 14, Goskhimizdat, 1960; or V. Alexeyev, *Course of Qualitative Chemical Semimicroanalysis*, Sec. 18, Goskhimizdat, 1962.

** In concentrated solutions of strong electrolytes, for reasons which cannot considered here, the activity coefficients may sometimes be greater than unity.

*** For values of μ not greater than 0.005 we can use:

$$\log f_a = -0.5z^2 \sqrt{\mu}$$

Here z is the ionic charge, and μ is the so-called *ionic strength of the solution*. This is a measure of the electrical field strength in the electrolyte, and is calculated from the formula:

$$\mu = \frac{1}{2}(C_1 z_1^2 + C_2 z_2^2 + \ldots + C_n z_n^2) \tag{4}$$

Here $C_1, C_2 \ldots C_n$ are the molar concentrations and $z_1, z_2 \ldots z_n$ are the charges of the individual ions present in solution. For example, the ionic strength of a solution containing 0.1 mole HCl and 0.2 mole $CaCl_2$ per litre is:

$$\mu = \frac{1}{2}(0.1 \times 1^2 + 0.2 \times 2^2 + 0.5 \times 1^2) = 0.7$$

Here 0.1 is the H^+ concentration, 0.2 is the Ca^{++} concentration, and 0.5 is the Cl^- concentration.

Thus, *the activities of the ions of any electrolyte depend not only on its concentration in solution but also on the concentrations and charges of all other ions present in solution.*

It is found experimentally that in dilute solutions of equal ionic strength the activity coefficients of most ions of equal charge are approximately the same. The values of these coefficients (to a degree of accuracy sufficient for practical purposes) are given in Table III.

Table III

Activity Coefficients

Ionic strength μ	Activity coefficient, f_a			
	Univalent ions	Bivalent ions	Trivalent ions	Quadri-valent ions
0.001	0.96	0.86	0.73	0.56
0.005	0.92	0.72	0.51	0.30
0.01	0.90	0.63	0.39	0.19
0.05	0.81	0.44	0.15	0.04
0.1	0.78	0.33	0.08	0.01

In returning to the question of salt effect, we must first note that the solubility product rule actually implies that it is not the product of the ionic concentrations but the product of ionic activities that is constant in a saturated solution. In the case of $PbSO_4$ this product is:

$$a_{Pb^{++}} a_{SO_4^{--}} = SP_{PbSO_4} = \text{constant} \tag{5}$$

But, in accordance with Equation (2) on p. 76:

$$a_{Pb^{++}} = [Pb^{++}]\, f_{Pb^{++}} \quad \text{and} \quad a_{SO_4^{--}} = [SO_4^{--}]\, f_{SO_4^{--}}$$

We therefore have:

$$[Pb^{++}][SO_4^{--}]\, f_{Pb^{++}} f_{SO_4^{--}} = SP_{PbSO_4}$$

Hence the product of the ionic concentrations in a saturated $PbSO_4$ solution is:

$$[Pb^{++}][SO_4^{--}] = \frac{SP_{PbSO_4}}{f_{Pb^{++}} f_{SO_4^{--}}}$$

The value of SP_{PbSO_4} in this equation is strictly constant for any given temperature. As was pointed out earlier, the activity coefficients decrease with increase of the ionic strength of the solution. Evidently any strong electrolyte, such as $NaNO_3$, KNO_3, etc., should decrease the values of $f_{Pb^{++}}$ and $f_{SO_4^{--}}$ when it is added to the solution. However, when the denominator of the fraction is decreased, the value of the whole fraction, and therefore the quantity equal to it—the product of the Pb^{++} and SO_4^{--} ion concentrations in the saturated solution—must increase. Since the molar concentration of the saturated solution is equal to the square root of this product, the solubility of $PbSO_4$ (and other sparingly soluble salts) should increase on addition of any strong electrolyte to the solution (the salt effect). This may be illustrated by the following numerical example.

Example 1. By how much is the solubility of $PbSO_4$ greater in 0.1 *M* KNO_3 solution than in pure water at room temperature?

Solution. To find the activity coefficients of the Pb^{++} and SO_4^{--} ions we must first calculate the ionic strength of the solution μ. The solution contains ions of two salts—KNO_3 and $PbSO_4$. But the solubility of the latter salt is low, and its ions are present in a very low concentration. Therefore, in calculation of the ionic strength μ we need consider only the concentrations and charges of the ions of the other salt, KNO_3. Therefore

$$\mu = \frac{1}{2}([K^+]\cdot 1^2 + [NO_3^-]\cdot 1^2) = \frac{1}{2}(0.1 + 0.1) = 0.1$$

In accordance with Table III, ionic strength corresponds to the following value for the activity coefficient of the bivalent ions:

$$f_{Pb^{++}} = f_{SO_4^{--}} = 0.33$$

We denote the required solubility of $PbSO_4$, in moles per litre, by x. Then

$$[Pb^{++}] = [SO_4^{--}] = x$$

$$SP_{PbSO_4} = [Pb^{++}][SO_4^{--}]\, f_{Pb^{++}} f_{SO_4^{--}} = x^2\,(0.33)^2 = 2.2 \times 10^{-8}$$

Hence

$$x = \frac{\sqrt{2.2 \times 10^{-8}}}{0.33} = 4.5 \times 10^{-4}\ M$$

We now find the solubility of $PbSO_4$ in water. In this case the ionic strength of the solution is due entirely to the presence of lead sulphate. Since its solubility is of the order of 1×10^{-4} *M*, the activity coefficients in this case can be taken as practically equal to unity. We can write:

$$[Pb^{++}][SO_4^{--}] = x^2 \approx 2.2 \times 10^{-8}$$

Hence

$$x \approx \sqrt{2.2 \times 10^{-8}} \approx 1.5 \times 10^{-4}\ M$$

It is clear from these results that in the presence of 0.1 mole of KNO_3 in 1 litre of solution the solubility of $PbSO_4$ is approximately 3 times its solubility in pure water (the salt effect).

This salt effect is produced by all strong electrolytes, including electrolytes having a common ion with the precipitate. In such a case, however, the salt effect which raises the solubility should be accompanied by the common ion effect, which lowers it. As a result the solubility is usually lowered, but not as much as is found by calculation from the simplified formula for the solubility product (i.e., without the activity coefficients taken into account).

For example, in the preceding section we calculated the loss due to solubility of $PbSO_4$ when this salt is precipitated with a 50% excess (over the calculated quantity) of precipitant. We now perform a more exact calculation in which we take into account the effect of excess precipitant on the activity coefficients of Pb^{++} and SO_4^{--} ions.

Example 2. Calculate the loss due to solubility of $PbSO_4$ in precipitation of Pb^{++} with 50% excess of H_2SO_4, with activity coefficients of the ions taken into account.

Solution. The earlier calculation (p. 73) shows that when Pb^{++} is precipitated with 50% excess of 0.5 *M* H_2SO_4 solution, the sulphuric acid concentration in the solution becomes 1×10^{-2} *M*. Assuming that at this dilution the acid is dissociated almost completely into H^+ and SO_4^{--} ions, we can write:

$$[SO_4^{--}] = 0.01 \text{ g-ion/litre and } [H^+] = 0.02 \text{ g-ion/litre}$$

Disregarding the small quantity of ions entering the solution from the $PbSO_4$ precipitate, we calculate the ionic strength of the solution:

$$\mu = \frac{1}{2}(0.02 \times 1^2 + 0.01 \times 2^2) = 0.03$$

Table III does not contain this value. Therefore, the corresponding activity coefficients must be found by interpolation. Table III shows that as the ionic strength increases from 0.01 to 0.05 (i.e., by 0.04) the activity coefficients of bivalent ions decrease from 0.63 to 0.44 (i.e., by 0.19). We find the decrease of f with increase of ionic strength from 0.01 to 0.03 (i.e., by 0.02) by proportion:

0.04 is to 0.19 as 0.02 is to x,

and hence

$$x = 0.09$$

Consequently

$$f_{Pb^{++}} = f_{SO_4^{--}} = 0.63 - 0.09 = 0.54$$

We denote the Pb^{++} ion concentration in the solution by x, and disregard the small quantity of SO_4^{--} ions entering the solution from the precipitate, in comparison with the much larger quantity introduced with the excess H_2SO_4. Then from the equation

$$[Pb^{++}]\,[SO_4^{--}]\, f_{Pb^{++}} f_{SO_4^{--}} = 2.2 \times 10^{-8}$$

we have:

$$x \times 10^{-2}\,(0.54)^2 = 2.2 \times 10^{-8}$$

and

$$x = 7.6 \times 10^{-6} \text{ g-ion/litre}$$

If all the Pb^{++} ions remaining in solution had been precipitated as $PbSO_4$, 100 ml of solution would have given $7.6 \times 10^{-6} \times 303 \times 0.1 = 2.3 \times 10^{-4}$ g of the salt.

Therefore, exact calculation, with activity coefficients of the ions taken into account, gives 0.00023 g for the loss due to solubility instead of the 0.00007 g found by approximate calculation.

It follows from all that has been said about the salt effect that its influence on losses due to solubility increases with the amount of precipitant taken. With a very large excess of precipitant, especially if it contains multivalent ions, the salt effect may be greater than the common-ion effect and the solubility of the precipitate may be raised rather than lowered. Therefore, even when there is no reason to expect that the solubility of the precipitate may be influenced by its amphoteric character, formation of complexes and acid salts, etc., addition of more than a 50% excess of precipitant is undesirable because the salt effect is excessively increased. However, precipitation is practically complete with a 50% excess of precipitant only if the solubility product of the precipitated (binary) compound is of the order of 10^{-8} or less. Therefore, compounds with solubility products greater than 10^{-8} are not generally used as precipitated forms in gravimetric analysis.

Evidently, the salt effect must be also taken into account in determination of a particular element in a solution containing large amounts of various extraneous strong electrolytes. This occurs in analysis of natural materials or industrial products, or when large amounts of various reagents (acids, alkalies, etc.) have to be added to the solution at different stages of analysis prior to precipitation. In such cases increase of the salt effect is one of the sources of error in gravimetric determinations.

To obtain sufficiently accurate results in calculations based on the rule that the solubility product is constant it is necessary to take into account the activity coefficients of the ions. However, in practice the solutions being investigated very often contain several different ions in concentrations which are not known exactly, and in such cases it is impossible to use activity coefficients. Therefore, in most cases these coefficients are conventionally assumed to be equal to unity, i.e., the calculations are performed with the simplified formula for the solubility product:

$$SP_{PbSO_4} \approx [Pb^{++}] [SO_4^{--}]$$

etc.

This simplification is quite admissible, because calculations based on the solubility product rule usually merely illustrate particular aspects of the theory. Qualitatively, such simplified calculations are nearly always in good agreement with experimental results.

In the rare cases (as in the above discussion of the salt effect) when there is no such agreement, the exact formula for the solubility product is used, with f_a taken into account.

21. Effect of Temperature on Completeness of Precipitation

As was shown earlier, the extent of precipitation is primarily determined by the value of the solubility product of the precipitate. However, this product remains constant only if the temperature is unchanged. If the temperature alters, the SP of the precipitate also changes.

In qualitative analysis it often happens that a precipitate formed in the cold (such as $KHC_4H_4O_6$) redissolves on warming. It is evident that in such cases temperature must have a very strong influence on completeness of precipitation. The effect of temperature on the solubility of precipitates often has to be taken into account even in cases when the precipitates are not dissolved completely on heating. For example, the solubility of AgCl at 100°C is nearly 25 times as high as at 10°C. The solubilities of most other precipitates also increase with temperature, although usually not to such a great extent. For example, the solubility of $BaSO_4$ is only doubled when the temperature is raised from 10°C to 100°C. Finally, in some instances the solubility of precipitates decreases with rise of temperature.

The change of solubility with temperature is associated with the heat effect of dissolution. When most salts dissolve the solutions become colder; i.e., heat is absorbed. By the Le Chatelier principle, the solubilities of such salts should increase with temperature. Conversely, if heat is liberated when a salt dissolves, its solubility decreases with rise of temperature.

If one crystalline hydrate is converted into another on rise of temperature, i.e., if the crystal lattice of the salt alters, it may happen that the different hydrates react differently to rise of temperature and the solubility would alter accordingly. For example let us consider the solubility of calcium sulphate. At room temperatures the aqueous solution is in equilibrium with a precipitate of the hydrate $CaSO_4 \cdot 2H_2O$, the solubility of which increases with temperature. However, at 60°C this hydrate loses part of its water of crystallization and is converted into the hydrate $CaSO_4 \cdot {}^1/_2H_2O$. In contrast to $CaSO_4 \cdot 2H_2O$, the hydrate $CaSO_4 \cdot {}^1/_2H_2O$ is less soluble at higher temperature, and therefore the solubility curve of calcium sulphate has a maximum at 60°C.

It will be shown later (Secs. 24 and 26) that it is usually advantageous to effect precipitation with heating, because this favours growth of crystals or (in the case of amorphous precipitates) coagulation of colloidal particles in the precipitate. However, whenever we deal with a precipitate the solubility of which increases appreciably with temperature, we must cool the solution completely before filtering off the precipitate. This is done, for instance, with precipitates of $MgNH_4PO_4$, $PbSO_4$, CaC_2O_4, etc. Conversely, if the solubility of a precipitate is very low and varies little with temperature, as in the case of $Fe(OH)_3$, it is preferable to filter the hot solution, as hot liquids filter more rapidly than cold.

In a number of cases the solubility increase can be suppressed sufficiently by the presence of excess precipitant in solution. It must be remembered, however, that this excess is removed when the precipitate is washed, so that the solubility rises again at the end of this process. This may lead to appreciable losses if hot water is used.

22. Effect of Hydrogen Ion Concentration (pH) on Completeness of Precipitation

One of the most important factors influencing the degree of precipitation is the H^+ ion concentration, i.e., the solution pH.* Let us consider the influence of this factor in some individual cases.

Precipitation of Sparingly Soluble Metal Hydroxides. In this case the precipitating ion is OH^-. Its concentration is related to the H^+ ion concentration as follows:

$$[H^+][OH^-] = K_{H_2O} = 10^{-14} \text{ (at 22°C)}^{**} \quad (1)$$

* It will be remembered that the hydrogen ion exponent pH is the logarithm of the H^+ ion concentration, with the sign reversed:

$$pH = -\log [H^+]$$

Similarly, the hydroxyl ion exponent $pOH = -\log [OH^-]$.

** Taking logarithms in Equation (1) and reversing the signs, we have:

$$pH + pOH = 14 \text{ (at 22°C)}$$

In neutral solutions pH = 7, in acid solutions $pH < 7$, and in alkaline solutions $pH > 7$. The pH value decreases with increasing acidity and increases with increasing alkalinity. This is discussed more fully in Sec. 58.

This equation shows that the OH^- ion concentration falls with increase of H^+ ion concentration, i.e., with decrease of solution pH. However, the OH^- ion concentration determines whether a given hydroxide is precipitated, and the extent of the precipitation. Evidently, the greater the solubility product of the hydroxide, the higher is the OH^- ion concentration required for complete precipitation, i.e., the higher the pH at which the precipitation must be performed.

The pH required for complete precipitation of any hydroxide is easy to calculate from its solubility product.

Let us perform this calculation for magnesium hydroxide. In this case we have:

$$[Mg^{++}]\,[OH^-]^2 = SP_{Mg(OH)_2} = 5 \times 10^{-12}$$

and hence

$$[OH^-] = \sqrt{\frac{SP_{Mg(OH)_2}}{[Mg^{++}]}} \qquad (2)$$

Since weighing on an analytical balance can be performed to a precision of about 10^{-4} g, and the average gram-molecular weight of various precipitates can be taken as 100 g, it may be assumed that the precipitation of any substance is practically complete if its molar concentration in solution at the end of precipitation is $10^{-4} : 100 = 10^{-6}$ *M*. This must therefore be the concentration of Mg^{++} ions at the end of precipitation. Accordingly, we have from Equation (2):

$$[OH^-] = \sqrt{\frac{5 \times 10^{-12}}{10^{-6}}} \approx 2 \times 10^{-3} \text{ g-ion/litre}$$

Therefore,

$$pOH = -\log 2 \times 10^{-3} = -(0.3 - 3) = 2.7$$

$$pH = 14 - pOH = 14 - 2.7 = 11.3$$

Therefore, Mg^{++} is completely precipitated as the hydroxide at pH = 11.3. If the pH > 11.3, the precipitation is even more complete, as the Mg^{++} ion concentration becomes less than 10^{-6} g-ion/litre. Conversely, at pH < 11.3 the precipitation is incomplete or may even not occur at all.

A similar calculation for the much less soluble ferric hydroxide $Fe(OH)_3$ ($SP = 3.8 \times 10^{-38}$) shows that precipitation is practically complete at pH $\gg 3.5$. Although, of course, such calculations are not exact, since activity coefficients of the ions are not taken into account and the solubility products of hydroxides are not always known exactly, they nevertheless provide a good illustration of the significance of solution pH in precipitation of hydroxides, and lead to a number of important practical conclusions. For example, a comparison of the pH values for $Mg(OH)_2$ and $Fe(OH)_3$ precipitation shows that by suitable regulation of pH it is possible to separate Mg^{++} ions from Fe^{+++} ions. It will be shown later that separation of ions by appropriate regulation of solution pH is widely used in quantitative analysis. We also met numerous instances of such separations in the work on qualitative analysis.

Precipitation of Sparingly Soluble Salts of Weak Acids. The pH is no less important in precipitation of sparingly soluble salts of weak acids; for example, carbonates, oxalates, phosphates, sulphides, etc. In such cases the precipitant ions are anions of the corresponding weak acids: CO_3^{--}, $C_2O_4^{--}$, PO_4^{---}, S^{--}, etc. However, these anions meet H^+ ions in solution and must evidently combine with them to form, first the anions HCO_3^-, $HC_2O_4^-$, HPO_4^{--}, $H_2PO_4^-$, and HS^-, and then undissociated molecules of H_2CO_3, $H_2C_2O_4$, H_3PO_4, and H_2S, as both the latter anions and the molecules have a low tendency to dissociation. It follows that the concentrations of anions such as CO_3^{--}, $C_2O_4^{--}$, PO_4^{---}, S^{--}, etc., in solution must depend very much on the H^+ ion concentration, decreasing with increase of the latter, i.e., with decrease of solution pH. Since this is so, the pH must also determine whether such salts are precipitated and the degree of precipitation.

As in the case of hydroxides, the pH required for practically complete precipitation of any sparingly soluble salt of a weak acid depends primarily on the solubility product of this salt. If the solubility product is small, a low concentration of the precipitant is required. Accordingly, a salt with a low SP can often be precipitated completely in a strongly acid medium, i.e., at a low pH value. For example, it is known in qualitative analysis that the sulphides of cations in Groups IV and V, the solubility products of which are less than 10^{-29}, are completely precipitated even in a relatively acid solution, at $pH = 0.5$. On the other hand, the solution must be neutral or alkaline ($pH \geqslant 7$) for precipitation of Group III sulphides, which have solubility products in the 10^{-15}-10^{-23} range.

In addition to SP, the dissociation constant of the weak acid is significant. The smaller this constant, the more completely do the precipitant ions combine with H^+ ions and the higher is the pH needed for practically complete precipitation of the salt. For example, carbonic acid ($K_1 = 4.3 \times 10^{-7}$; $K_2 = 5.6 \times 10^{-11}$) is much weaker than oxalic acid, $H_2C_2O_4$ ($K_1 = 5.9 \times 10^{-2}$; $K_2 = 6.5 \times \times 10^{-5}$); therefore Ca^{++} should be precipitated as $CaCO_3$ at a much higher pH value than in precipitation as CaC_2O_4, although their solubility products are of the same order of magnitude (4.8×10^{-9} for $CaCO_3$ and 2.6×10^{-9} for CaC_2O_4). This can be easily confirmed by calculations similar to those given above for hydroxides. The calculations are somewhat complicated by the fact that the precipitated compounds are salts of dibasic acids. In accordance with the stepwise dissociation of these acids, the recombination of their anions with H^+ also occurs in stages; for example:

$$CO_3^{--} + H^+ \rightleftarrows HCO_3^- \quad (K_2 = 5.6 \times 10^{-11})$$

$$HCO_3^- + H^+ \rightleftarrows H_2CO_3 \quad (K_1 = 4.3 \times 10^{-7})$$

Since the dissociation constant of the HCO_3^- ion is considerably smaller than that of the acid H_2CO_3 itself, the greater proportion of the CO_3^{--} ions introduced with the excess reagent is converted into HCO_3^- ions, and usually only a small proportion of the latter is converted further into undissociated H_2CO_3 molecules. This proportion can be estimated from the equation

$$K_1 = \frac{[H^+]\,[HCO_3^-]}{[H_2CO_3]}$$

or

$$\frac{K_1}{[H^+]} = \frac{[HCO_3^-]}{[H_2CO_3]} \tag{3}$$

Equation (3) shows that when $K_1 \gg [H^+]$ the HCO_3^- ion concentration must be very much higher than the concentration of undissociated H_2CO_3 molecules. In this case the formation of H_2CO_3 molecules may be disregarded without any appreciable error; i.e., it may be assumed that

$$[CO_3^{--}] + [HCO_3^-] \approx C \tag{4}$$

where C is tle total concentration of the precipitant in solution at the end of the precipitation.

Therefore, problems of this kind may be solved by the following procedure. First, we use the equation for K_2 of the acid and Equation (4) and find the $[H^+]$ and pH of the solution. We then substitute the value found for $[H^+]$ into Equation (3) and check the assumption that formation of H_2CO_3 molecules may be disregarded. If it is found that $K_1 \gg H^+$, the value found for the pH may be taken as correct.

The foregoing is illustrated by the following numerical examples.

Example 1. Find the pH at which Ca^{++} is precipitated practically completely as $CaCO_3$ from a solution containing 0.01 g-eq (i.e., 0.005 g-ion) of Ca^{++}, if 50% excess of precipitant is used and the total volume of the solution is 100 ml.

Solution. First we find C, the excess of precipitant in solution, in moles per litre. The precipitation of 0.005 g-ion of Ca^{++} requires the same number of moles of precipitant, for example, $(NH_4)_2CO_3$, and with 50% excess the amount is 0.0075 mole. Therefore, the excess of precipitant is 0.0025 mole in 100 ml. Calculated as moles per litre, this is $0.025 = 2.5 \times 10^{-2}$ M. This is the concentration of the precipitant at the end of the precipitation. This would also be the concentration of CO_3^{--} ions in solution if they all remained free. However, in reality some are converted into HCO_3^- anions and some into H_2CO_3 molecules.

Disregarding formation of H_2CO_3 molecules, we can write:

$$[CO_3^{--}]+[HCO_3^-]\approx 2.5\times 10^{-2}\text{ g-ion/litre}$$

For practically complete precipitation of Ca^{++} the concentration of CO_3^{--} ions must not be less than:

$$[CO_3^{--}]=\frac{SP_{CaCO_3}}{[Ca^{++}]}=\frac{4.8\times 10^{-9}}{10^{-6}}=4.8\times 10^{-3}\text{ g-ion/litre}$$

Substituting the value found for $[CO_3^{--}]$ into the above equation, we have

$$[HCO_3^-]=2.5\times 10^{-2}-4.8\times 10^{-3}=2\times 10^{-2}\text{ g-ion/litre}$$

Knowing the concentrations of the CO_3^{--} and HCO_3^- ions, we find the required $[H^+]$ ion concentration from the equation for the second-stage dissociation constant of H_2CO_3:

$$K_2=\frac{[H^+][CO_3^{--}]}{[HCO_3^-]}=5.6\times 10^{-11}$$

We then have:

$$[H^+]=\frac{5.6\times 10^{-11}[HCO_3^-]}{[CO_3^{--}]}=\frac{5.6\times 10^{-11}\times 2\times 10^{-2}}{4.8\times 10^{-3}}=2.3\times 10^{-10}\text{ g-ion/litre}$$

Consequently:

$$pH=-\log 2.3\times 10^{-10}=-(0.4-10)=9.6$$

Thus, for complete precipitation of $CaCO_3$ the medium must be alkaline at $pH=9.6$.

We now check whether formation of undissociated H_2CO_3 molecules could be disregarded:

$$\frac{K_1}{[H^+]}=\frac{[HCO_3^-]}{[H_2CO_3]}$$

or

$$\frac{4.3\times 10^{-7}}{2.3\times 10^{-10}}=\frac{[HCO_3^-]}{[H_2CO_3]}\approx 2{,}000$$

Thus, at the given pH the HCO_3^- ion concentration is approximately 2,000 times the concentration of H_2CO_3 molecules. It was therefore quite permissible to disregard formation of H_2CO_3 molecules.

Example 2. Solve the problem analogous to that given in Example 1, for precipitation of Ca^{++} as CaC_2O_4.

Solution. The concentration of precipitant at the end of the precipitation is, as before 2.5×10^{-2} *M*. Therefore, disregarding formation of $H_2C_2O_4$ molecules, we may write:

$$[C_2O_4^{--}]+[HC_2O_4^-]\approx 2.5\times 10^{-2}\text{ g-ion/litre}$$

The condition for practically complete precipitation is:

$$[C_2O_4^{--}]=\frac{SP_{CaC_2O_4}}{[Ca^{++}]}=\frac{2.6\times 10^{-9}}{10^{-6}}=2.6\times 10^{-3}\text{ g-ion/litre}$$

Consequently

$$[HC_2O_4^-]=2.5\times 10^{-2}-2.6\times 10^{-3}=2.2\times 10^{-2}\text{ g-ion/litre}$$

Therefore

$$[H^+]=\frac{K_2[HC_2O_4^-]}{[C_2O_4^{--}]}=\frac{6.4\times 10^{-5}\times 2.2\times 10^{-2}}{2.6\times 10^{-3}}\approx 5\times 10^{-4}\text{ g-ion/litre}$$

and

$$pH = -\log 5 \times 10^{-4} = -(0.7-4) = 3.3$$

Therefore, CaC_2O_4 is completely precipitated even in a moderately acid medium (at pH $\geqslant$ 3.3). This result is fully justified in practice: CaC_2O_4 is usually precipitated at pH = 4.

We check our result:

$$\frac{K_2}{[H^+]} = \frac{[HC_2O_4^-]}{[H_2C_2O_4]} = \frac{5.9 \times 10^{-2}}{5 \times 10^{-4}} \approx 100$$

Here again the solution can be regarded as sufficiently accurate, since at pH = 3.3 the concentration of $HC_2O_4^-$ anions is approximately 100 times the concentration of undissociated $H_2C_2O_4$ molecules.

The above calculations demonstrate the significance of the dissociation constants of the weak acid a salt of which is precipitated. The smaller the dissociation constants, i.e., the weaker the acid, the higher is the pH required for practically complete precipitation of the salt. The calculations also show that an acceptable result can often be obtained relatively simply, with formation of undissociated molecules of the weak acid disregarded. However, this simplification is not possible in every instance. The following examples illustrate the procedure when it is not possible.

Example 3. Find the pH for practically complete precipitation of Fe^{++} ions by hydrogen sulphide. The conditions are the same as in the preceding examples.

Solution. As before, we take the excess of precipitant to be 2.5×10^{-2} *M*. If we calculate the required $[H^+]$ ion concentration as described above, from $SP_{FeS} = 3.2 \times 10^{-18}$ and the dissociation constants of hydrogen sulphide $K_1 = 5.7 \times 10^{-8}$ and $K_2 = 1.2 \times 10^{-15}$, disregarding the formation of undissociated molecules H_2S we have $[H^+] = 9.4 \times 10^{-6}$ g-ion/litre and pH = 5.0. However, we must check whether formation of H_2S molecules may be disregarded:

$$\frac{[HS^-]}{[H_2S]} = \frac{[K_1]}{[H^+]} = \frac{5.7 \times 10^{-8}}{9.4 \times 10^{-6}} = 6 \times 10^{-3} = 0.006$$

This means that many more H_2S molecules than HS^- ions are formed, and it was not permissible to disregard the formation of these molecules. Conversely, the formation of HS^- ions could be disregarded. In that case we have:

$$[S^{--}] + [H_2S] = 2.5 \times 10^{-2}$$

But $[S^{--}]$ is much less than 2.5×10^{-2};

$$[S^{--}] = \frac{SP_{FeS}}{[Fe^{++}]} = \frac{3.2 \times 10^{-18}}{10^{-6}} = 3.2 \times 10^{-12} \text{ g-ion/litre}$$

Therefore

$$[S^{--}] + [H_2S] \approx [H_2S] = 2.5 \cdot 10^{-2} \text{ g-ion/litre}$$

From the values found for $[S^{--}]$ and $[H_2S]$ and from the equation

$$\frac{[H^+]^2 [S^{--}]}{[H_2S]} = K_1K_2 = 6.8 \times 10^{-23}$$

we have

$$[H^+] = \sqrt{\frac{6.8 \times 10^{-23} \times 2.5 \times 10^{-2}}{3.2 \times 10^{-12}}} = 7.3 \times 10^{-7} \text{ g-ion/litre}$$

and

$$pH = -\log 7.3 \times 10^{-7} = -(0.86 - 7.0) = 6.14$$

Since this pH value is very different from the value found previously, it is advisable to check again whether formation of HS^- ions may be disregarded:

$$\frac{[HS^-]}{[H_2S]} = \frac{K_1}{[H^+]} = \frac{5.7 \times 10^{-8}}{7.3 \times 10^{-7}} = 0.078$$

Since at pH = 6.14 the $[HS^-]$ concentration is again considerably less than the H_2S concentration, the assumption is justifiable and the result is acceptable.

Example 4. Solve the problem analogous to that given in Example 3, for precipitation of MnS (SP = 1.4×10^{-15}).

Solution. Taking the excess of precipitant to be 2.5×10^{-2} *M*, and disregarding formation of undissociated H_2S molecules, we have

$$[S^{--}] + [HS^-] = 2.5 \times 10^{-2}$$

From this we find by the same method as before, that $[H^+] = 2.1 \times 10^{-8}$ and pH = 7.68.

We now check whether formation of undissociated H_2S molecules could be disregarded:

$$\frac{[H_2S]}{[HS^-]} = \frac{[H^+]}{K_1} = \frac{2.1 \times 10^{-8}}{5.7 \times 10^{-8}} = 0.37$$

Therefore, here again it is not permissible to disregard formation of undissociated H_2S molecules. However, in distinction from Example 3, here we may not disregard formation of HS^- ions either, as the amount of these ions formed is about three times the amount of H_2S molecules. In such cases different procedures are possible.

1. It follows from the equation given above that $[H_2S] = 0.37\,[HS^-]$. We can therefore write:

$$[S^{--}] + [H_2S] + [HS^-] = [S^{--}] + [HS^-] + 0.37\,[HS^-] = 2.5 \times 10^{-2}$$

where

$$[S^{--}] = \frac{SP_{MnS}}{[Mn^{++}]} = \frac{1.4 \times 10^{-15}}{10^{-6}} = 1.4 \times 10^{-9} \text{ g-ion/litre}$$

Hence $0.37\,[HS^-] = 2.5 \times 10^{-2}$ and $[HS^-] = 1.8 \times 10^{-2}$ g-ion/litre.

Substituting this value into the equation for K_2 of hydrogen sulphide we find as a second approximation:

$$[H^+] = \frac{K_2\,[HS^-]}{[S^{--}]} + \frac{1.2 \times 10^{-15} \times 1.8 \times 10^{-2}}{1.4 \times 10^{-9}} = 1.5 \times 10^{-8}$$

and

$$pH = 7.8$$

2. It is also possible to perform a more exact calculation without any simplifying assumptions. For this, we find $[S^{--}]$, which is in this instance $1.4 \cdot 10^{-9}$ g-ion/litre, and express $[HS^-]$ and $[H_2S]$ in terms of this value and of the required $[H^+]$ ion concentration:

$$[HS^-] = \frac{[H^+][S^{--}]}{K_2} = \frac{[H^+]\,1.4 \times 10^{-9}}{1.2 \times 10^{-15}} = 1.17 \times 10^{6}\,[H^+] \quad (1)$$

$$[H_2S] = \frac{[H^+]^2[S^{--}]}{K_1K_2} = \frac{[H^+]^2\,1.4 \times 10^{-9}}{6.8 \times 10^{-23}} = 2.06 \times 10^{13}\,[H^+]^2 \quad (2)$$

Putting the values found for $[S^{--}]$, $[HS^-]$, $[H_2S]$ in the equation

$$[S^{--}]+[HS^-]+[H_2S]=2.5\times 10^{-2}$$

we have:

$$1.4\times 10^{-9}+1.17\times 10^6[H^+]+2.06\times 10^{13}[H^+]^2=2.5\times 10^{-2}$$

After rearranging and dividing every term in the equation by 2.06×10^{13}, the coefficient of $[H^+]^2$, we obtain the following quadratic equation:

$$[H^+]^2+5.68\times 10^{-8}[H^+]+1.21\times 10^{-15}=0 \quad (3)$$

Solving this equation, we have

$$[H^+]=-2.84\times 10^{-8}+\sqrt{8.10\times 10^{-16}+1.21\times 10^{-15}}=$$

$$=1.65\times 10^{-8}\text{ g-ion/litre}$$

and

$$pH=7.78$$

Thus, the more exact calculation gave almost the same result as the approximate calculation, with formation of H_2S taken into account.

Of course, even here all the calculated results are only approximate, as the activity coefficients of the ions are not taken into account. Moreover, the solubility products of some salts are not known with sufficient accuracy. Nevertheless, the pH values are of the right order, and therefore such calculations are useful in analytical practice. It must be remembered that the calculations give only the *lowest* pH values for practically complete precipitation. At higher pH values it is usually (although not always) even more complete.

Precipitation of Sparingly Soluble Salts of Strong Acids. Sparingly soluble salts of strong monobasic acids, such as AgCl, AgBr, AgI, etc., are precipitated by the corresponding anions, namely, Cl^-, Br^-, I^-, etc. These anions evidently do not combine with H^+ ions, because HCl, HBr, HI, etc., are strong acids and are almost completely dissociated in aqueous solution. Therefore, the degree of precipitation of sparingly soluble salts of these acids (in contrast to salts of weak acids) is almost independent of the solution pH. If the influence of excess acid in solution must be taken into account in such cases, this is only because in the presence of excess acid the salt effect increases, or in some cases complexes are formed from the salt cations and acid anions; for example,

$$AgCl+HCl=H[AgCl_2]$$

and the solubility of the salt (AgCl) therefore increases.

The situation is somewhat different in precipitation of sparingly soluble sulphates, as the dissociation of H_2SO_4 is almost complete only at the first stage, with formation of H^+ and HSO_4^- ions. The second stage of dissociation

$$HSO_4^-=H^++SO_4^{--}$$

proceeds to a very considerable extent, since K_2 has a high value (1.2×10^{-2}), but not to completion. It follows that, if the SP of the precipitate is not too small and the H^+ ion concentration is high enough, these ions may combine with SO_4^{--} ions to give HSO_4^- anions. This means that the solution pH cannot be ignored in precipitation of sulphates. Precipitation of sparingly soluble sulphates should be less complete in acid solutions than in neutral or alkaline solutions. This effect is most pronounced with the more soluble sulphates, such as $CaSO_4$ (SP $= 6.1 \times 10^{-5}$), $SrSO_4$ (SP $= 2.8 \times$ $\times 10^{-7}$) and $PbSO_4$ (SP $= 2.2 \times 10^{-8}$). The solubility is increased noticeably by H^+ ions even in the case of the least soluble sulphate, $BaSO_4$ (SP $= 1.1 \times 10^{-10}$). Data on the solubility of $BaSO_4$ in HNO_3 solutions are given below.

HNO_3 concentration (M)	0.05	0.1	0.5	1.0	2.0
Solubility of $BaSO_4$ (millimoles per litre) at 19°C	0.9	1.2	3.9	7.7	11.9
Ditto, at 100°C	7.7	—	26.5	41.6	—

Despite this, $BaSO_4$ is precipitated from acid solutions as this gives larger crystals in the precipitate (Sec. 25). The increased solubility due to the presence of acid is eliminated at the end of the precipitation by the addition of excess precipitant.

23. Effect of Complex Fornation on Completeness of Precipitation. Masking

It was shown above that the influence of pH on precipitation of sparingly soluble electrolytes depends on the decrease in the concentration of the precipitant ions owing to combination with H^+ ions. If this decrease is so great that the solubility product of the required precipitate is not reached, precipitation does not occur at all.

However, the equation for the solubility product contains the concentration of the ion being precipitated as well as of the precipitant ion. If the concentration of the former is reduced by incorporation in a complex ion of a low degree of dissociation, it is evidently possible to render the precipitation incomplete or even to prevent it entirely. For this the product of the respective ion concentrations in solution must be less than the solubility product of the compound being precipitated.

Prevention of the precipitation of any given ion by combining it in a complex of a low degree of dissociation is known as masking. Masking is widely used in analytical practice.

Masking is often used in qualitative analysis in cases where the detection of a particular ion has to be performed in the presence of ions interfering with the reaction. If such ions are combined in complexes, their concentration can be reduced to a level at which they no longer interfere with detection of the ion in question. For example, when Co^{++} is detected as the complex thiocyanate $[Co(CNS)_4]^{--}$ the solution must be free from Fe^{+++} ions, which give an intensely coloured compound with CNS^- ions. Therefore, if Fe^{+++} ions are present, NH_4F (or NaF) is added to form the stable complex. It is also possible to remove Fe^{+++} ions by addition of tartaric or citric acids, which form fairly stable complexes (i.e., of a low degree of dissociation) with Fe^{+++} ions.

Similar masking of interfering ions is widely used in quantitative analysis. For example, as Ni^{++} is precipitated with dimethylglyoxime in an alkaline medium, Fe^{+++} ions interfere with determination of nickel, as they form a precipitate of $Fe(OH)_3$ under these conditions. To avoid formation of this hydroxide, the precipitation is performed in the presence of a sufficient quantity of tartaric acid. Tartaric (or excess oxalic) acid is also added for masking Fe^{+++} in determination of Ca^{++}, etc.

Evidently, masking achieves the same aim as precipitation of the interfering ion in the form of an insoluble compound: the concentration of that ion is lowered to such an extent that it is not precipitated by the given reagent and therefore does not interfere with the determination. However, masking achieves this aim much more easily and quickly, as it is not necessary to filter the solution and wash the precipitate; all that is needed is to add the appropriate "masking agent", such as NaF, tartaric acid, etc. Let us now consider what factors determine the possibility of masking any particular ion. First, we must note the influence of the same two factors as were considered in the effect fn pH on the completeness of precipitation; namely, the solubility product of the precipitated compound and the dissociation constants of the reaction product, i. e., of the complex ion formed.

It is obvious that the greater the solubility product of the compound the precipitation of which we want to prevent, the easier it is to do so, because the concentration of the ion combined in the complex needs to be reduced to a lesser extent before the solubility product becomes unattainable. Conversely, if the solubility of the unwanted precipitate is very low, the concentration of the corresponding ion must be very greatly reduced.

On the other hand, the extent to which the concentration of a particular ion is reduced by addition of any masking agent depends on the degree of dissociation of the complex ion formed. The dissociation of a complex may be characterized by its instability constant

(K_{inst}). For example, the complex ions $[Ag(NH_3)_2]^+$ and $[Ag(CN)_2]^-$ which dissociate as follows

$$[Ag(NH_3)_2]^+ \rightleftarrows Ag^+ + 2NH_3$$

$$[Ag(CN)_2]^- \rightleftarrows Ag^+ + 2CN^-$$

have the following instability constants:

$$K_{inst.} = \frac{[Ag^+][NH_3]^2}{[Ag\,(HN_3)_2]^+} = 6.8 \times 10^{-8}$$

$$K_{inst.} = \frac{[Ag^+][CN^-]^2}{[Ag(CN)_2]^-} = 1 \times 10^{-21}$$

Comparison of the instability constants of the two complexes shows that the concentration of Ag^+ ions in a solution of a silver salt is lowered much more by addition of potassium cyanide than ammonia under the same conditions. In other words, the masking effect of KCN is much greater than that of NH_3. Experiment confirms this supposition. Thus, by addition of KCN we can prevent precipitation of AgCl, AgBr, and AgI, and only the least soluble silver salt (Ag_2S) is precipitated in the presence of KCN. If NH_3 is added the precipitation of silver chloride only is prevented, as it is the most soluble of these salts. The other salts, i.e., AgBr, AgI, and Ag_2S, are precipitated even in the presence of ammonia.

In addition to these factors, the effect of excess of masking agent should be noted. The higher its concentration in solution, the lower is the degree of dissociation of the complex, and therefore the lower is the resultant concentration of the combined ion. For example, calculation shows that, if the amount of KCN corresponding to the reaction equation is used, AgI should be precipitated by addition of KI. It is only because in fact KCN is always added in some excess that the Ag^+ ion is masked.

Finally, the solution pH is important in masking, as in precipitation. This applies to all cases where the ligands in a given complex ion are molecules or ions capable of combining with H^+ ions. These include ammonia molecules, which form NH_4^+ cations with H^+ ions, and anions of weak acids such as hydrocyanic, tartaric, citric, dimethylglyoxime, etc. In all these cases increase of hydrogen ion concentration, i.e., decrease of solution pH, leads to decomposition of the complex and makes masking of the corresponding cations impossible. For example, if an ammoniacal solution containing the complex salt $[Ag(NH_3)_2]Cl$ is acidified, the complex ion is decomposed by the reaction

$$[Ag(NH_3)_2]^+ + 2H^+ \rightleftarrows Ag^+ + 2NH_4^+$$

Since the solution also contains Cl^- ions, the solubility product of AgCl is exceeded and the salt is precipitated. This effect is, of course, used in detection of Ag^+ and Cl^- ions. Similarly, if the deep blue solutions of complex salts of copper with ammonia, tartaric acid, or glycerol are acidified, the colour disappears and is replaced by the pale blue colour due to Cu^{++} cations. This shows that the complex ions are decomposed by the action of H^+ ions. It is therefore evident that in all these cases the pH must be sufficiently high to ensure masking.

It has already been pointed out that masking of interfering ions makes analysis very much easier, because it is not necessary to remove them by precipitation, which takes much labour and time. However, complex formation may also cause difficulties in analysis. Such is the case, for instance, if the solution contains any substances or ions which can form complexes with the ion which is being determined, and thus prevent its precipitation. Many organic substances containing hydroxyl or carboxyl groups in their molecules, such as certain organic acids (oxalic, tartaric, citric, etc.), various sugars, and so on, are of this type. If such substances are present in the solution, they must be removed by oxidation to CO_2 and H_2O. Another instance of the adverse effect of complex formation on gravimetric determinations has already been given (p. 73). This is increase of solubility of the precipitated compound as the result of complex formation with excess precipitant ion. In some cases this effect is very pronounced. For example, Fig. 13 shows that in precipitation of HgI_2 the solubility of the precipitate increases on addition of the slightest excess of precipitant. Because of this, HgI_2 cannot be used in gravimetric analysis. The same figure shows a curve representing changes in the solubility of $BaSO_4$ in presence of excess precipitant. In this case no complexes are formed and the solubility of $BaSO_4$ decreases in accordance with the solubility product rule. In most cases found in practice these curves are of the form represented by the dash line in Fig. 13. For most precipitates the solubility first decreases in presence of excess precipitant (although less than is indicated by the solubility product rule in

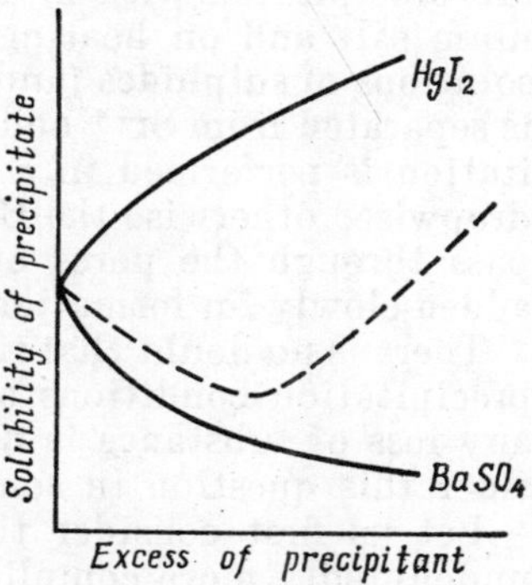

Fig. 13. Effect of excess precipitant on the solubility of precipitates

its simplified form); it then reaches a minimum and begins to increase again owing to complex formation, the salt effect, and other causes.* The empirical rule according to which a precipitant is added in 50% excess is based on this course of the curve. However, the example of HgI_2 shows that it is not always applicable.

24. Amorphous and Crystalline Precipitates

Care must be taken even in qualitative analysis to conduct precipitation under definite conditions. For example, Group III cations are precipitated with ammonium sulphide in presence of an ammonium salt and on heating, in order to avoid formation of colloidal solutions of sulphides (and hydroxides). In the same way, when Ba^{++} is separated from Sr^{++} and Ca^{++} by the action of $K_2Cr_2O_7$, the precipitation is performed in a hot solution and the precipitant is added dropwise; otherwise the $BaCrO_4$ crystals may be so small that they pass through the pores of the filter. The precipitant must also be added slowly for formation of crystalline $MgNH_4PO_4$ precipitate, etc.

There is no doubt that in quantitative determinations the optimum precipitation conditions are even more important, as in such cases any loss of substance is quite inadmissible. Therefore we must consider this question in some detail.

Let us first consider the process of precipitate formation. It is undoubtedly more complicated than the chemical reaction equation would suggest. For example, the equation

$$Ba^{++} + SO_4^{--} = \downarrow BaSO_4$$

suggests that all that is necessary for formation of barium sulphate is that two ions, Ba^{++} and SO_4^{--}, should meet in solution. But, of course, this is not so. $BaSO_4$ is precipitated in the form of crystals, and a crystal lattice cannot be built out of two ions. Therefore, not two but a fairly large number of these ions must meet simultaneously, and they must be in the correct proportions and in the right configuration in space. Of course, the crystals formed in the first instant are not the relatively large crystals, consisting of enormous numbers of ions, which are precipitated; they are extremely minute *crystal nuclei* or *primary particles* of a size characteristic of colloidal systems (1-100 mμ).** Such small particles are not precipitated. The particles must grow in size for precipitation to occur.

The primary particles may increase in size in two different ways, in accordance with the individual properties of the precipitated

* See, for example, the data on the solubility of AgCl in NaCl solutions (p. 74).

** It will be remembered that 1 mμ (millimicron) is 10^{-6} mm.

compounds, primarily their solubility, and also in accordance with the precipitation conditions. Either crystalline or amorphous precipitates may be formed.

In formation of crystalline precipitates addition of each portion of precipitant does not cause immediate formation of crystal nuclei, and the substance being precipitated remains for some time in supersaturated solution. As the precipitant is gradually added the substance separates out of the supersaturated solution mainly on the surfaces of the crystal nuclei previously formed; these gradually grow so that eventually a crystalline precipitate consisting of a comparatively small number of relatively large crystals is formed.

This is the usual course of precipitation when the solubility of the precipitate is not too low, especially if steps are taken to raise it by heating or by addition of suitable reagents such as acids.

The formation of amorphous precipitates occurs in a different manner. In this case addition of each portion of precipitant causes rapid formation of an enormous number of very minute crystal nuclei in the liquid; these grow not by deposition of the substance on their surfaces but by joining to form larger aggregates which sink by gravity to the bottom of the vessel. In other words, in this case *coagulation of an initially formed colloidal solution takes place*. Amorphous precipitates formed in this way have an enormous total surface area and therefore adsorb various extraneous substances from solution much more than crystalline precipitates do. On the other hand, since the bonds between the individual crystal nuclei in the aggregates are relatively weak, the aggregates may break up again to give a colloidal solution.

It follows that it is not quite correct to describe such precipitates as amorphous. It would be more accurate to call them "cryptocrystalline", since they consist of crystals, although these are extremely minute. In fact, the existence of crystal lattices in amorphous precipitates can in most cases be proved experimentally by X-ray investigation, and sometimes by means of the microscope.

Substances of very low solubility form amorphous precipitates especially readily. These include metal sulphides and hydroxides, silicic acid, etc. Because of the very low solubility, the solubility product is greatly exceeded by addition of even small amounts of precipitant, and this favours the rapid formation of numerous crystal nuclei. Conversely, with precipitates of higher solubility the solubility product is not exceeded as much. This favours formation of a supersaturated solution and leads, as we showed earlier, to deposition of a crystalline precipitate.

The type of precipitate formed depends not only on the individual properties of the substance but also on the precipitation conditions. For example, $BaSO_4$ is precipitated in crystalline form out of dilute aqueous solutions. However, if it is precipitated out of a mixture of water with 30-60% of alcohol, which greatly reduces the solubility of barium sulphate, a colloidal solution or an amorphous precipitate is formed. On the other hand, by precipitating sulphides in presence of pyridine (C_5H_5N), E. Ostroumov obtained some of them in crystalline form. These investigations proved experimentally that any substance can be obtained either as a crystalline or as an amorphous precipitate. However, the precipitation of one of these forms usually involves conditions which are unacceptable in quantitative determinations. Therefore, in accordance with the individual properties of the compounds formed, some are obtained in analysis as crystalline and others as amorphous precipitates. The analyst's task is to provide conditions in which the precipitate is the most suitable for the subsequent treatments of filtration and washing.

The optimum precipitation conditions for amorphous and crystalline precipitates respectively are very different. We shall first consider the conditions for formation of crystalline precipitates.*

25. Conditions for Formation of Crystalline Precipitates

As has already been pointed out, many crystalline precipitates (such as $BaCrO_4$, $BaSO_4$, CaC_2O_4, etc.) are sometimes so fine that their particles pass through the filter pores and a turbid filtrate is obtained. Often this turbidity cannot be removed even by repeated filtration through the same filter. In order to prevent passage of the precipitate through the filter and to avoid the attendant losses, it is necessary to create such conditions that the crystals in the precipitate are sufficiently large.

This is also convenient in other respects; such precipitates settle rapidly, do not clog the filter pores and, being of small surface area, adsorb extraneous substances from solution to a lesser extent than microcrystalline and especially amorphous precipitates.

What are the conditions favouring deposition of coarse-grained crystalline precipitates?

This question is not difficult to answer in the light of what has been said in Sec. 24 about the formation mechanism of crystalline precipitates. Evidently *the precipitation must be performed in such a manner that the supersaturation of the solution with respect to the precipitated compound is kept as low as possible*, i.e., so that its solubility product is not exceeded too much. Considerable supersaturation of the solution favours rapid formation of numerous new crystal nuclei; naturally, these cannot grow sufficiently before the end

---

* The theory of this process was first worked out at the end of the 18th century by the Russian scientist T. Löwitz.

of the precipitation. Conversely, in precipitation from a slightly supersaturated solution few new crystal nuclei are formed by addition of each portion of precipitant, but on the other hand most of the substance is deposited on the surfaces of the crystal nuclei formed earlier. As a result, a relatively coarsely crystalline precipitate is formed.

To keep the supersaturation of the solution during precipitation as low as possible it is necessary:

(1) to perform the precipitation from fairly dilute solution, with a dilute solution of precipitant;

(2) to add the precipitant *very slowly*, drop by drop (especially at the start of precipitation);

(3) to stir the solution continuously with a glass rod in order to avoid high local supersaturations as the precipitant is added.

It will be shown later that in formation of crystalline precipitates slow addition of the precipitant is also necessary in order to reduce, as much as possible, contamination of the precipitates with extraneous impurities (p. 109).

Clearly, the degree of supersaturation depends not only on the concentration of the ions of the precipitated compound, but also on its solubility. The higher the solubility, the less must the degree of supersaturation be under given conditions. *In formation of crystalline precipitates it is therefore advantageous to raise the solubility of the precipitate during the operation.*

Of course, at the end of precipitation this higher solubility must be *lowered again* by addition of excess precipitant or by some other means, as otherwise the precipitation would be incomplete.

Consequently, formation of coarse-grained crystalline precipitates is also favoured by:

(4) precipitation from hot solution by a hot solution of precipitant, as the solubility of most precipitates rises with temperature;

(5) addition of substances which raise the solubility of the precipitate; for example, in precipitation of barium sulphate HNO_3 is added, because it raises (see p. 90) the solubility of $BaSO_4$ by formation of HSO_4^- ions. Towards the end of precipitation this raised solubility of $BaSO_4$ is lowered again by the addition of a moderate excess of precipitant.

With the same aim in view Ca^{++} is precipitated as $CaC_2O_4 \cdot H_2O$ from acid and not neutral solution, as calcium oxalate is a sparingly soluble salt of a relatively weak acid and therefore it is considerably more soluble in an acid medium than in water. This makes conditions favourable for formation of relatively large crystals, but at the same time the precipitation becomes incomplete.

For practically complete precipitation of Ca^{++} ions it is evidently necessary to lower the acidity of the solution towards the end of precipitation to pH $\geqslant$ 3.3 (p. 87) by dropwise addition of NH_4OH solution. As the acid is neutralized the solubility of CaC_2O_4 gradually decreases and fresh amounts of it are precipitated. However, if the ammonia is added slowly this occurs mainly by growth of crystals already formed.

In conformity with theoretical considerations, experience shows that $CaC_2O_4 \cdot H_2O$ precipitated in this way is easy to filter off, whereas if it is precipitated from neutral or alkaline solution it can pass very easily through the filter pores.

In formation of crystalline precipitates, quite often the precipitation of the substance from supersaturated solution takes a considerable time. Moreover, the analyst's aim—to obtain a sufficiently coarse-grained precipitate—is only partially achieved under all the precipitation conditions listed above, as in addition to the large crystals a certain amount of very fine crystals is usually formed, and these can subsequently pass through the filter pores. Therefore, in most cases *the precipitate must be left to stand for several hours (usually overnight) after addition of the precipitant*. When left to stand, precipitates undergo the so-called *ripening* or *ageing*, accompanied by particle growth. The cause of this growth *is the higher solubility of very fine crystals of a substance in comparison with larger crystals* under the same conditions. For example, it was found experimentally that the solubility of the smallest $BaSO_4$ crystals (0.04 μ in diameter) is almost 1,000 times the solubility of large crystals at the same temperature.* This increase of solubility with decrease of crystal size, which is also observed with other substances, is attributable to surface tension, which tends to minimize the area of contact between the solution and the precipitate. In this instance this can be achieved only *by dissolution of the fine crystals of the precipitate and growth of the larger crystals at their expense*. This is the "recrystallization" process which takes place during ripening of a precipitate. Its mechanism may be represented as follows. Because of the lower solubility of the large crystals, the solution saturated with respect to these crystals is still unsaturated with respect to the small crystals and should dissolve them. As a result, it becomes

* It follows from this that the particle size of a precipitate also affects its solubility product. A coarse-grained precipitate always has a lower SP than a microcrystalline precipitate of the same substance at the same temperature. The characteristic constant of a given substance is taken to be the product of the activities of the ions of the sparingly soluble electrolyte in a saturated solution in contact with a *coarse-grained crystalline* precipitate of this electrolyte. It is this constant which is the solubility product of the electrolyte (see Appendix III)

supersaturated with respect to the large crystals and the dissolved substance is deposited on the latter. In consequence, the solution again becomes unsaturated with respect to the small crystals, which continue to dissolve, and so on.

The course of all these processes, represented schematically in Fig. 14, is evidently associated with diffusion of the dissolved substance from the small to the large crystals. However, diffusion is very slow at room temperature. Rise of temperature increases the rate of diffusion, and ripening of precipitates is therefore accelerated. Stirring of the solution has the same effect. It is therefore advantageous to place the beaker with the precipitate in a warm place (for example, on a boiling water bath) and to stir its contents from time to time.

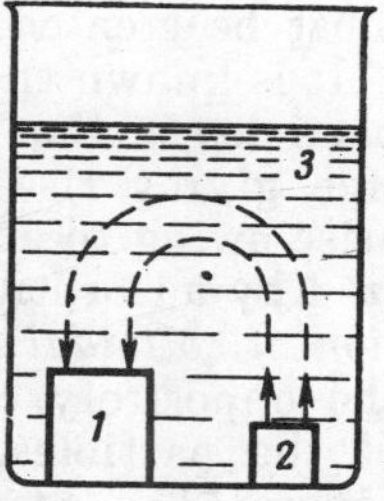

Fig. 14. Diagram of processes taking place during ripening of crystalline precipitates:
1—large crystals; *2*—small crystals; *3*—solution

The precipitates formed after ripening *are not only easier to filter off, but also purer*. The reasons for this are: (1) adsorption is decreased owing to increase of the particle size; (2) recrystallization converts less perfect crystals into crystals of more regular form, corresponding to a more stable ionic configuration. This is accompanied by partial liberation of the impurities trapped by the precipitate from solution.

It was found in one experiment that the amount of Na_2SO_4 trapped from solution by 2 g of $BaSO_4$ precipitate decreased as follows during ripening:

Amount of Na_2SO_4 in precipitate, mg	22.6	19.0	17.4	14.0	10.4	8.2	7.6
Ripening time	15 min.	3.0 hr.	18 hr.	2 days	48 days	5 mth.	7 mth.

It must be pointed out, however, that in some cases the precipitate may not be freed of impurities by ripening. For example, if an impurity forms a chemical compound with the precipitate, the amount of the impurity present may even increase with time. For example, it was found in one experiment that the amounts of Zn^{++}, Co^{++}, and Ni^{++} taken out of solution by a $Fe(OH)_3$ precipitate increased with time. This is probably due to gradual formation of chemical compounds (ferrites) between ferric hydroxide and these cations.

Ripening of a precipitate may sometimes be accompanied by *postprecipitation* of various impurities; this is considered more fully in Sec. 27.

26. Conditions for Formation of Amorphous Precipitates

In formation of amorphous rpecipitates it must first be taken into account that they are produced by coagulation of a colloidal solution initially formed, and can be redissolved. It is therefore evident that conditions favouring coagulation of colloidal solutions must be created.

It is known that one of the factors preventing cohesion of colloidal particles is the presence on them of electrical charges of the same sign giving rise to forces of electrostatic repulsion. These charges arise owing to adsorption of ions from solution, and can be neutralized by adsorption of ions of the opposite sign. Accordingly, *coagulation of colloidal solutions can be induced by addition of an electrolyte* the oppositely charged ions of which are adsorbed on the surface of the particles, neutralize their charges, and so enable them to cohere. The coagulating concentration of the electrolyte (i.e., the minimum concentration needed to coagulate a given colloidal solution) increases rapidly with decreasing valence of the ion of a charge opposite to the particles. For example, in the case of As_2S_3 sol, the particles of which are negatively charged, coagulation is caused by adsorption of cations, and the coagulating concentrations of Al^{+++}, Ba^{++}, and K^+ ions are in the proportion of 1 : 20 : : 1,000.

Another factor in the stability of colloidal systems is solvation (hydration) of colloidal particles, i.e., adsorption of solvent molecules. As a result, the colloidal particles become surrounded by solvation layers which prevent them from approaching closely enough to form larger aggregates. Therefore, when we have a sol of a substance the particles of which have a high tendency to solvation, it is not enough to neutralize the particle charges in order to induce coagulation; the solvation layers must be destroyed as well. This can also be done by addition of electrolytes if their concentration is high enough. At high concentrations the electrolyte ions remove solvent molecules from the colloidal particles in becoming solvated themselves and, moreover, discharge the colloidal particles. These processes lead to coagulation of the sol (in this case, it is known as *salting-out*).

In many cases coagulation is also assisted by increase of the solution temperature. This decreases adsorption of the ions which confer charges on the particles, and assists destruction of their solvation layers.

It should be noted that coagulation may occur also if a solution contains colloidal particles with unlike charges; for example, when a negatively charged silicic acid sol is mixed with a positively charged gelatin sol, etc. This is now used for rapid determinations of SiO_2 in various materials.*

It follows from all this that in order to prevent formation of colloidal systems *amorphous substances should be precipitated*: (*a*) *from hot solutions*; (*b*) *in the presence of a suitable coagulating electrolyte.* Either various ammonium salts, or acids (if their presence does not cause a considerable increase of the solubility of the precipitate), are used for this purpose.

The properties of amorphous precipitates, in particular their density and the associated surface area and settling rate, depend on the solution concentration in precipitation.

It is found in practice that if precipitates such as $Al(OH)_3$, $Fe(OH)_3$ etc., are formed from dilute solutions they are loose and bulky, settle extremely slowly, and, because of their enormous surface area, they strongly adsorb impurities.

Conversely, when formed from concentrated solutions such precipitates are much denser, of smaller surface area, settle more rapidly, and are easier to wash free of impurities. Therefore, on N. Tananayev's recommendation, *such substances are precipitated from concentrated solutions by concentrated solutions of precipitants,* which may be added rapidly.

It should be taken into account, however, that although adsorption is decreased because the total surface area of the precipitate is reduced, it is at the same time intensified owing to increased concentrations of the adsorbed ions in solution. To avoid this intensification of adsorption, a large volume (about 100 ml) of hot water is added immediately after the end of precipitation and the liquid is stirred. This disturbs the adsorption equilibrium and some of the adsorbed ions pass from the surface of the precipitate back into solution.

In contrast to crystalline precipitates, amorphous precipitates are not left to stand after precipitation but are immediately transferred to the filters and washed.

In such cases the precipitate should not be left for a long time in contact with the solution, as it may become so dense that washing becomes difficult. Furthermore, amorphous precipitates are often formed by the action of alkalies. These act on glass, so that the precipitate becomes contaminated with non-volatile impurities (such as SiO_2) leached out of the glass.

It follows that the most favourable conditions for formation of crystalline and amorphous precipitates respectively are in many ways opposite to each other.

---

* Fuller details on colloidal solutions and their coagulation are given in the books of V. Alexeyev, *Qualitative Analysis*, Sec. 41, Goskhimizdat, 1960, and *Course of Qualitative Chemical Semimicroanalysis*, Sec. 44, Goskhimizdat, 1962.

27. Coprecipitation

It has already been repeatedly pointed out that the precipitates formed during analysis carry down with them various impurities, which are often quite soluble by themselves. For example, if sulphuric acid is added to a solution containing a mixture of $BaCl_2$ and $FeCl_3$, we would expect only $BaSO_4$ to be precipitated, since the other salt which might be formed, $Fe_2(SO_4)_3$, is soluble in water. However, in reality this salt is partially precipitated too. This can be seen if the precipitate if filtered off, washed, and ignited. The residue is not white (the colour of $BaSO_4$) but is coloured brownish by ferric oxide which is formed by decomposition of $Fe_2(SO_4)_3$ on heating:

$$Fe_2(SO_4)_3 = Fe_2O_3 + \uparrow 3SO_3$$

The precipitation of any extraneous substances, which are not generally precipitated under the given conditions by the precipitant used, is known as *coprecipitation*.

Coprecipitation of soluble substances may be illustrated by the following experiment.

To a mixture of $BaCl_2$ and $KMnO_4$ solutions an excess of H_2SO_4 (to a strongly acid reaction) is added by small portions, and the $KMnO_4$ remaining in solution is then reduced by addition of Na_2SO_3. The reduction proceeds in accordance with the equation:

$$2KMnO_4 + 5Na_2SO_3 + 3H_2SO_4 = 2MnSO_4 + K_2SO_4 + 5Na_2SO_4 + 3H_2O$$

The solution becomes colourless, but the precipitate is found to be of a violet colour, indicating that some $KMnO_4$ is coprecipitated together with $BaSO_4$.

Coprecipitation should be distinguished from ordinary (chemical) precipitation of sparingly soluble impurities, together with the main substance, when their solubility products are exceeded on addition of the precipitant. For example, if Al^{+++} is precipitated from a solution also containing Fe^{+++} ions by NH_4OH solution, ferric hydroxide must always be precipitated together with $Al(OH)_3$ because its solubility product is exceeded. However, this effect cannot be regarded as coprecipitation of $Fe(OH)_3$, because that compound would have been precipitated by ammonia even in absence of Al^{+++}. Nevertheless in some instances one speaks of coprecipitation of sparingly soluble substances if the experimental conditions are such that these substances could not be precipitated by the action of the precipitant in absence of the main substance. This happens, for example, when the concentration of such extraneous ions in solution is very low, or if the solution contains any substances which interfere with their normal precipitation, etc.

Thus, despite the very low solubility of $BaSO_4$, the precipitation of this substance together with $BaSO_4$ by the action of H_2SO_4 must be regarded as coprecipitation, because the Ra^{++} ion concentration in solutions is usually so low that these ions are not precipitated by sulphuric acid in absence of Ba^{++}. Partial precipitation of nickel and cobalt hydroxides together with $Fe(OH)_3$ by excess NH_4OH must also be regarded as coprecipitation, because these hydroxides are soluble in ammonia and should remain in solution as complex $[Co(NH_3)_6]^{++}$ and $[Ni(NH_3)_6]^{++}$ ions.

Coprecipitation is of great importance in analytical chemistry. Primarily, it is one of the most important sources of error in gravimetric determinations, because a precipitate (weighed form) containing coprecipitated impurities is no longer a pure substance with a perfectly definite formula; unless this formula is known, exact calculation of the amount of the element being determined is impossible. Therefore, the analyst performing gravimetric determinations must constantly take steps to diminish coprecipitation of impurities and of the precipitant itself.

However, coprecipitation may also play a very important positive role in analysis. It happens quite often in analytical practice that the concentration of a particular substance in solution is so low that it cannot be precipitated in the usual way. Coprecipitation of such a *microcomponent* (i.e., component present in a very low concentration) with a suitable *collector* (carrier) may be induced in such cases.

For example, determination of lead content is important in water analysis. However, the concentration of Pb^{++} ions in water is so low that the solubility product of even the least soluble lead compound, PbS, cannot be reached.

The Pb^{++} concentration in solution must be greatly increased before it is precipitated. This might be achieved by evaporation of 10 litres of water down to about 100 ml. However, such evaporation would take a great deal of time and heat, and would also increase the concentrations of all the other components in solution, which might complicate the subsequent analysis.

Microcomponents can be concentrated much more rapidly and simply by coprecipitation with suitable collectors. In the case in question the collector used is $CaCO_3$ precipitate formed by addition of Na_2CO_3 solution to the water. Practically all the Pb^{++} ions present in the water are precipitated together with $CaCO_3$. If the small precipitate is filtered off and dissolved in the smallest possible amount of HCl or CH_3COOH a solution is obtained in which the Pb^{++} ion concentration is thousands or tens of thousands of times higher than in the original water. Determination of Pb^{++} in such a solution presents no difficulties.

Coprecipitation of microcomponents with collectors is used very frequently. It is especially important in the chemistry of rare elements.

Coprecipitation is also used for other purposes; for example, to raise the sensitivity or selectivity of reactions, to improve precipitation conditions, to remove substances which interfere in analysis, etc.

Because of the great practical importance of coprecipitation, it has been the subject of numerous experimental investigations for a hundred years (since the middle of the 19th century). Important progress was achieved in this field only after the highly sensitive methods of the chemistry of the radioactive elements had been applied to studies of coprecipitation, which is especially important for the chemistry of these elements. Concentrations of radioactive elements are usually extremely low, and therefore in most cases such elements are isolated by coprecipitation with suitable collectors.

Experimental investigations have shown that several different types of coprecipitation exist. From the point of view of analytical chemistry they are most conveniently divided into two groups, depending on the location of the coprecipitated component—on the surface or within the particles of the precipitate. Accordingly, a distinction is made between adsorption and occlusion.

Adsorption. Adsorption is the term used to describe the changes in concentration of substances or ions at the interface between two phases; for example, between a solid phase (precipitate) and solution, a solid phase and a gas, etc. The dissolved substance or gas usually becomes concentrated at the surface of the solid, which is then termed the *adsorbent*. Adsorption of dissolved substances from solutions, discovered by T. Löwitz at the end of the 19th century, is especially important in analytical chemistry.

The explanation of adsorption is that ions or molecules on the surface of a substance are not under the same conditions as particles within that substance. Whereas particles within the substance are bound with their neighbours in all directions, so that the forces between them are mutually balanced, in a surface layer only the forces directed into the substance and in the plane of the surface itself are balanced. Therefore, a free field of force arises at the surface and the particles can attract ions or molecules of dissolved substances or gases.

Adsorption is a reversible process, because it is accompanied by the opposite process of desorption, i.e., passage of adsorbed ions or molecules from the adsorbent surface into solution. The simultaneous occurrence of these two mutually opposed processes leads, as always, to a state of dynamic equilibrium, known in this case as *adsorption equilibrium*.

The position of adsorption equilibrium depends on numerous factors; the following must be considered in detail.

Effect of the Adsorbent Area. Since substances or ions are adsorbed on the surface of the adsorbent, the amount of a substance adsorbed by a given adsorbent is directly proportional to the total surface area of the adsorbent. It follows that adsorption becomes most significant in analysis when one deals with amorphous precipitates, as the particles in such precipitates are formed by aggregation of large numbers of small primary particles and therefore have enormous surface areas (Sec. 24).

On the other hand, with crystalline and especially with coarse-grained crystalline precipitates, which have much smaller surface areas, adsorption is usually insignificant by comparison with other types of coprecipitation.

Effect of Concentration. Adsorption of various substances or ions increases with increase of their concentration in solution; however, the increase is not proportional to the concentration but slower (Fig. 15).

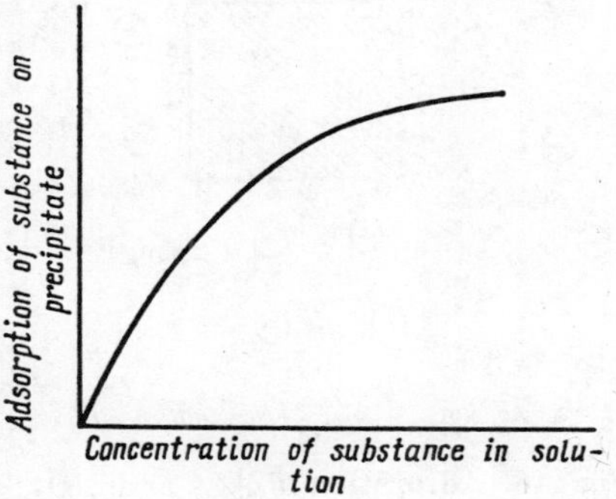

Adsorption of substance on precipitate

Concentration of substance in solution

Fig. 15. Variation of the adsorption of a substance with concentration

Effect of Temperature. Adsorption is an exothermic process, and it should therefore be favoured by decrease of temperature. Rise of temperature favours desorption, so that the amount of substance adsorbed decreases.

Effect of the Nature of the Adsorbed Ions. Adsorption is characterized by a high degree of selectivity: a particular adsorbent adsorbs some ions (or substances) in preference to others under the same conditions. The following rule holds: *adsorbents with ionic crystal lattices preferentially adsorb ions which form sparingly soluble or weakly dissociated compounds with oppositely charged ions in the lattice*; *in particular, ions common with the precipitate*. For example, $BaSO_4$ precipitate preferentially adsorbs its own common ions, Ba^{++} and SO_4^{--}, dependent on which is present in the solution in excess. Among extraneous ions, NO_3^- ions are adsorbed more than Cl^- ions because $Ba(NO_3)_2$ is less soluble than $BaCl_2$, etc.

Similarly, AgI precipitate preferentially adsorbs Ag^+ and I^- ions, etc.

Adsorption of any ions by a precipitate confers the corresponding electric charge on the precipitate particles; accordingly, each particle attracts oppositely charged ions (counter-ions or "gegenions').

For example, if an AgI precipitate is in contact with $AgNO_3$ solution, then the precipitate particles become positively charged by adsorbing Ag^+ ions and attract NO_3^- ions as counter-ions. In other words, the AgI precipitate becomes contaminated with adsorbed $AgNO_3$. Conversely, if an AgI precipitate is in contact with KI solution, its particles become negatively charged owing to adsorption of I^- ions and retain K^+ cations as counter-ions.

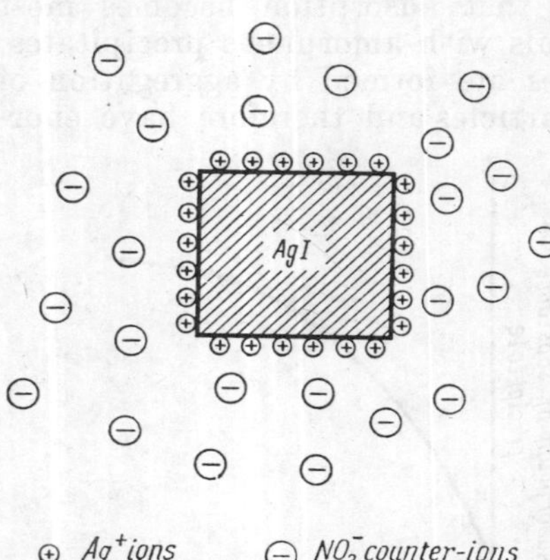

Fig. 16. Adsorption of Ag^+ and NO_3^- ions by crystals of AgI precipitate

It follows from all this that a distinction must be made between two types of adsorption: primary and secondary.

In *primary adsorption* the precipitate adsorbs either its own ions or ions which can replace them isomorphously.* In this case the adsorbed ions form a single layer on the precipitate particles and confer a positive or negative charge on them. A consequence of this is *secondary adsorption* of ions of the opposite sign (counter-ions) by the particles; these ions remain in solution and form the so-called diffuse layer (Fig. 16) near the particle surfaces.

Secondary adsorption increases very rapidly with increasing charge of the adsorbed ions and with decreasing solubility of the adsorption compound formed.

Effect of Precipitation Conditions. Adsorption is very much influenced by the experimental conditions. For example, the concentrations of the reacting solutions are very significant. It was pointed out in Sec. 26 that it is more convenient to precipitate amorphous substances such as $Fe(OH)_3$, $Al(OH)_3$, etc., from concentrated solutions, because denser precipitates of smaller surface area are formed and they adsorb far fewer extraneous ions. Conversely, it is preferable to precipitate crystalline substances from dilute solutions, as larger crystals are formed, with a smaller surface area than the same weight of small crystals.

Since ageing of crystalline precipitates involves an increase of particle size and recrystallization of the particles with formation of more perfect crystals, ageing should result in partial removal of adsorbed impurities from precipitates. This is found to be the

---

* See p. 109.

case (for example, see the data on p. 99 concerning the amounts of Na_2SO_4 held by a $BaSO_4$ precipitate during ageing).

As has already been stated, substances or ions adsorbed by a precipitate are in dynamic equilibrium with the same substances (or ions) present in solution. When a precipitate is washed, the solution permeating it is gradually replaced by pure water, the adsorption equilibrium is disturbed, and the adsorbed substances or ions pass from the precipitate surface into solution. In other words, adsorbed ions can be removed by washing the precipitate.

Occlusion. Occlusion differs from surface adsorption in that the coprecipitated impurities *are within the precipitate particles and not on the surface*. Therefore, occluded impurities cannot be removed from a precipitate by washing. The whole precipitate must de dissolved to bring them into solution. Occlusion may occur due to various causes, namely: entrainment of impurities, in particular, the mother liquor during crystallization (mechanical occlusion), adsorption during crystallization (adsorptive occlusion or "internal adsorption"), formation of mixed crystals (occlusion due to isomorphism) and formation of chemical compounds of the precipitate with coprecipitated impurities (chemical occlusion).

Mechanical Occlusion. Crystals grown under practical conditions are hardly ever "ideal", i.e., do not form quite regular crystal lattices. They contain minute cracks and cavities filled with the mother liquor. Very small crystals are apt to aggregate, entraining the mother liquor. The faster crystallization occurs, the more of such impurities will be entrained, because on fast crystallization the ions do not have time, as it were, to form a regular crystal lattice. This case of coprecipitation is known as mechanical occlusion.

Adsorptive Occlusion. In chemical analysis a precipitate is not put into a solution as such, but is formed as the precipitant is added. At first very small crystal nuclei are formed; these gradually grow and their surface is continuously renewed by deposition of new layers of the substance. This constantly renewing crystal surface continuously adsorbs various impurities from solution. As the crystal grows, these impurities are gradually displaced by the ions which constitute the crystal lattice of the precipitate. However, usually this displacement is incomplete. In accordance with the precipitation conditions some part of the impurities, initially present on the particle surface, becomes separated from the solution by the newly deposited layers of substance. This trapping of initially adsorbed substances within growing crystals is known as adsorptive occlusion*

* Some authors call this case of coprecipitation "internal adsorption". However, as was indicated above (p. 104), adsorption is a surface phenomenon. In this case the impurities also settle on the crystal surfaces, but since this occurs in the course of crystallization, before the crystals are completely

Internal adsorption conforms to the same laws as adsorption. For example, the effect of the concentration of an impurity on internal adsorption is represented by a curve similar to that for adsorption (see Fig. 15). As in adsorption, the solubility and degree of dissociation of the compounds formed have a strong influence on this type of occlusion. For example, a $BaSO_4$ precipitate adsorbs NO_3^- ions much more strongly than Cl^- ions, because $Ba(OH)_2$ is less soluble than $BaCl_2$.

The sequence of addition of the solutions is very significant in adsorptive occlusion. Suppose, for example, that we precipitate $BaSO_4$ by dropwise addition of H_2SO_4 solution to $BaCl_2$ solution. The crystals of the precipitate then grow in a medium containing Ba^{++} ions in excess, and these ions become adsorbed by the precipitate and confer positive charges on its crystals. As a result, Cl^- anions are held as counter-ions. As new portions of precipitant are added, these counter-ions are displaced by the SO_4^{--} ions, which are common to the precipitate and are more readily adsorbed. However, since this displacement is incomplete, the precipitate occludes some Cl^- anions. In other words, we obtain not a pure $BaSO_4$ precipitate but an indefinite mixture containing a small amount of $BaCl_2$. If the solution contained some other anions such as Br^-, I^-, NO_3^-, etc., instead of Cl^-, these would also be occluded; the more so the lower the solubility of the corresponding barium salt. On the other hand, extraneous cations present in the solution are not occluded to any appreciable extent by barium sulphate during precipitation under these conditions.

The situation is different if the order of precipitation is reversed, i.e., if $BaCl_2$ solution is added dropwise to H_2SO_4 solution. In this case the $BaSO_4$ crystals grow in a medium containing SO_4^{--} ions in excess. As the crystals adsorb the anions, they become negatively charged, and therefore attract cations (H^+ ions in this case) as counter ions. This means that as the result of occlusion the precipitate would contain an admixture of H_2SO_4 or of various sulphates, such as Na_2SO_4, K_2SO_4, etc. (if the corresponding cations were present in the solution).

It follows from all this that *to diminish internal adsorption of extraneous cations precipitation should be performed so that the crystals of the precipitate grow in a medium containing its own cations in excess. Conversely, if it is required to obtain a precipitate as free of occluded extraneous anions as possible, the precipitation should be*

---

formed, the adsorbed impurities become coated with fresh layers of the precipitating substance, i.e., become embedded or "occluded" in the crystal. For this reason it is more correct to call this case of coprecipitation "adsorptive occlusion".

performed in a medium containing anions of the precipitated compound in excess.

The following example shows how strongly internal adsorption is influenced by the sequence of addition of the solutions. In a certain experiment sulphuric acid was added slowly to $BaCl_2$ solution, and a precipitate containing 1.6% of chlorides was obtained. When the sequence of addition was reversed, under the same conditions of temperature, concentration, etc., the precipitate contained only 0.13% of chlorides or one-twelfth of the previous amount.* Of course, by decreasing adsorptive occlusion of anions with this sequence of precipitation we make the conditions more favourable for internal adsorption of cations.

In addition to these factors, the *rate at which the precipitant is added* also influences adsorptive occlusion. If the precipitant is added in excess at once, the precipitate crystals grow in a medium containing an excess of the precipitating ion. In other words, the conditions are similar to those produced when the sequence of addition is reversed. However, apart from this indirect influence, the rate of precipitant addition can apparently influence adsorptive occlusion more directly. It is known that purer precipitates are usually obtained if the precipitant is added slowly. This may be partly because a more coarse-grained precipitate, of smaller surface area, is formed by slow precipitation. However, since adsorption plays a relatively small part in formation of crystalline precipitates, it is more probable that slow growth of the crystals favours a decrease of adsorptive occlusion, because under such conditions replacement of adsorbed impurities on the crystal surface by the ions of the precipitate is easier.

The mechanism of adsorptive occlusion which has been discussed above explains one of the characteristics of coprecipitation, namely, that *in most cases coprecipitation occurs only while the precipitate is being formed.*

Formation of Mixed Crystals (Isomorphous Coprecipitation). Studies of coprecipitation phenomena have shown that isomorphism of a precipitate with the coprecipitated impurity is also of great importance in coprecipitation. It will be remembered that *substances are said to be isomorphous if they can crystallize with formation of a joint crystal lattice; so-called mixed crystals are formed in the process.*

The various alums are typical examples of isomorphous substances. If a mixture of the colourless potash alum $KAl(SO_4)_2 \cdot 12H_2O$ and the deep violet chrome alum $KCr(SO_4)_2 \cdot 12H_2O$ is dissolved in water and left to crystallize, mixed crystals containing both potash alum

* A. Babko and I. Pyatnitsky, ***Quantitative Analysis***, Goskhimizdat, 1956, p. 79.

and chrome alum are formed. The higher the concentration of chrome alum in solution, the deeper the violet colour of these crystals. By variation of the concentrations of the two alums it is possible to obtain a continuous range of crystals, from those consisting of $KAl(SO_4)_2 \cdot 12H_2O$ only to crystals containing $KCr(SO_4)_2 \cdot 12H_2O$ only.

Isomorphous substances have formulas of the same type. These substances usually crystallize in the same form (see Fig. 17); this is the origin of the term "isomorphous", which means "having the same form".

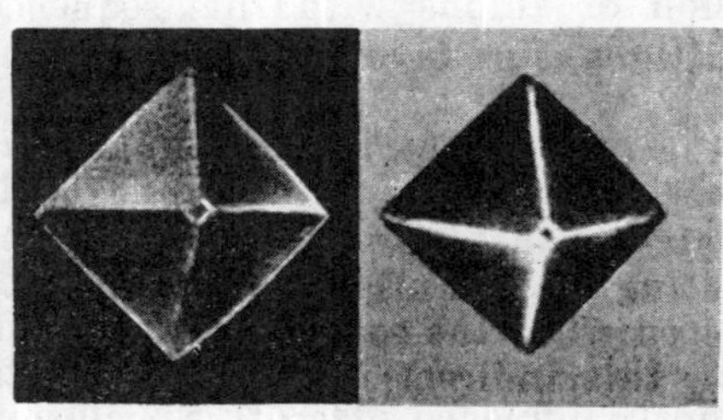

Fig. 17. Crystals of potash and chrome alums

The principle of isomorphism is that ions of the same coordination number and similar radii can replace each other in the crystal lattice without disturbing its stability. For example, since the radius of the Ra^{++} ion (1.52 Å)* is close to the radius of the Ba^{++} ion (1.43 Å), $RaSO_4$ and $BaSO_4$ are isomorphous. Therefore, when $BaSO_4$ is precipitated from a solution containing even minute traces of Ra^{++} ions the latter are incorporated with Ba^{++} ions in the crystals of the precipitate formed. In other words, radium sulphate is *isomorphously precipitated* with barium sulphate.

In contrast to the Ba^{++} ion, the Ca^{++} ion has a much smaller radius (1.06 Å) than the Ra^{++} ion. Accordingly, Ca^{++} and Ra^{++} cannot both enter the same crystal lattice or isomorphously replace each other. Therefore, Ra^{++} ions are not coprecipitated with $CaSO_4$, despite the low solubility of $RaSO_4$.

The significance of isomorphism in coprecipitation was demonstrated first by V. Khlopin (1924) and later by O. Hahn (1926). One example of isomorphous coprecipitation is provided by the experiment, described above, on the coprecipitation of $KMnO_4$ and $BaSO_4$, which are isomorphous.**

The amount of an impurity coprecipitated during formation of mixed crystals depends on the relative concentrations of the impurity and the precipitated ions in solution. The quantitative laws of isomorphous precipitation were established by the work of

* Å is the angstrom unit, 10^{-8} cm.

** It must be noted that here we have a special type of isomorphism. Unlike the usual case when one type of ion in the precipitate is replaced by another, here a pair of ions (Ba^{++} and SO_4^{--}) is replaced by another pair (K^+ and MnO_4^-), comparable in size to the first pair.

V. Khlopin and his school, and of O. Hahn and his associates, and proved to depend on the experimental conditions.

For example, if a precipitate is formed from a strongly supersaturated solution with prolonged stirring in order to accelerate recrystallization of the precipitate particles, eventually a state of equilibrium is reached when the ratio of the amounts of Ra^{++} and Ba^{++} in the precipitate is proportional to their concentrations in solution.

This law, known as the *distribution law*, may be represented by the equation

$$\frac{x}{y} = D\frac{a-x}{b-y}$$

or

$$\frac{x}{a-x} = D\frac{y}{b-y} \tag{1}$$

Here x and y are the amounts of radium and barium in the precipitate;
a and b are their initial concentrations in solution;
D is the constant, known as the distribution (or enrichment) coefficient.

If $D > 1$, it means that the coprecipitated ion passes from solution into the precipitate and the mixed crystals formed are richer in this ion than the solution. This is usually the case when the solubility of the coprecipitated substance is less than the solubility of the compound with which it is coprecipitated. In this example radium sulphate is less soluble than barium sulphate. Accordingly, $D > 1$ and the precipitate is enriched with radium.

In this example of isomorphous coprecipitation the coprecipitated impurity (Ra^{++}) is distributed quite uniformly in the mixed crystals formed. However, under other precipitation conditions the distribution may not be uniform. For example, if $BaCl_2 \cdot 2H_2O$ is crystallized out very slowly by evaporation of a saturated solution of this salt containing an admixture of a radium salt, the precipitate crystals are formed so slowly that there is time for equilibrium to be reached between the precipitate and the solution during the precipitation. Since Ra^{++} has a greater tendency to separate out of solution than Ba^{++}, the solution becomes progressively poorer in radium as crystallization proceeds. It follows that the inner layers of the crystals, deposited from a solution richer in radium, should contain more radium than the outer layers which were deposited later. The quantitative relationships in this case are also different. Instead of Equation (1), the following logarithmic formula is valid in this case:

$$\ln\frac{x}{a-x} = \lambda \ln\frac{y}{b-y} \tag{2}$$

Here x, y, a and b have the same significance as in Equation (1). The quantity λ is a constant. If, as in this instance, $\lambda > 1$, the coprecipitated ion is concentrated in the precipitate crystals.

In contrast to adsorptional coprecipitation, which is highly sensitive to the slightest variations in the experimental conditions, isomorphous coprecipitation is influenced relatively little by such variations. This makes it possible to distinguish experimentally between these two forms of coprecipitation.

Formation of Chemical Compounds. Formation of chemical compounds can also cause occlusion of various impurities. For example, precipitation of Pb^{++} or Hg^{++} with hydrogen sulphide is accompanied by coprecipitation of Cl^-, Br^-, and I^- anions. This is due to formation of various complex ions in solution, such as $[HgCl]^+$, $[PbI]^+$, etc., so that $[HgCl]_2S$ (white), $[PbI]_2S$ (reddish brown), etc., may be precipitated.

It should be noted that formerly most coprecipitation effects were attributed to formation of new chemical compounds; however, such explanations were in most cases disproved by detailed investigations.

In addition to coprecipitation, the analyst has to deal with an effect known as *postprecipitation*. This is the gradual deposition of an impurity from solution when the solution and precipitate are left in contact. For example, in the separation of Group IV and Group III cations by hydrogen sulphide in an acid medium the precipitate initially formed is free from zinc sulphide. However, if the filtration is performed some time after precipitation the precipitate is contaminated with ZnS owing to postprecipitation during standing.

Postprecipitation of zinc sulphide is caused by adsorption of S^{--} ions from solution by particles of the Group IV sulphide precipitate, so that the concentration of these ions becomes higher on the particle surfaces than in solution. Since the rate of precipitation depends on the concentrations of the reacting ions, it is not surprising that separation of ZnS from supersaturated solution occurs most easily on precipitated particles of other sulphides.

Similarly, if a calcium oxalate precipitate is left in contact with a mother liquor containing Mg^{++} ions, magnesium oxalate MgC_2O_4 is postprecipitated owing to the presence of adsorbed $C_2O_4^{--}$ ions on the particles of the CaC_2O_4 precipitate.

It follows that the recommended ripening of crystalline precipitates is not always advantageous, because it may be accompanied by contamination of the precipitates owing to postprecipitation of impurities.

28. Decrease of Coprecipitation

When a precipitate is contaminated with impurities, the composition of the precipitate (weighed form) cannot be represented by a definite chemical formula, so that it is impossible to calculate exactly the content of any particular element in it. Therefore, coprecipitation is one of the most serious sources of error in gravimetric analysis, and the analyst must take steps to diminish its effects on the analytical results.

Coprecipitation can be reduced, first of all, by appropriate choice of analytical procedure. If it is required to determine any particular impurities (microcomponents) it is obviously inappropriate to precipitate the main constituent first. Being present in a very large amount, it would give a very bulky precipitate, and most (or even practically all) of the microcomponent would be coprecipitated with it, so that an erroneous result would be obtained in the determination. Evidently, in this case the microcomponent must be precipitated first. Further, coprecipitation can be decreased by suitable choice of precipitant. For example, it is found in practice (see Sec. 35) that coprecipitation of impurities is much less with organic than with inorganic precipitants.

Coprecipitation can also be diminished by suitable adjustment of the precipitation conditions, especially in the case of adsorptional coprecipitation.

As was pointed out in Sec. 27, such conditions as the sequence of addition of the solutions, their concentrations, temperature, rate at which the precipitant is added, etc., have a very strong influence on adsorption. Partial removal of coprecipitated impurities during the ripening of crystalline precipitants is also significant.

Since both adsorptional and isomorphous coprecipitation greatly depend on the nature of the ions in question, coprecipitation can sometimes be diminished considerably by replacement of certain ions with others. For example, if Ba^{++} ions have to be precipitated in presence of Fe^{+++} ions, the latter should first be reduced to Fe^{++} ions, which are coprecipitated much less with $BaSO_4$. Similarly, coprecipitation can be decreased if the coprecipitated ions are bound in the form of some fairly stable and less coprecipitated complex.*

A precipitate must be washed thoroughly after every precipitation in order to remove adsorbed impurities and residual mother liquor. However, it is impossible to remove occluded impurities in this manner, because they are contained inside the precipitate particles. *Reprecipitation* is often used in quantitative determinations for removal of such impurities, and of adsorbed impurities which are difficult to remove by washing. This operation is explained by the following example.

It is known that in gravimetric analysis Ca^{++} is usually precipitated as calcium oxalate, $CaC_2O_4 \cdot H_2O$. If the solution also contains Mg^{++} (which is usually the case in analysis of natural materials and industrial products), the precipitate formed is strongly contaminated with MgC_2O_4 as the result of coprecipitation and postprecipitation. To remove this impurity the precipitate is filtered off, washed, and dissolved in HCl. The resultant solution contains all the calcium from the original substance and a small proportion

---

*** For example, the best method of obtaining a $BaSO_4$ precipitate free from iron is by precipitation in the presence of the sodium salt of ethylenediamine tetraacetic acid, which forms a stable complex with Fe^{+++}**

of the magnesium, because only a relatively small amount of magnesium was coprecipitated. The acid is neutralized and the precipitation of CaC_2O_4 is repeated; in this reprecipitation the concentration of Mg^{++} ions is very much lower than before. Therefore, the CaC_2O_4 precipitate is now almost free of the MgC_2O_4 impurity. This procedure is used with success for preparation of pure precipitates in many other cases too.

However, if for some reason it cannot be used (for example, if the precipitate, such as $BaSO_4$, is not soluble in acids or other solvents), the coprecipitated ions must first be separated from the ions which are to be determined. Of course, such separation may not always be possible because of serious complications due to coprecipitation effects.

If it is not possible to diminish coprecipitation sufficiently or to separate the coprecipitated impurity then the impurity is determined quantitatively in the precipitate at the end of the analysis, and the appropriate correction is applied to the analytical result.

29. Filtration

Filtration and washing of precipitates are very important operations; the accuracy of analytical results depends to a considerable extent on the thoroughness with which they are carried out.

In gravimetric analysis the so-called *ashless filters* are used for filtration; these are filter papers from which most mineral matter has been removed by washing with hydrochloric and hydrofluoric acids. Such filter papers are available commercially. When burnt, they leave very little ash; the ash weight is shown on the packet. It is usually so low that it can be neglected; if it exceeds 0.0002 g it must be subtracted from the weight of the precipitate.

Ashless filter papers are made in various density grades in accordance with the particle sizes of the precipitates for which they are intended. Thus, the least dense, rapid filter papers are used for separation of gelatinous amorphous precipitates, which are especially difficult to filter off. Packets of such papers are distinguished by a a red (or black) paper band. Most precipitates can be filtered off on papers of moderate density (white band); finally, the densest, so-called "baryte" papers (blue band) are used with the finest precipitates such as $BaSO_4$ or CaC_2O_4.

Sometimes a small amount of "paper pulp" is first put on the filter to avoid excessive clogging of the filter pores with particles of the precipitate (especially in the case of gelatinous precipitates). To prepare the paper pulp, ashless filter paper is treated with concentrated HCl (for not more than 2-3 minutes); water is then added to the acid and the mixture is stirred until the paper disintegrates into separate fibres. The paper pulp is filtered off, washed thoroughly to remove all the acid, and kept in the form of a suspension in water.

In filtration it is most important to choose the right size of filter; *this choice must be guided by the amount of precipitate and not by the volume of liquid to be filtered.* The precipitate must not occupy more than half the filter, because otherwise it cannot be washed thoroughly. However, the filter papers must not be too large either, because they would require longer washing to remove substances adsorbed from solution. The funnel is so chosen that the paper ends 5-15 mm from its edge.

Filter funnels usually have a cone angle of 60°. For a filter paper to fit well into such a funnel the paper must be folded in half, and then in half again with the second fold at right angles to the first. If the funnel angle is not 60° (as occasionally happens), the second fold must not be exactly at right angles to the first, but a more or less obtuse angle must be formed. This angle is varied and either the smaller or the larger of the resultant folds is opened out until the filter fits closely to the inside of the funnel (which must be absolutely dry). The filter is then filled with distilled water and pressed carefully against the funnel with a clean finger in order to press out the air bubbles formed between the paper and the funnel. If the paper is fitted properly, the funnel tube during filtration usually becomes filled with the filtrate, which pulls the liquid in the funnel by its weight, so that filtration is greatly accelerated.* Otherwise air bubbles enter the funnel tube and the flow of liquid through it is greatly retarded.

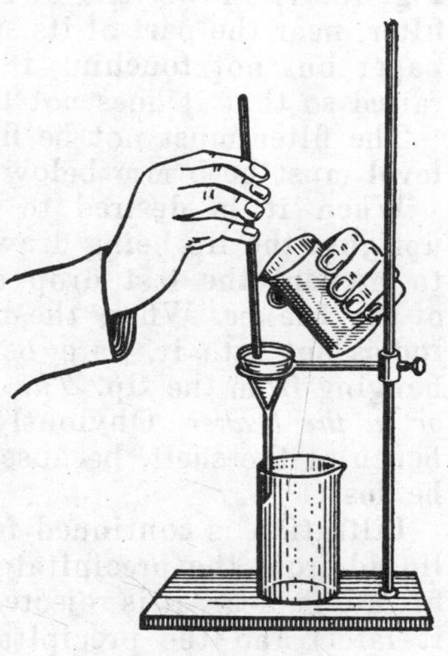

Fig. 18. Filtration

The filter funnel is placed in a ring on a stand, with a clean beaker underneath so that the bevelled tip of the tube touches the side of the beaker (Fig. 18). This is done to avoid splashing of the liquid in filtration. It is useful to rub the outside lip of the beaker containing the precipitate lightly with the finger. It is then not wetted

* If the funnel tube does not fill with liquid, the following procedure may be used. The filter is filled with distilled water and the lower end of the tube is closed with the finger. The part of the filter consisting of three layers of paper is pressed (under water) against the funnel with the index finger of the other hand, and the paper is shifted upwards very slightly in order to let the air out of the tube. When the tube is completely filled with liquid the paper is returned to its original position and pressed firmly against the glass.

by water and drops of the liquid will not run down the outside of the beaker.

The liquid is first *decanted*, or poured carefully into the filter without disturbing the precipitate, so that the filter pores remain unclogged by the precipitate particles as long as possible. To avoid splashing, *this must be done with the aid of a glass rod* as shown in Fig. 18. The lower end of the rod must be kept in the middle of the filter, near the part of its surface where it consists of three layers of paper but not touching it. As the filter becomes filled the rod is raised so that it does not touch the liquid.

The filter must not be filled to its brim with liquid. The liquid level must be 5 mm below the paper edge.

When it is desired to stop decantation, the beaker is turned upright, the lip being drawn upwards along the glass rod. This is to prevent the last drop of liquid from running down the outside of the beaker. When the beaker is in a vertical position, the glass rod is put into it, care being taken not to lose the drop of liquid hanging from the tip. *The rod must always be either above the filter or in the beaker.* Obviously the rod must not be put down on the bench or the shelf, because adhering particles of precipitate would be lost.

Filtration is continued for as long as it is possible to decant the liquid from the precipitate. After it has been ascertained that the filtrate is clear, it is rejected (unless it is the intention to investigate it later) and the precipitate is washed.

Filtration Through Glass Crucibles. Instead of ordinary filter paper, it is very convenient to use special sintered glass crucibles or tubes (or funnels) for filtration. These crucibles, which are now widely used in laboratory practice, are small glass vessels with sealed-in porous glass plates which serve as the filtering layers instead of paper. These plates are of different porosities; accordingly, four grades of sintered glass crucibles, denoted by numbers (from No. 1 to No. 4) are available. The pore size decreases with increasing number. The most fine-pored crucibles (No. 3 and No. 4) are used for analytical work.

The filtration is performed under reduced pressure. The sintered glass crucible *1* (Fig. 19) is inserted with the aid of a rubber ring in the neck of a suction flask *2*, the side tube of which is connected to a water-jet pump (or some other type of vacuum pump) *3* with an intermediate flask *4*. When a vacuum is produced in the filter flask, atmospheric pressure forces the liquid through the pores in the glass filter while the precipitate is retained.

Instead of sintered glass crucibles, *Gooch crucibles* are sometimes used; here the filtering medium is a layer of asbestos deposited on the porous bottom of the filter.

Porcelain crucibles with porous bottoms are also used for filtration, in the same way as glass filter crucibles. In contrast to glass

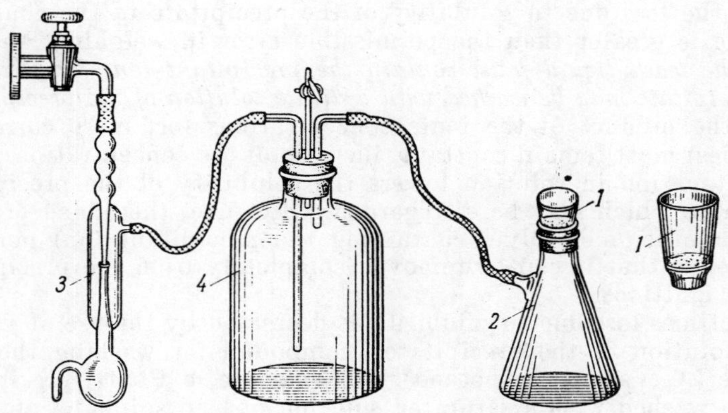

Fig. 19. Filtration through a sintered glass crucible:
1—sintered glass crucible; 2—suction flask; 3—vacuum pump; 4—intermediate flask

crucibles, porcelain crucibles can be heated to very high temperatures but are more hygroscopic.

30. Washing of Precipitates

The purpose of washing a precipitate is to remove adsorbed impurities and the mother liquor which permeats the precipitate. Adsorbed impurities are in equilibrium with the corresponding ions in solution. Therefore, when this solution is replaced by pure water (or some other wash liquid), in which the concentration of these ions is zero, desorption of these ions predominates overadsorption. As a result, the adsorbed impurities are gradually removed from the precipitate in the course of washing, and eventually the precipitate becomes quite pure.*

Composition of Wash Liquids. The choice of liquid used for washing a particular precipitate is important. The following four cases must be distinguished.

---

* It will be remembered that *only impurities adsorbed on the surface of the precipitate can be removed by washing.* If the impurities are occluded, i.e., are contained within the precipitate particles, owing to internal adsorption, isomorphous coprecipitation, or other causes, other methods must be used for obtaining pure precipitates. These methods were considered in Sec. 28.

Washing with a Solution of the Precipitant. It is only very rarely (see Sec. 18) that the solubility of a precipitated compound is so low that it can be disregarded. In most cases, unless special measures are taken, the loss due to solubility of the precipitate in the course of washing is greater than the permissible error in weighing. In such cases *the wash liquid must contain the precipitant ion; for example, the precipitate may be washed with a dilute solution of the precipitant.* Since the product of the ionic concentrations (or, more correctly, activities) must remain constant, increase of the concentration of the precipitant ion in solution lowers the solubility of the precipitate to a value which may be disregarded. Of course, the added precipitant (or other electrolyte containing the precipitant ion) must be volatile, so that it can be removed completely from the precipitate during ignition.

Sometimes loss due to solubility is decreased by the use of a saturated solution of the precipitated compound for washing the precipitate (A. Vasilyev's method). For example, a $PbSO_4$ precipitate is often washed with a saturated solution of lead sulphate, etc.

Some specimen calculations of the solubility losses when precipitates are washed with pure water and with dilute solutions of precipitant are given below.

Example 1. Find the loss due to solubility when 0.1 g of CaC_2O_4 precipitate is washed with 200 ml of water.

Solution. First find the solubility in moles of CaC_2O_4 per litre (SP = $2.6 \cdot 10^{-9}$). Denoting this by x we have:

$$[Ca^{++}] = x; \ [C_2O_4^{--}] = x$$

and

$$[Ca^{++}]\,[C_2O_4^{--}] = x^2 = 2.6 \times 10^{-9}$$

Hence:

$$x = \sqrt{2.6 \times 10^{-9}} = \sqrt{26 \times 10^{-10}} = 5.1 \times 10^{-5}\,M$$

Therefore, the amount of CaC_2O_4 dissolved* in 200 ml of water is

$$5.1 \times 10^{-5} \times 128 \times 0.2 \approx 0.0013 \text{ g}$$

The percentage error due to dissolution of the precipitate during washing is found by proportion:

$$0.1 - 100\%$$

$$0.0013 - y$$

$$y = \frac{0.0013 \times 100}{0.1} = 1.3\%$$

Example 2. What is the loss if, in Example 1, the CaC_2O_4 precipitate is washed with 0.01 M $(NH_4)_2C_2O_4$ solution instead of water?

Solution. Denoting, as before, the solubility of CaC_2O_4 in moles per litre by x, we write:

$$[Ca^{++}] = x; \ [C_2O_4^{--}] = 0.01 + x$$

---

* 128 is the approximate molecular weight of CaC_2O_4.

Since x is small by comparison with 0.01, it can be disregarded; therefore

$$[Ca^{++}][C_2O_4^{--}] = x \times 0.01 = 2.6 \times 10^{-9}$$

or

$$x = 2.6 \times 10^{-7}$$

Hence the solubility loss is:*

(a) in grams:

$$2.6 \times 10^{-7} \times 128 \times 0.2 = 0.0000067 \text{ g}$$

(b) as a percentage:

$$y = \frac{0.0000067 \times 100}{0.1} = 0.0067\%$$

Comparison of these results shows that when water is used the loss due to solubility of CaC_2O_4 is nearly 7 times the permissible error in weighing, whereas when a solution of a salt with a common ion is used the loss is negligibly small.

Washing with Electrolyte Solution. When pure water is used for washing, many precipitates are *peptized*, i.e., converted into the colloidal state, so that part of the precipitate passes through the filter. To explain this it should be taken into account that the coagulant electrolyte added in the precipitation and all other electrolytes are gradually washed out of the precipitate. Therefore, the colloidal particles which had been coagulated become charged again and begin to repel each other. As a result, the large aggregates disintegrate again into minute colloidal particles which pass freely through the filter pores.

To prevent this undesirable effect, the precipitate must be washed with a dilute solution of an electrolyte rather than with pure water. The adsorbed ions removed from the precipitate are then replaced by ions of the electrolyte used for the washing, i.e., *exchange adsorption* occurs. Peptization of the precipitate is therefore prevented. The electrolyte must, of course, be a volatile substance which is removed completely from the precipitate by ignition.

In practice, either volatile acids (if they do not dissolve the precipitate) or ammonium salts are used for this purpose. Of course, there is no need to ensure that the coagulant electrolyte contains an ion in common with the precipitate, because in this case its purpose is quite different from that discussed earlier.

Washing with Substances Which Suppress Hydrolysis of the Precipitant. Sometimes precipitants undergo hydrolysis when washed with pure water; this may raise the solubility of the precipitate, or the weighed form may no longer be an individual substance with a definite chemical formula. This can be prevented by the use of a solution of a substance which suppresses hydrolysis of the precipi-

* This calculation is approximate, as the activity coefficients of the ions were not taken into account. A more precise calculation can be carried out as described in Sec. 20 (Example 2).

tate. For example, $MgNH_4PO_4$ precipitate, which gives NH_4OH as one of its hydrolysis products,

$$MgNH_4PO_4 + H_2O \rightleftarrows MgHPO_4 + NH_4OH$$

is washed with dilute ammonia solution.

The ammonia present in the wash liquid shifts the hydrolysis equilibrium to the left, i. e., decreases the degree of hydrolysis of $MgNH_4PO_4$.

Washing with Water. If there is no danger either of solubility loss, or of formation of colloidal solutions, or of hydrolysis, precipitates are simply washed with distilled water.

It is preferable to use hot wash liquids, because hot liquids filter more rapidly than cold owing to the decrease of viscosity with the rise of temperature. For example, water at 100°C filters approximately twice as fast as at 20°C, and four times as fast as at 0°. Moreover, adsorption is also less at high temperatures.

It must be taken into account, however, that losses due to solubility of the precipitate increase with rise of temperature (Sec. 21). Therefore, if the solubility of a precipitate increases with temperature, it must be washed with cold and not hot wash liquid.

Washing Technique. Washing is first performed by decantation,* and the precipitate is washed on the filter only at the end. When a precipitate is washed by decantation, a certain amount of wash liquid is poured into the beaker containing the precipitate, stirred thoroughly, and the particles are allowed to settle; then as much of the liquid as possible is poured down a glass rod into the filter before a fresh portion of wash liquid is put into the beaker. It is easy to see that impurities are washed out much more rapidly in this way.

Suppose, for example, that the amount of impurity to be washed out is 0.1 g, and 20 ml of liquid is used in each decantation, 90% (18 ml) being poured onto the filter and 10% (2 ml) remaining in the beaker; then

	Removed g	Remains g
In first decantation	0.09	0.01
In second decantation	0.009	0.001
In third decantation	0.0009	0.0001

The amount of impurity is seen to decrease in a geometrical progression with a common ratio of 0.1. If 10 ml was left each time in the beaker instead of 2 ml, the common ratio of the progression would be 0.5 and the washing would take much longer.**

* It will be remembered that decantation is careful pouring of the liquid from the settled precipitate onto the filter (p. 116).

** These figures suggest that 3 to 4 washings should be enough to remove impurities from the precipitate. In reality, however, more washings are needed because impurities are retained in the precipitate by adsorption forces.

The advantage of washing by decantation is obvious: the precipitate is mixed very thoroughly with the wash liquid, and there is very little clogging of the filter pores.

Decantation is repeated several times and the precipitate is then transferred "quantitatively" (i.e., completely, without loss) to the filter. To do this, the precipitate is stirred up in a small amount of the wash liquid and the suspension is poured carefully into the filter down a rod. *This is a very important stage in the work: the loss of a single drop of the turbid liquid may make the result of the analysis quite wrong.* The beaker is rinsed out with small portions of the wash liquid from a wash bottle; each portion is poured off together with the particles of precipitate into the filter, so that the precipitate is transferred to the filter as completely as possible. At the end, all the particles of precipitate adhering to the sides of the beaker are removed on a small piece of ashless filter paper which is moved inside the beaker by a glass rod. The rod itself is wiped with a similar piece and both pieces are put in the filter. Another way of removing particles of precipitate from the walls of the beaker and the glass rod is to rub them off by means of another glass rod provided with a rubber tip and rinse them down with a stream of water from the wash bottle.

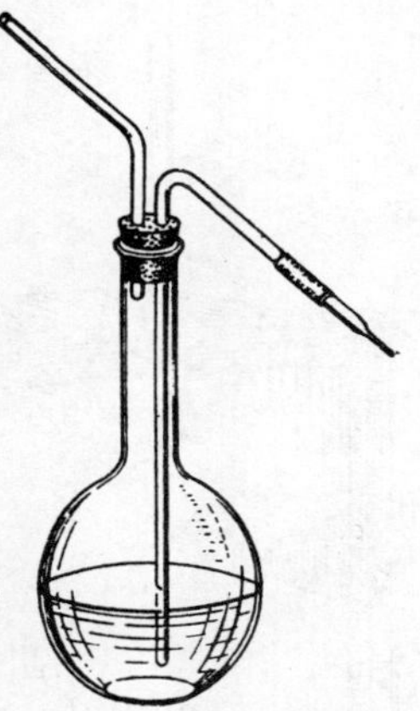

Fig. 20. Wash bottle

When no more particles remain either in the beaker or on the rod, the precipitate is finally washed on the filter. This is most conveniently done with the aid of a wash bottle (Fig. 20). To avoid splashing, the jet of liquid from the wash bottle should not be directed at the precipitate itself, at the centre of the filter, but at the side, nearer to the upper edge. The drawnout tip of the wash bottle tube is moved around the filter so as to wash the precipitate down gradually to the bottom of the filter. *Here, as in decantation, before a new portion of liquid is added to the filter the preceding portion must be allowed to drain completely.*

When it seems probable that the impurities have been completely washed out, *a test for completeness of washing* is carried out.

The beaker under the funnel is replaced by a clean test tube or watch glass, a few millilitres of filtrate are collected, and tested with a suitable reagent for the ion which is being washed out. Washing is continued until the test is negative.

It should be remembered that *filtration and washing must be completed during a single session*, because otherwise the precipitate dries and cracks and becomes impossible to wash.

31. Drying and Ignition of Precipitates

The funnel containing the washed precipitate is covered with a piece of filter paper (not ashless), moistened with distilled water.* The paper projecting beyond the rim of the funnel is pressed firmly against the outside of the funnel and torn off. This forms a close-fitting lid which protects the precipitate against dust, currents of air, etc. The funnel with the precipitate is then put for 20-30 minutes into a drying oven at about 90-105°C (not any higher, because the paper would be charred and fall to pieces when taken out of the funnel).

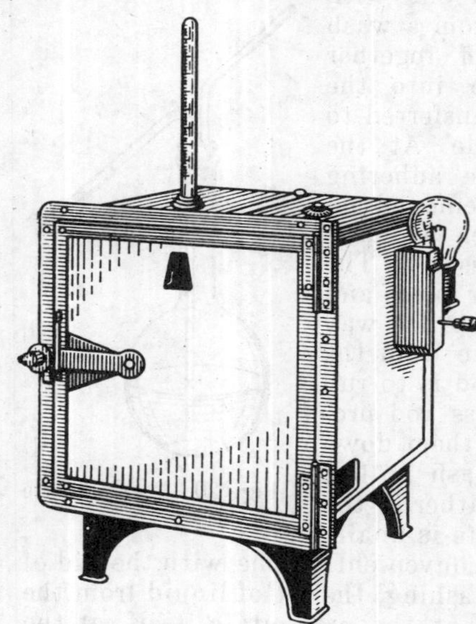

Fig. 21. Electric drying oven with thermoregulator

Electric drying ovens (Fig. 21) are generally used in laboratories. The lower part of the oven contains several heating coils covered with a perforated metal sheet. The outside of the oven is provided with switches for the separate coils so that the temperature can be regulated. An oven fitted with a thermoregulator, which maintains the required temperature automatically, is especially convenient. The oven has shelves with holes into which the funnels containing the precipitates are inserted.

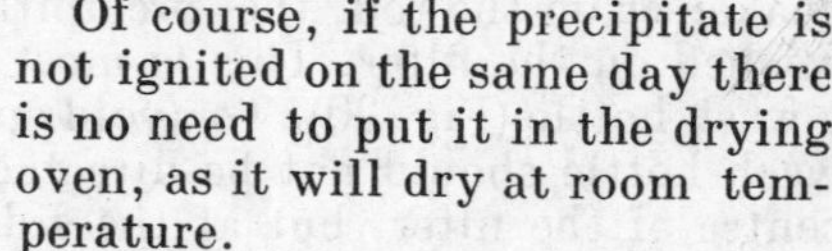

Of course, if the precipitate is not ignited on the same day there is no need to put it in the drying oven, as it will dry at room temperature.

Precipitates are ignited in porcelain or platinum crucibles. Before the ignition the weight of the empty crucible must be known, and it is necessary to be sure that this weight will not alter during the ignition. *The crucible is therefore first heated to constant weight*, i.e., until its weight ceases to change.

The crucible is heated under the same conditions as in the subsequent ignition of the precipitate; this is done in good time, during the preceding stages of analysis. A clean and absolutely dry crucible is put in a porcelain triangle resting on a tripod (Fig. 22) and heated

* The student should write his name and the formula of the precipitate on this piece of paper in ordinary (not "indelible") pencil, so that it can be identified.

in the burner flame so that the blue cone of the flame is a few millimetres below the bottom of the crucible. It will be remembered that when gas burners are used the air supply must be carefully adjusted. With excess air the flame may "strike back" or go out, while with a deficiency of air a smoky flame at a low temperature is obtained.

After 15-20 minutes the burner is turned out; the hot crucible is allowed to cool in air for 1-2 minutes and then put into a desiccator (Fig. 5) for final cooling so that the crucible does not absorb moisture from the air and so increase in weight. The desiccator lid is moved sideways (not raised upwards) and removed; the crucible is then lifted by means of crucible tongs (Fig. 23) into one of the sockets in the porcelain plate of the desiccator. *The lid of the desiccator should not be replaced immediately, but only after a few minutes,* because otherwise a vacuum is produced and the lid is difficult or even impossible to remove. The desiccator with the crucible should then be taken to the balance room and left there for at least 20-25 minutes to allow the crucible to cool down to the temperature of the balance so as to ensure correct weighing.

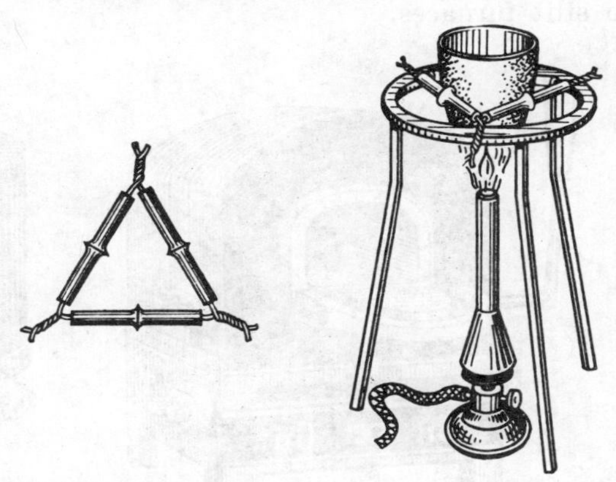

Fig. 22. Porcelain triangle and ignition of crucible

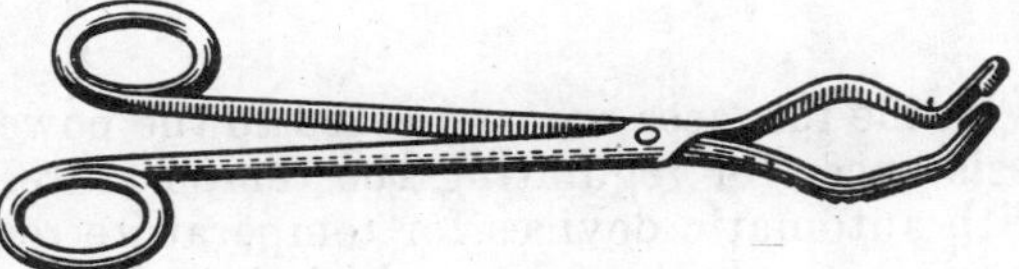

Fig. 23. Crucible tongs

The crucible is weighed, the weight is noted down, and the crucible is then heated again, cooled in the desiccator, and weighed. If the second weighing does not differ from the first by more than 0.0002 g, it may be assumed that the weight is now constant. Otherwise the heating and weighing is repeated as necessary.

Of course, all consecutive weighings, even if their results are the same, must be written down in the laboratory note book. Very often it is preferred to ignite precipitates in a special electric furnace and not in a gas burner flame. Generally either a muffle furnace (Fig. 24), which can hold from 12 to 25 crucibles at once, is used, or a crucible furnace (Fig. 25) which holds only one crucible and which uses much less electricity.

High temperatures are usually produced in electric furnaces by means of high-resistance wire wound on a ceramic support. Temperatures of the order of 800-1000°C are attained with the use of Nichrome wire, while for temperatures of 1100-1200°C certain special alloys are used. Instead of metal wire, the so-called silit rods are also used in electric furnaces; temperatures of 1350-1400°C can be reached in silit furnaces.

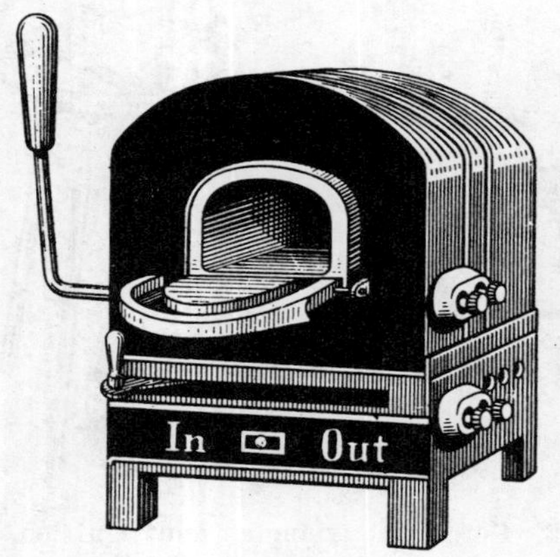

Fig. 24. Muffle furnace

Fig. 25. Crucible furnace

Muffle furnaces are connected to the power supply through variable resistances for regulating the temperature. Some furnaces are fitted with automatic devices for temperature regulation. Of course, if the precipitate obtained in analysis is to be ignited in a muffle (or crucible) furnace, the empty crucible must be heated in the same furnace.

Ignition Technique. *Ignition of Precipitates on the Filter.* The filter is taken out of the funnel by means of a pointed glass rod (or a clean quill toothpick), the edges are turned over so that the precipitate is completely surrounded by paper, and the filter is placed, tip upwards, in a crucible which has been heated to constant weight.

All these operations must be performed very carefully, so as not to blow away and lose any of the precipitate. The filter should be handled by its outer surface in the region where it consists of three layers of paper. To avoid loss by powdering, it is best to remove the filter from the funnel while it is still slightly moist.

The crucible with the precipitate is put in a triangle on a tripod and heated very carefully over a small flame so that the filter first dries completely and then chars slowly without catching fire (minute particles of the precipitate may be blown away in a flame). If the paper should catch fire, the burner must be removed and the flame allowed to go out (but it must not be blown out). When the filter has charred and smoking has ceased, the burner flame is gradually increased. Care must be taken not to allow the inner blue cone of the flame to touch the bottom of the crucible.

At this stage, in order to allow better access of air, the crucible should be placed in a slanting position in the triangle and turned with the tongs from time to time to allow the carbon deposit on the side of the crucible to burn away, and to convert the filter itself completely into ash. When all the carbon has burned away the ignition is continued for a further 15-20 minutes; the crucible is then transferred to a desiccator, cooled, and weighed. To confirm that the chemical changes taking place during the ignition have been completed, the crucible is ignited again for 15-20 minutes and weighed, this is repeated to constant weight.

When an electric furnace is used, the filter is first charred by means of a gas burner (or on an electric hot-plate), and the crucible is put in the furnace only when smoking has stopped.

Ignition of Precipitates Separately from the Filter. Many precipitates are partially reduced by carbon and by products of incomplete combustion of the filter. Therefore, the procedure described above cannot be used for ignition in such cases. The precipitate is then transferred as completely as possible onto a sheet of glazed paper, the filter is ashed in the crucible, and the precipitate is then transferred to the crucible and ignited.

In practice, this procedure is complicated by the fact that the precipitate cannot be removed completely from the filter. The part which remains on the filter becomes reduced when the filter is ashed. Therefore, before the main bulk of the precipitate is put into the crucible, the contents of the latter must be converted back into the required compound by means of suitable reagents. For example, the part of an AgCl precipitate which has been reduced to metallic silver by the carbon in the filter is treated with a few drops of HNO_3 and HCl. The following reactions then take place:

$$Ag + 2HNO_3 = AgNO_3 + H_2O + NO_2\uparrow$$

$$AgNO_3 + HCl = \downarrow AgCl + HNO_3$$

The excess acids are removed by evaporation, the remaining part of the precipitate is transferred to the crucible and carefully ignited.*

* Or, more correctly, heated to fusion (AgCl decomposes on stronger heating).

These complications can usually be avoided if ignition is replaced by drying of the precipitate to constant weight. In such cases a glass filter crucible (p. 116) is used instead of a paper filter. Of course, the filter crucible must first be brought to constant weight at the same temperature.

This procedure is sometimes advantageous also because a more convenient weighed form can be obtained. For example, if a $CaC_2O_4 \cdot H_2O$ precipitate is ignited, the weighed form obtained is CaO, which is difficult to weigh accurately because it absorbs water vapour and CO_2 from the air. Ignition may be replaced by drying of the precipitate (at a lower temperature) to constant weight in a glass filter crucible. The weighed form is then not calcium oxide but calcium oxalate $CaC_2O_4 \cdot H_2O$ which is free from the above-mentioned properties and also has a higher molecular weight.

Another reason why it is preferable to dry AgCl precipitates to constant weight is that unless care is taken the precipitates partially decompose during ignition. This risk is avoided if AgCl is dried.

32. Calculation of Gravimetric Results

In analysis by the precipitation method the substance weighed is usually not the substance the amount of which is to be determined, but an equivalent amount of another substance—the weighed form. For example, in determination of barium in barium chloride the substance weighed is not barium element but its compound, $BaSO_4$, obtained in the course of analysis. Similarly, CaO or $CaC_2O_4 \cdot H_2O$ is weighed in determination of calcium, $Mg_2P_2O_7$ in determination of magnesium, etc.

Therefore, at the end of a determination it is necessary to calculate the amount of substance which is to be determined from the amount of the weighed form (found from the difference between the constant weights of the crucible with precipitate and the empty crucible).

All such calculations are performed by proportion, which may be represented in the following general form:

$$M_w : M_d$$

$$a : x$$

Here M_d is the molecular (or atomic) weight of the substance (or element) being determined;

M_w is the molecular weight of the weighed form;

a is the weight of the weighed form found by analysis.

Examples. The weight of an AgCl precipitate is 0.1290 g; find the amount of chlorine. By proportion:

$$AgCl : Cl$$
$$143.3 : 35.45$$
$$0.1290 : x$$
$$x = 0.1290 \times \frac{35.45}{143.3} = 0.03192 \text{ g}$$

Similarly, to find the weight of magnesium corresponding to an $Mg_2P_2O_7$ precipitate weighing 0.3515 g, we write:

$$Mg_2P_2O_7 : 2Mg$$
$$222.6 : 2 \times 24.31$$
$$0.3515 : x$$
$$x = 0.3515 \times \frac{2 \times 24.31}{222.6} = 0.07676 \text{ g}$$

If it was required to find the weight of $MgSO_4 \cdot 7H_2O$ which gives 0.3515 g $Mg_2P_2O_7$ we would have the proportion:
$Mg_2P_2O_7$ is obtained from $2MgSO_4 \cdot 7H_2O$

$$222.6 : 2 \times 246.5$$
$$0.3515 : x$$
$$x = 0.3515 \times \frac{2 \times 246.5}{222.6} = 0.7782 \text{ g}$$

These examples show that x, the required amount of substance (or element) being determined, is the product of two factors. One of these, the weight of precipitate found in the analysis, (a), is a variable quantity which depends on the weight of the original sample. The other factor, however, the ratio of the molecular (or atomic) weight of the substance (or element) being determined to the molecular weight of the precipitate (weighed form), is independent of the sample weight, and is a constant which can be calculated once and for all, and used in all analyses of the same type. This factor is known as the *analytical factor* or *conversion factor* and is represented by the symbol F. Therefore

$$x = aF \tag{1}$$

Of course, F is constant only if neither the weighed form nor the substance being determined are changed. For example, no matter how many times magnesium is determined from the weight of an $Mg_2P_2O_7$ precipitate, the weight of the precipitate found by analysis must always be multiplied by the same ratio:

$$F = \frac{2Mg}{Mg_2P_2O_7} = \frac{2 \times 24.31}{222.6} = 0.2183$$

However, if we wanted to find the amount of $MgSO_4 \cdot 7H_2O$ in an analysed substance, the conversion factor would evidently be different, namely:

$$F = \frac{2(MgSO_4 \cdot 7H_2O)}{Mg_2P_2O_7} = \frac{2 \times 246.5}{222.6} = 2.175$$

The student must firmly grasp that for calculation of the conversion factor:

1. The molecular (or atomic) weight of the substance (or element) being determined must be divided by the molecular weight of the weighed form, i.e.,

$$F = \frac{M_d}{M_w}$$

2. The molecular (or atomic) weights *must be taken with the appropriate coefficients to make them equivalent to each other*; i.e., so that they contain equal numbers of atoms of the elements in question.

In the examples given above, in calculations of F the atomic weight of Mg (or the molecular weight of $MgSO_4 \cdot 7H_2O$) had to be doubled, because the $Mg_2P_2O_7$ molecule contains two Mg atoms.

It is easy to understand the physical meaning of the conversion factor; we need only put $a = 1$ in Formula (1). Then $x = F$. Therefore, the conversion factor represents the number of grams of the substance (or element) being determined which corresponds to 1 g of the weighed form.

Conversion factors (and the corresponding logarithms) for the most important gravimetric determinations are given in chemical reference books. Conversion factors make calculations much simpler; this is especially important for industrial laboratory work, where numerous determinations of the same elements are carried out. However, students learning quantitative analysis should not use tables, but should calculate the conversion factors independently.

In analytical instruction a student often has to find the absolute weight of a particular element, in grams, contained in a given solution. In such cases the analytical calculation is reduced to multiplication of the weight of the precipitate found by the appropriate conversion factor.

In analyses of practical importance, on the other hand, usually the percentage content of some element (or compound) in a given substance is required, rather than the absolute content. Therefore, if the required percentage is denoted by p and the weight of substance taken by g, we can write: g grams of original substance contains aF g of the substance sought; 100 grams of original substance contains p g of the substance sought

$$p = \frac{aF \times 100}{g} \% \qquad (2)$$

It must be remembered that, since the weight of the precipitate is found to four significant figures, the conversion factor and all the analytical results must also be taken to four significant figures (Sec. 15).

Tables of four-figure logarithms and antilogarithms (given at the end of this book) should be used for the calculations.

33. Taking the Sample

Above we discussed all the most important and characteristic operations of gravimetric analysis by the precipitation method. If we have to analyse a solution which does not contain any interfering ions, the whole analysis is reduced to those operations. In the more general case, the analyst must prepare the solution himself before performing the precipitation.

It follows that precipitation of an ion to be determined must nearly always be preceded by certain preliminary operations, namely: (a) taking the sample; (b) dissolving the sample; (c) preparation of the solution for analysis.

First we must consider the weight of the sample to be taken. It is easy to see that the sample must not be either too large or too small. In the former case a large amount of precipitate would be obtained, and it would be impossible to wash it thoroughly. If the sample is too small, the inevitable errors in weighing and other analytical operations will be too high a percentage of the final result, and the precision of the analysis is diminished.

It has been found by experience that in macroanalysis *the optimum amount of precipitate* (*weighed form*) *is about 0.5 g with crystalline precipitates*, *and about 0.1-0.3 g with bulky amorphous precipitates.*

It has already been said that in most cases not only the qualitative composition of the analysed substance but also the approximate quantitative content of the component to be determined is known. Therefore, it is usually possible to calculate the most suitable sample weight. These calculations are illustrated by the following examples.

Example 1. Find the weight of alum, $KAl(SO_4)_2 \cdot 12H_2O$, which should be taken for determination of aluminium as Al_2O_3.

Solution. Since Al^{+++} is precipitated as $Al(OH)_3$, which is bulky and relatively difficult to filter off and wash, we should aim at the minimum amount of the weighed form (0.1 g). By proportion:

$$2 \times 474 \text{ g } KAl(SO_4)_2 \cdot 12H_2O \text{ gives } 102 \text{ g } Al_2O_3$$

$$x \text{ g } KAl(SO_4)_2 \cdot 12H_2O \text{ gives } 0.1 \text{ g } Al_2O_3$$

$$x = \frac{0.1 \times 948}{102} \approx \frac{0.1 \times 900}{100} \approx 0.9 \text{ g}$$

There is obviously no sense in trying to weigh out the exact amount of substance as found by calculation. This calculation is only rough, and should be performed approximately (Sec. 15). The weighing itself, of course, must be performed accurately.

Example 2. Find the weight of Б-16 babbitt which should be taken for determination of its Pb content as $PbSO_4$, if by the GOST (USSR Standard) the lead content of this babbitt grade is 65-67%.

Solution. First we calculate the amount of metallic lead which gives the optimum weight of $PbSO_4$ precipitate. As this precipitate is crystalline, we have the proportion:

$$207 \text{ g Pb gives } 303.0 \text{ g } PbSO_4$$

$$x \text{ g Pb gives } 0.5 \text{ g } PbSO_4$$

$$x = \frac{207 \times 0.5}{303}$$

From the average Pb content (66%) of this alloy we now calculate the weight of alloy (y) which contains the required weight of lead (x):

$$66 \text{ g Pb is contained in } 100 \text{ g of alloy}$$

$$x \text{ g Pb is contained in } y \text{ g of alloy}$$

$$y = \frac{100x}{66} = \frac{207 \times 0.5 \times 100}{66 \times 303} \approx \frac{200 \times 0.5 \times 100}{70 \times 300} \approx 0.5 \text{ g}$$

How precisely should the sample be weighed? Evidently the error in this operation should not exceed the permissible error of the determination as a whole. Since the latter error is usually some tenths of 1%, we may assume that the error in weighing the sample must not exceed 0.1%. It follows that small samples should be weighed on an analytical balance to the fourth decimal place. Larger samples (about 10 g or more) may be weighed on a technical balance to within 0.01 g.

The sample is weighed on a watch glass, or in a weighing bottle, test tube, etc.

Technique of Sample Weighing. *First Method.* An empty watch glass (or weighing bottle) is weighed first; the required amount of substance to be analysed is then put on it and it is weighed again. The difference between the two weighings is the weight of the sample. The weighed sample is carefully transferred into a beaker (or flask) where it is to be dissolved; any grains remaining on the glass are rinsed down with a jet of water from a wash bottle (or brushed down with a fine brush).

Second Method. The required amount of substance is placed on a watch glass and weighed. The substance is then carefully tipped out into a beaker and the glass with residual grains is weighed again. The difference between the two weighings is the weight of the sample. This method is especially convenient if several samples of the same substance have to be taken. A test tube (or weighing bottle) is filled with enough substance for all the samples, and these are then weighed out one after the other; each weighed portion is tipped out into a prepared vessel and the tube with the remaining substance is weighed each time.

34. Dissolution. Fusion

When a sample has been weighed out, it is dissolved (or decomposed). The usual solvents are water, acids (or acid mixtures), alkalies, or oxidizing agents.

If the substance under investigation is soluble in water, it is dissolved in water; the solution is acidified if extensive hydrolysis is expected. If the substance is insoluble in water, other solvents are used, or fusion may be necessary. Of course, the solvent must be chosen beforehand with the aid of qualitative tests which must be guided both by the solubilities of the compounds formed and by the nature of the reaction caused by the particular reagent.

For example, if a lead alloy has to be dissolved, nitric and not hydrochloric or sulphuric acid should be used, because $PbSO_4$ and $PbCl_2$ are sparingly soluble in water. On the other hand, nitric acid must not be used to dissolve metallic tin, because the sparingly soluble metastannic acid $(H_2SnO_3)_5$ is formed.

To dissolve $CaCO_3$ hydrochloric acid is the most convenient, but not sulphuric acid, because $CaSO_4$ is sparingly soluble in water. It is also obvious that there is no sense in using HNO_3 or aqua regia (a mixture of 1 volume of concentrated HNO_3 with 3 volumes of concentrated HCl), because there cannot be any oxidation-reduction process in this case. However, in analysis of native sulphide ores oxidizing agents (such as a mixture of HNO_3 with HCl) should be used to convert the sulphur into SO_4^{--} ions.

The subsequent course of analysis must also be taken into account when the solvent is chosen. For example, aluminium alloys can be dissolved either in acids or in alkalies. However, it is often more convenient to dissolve them in alkalies, because then only aluminium and zinc (forming AlO_2^- and ZnO_2^{--} ions) go into solution, while such alloy components as Mg, Cu, Mn, Fe, Ca, etc., remain undissolved and can easily be separated off.

In the same way, when sulphur is determined in iron or steel, either HCl or HNO_3 could be used as the solvent. The choice depends on the method to be used for the determination. If sulphur is to be separated in the form of H_2S gas, obviously the use of HNO_3, which oxidises H_2S, is inadmissible and the iron (or steel) sample must be treated with HCl (or H_2SO_4). Conversely, if it is intended to presipitate sulphur as $BaSO_4$, nitric acid must be used in order that all the sulphur should be oxidized to SO_4^{--} anions, but HCl or H_2SO_4 cannot be used.

When a substance is dissolved in acid, gases (CO_2, H_2, H_2S, etc.) may be evolved and carry out droplets of solution with them. This leads to losses of the substance. Therefore, the dissolving must be performed very carefully; the beaker in which the substance is dissolved must be covered with a watch glass. The drops of liquid on the glass are rinsed down into the beaker with a jet of water from a wash bottle when the dissolution is complete. If the substance is dissolved in a flask, a funnel is inserted in its neck to retain any splashes.

Of course, it is not always possible to find a suitable solvent. Sometimes the substance has to be fused (or sintered) with suitable fluxes to decompose it and to bring into solution the component which is to be determined. Fusion produces new compounds which, unlike the original substance, may be soluble in water or in acids. Various fluxes are used, depending on the chemical nature of the substance analysed. For example, the acid-insoluble modification of Al_2O_3 can be fused with either alkaline or acidic fluxes, because of its amphoteric character, in order to convert it into a soluble form.

In the former case Al_2O_3 is fused with caustic soda, when the following reaction takes place:

$$Al_2O_3 + 2NaOH = 2NaAlO_2 + H_2O$$

In the latter case the flux used is $KHSO_4$. The following reactions take place in the fusion:

$$6KHSO_4 = 3K_2SO_4 + 3H_2O + 3SO_3$$
$$Al_2O_3 + 3SO_3 = Al_2(SO_4)_3$$
$$Al_2O_3 + 6KHSO_4 = Al_2(SO_4)_3 + 3K_2SO_4 + 3H_2O\uparrow$$

Silicates, which are usually salts of various polysilicic acids of the general formula $m\mathrm{SiO_2}\cdot n\mathrm{H_2O}$, are fused with a mixture of Na_2CO_3 and K_2CO_3 to bring them into solution. It is an advantage to use a mixture of these compounds rather than either one singly, because mixtures melt at lower temperatures than pure substances.

The effect of fusion is to replace the acidic oxide SiO_2 in the silicate by CO_2. However, since many of the carbonates so formed readily decompose at high temperatures, metal oxides and the silicates of potassium and sodium are usually obtained instead.*

* Another method used for decomposition of silicates is to boil them with a mixture of hydrofluoric and sulphuric acids, when silicon is removed as gaseous silicon fluoride, SiF_4:

$$2KAlSi_3O_8 + 24HF + 4H_2SO_4 = K_2SO_4 + Al_2(SO_4)_3 + \uparrow 6SiF_4 + 16H_2O$$

Insoluble sulphates such as $BaSO_4$, $SrSO_4$, and $CaSO_4$ are also fused with Na_2CO_3 and K_2CO_3 to convert them into carbonates.

When such substances as Cr_2O_3 or chrome iron ore ($FeO \cdot Cr_2O_3$) have to be dissolved, oxidizing fluxes should be used to convert the Cr^{III} into Cr^{IV}. Fluxes used for this purpose include a mixture of Na_2CO_3 and $NaNO_3$, sodium peroxide Na_2O_2, etc.

Crucibles made of various materials are used for fusion. Platinum crucibles are the most resistant; they are widely used, especially for fusing silicates. It must be remembered, however, that alkalies and oxidizing fluxes attack platinum, and some metals form alloys with it (p. 46). This restricts the uses of platinum crucibles. Instead, silver crucibles are used for fusion with alkaline fluxes, and nickel or iron for fusion with oxidizing fluxes. Of course, part of the crucible material passes into solution as the result of fusion.

For fusion, a weighed sample of the substance is mixed thoroughly with about 5 times its own weight of a suitable flux,* put into a crucible, covered with a lid, and heated. At first the heating is done very slowly and cautiously, because on strong heating the crucible contents may be ejected by the gases or vapours evolved. After about 10-15 minutes the heating is intensified and the crucible contents are gradually melted. When the fusion is complete, the mass is left to cool completely, and the crucible contents are then leached out with water or dissolved in dilute acid. The solution is then analysed in the usual way.

After the substance has been dissolved, in most cases the solution must be suitably prepared for analysis before the determination is started. Such preparation includes a whole series of operations, different in different cases. They include evaporation of the solution to increase its concentration or to remove interfering acids (usually HNO_3), neutralization of acids and adjustment of the pH to the value required in precipitation, addition of complexing agents to mask interfering ions, etc. Finally, if the difficulties caused by the presence of interfering ions cannot be resolved either by suitable adjustment of pH or by masking, such ions are previously separated. Separation of ions is an important operation both in qualitative and in quantitative analysis, and it must therefore be discussed in detail.

35. Separation of Ions in Quantitative Analysis

Various methods of ion separation are used in quantitative analysis. Let us consider the most important of these methods.

I. Chemical Methods. As in qualitative analysis, chemical methods are usually based on precipitation of some ions in the form of insol-

* Excess flux is necessary in order to make the reaction as complete as possible.

uble compounds while the ions which are to be separated from them remain in solution. The precipitate is filtered off and washed, and the ions are thus separated.

In practice, this operation is much more complicated in quantitative than in qualitative analysis. Whereas in qualitative detection of a particular ion in the filtrate obtained after separation it is only necessary to obtain the reactions for that ion, in quantitative analysis the separation should be complete, which is much more difficult to achieve.

For example, when a precipitate is washed in qualitative analysis the washings are usually rejected and only the filtrate is investigated.

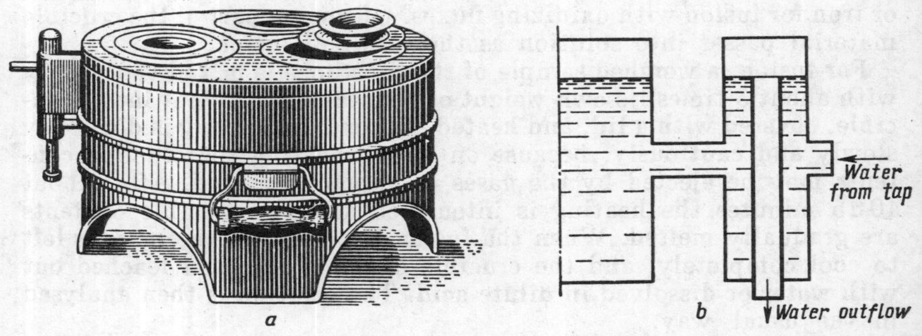

Fig. 26. Water bath (*a*) and automatic constant level device (*b*)

In quantitative analysis, if the ion to be determined remains in solution, it is evident that the analysis cannot be restricted to the filtrate. The washings must be collected and added to the filtrate, because if they were discarded there would be a considerable loss. In many cases the solutions obtained in this way are too dilute and they must be concentrated by evaporation.

This operation, too, must be performed differently in quantitative analysis. In qualitative analysis it is permissible to put the solution in a porcelain basin and boil it on a wire gauze; such boiling is quite inadmissible in quantitative analysis, because it causes inevitable losses due to splashing. Therefore, in quantitative analysis a water bath must be used for evaporation.

The water bath (Fig. 26*a*) is a metallic vessel with one or several openings (closed by lids of different diameters) for the basins. It contains water which is heated to boiling by gas burners or by electricity.

When a basin with solution is placed in a nest of the water bath, the solution is heated by steam to nearly 100°C, but cannot boil. Therefore, although the evaporation is somewhat slower, it is quiet and there is no risk of any loss. Care must be taken that the bath does not boil dry and that all free nests are covered. Baths with a constant level device, like that shown in Fig. 26, are especially convenient. The principle of the device is clear from Fig. 26*b*. Water flows slowly from the tap into the bath all the time, and the excess runs to waste.

Coprecipitation effects cause particularly serious difficulties in quantitative separation of ions. Therefore, all available steps to diminish coprecipitation should be taken. As was pointed out in Sec. 27 and Sec. 28, in many cases coprecipitation can be diminished considerably by correct choice of precipitation conditions, such as the sequence and rate of addition of the solutions, temperature, concentration, etc. However, in most cases sufficiently pure precipitates cannot be obtained by single precipitation; therefore, in quantitative separations it is very often necessary to use reprecipitation (p. 113). Of course, this considerably lengthens the time needed for the analysis because, firstly, precipitation, filtration, and washing all have to be done twice; and secondly, the substances remaining in solution are contained in a larger volume, obtained by combination of both filtrates and the corresponding washings.

It is therefore evident that ion separation in quantitative analysis is a very lengthy and laborious operation. Therefore, it is used only if it is absolutely necessary, i.e., when no suitable, sufficiently specific, and convenient precipitants are available and the interfering effects of extraneous ions cannot be prevented by pH regulation or masking.

Let us now consider some inorganic and organic precipitants which are most commonly used for ion separation by precipitation.

Inorganic Precipitants. Most of the insoluble inorganic compounds used in gravimetric determinations and ion separation are either salts of weak acids or metal hydroxides. Among the former, *sulphides* (salts of hydrogen sulphide, H_2S) are the most widely used both in qualitative and in quantitative analysis. Despite the well-known disadvantages of hydrogen sulphide, the properties of sulphides are so useful in analysis that these disadvantages must be disregarded.

We should note the extremely low solubilities of many sulphides. They are the least soluble compounds of a number of metals. It is therefore possible to precipitate sulphides of these metals at so low concentrations of the corresponding cations at which other sparingly soluble compounds are not precipitated. Because of their very low solubilities, many sulphides are formed in the presence of masking agents which prevent formation of hydroxides or certain salts. For example, whereas the presence of tartaric acid in solution prevents precipitation of iron or copper as the hydroxides, the sulphides of these metals are precipitated in its presence. The precipitation of these sulphides is prevented only by the presence of excess CN^- ions in solution. On the other hand, Cd^{++}, which forms a less stable complex $[Cd(CN)_4]^{--}$ with CN^- ions, is precipitated by hydrogen sulphide even in presence of KCN; this is used in analysis for separation of copper and cadmium.

The fact that the solubility products of different sulphides differ very greatly is extremely important. Because of this, it is possible to separate different metal cations by precipitation as sulphides, with suitable regulation of the solution pH. For example, in qualitative analysis the sulphides of Groups IV and V are precipitated by hydrogen sulphide in acid solution at pH = 0.5, i.e., at $[H^+] = 0.3$ g-ion/litre, as their solubility products are very low (of the order of 10^{-29} or less). On the other hand, the Group III sulphides (SP of the order of 10^{-15}-10^{-23}) are precipitated by hydrogen sulphide or ammonium sulphide in alkaline solution (at pH $\approx$ 9). Analogous methods are often used in quantitative analysis; for example, to separate copper, bismuth, tin, and other metal cations from iron, etc. By regulating the solution acidity in precipitation of sulphides we can also effect quantitative separation of cations belonging to the same analytical group. For example, in presence of acetic acid zinc can be separated quantitatively from iron; in presence of 10 *N* HCl arsenic can be separated from tin and antimony, etc.

It is known that H_2S is very easily oxidized (usually to free sulphur) and is therefore an active reducing agent. It follows that when sulphides are precipitated in acid solution, the solution should not contain oxidizing agents, including large amounts of Fe^{+++}; these ions are previously reduced to Fe^{++} by means of SO_2.

In addition to sulphide formation, precipitation of various cations in the form of insoluble *hydroxides* is widely used for ion separation in quantitative analysis. The separation is based either on the amphoteric character of certain ions, or on solubility differences between various hydroxides. To separate iron from vanadium, molybdenum and aluminium, the solution is treated with excess caustic alkali. The non-amphoteric ferric hydroxide is precipitated whereas the other above-mentioned metals remain in solution in the form of anions (VO_3^-, MoO_4^{--}, and AlO_2^-) because their hydroxides are acidic or amphoteric.

It was shown in Sec. 22 that differences of hydroxide solubility can be utilized for separating cations, by adjustment of the solution pH. For example, it was shown that the solution must be alkaline (pH $\geqslant$ 11.3) for complete precipitation of magnesium hydroxide (SP = 5×10^{-12}), the far less soluble ferric hydroxide $Fe(OH)_3$ (SP = 3.8×10^{-38}) is precipitated almost completely even in moderately acid solution (pH $\geqslant$ 3.5). Aluminium hydroxide

$Al(OH)_3$ ($SP = 1.0 \times 10^{-32}$) is also precipitated in acid solution (at $pH \leqslant 5$). Accordingly, in analysis of many ores, slags, limestones, etc., aluminium and iron are separated from magnesium, calcium, and certain other bivalent elements by precipitation as the hydroxides $Al(OH)_3$ and $Fe(OH)_3$. The precipitation is effected by the action of weak bases, such as a solution of ammonia, NH_4OH, in presence of an ammonium salt which suppresses the dissociation of NH_4OH and therefore lowers the solution pH so much that the solubility products of the bivalent-metal hydroxides are not reached. Instead of NH_4OH, a solution of pyridine (C_5H_5N) is also used; this is a weak base which makes the solution pH about 6.5.

Sometimes hydroxides are also precipitated by addition of a suspension of a sparingly soluble hydroxide, such as zinc hydroxide. It follows from the solubility product rule that any given hydroxide precipitates all hydroxides less soluble than itself, but not any that are more soluble.

Precipitation with ammonium hydroxide does not give precise separation of the ions, because this reagent usually contains some ammonium carbonate $(NH_4)_2CO_3$ as an impurity; this precipitates certain bivalent cations, such as Ca^{++}, which should remain in solution. Moreover, some $Al(OH)_3$ dissolves in excess NH_4OH to form aluminate (AlO_2^- ions). Precipitation by suspensions of metal hydroxides is free from these disadvantages, and that is one of the reasons for its use.

In addition to these methods, and for the same reasons, it is sometimes preferred to separate cations by precipitation of some of them as hydroxides or basic salts formed by hydrolysis. For example, in analysis of various ores, slags, certain alloys, and similar materials Fe^{+++} and Al^{+++} ions are sometimes precipitated by the action of sodium acetate on a previously neutralized boiling solution. In the case of Fe^{+++} the reaction is

$$Fe^{+++} + 3CH_3COO^- + 2H_2O = Fe(OH)_2CH_3COO + 2CH_3COOH$$

Basic aluminium acetate, $Al(OH)_2CH_3COO$, is precipitated together with $Fe(OH)_2CH_3COO$. If the solution contains PO_4^{---}, this is also precipitated as $FePO_4$ and $AlPO_4$.

Instead of sodium acetate, salts of other weak acids, such as ammonium benzoate $C_6H_5COONH_4$, etc., are often used in hydrolytic precipitation. There is also the method, mentioned on p. 68, for hydrolytic precipitation of Al^{+++} in presence of Fe^{+++} by the reaction:

$$2Al^{+++} + 3S_2O_3^{--} + 3H_2O = \downarrow 2Al(OH)_3 + \downarrow 3S + 3SO_2$$

Certan other analogous methods are also used.

Organic Precipitants. The first to use organic reagents in qualitative and quantitative inorganic analysis was the Russian scientist M. Ilyinsky (1855-1941), who proposed (in 1884) the use of the organic compound α-nitroso-β-naphthol as a reagent for the Co^{++} ion. However, the extensive use of organic reagents began after the classic work of L. Chugayev (1873-1922), who proposed (in 1905) his well-known dimethylglyoxime reaction for Ni^{++} and who initiated studies of the analytical properties of complex salts. Chugayev's work marked the beginning of a new and most fruitful trend in analytical chemistry, marked by the extensive use of organic compounds as reagents for various ions. During the period of more than 50 years since that time an enormous number of valuable organic reagents which are widely used in both qualitative and quantitative analysis have been discovered. The main reason for the growing use of organic reagents in analytical practice is that they have a number of advantages over inorganic reagents. Of these advantages, the following must be noted.

1. The compounds formed by the action of organic reagents very often have extremely low solubility in water, so that solubility losses can be avoided in precipitation and washing.
2. Coprecipitation is much less pronounced with organic than with inorganic precipitants.
3. Organic precipitants usually have high molecular weights. Therefore, the percentages of the elements to be determined in the precipitates formed are lower than with inorganic precipitants. Consequently, if such a precipitate is the weighed form the conversion factor is relatively small and the precision is higher.
4. The products formed with organic reagents are often intensely coloured. This makes it possible to detect, and to determine colorimetrically, ions at extremely low concentrations.

The reactions which take place with organic reagents belong to various types. Formation of internal complexes is of particular interest in analysis.

The salt-forming properties of organic compounds depend on the presence of definite groups with acidic properties, such as —COOH, $—SO_3H$, —OH, =NOH, =NH, $—NH_2$, etc., in their molecules. Under certain conditions the hydrogen atoms in these groups can be replaced by metal ions. If, in addition to such an *acidic group*, the organic molecule also contains a *complex-forming group*, which can act as a ligand for a given cation, then the latter, in replacing the hydrogen atom in the acidic group, can also form coordination bonds with the complex-forming group. Salts formed in this manner are known as *internal complexes, or chelates*.

One of the simplest examples of an internal complex is the copper salt of aminoacetic acid (glycine),

$$NH_2-CH_2-C\begin{matrix}\nearrow O\\ \searrow OH\end{matrix}$$

Its structure* is

$$\begin{matrix} O=C & - & O & & & O & - & C=O \\ | & & & \searrow & \swarrow & & & | \\ & & & & Cu & & & \\ | & & & \nearrow & \nwarrow & & & | \\ H_2C & - & H_2N & & & NH_2 & - & CH_2 \end{matrix}$$

The Cu^{++} ion in this compound has all the properties of a fully coordinated ion.

The compound of Ni^{++} with dimethylglyoxime is also an internal complex. Its formation may be represented by the following equation:

$$2\begin{matrix} CH_3-C=N-OH \\ | \\ CH_3-C=N-OH \end{matrix} + Ni(OH)_2 = \begin{matrix} & O\ldots H-O & \\ & \uparrow \qquad | & \\ CH_3-C=N & & N=C-CH_3 \\ | & \searrow Ni \swarrow & | \\ CH_3-C=N & \nearrow \quad \nwarrow & N=C-CH_3 \\ & | \qquad \downarrow & \\ & O-H\ldots O & \end{matrix} + 2H_2O$$

Dimethylglyoxime **Dimethylglyoxime nickel salt**

This equation shows that, in addition to replacing two hydrogen atoms in $=N-OH$ groups of two dimethylglyoxime molecules, the Ni^{++} ion also forms coordination bonds with nitrogen atoms in two more such groups. Therefore, the $=N-OH$ groups are simultaneously acidic and complex-forming.

It follows from these examples that molecules of internal-complex salts have a cyclic (ring) structure. As in the examples considered above, they usually have five- or six-membered rings, which are very stable. In general, internal-complex salts *have low solubilities in water, are brightly coloured, and have very low degrees of dissociation.*

It is especially important that individual properties of cations which are not manifested in normal salt formation are often very pronounced in formation of internal complexes. This is a factor in the specific action of organic reagents.

It is found that Ni^{++} forms characteristic precipitates, in most cases red, not only with dimethylglyoxime but also with certain other organic compounds (dioximes) containing the following grouping in their molecules:

$$\begin{matrix} -C=NOH \\ | \\ -C=NOH \end{matrix}$$

---

* Arrows in the formula represent coordination valence bonds.

This is therefore a *specific group* for the Ni^{++} ion; its presence is responsible for the formation of insoluble and intensely coloured compounds with Ni^{++}. Other groups are specific for other cations. For example, the group

$$\begin{array}{cc} =\!C- & C- \\ | & \| \\ HO & NOH \end{array}$$

is specific for Cu^{++}; the group

$$\begin{array}{ccc} S=C- & NH- & C= \\ | & & | \end{array}$$

is specific for Ag^{+}, etc.

The presence of a specific group determines the reactivity of a particular organic reagent. Its analytical value, associated with the solubility of the compound formed and the intensity of its colour, the degree of specific action, etc., depends to a considerable extent on the other atomic groups (radicals) joined to the specific group. Therefore, the properties of a particular reagent can often be considerably improved and its sensitivity or specificity increased by varying these radicals.

Organic precipitants must be used under definite conditions; in particular, at an appropriate solution pH. The reason for this is easy to see. It was stated earlier that when internal-complex salts are formed hydrogen atoms in the acidic groups of the reagent are replaced by metal ions; hydrogen ions then pass into solution, as can be seen, for example, in the above equation for the reaction between Ni^{++} and dimethylglyoxime. Clearly, the equilibrium must depend on the H^{+} ion concentration, i.e., on the solution pH. Dimethylglyoxime, like other similar organic reagents, behaves like a weak acid. Therefore, everything that was said about the significance of pH in the precipitation of sparingly soluble salts of weak acids (p. 84) must apply to this reaction. Here again, if the solubility product of the precipitate and the acidic dissociation constant of the reagent are known, we can calculate the pH at which precipitation is complete.

When Ni^{++} is precipitated with dimethylglyoxime, as in other precipitations of internal complexes, H^{+} ions accumulate in solution and must be removed in order to displace the reaction equilibrium to the right. Therefore, it would seem that the higher the solution pH the more complete is the precipitation. In practice, however, we have to take into account certain side reactions which might make an excessive increase of pH disadvantageous. For example, compounds formed by the reagent with other cations present in solution might be precipitated. In the case of cations which form amphoteric hydroxides increase of pH would convert them into the corresponding anions such as AlO_2^{-}, MoO_4^{--}, etc., and precipitation of the internal complex might become impossible. Finally, organic precipitants are often used in presence of various masking agents, such as tartaric acid, the action of which also depends on the solution pH.

For all these reasons, there is usually an upper as well as a lower pH limit in the use of organic precipitates. For example, the pH in precipitation of Ni^{++} with dimethylglyoxime should be between 5 and 10.

Most organic precipitants are sparingly soluble in water. Therefore, they often have to be used in the form of solutions in alcohol, acetone, and other non-aqueous solvents. However, the presence of these solvents during precipitation raises the solubility of the precipitates so that the precipitation is less complete. Therefore, a large excess of precipitant should be avoided.

Finally, let us consider a few of the commonest organic precipitants.

i. *Dimethylglyoxime.* The structural formula of dimethylglyoxime was given earlier (p. 139). This compound is a very important reagent for detection and determination of Ni^{++} and for separation of nickel from other cations. Dimethylglyoxime also forms a red but soluble complex compound with Fe^{++} and with certain other cations.

ii. *Hydroxyquinoline* C_9H_7ON, also known as "oxine" (the correct name is 8-hydroxyquinoline) has the following structure:

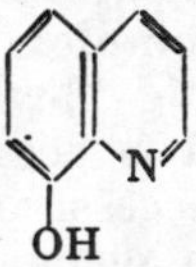

N
OH

Hydroxyquinoline is amphoteric. The presence of a hydroxyl group in the benzene nucleus confers acidic properties on it, while its basic properties are due to the presence of a tertiary nitrogen atom.* It precipitates a large number of different cations, which replace the hydrogen atoms in its hydroxyl groups and also form coordination bonds with its nitrogen atoms. This may be represented as follows:

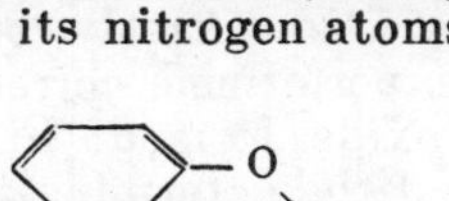

O
N → Me/*n*

Here *n* (the cation charge) shows that the metal cation is combined not with one but with *n* univalent hydroxyquinoline radicals.

* A nitrogen atom is said to be tertiary if all its three valence bonds are attached to other atoms or radicals, as in tertiary amines such as $(CH_3)_3N$, $(C_2H_5)_3N$, etc. The basic properties of hydroxyquinoline make it capable of forming salts with acids such as CH_3COOH. Therefore, although it is sparingly soluble in water, it is much more soluble in presence of CH_3COOH.

Although hydroxyquinoline forms insoluble internal complexes with a large number of different cations, the solubility products of these complexes vary considerably (between 10^{-12} and 10^{-30}, according to A. Babko), so that they are precipitated at different pH values, the pH ranges in which precipitation of certain metal complexes with hydroxyquinoline is practically complete are given below.

Metal	Fe^{III}	Cu^{II}	Mo^{VI}	Al^{III}	Ti^{IV}	Zn^{II}	Cd^{II}	Mg^{II}
pH	3-12	3-14	4-7	4-10	5-10	5-13	5-14	8-13

The fact that different complexes of hydroxyquinoline are precipitated at different pH values is used in the separation of certain cations. For example, to separate aluminium and magnesium, hydroxyquinoline is first added in presence of acetate buffer mixture ($CH_3COOH + CH_3COONa$), which maintains the solution pH constant at about 5. The above figures show that only the aluminium complex is precipitated at this pH, while Mg^{++} remains in solution. After separation of the precipitate ammonia is added to the filtrate, and the magnesium complex is then precipitated.

In other separations with hydroxyquinoline, in addition to adjustment of pH to a definite value, complex-formers which prevent the precipitation of some cations are added to the solution while other cations are precipitated. For example, in precipitation with hydroxyquinoline in presence of tartaric acid it is possible to separate Al^{+++}, which forms a stable complex with this acid, from a number of cations (Cu^{++}, Cd^{++}, Zn^{++}, Mg^{++}) which are precipitated by hydroxyquinoline in its presence. It is possible to isolate cations such as Fe^{+++}, Ti^{++++}, Al^{+++}, etc., successively from a solution in presence of malonic acid as a masking agent by precipitation with hydroxyquinoline, with appropriate adjustment of pH.

In precipitation with hydroxyquinoline the solutions are usually heated. The precipitated complexes are crystalline and easy to filter off and wash. The final stages of the determination consist either in drying and weighing the precipitated hydroxyquinoline complex, which should have a composition exactly corresponding to its formula if the precipitation was performed correctly, or in ignition and weighing of the metal oxide formed. Finally, the precipitate is often dissolved in HCl and the determination is completed by titration of the solution with $KBrO_3$ solution in presence of KBr (see p. 385).

iii. *Cupferron* $C_6H_9O_2N_3$ is the ammonium salt of nitrosophenylhydroxylamine and has the following structural formula:

NO
—N<
ONH$_4$

This reagent precipitates internal complexes of a number of metals. The metal cation replaces the ammonium in the reagent molecule and also forms a coordination bond with the nitrogen atom of the —NO group. The structure of the metal complexes is therefore represented by the formula:

N
—N Me/n
O

Originally this reagent was proposed for precipitation of copper, which accounts for its name (Kupfer is the German for copper). However, it is now used not for determination of copper but for precipitation of other metal cations, such as iron, vanadium, zirconium, titanium, tin, tantalum, niobium, quadrivalent uranium, etc. Accordingly, cupferron is widely used in analysis of various ores and alloys containing these metals.

Many other organic reagents are used in analytical practice. Some of them are used in the study of qualitative analysis. We shall not discuss them in greater detail here.

Separation of Ions by Extraction. In addition to the precipitation method discussed above, extraction is sometimes used for separating ions in quantitative analysis. In this method a particular component is dissolved out of solution by shaking with a water-insoluble organic solvent in which this component is more soluble than in water.

For example, Fe^{+++} ions are sometimes removed by extraction of $FeCl_3$ from concentrated hydrochloric acid solution with ether. Various thiocyanates, hydroxyquinoline complexes, and similar compounds are also often extracted.

The advantage of extraction over precipitation is that the interfacial area is very small. Therefore, adsorption effects, which greatly complicate separation by precipitation, have no significance in extraction. In practice extraction is used especially often in colorimetric analysis (p. 385).

Chromatographic Methods of Separation. Chromatographic methods of ion separation have become particularly important in recent years. As is well known,* chromatographic analysis was first introduced into science in 1903 by the eminent Russian botanist M. Tsvet. The method is based on selective adsorption of various substances or ions by particular adsorbents. For example, specially prepared (activated) aluminium oxide Al_2O_3 in powder form is put

---

* See V. Alexeyev, *Course of Qualitative Chemical Semimicroanalysis*, Goskhimizdat, 1962, Secs. 1 and 12.

in a glass tube (Fig. 27) and the solution under investigation is passed through this adsorption column. The substance or ion which is the most strongly adsorbed is adsorbed first (at the top of the column) while less adsorbable substances are adsorbed in lower layers. In this way the various components of the solution are separated in space, forming separate zones in the column. These zones are usually identified by their characteristic colours, which is why this method is called chromatography.

Consider the following example. If a solution containing Cu^{++} and Co^{++} ions is passed through a column containing Al_2O_3, and the column is then rinsed through lightly with water, a "chromatogram" is formed, with two zones of different colours: an upper pale blue Cu^{++} zone, and a lower pink Co^{++} zone (see Fig. 27). If the substances or ions separated are colourless, the chromatogram is "developed" by means of a suitable reagent. For example, if a solution containing the colourless Pb^{++} and Hg^{++} ions is passed through the column, to reveal the zones a solution of KI is drawn through the column. A yellow PbI_2 zone then appears at the top, with a red HgI_2 zone below.

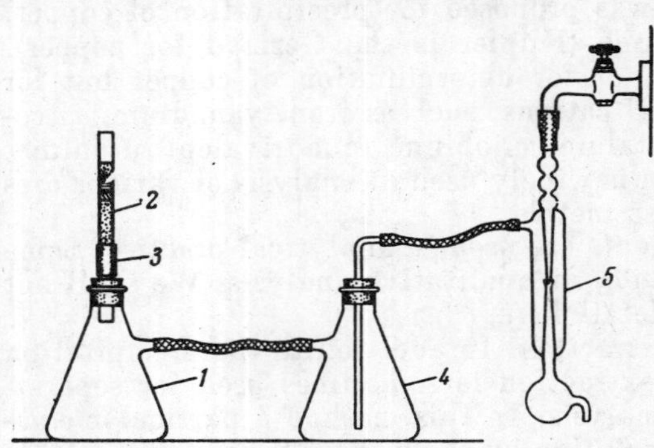

Fig. 27. Chromatographic column, showing separation of Cu^{++} and Co^{++} ions:
1—Bunsen flask; 2—chromatographic column with adsorbent; 3—rubber tube; 4—Bunsen flask; 5—water-jet pump

For quantitative determination of the individual substances or ions the chromatographic column can be taken out of the tube and cut into portions containing separate zones. The portions are then treated with suitable reagents to dissolve the adsorbed substances, and the solutions are analysed.

Alternatively, it is also possible to draw a suitable solvent (for example, an acid solution) through the column and to wash out all the zones successively; the separate portions of the liquid flowing out of the column are collected and analysed.

In addition to the adsorption chromatography described above, precipitation chromatography is also used. Here the separation of ions in the column is based on different solubilities of the compounds which they form with a precipitant mixed with the adsorbent; for example, with hydroxyquinoline, cupferron, etc. Zones of less soluble compounds are then formed at the top of the column and zones of more soluble compounds lower down.

Ion-exchange chromatography is especially important in analysis of inorganic compounds. *Ion exchangers* are used as adsorbents in this method. Ion exchangers are substances which are insoluble in water and which are able to exchange some of their surface ions for ions present in solution. They include permutite, which is widely used in technology for water softening, sulphonated coal, various synthetic ion-exchange resins, etc. Ion exchangers are classified as cation exchangers, which exchange cations with solutions, and anion exchangers.

If a cation exchanger containing exchangeable H^+ ions is denoted by RH, and the salt present in solution is written as MeA, then cation exchange can be represented by the equation:

$$RH + MeA \rightleftarrows RMe + HA$$

or

$$RH + Me^+ \rightleftarrows RMe + H^+ \quad (1)$$

This process is reversible. Thus, when a solution of a salt is passed through a cation-exchange column, its cations (Me^+) are adsorbed, and an equivalent amount of acid (H^+ ions) is released into solution. Conversely, if the exchanger in the Me form is now treated with a solution of an acid, its H^+ ions displace the previously adsorbed Me^+ cations, i.e., the cation exchanger is regenerated.

Analogously, anion exchange can be represented as follows:

$$ROH + A^- \rightleftarrows RA + OH^- \quad (2)$$

When alkali is passed through the column, the A^- anions previously adsorbed are replaced by OH^- ions and the ROH exchanger is regenerated.

Ion-exchange chromatography has numerous applications in quantitative analysis. For example, it is used for increasing the ion concentrations of very dilute solutions. Such a solution is passed through an ion-exchange column and the adsorbed ions are then displaced by a relatively small amount of a suitable reagent (e.g., acid). This gives a much more concentrated solution for analysis.

Ion exchangers can be used for determining the concentration of many salts in solutions. The salt solution is passed through a column containing a cation exchanger in the H form; the salt cations are then removed and the equivalent amount of acid appears in the solution (see Equation 1). The acid is titrated with alkali, and the amount of the salt (or the corresponding cation) in the unknown solution is easily calculated from the result. Cation exchangers can also be used for removing Cu^{++}, Ni^{++}, and other cations which interfere with determinations of certain anions (such as PO_4^{---}, SO_4^{--}, etc.). The solution is passed through a cation-exchange column in the Na form, which removes Cu^{++}, Ni^{++}, and other cations and replaces them by Na^+ ions, which do not interfere in the determination.

Ion-exchange chromatography is also used for separating certain cations. For example, it is possible to use differences between the properties of the corresponding hydroxides. In chromatographic separation of Fe^{+++} and Al^{+++} the solution is first passed through a cation exchanger which adsorbs these ions, and a solution of alkali is then run through the column. Iron remains in the column as $Fe(OH)_3$ whereas aluminium, the hydroxide of which is amphoteric, is washed out as AlO_2^- anions. Similar methods are used for separating iron from zinc, tin, tungsten, molybdenum, etc.

In other methods of separating cations by ion exchange, complex formation is used. For example, to separate Bi^{+++} from Cu^{++} and Pb^{++} these ions are adsorbed in a cation-exchange column which is then treated with KI solution. The Bi^{+++} ions form the stable $[BiI_4]^-$ complex and are washed out of the column in that form, while Cu^{++} and Pb^{++} remain in the column.

Similarly, chromatographic separation of rare earth elements can be based on differences in the stabilities of their citrate complexes. The stabilities can be varied by suitable adjustment of the solution pH.

The use of ion exchangers in analysis becomes difficult if large amounts of various extraneous ions are present in solutions. Other complications arise in connection with the presence of H^+ ions. Ion-exchange chromatography is most suitable for analysis of dilute solutions in absence of considerable amounts of extraneous ions.

QUESTIONS AND PROBLEMS
(on Secs. 16-35)

1. What are the principles of gravimetric determination (a) by precipitation; (b) by volatilization?

2. Define the precipitated and weighed forms. State the requirements to which they must conform in gravimetric analysis.

3. Which of the following calcium salts is the most suitable as the precipitated form: $CaSO_4 \cdot 2H_2O$ (SP = 6.1×10^{-5}), $CaCO_3$ (SP = 4.8×10^{-9}), or $CaC_2O_4 \cdot H_2O$ (SP = 2.6×10^{-9})?

4. Are such compounds as $Al(OH)_3$, $Cu(OH)_2$, etc., suitable as weighed forms?

Why are they ignited in analysis? Why are $CaSO_4$ and $CaCO_3$ more convenient weighed forms than CaO?

5. Phosphorus may be determined either as $Mg_2P_2O_7$ or as $(NH_4)_3PO_4 \cdot 12MoO_3$.

In which case would the loss of the same weight of precipitate have the greater effect on the result? Make the calculation for the loss of 1 mg of the weighed form.

6. Why is calcium precipitated with $(NH_4)_2C_2O_4$ and not with $Na_2C_2O_4$ in gravimetric analysis? Is NaCl or HCl solution the better precipitant for Ag^+ ions?

7. State the solubility product rule in its exact and approximate forms. Illustrate it by the appropriate formulas for $CaCO_3$.

8. Explain the terms *activity* and *activity coefficient*. When can the latter be taken as unity?

9. What are the values of $a_{Fe^{+++}}$ and a_{Cl^-} in 0.0083 *M* $FeCl_3$ solution if $f_{Fe^{+++}} = 0.20$; $f_{Cl^-} = 0.80$?

Answer: $a_{Fe^{+++}} = 0.0017$ g-ion/litre; $a_{Cl^-} = 0.020$ g-ion/litre.

10. What is the ionic strength of a solution? Calculate the ionic strength of the following solutions containing in 1 litre: (a) 0.1 *M* KCl; (b) 0.1 *M* K_2SO_4; (c) 0.1 *M* $MgSO_4$; (d) 0.1 *M* $AlCl_3$; (e) 0.01 *M* K_2SO_4 + 0.01 *M* $Al_2(SO_4)_3$?

Answer: (a) 0.1; (b) 0.3; (c) 0.4; (d) 0.6; (e) 0.18.

11. Calculate the activities of Ca^{++} and Cl^- ions in 0.01 *M* $CaCl_2$ solution.

Answer: $a_{Ca^{++}} = 0.0054$ g-ion/litre; $a_{Cl^-} = 0.017$ g-ion/litre.

Hint. To solve this problem, first calculate the ionic strength of the solution and from it find the activity coefficients of the ions from Table III (p. 77).

12. The solubilities of $PbSO_4$ and PbI_2 are 0.045 g and 0.300 g per litre respectively. Calculate the solubility products of these salts. Why has the less soluble salt the greater solubility product in this case? Would this be the case for such pairs of salts as $PbSO_4$ and $SrSO_4$, or Ag_2CrO_4 and $Ag_2C_2O_4$?

Answer: 2.2×10^{-8} and 1.1×10^{-9}; no.

13. The solubility of $AgNO_2$ is 4.15 g/litre. Calculate its solubility product, taking the activity coefficients of the ions into account.

Answer: SP = 5.4×10^{-4}.

14. How much is the solubility* of CaC_2O_4 in 0.01 *M* $(NH_4)_2C_2O_4$ solution less than in pure water?

Answer: (a) About 200 times by the approximate SP formula; (b) about 78 times with the activity coefficients taken into account.

15. How is the solubility of CaC_2O_4 influenced by the presence of 0.1 *M* KCl in solution?

Answer: The solubility is increased approximately 3-fold.

16. State the conditions under which a $CaCO_3$ solution is (a) unsaturated; (b) saturated; (c) supersaturated. How can an unsaturated solution be made saturated and supersaturated with respect to $CaCO_3$ without addition of the solid salt?

17. Using the solubility product rule, formulate the conditions in which (a) a precipitate is formed; (b) a precipitate is dissolved.

18. The solubility of $CaSO_4$ is 2 g/litre. A saturated calcium sulphate solution is mixed with an equal volume of ammonium oxalate solution containing 0.0248 g of $(NH_4)_2C_2O_4$ per litre. Calculate the product of the Ca^{++} and $C_2O_4^{--}$ ion concentrations in the solution and determine whether a precipitate of CaC_2O_4 is formed.

Answer: $[Ca^{++}][C_2O_4^{--}] = 7.5 \times 10^{-7}$. A precipitate is formed.

* Numerical values of the solubility products are given in Appendix III

19. Use the solubility products of silver chloride and bromide (see Appendix III) to find the difference between the amount of silver remaining in 200 ml of saturated solution of each salt.

Answer: 0.00031 g.

20. Calculate the number of ml of 0.25 *M* $(NH_4)_2C_2O_4$ needed for precipitation of Ca^{++} from a solution obtained from 0.7 g $CaCO_3$.

Answer: About 28 ml (about 42 ml with 50% excess).

21. Find the number of ml of ammonia solution (sp. gr. 0.99), containing 2.5% NH_3 by weight, which must be taken for precipitation of iron from a solution formed from 1 g of $(NH_4)Fe(SO_4)_2 \cdot 12H_2O$.

Answer: About 4.3 ml (about 6 ml with 50% excess)

22. Find the weight of $BaSO_4$ (SP $\approx 1 \times 10^{-10}$) remaining in 200 ml of solution when $BaCl_2$ is precipitated by an equivalent amount of H_2SO_4. Can the precipitation be regarded as practically complete?

Answer: About 0.0005 g; no.

23. What is the solubility loss of $BaSO_4$ if, under the conditions of Problem 22, excess H_2SO_4 is added to raise the SO_4^{--} ion concentration to 0.001 g-ion/litre?

Answer: 0.000005 g.

24. In precipitation of silver from 100 ml of a solution containing 0.3398 g $AgNO_3$ 17 ml of 0.1 *M* HCl solution was used. Calculate the amount of silver (in moles) remaining unprecipitated, and find the percentage error.

Answer: About 3×10^{-4} *M*; about 15%.

25. What would be the percentage error in Problem 24 if 21 ml and not 17 ml of 0.1 *M* HCl had been used?

Answer: About 0.08%.

26. What is the purpose of using excess precipitant in precipitation? Why must not the excess be too great?

27. 50 ml of 0.03 *M* K_2SO_4, which was 50% excess, was added to 50 ml of 0.02 *M* $CaCl_2$ solution. How much $CaSO_4$ remained in solution? Are precipitates like $CaSO_4$ suitable precipitated forms in gravimetric analysis*?

Answer: 0.0775 g; not suitable.

28. Explain the influence of solution pH on the completeness of precipitation of sparingly soluble electrolytes. When is this influence strong, and when is it negligible?

29. Find the pH at which precipitation of $Al(OH)_3$ is practically complete.

Answer: At pH = 5.3.

30. Find the pH for practically complete precipitation of (a) $Cu(OH)_2$; (b) $Cd(OH)_2$.

Answer: (a) At pH = 7.4; (b) at pH = 10.0.

31. What factors determine the pH required for practically complete precipitation of sparingly soluble salts of weak acids? Give examples.

---

* In solving this problem do not disregard the amount of SO_4^{--} ions entering the solution from the $CaSO_4$ precipitate.

32. Find the pH values for complete precipitation of Ba^{++} (a) by the action of $(NH_4)_2C_2O_4$; (b) by the action of $(NH_4)_2CO_3$, if the concentration of the precipitant at the end of the precipitation is 0.1 *M*.

Answer: (a) At pH = 4.3; (b) at pH = 9.1.

33. Find the pH for practically complete precipitation of ZnS from a 0.1 *M* solution of a zinc salt with 50% excess of $(NH_4)_2S$ as precipitant.

Answer: At pH = 3.3.

34. What is masking? What is its significance in analysis? What factors determine the possibility of masking of a given ion by a particular masking agent? What is the significance of using an excess of masking agent? When does pH influence masking? Give examples.

35. How does the solubility of precipitates usually change with increasing excess of precipitant? Is the rule by which a 50% excess of precipitant is added for precipitation of sparingly soluble electrolytes always valid?

36. What are the aims in providing definite conditions in the formation of crystalline precipitates? What are these conditions? In such cases, what is the role of the degree of supersaturation of the solution with respect to the precipitated compound?

37. Name the processes taking place during the ripening of crystalline precipitates. Explain why such ripening is advantageous in analysis.

38. What are colloidal solutions, and why should their formation be prevented in analysis? What is coagulation? How is it caused?

39. In what conditions is precipitation of amorphous precipitates performed? Why is it more advantageous to use concentrated solutions? What is achieved by subsequent addition of hot water to the solution?

40. What is coprecipitation? How does it differ from ordinary (chemical) precipitation of impurities together with a given compound? Why must coprecipitation be prevented in gravimetric analysis?

41. What is the significance of coprecipitation in determination of very small amounts ("traces") of various impurities? What is precipitation with a collector?

42. When Cu^{++} ions are present in a solution in a very low concentration they are not precipitated by the action of H_2S, but if a mercuric salt is added first, CuS is precipitated together with HgS. How does HgS act in this case?

43. What is adsorption? What causes adsorption on the surface? Do crystalline or amorphous precipitates adsorb more dissolved substances? What is the explanation.

44. How does (a) temperature, (b) the concentration of an adsorbed substance in solution, influence adsorption? How is selective adsorption manifested? What ions are adsorbed better than others by a given crystal lattice? What is internal adsorption?

45. Given that silver acetate is less soluble than silver nitrate, state which of these salts gives the purer AgCl precipitate by the action of Cl^- ions.

46. A precipitate of $Fe(OH)_3$ was formed (a) in a solution containing excess NaOH; (b) in a solution containing excess $FeCl_3$. Describe the primary and secondary adsorption processes in each case.

47. What is occlusion? Name different types of occlusion.

48. Describe how the precipitation of CaC_2O_4 should be performed if it is required to diminish adsorption (a) of extraneous cations, (b) of extraneous anions, as much as possible.

49. What is isomorphism? What are mixed crystals? Give examples. Explain the role of isomorphism in coprecipitation.

50. In what cases is isomorphous substitution of ions possible in the formation of a crystal lattice?

51. Crystals of KCl and KBr are isomorphous, but KCl and NaCl crystals are not. Explain this difference.

52. Name the various methods used to decrease coprecipitation. What is reprecipitation, and how is it performed?

53. What are the aims in washing of precipitates? What are the guiding considerations in the choice of a washing liquid?

54. A precipitate containing 0.3 g $CaCO_3$ was washed with 300 ml of water. Assuming that equilibrium was reached between the precipitate and the washing liquid, calculate the weight of $CaCO_3$ dissolved in the process and find the percentage loss of the precipitate due to solubility.

Answer: 0.0021 g; 0.70%.

55. Solve Problem 54 for a case in which the precipitate was washed with 0.1 *M* $(NH_4)_2CO_3$ solution.

Answer: 1.44×10^{-6} g; ~0.0005%.

56. What causes a precipitate to pass through the filter in prolonged washing with pure water? How can this effect be prevented?

57. How are precipitates washed by decantation? What are the advantages of this method over washing on the filter?

58. Explain why, when a precipitate is washed, should the previous portion of liquid be allowed to drain before the next portion is added.

59. Which is the more effective in washing a precipitate: the use of 2 portions of washing liquid of 50 ml each, or 10 portions of 10 ml?

60. What is ashless filter paper? What grades are used in gravimetric analysis? What are the advantages of filter crucibles?

61. When are precipitates ignited with the filter and when are they ignited separately?

62. What is a conversion factor? What does it indicate? Calculate the conversion factors for finding (a) the amount of sulphur from the weight of $BaSO_4$; (b) the amount of silver from the weight of Ag_2S; (c) the amount of zinc from the weight of $Zn_2P_2O_7$.

Answer: (a) 0.1374; (b) 0.8706; (c) 0.4288.

63. Calculate the conversion factors for finding: (a) the amount of $BaCl_2 \cdot 2H_2O$ from the weight of $BaSO_4$; (b) $Ca_3(PO_4)_2$ from CaO; (c) $Ca_3(PO_4)_2$ from $Mg_2P_2O_7$; (d) Cr_2O_3 from $PbCrO_4$.

Answer: (a) 1.047; (b) 1.844; (c) 1.393; (d) 0.2352.

64. Find the percentage of silver in $AgNO_3$ if precipitation from a solution containing 0.5000 g of this salt gave 0.4216 g AgCl. Check the accuracy of the analysis by comparing the result with the percentage of silver corresponding to the formula $AgNO_3$.

65. What weight of ferrous sulphate $FeSO_4 \cdot 7H_2O$ should be taken for determination of iron as ferric oxide Fe_2O_3 if the optimum weight of the latter is 0.2 g?

Answer: about 0.7 g.

66. What weight of an alloy containing about 20% zinc should be taken for determination of zinc as $Zn_2P_2O_7$? The precipitated form in this case is crystalline $ZnNH_4PO_4$.

Answer: About 1 g.

67. By what considerations is the choice of a solvent guided?

68. Name the most important types of fluxes used for fusion of precipitates. Write the equations for the reactions taking place in the fusion of: (a) Al_2O_3

with $KHSO_4$; (b) SiO_2 with a mixture of Na_2CO_3 and K_2CO_3; (c) Cr_2O_3 with a mixture of Na_2CO_3 and KNO_3; (d) Cr_2O_3 with Na_2O_2.

69. When is separation of different ions necessary? Why is this operation more laborious and complicated in quantitative than in qualitative analysis?

70. Name the most important inorganic precipitants used for ion separation, and give examples of their use. What are the advantages of organic over inorganic precipitates?

71. What are internal-complex salts? Give examples. What properties of internal-complex salts are valuable in analysis? What variable factors can be used for influencing the course of ion separation by precipitation in the form of complexes?

72. What is extraction? How is it applied to ion separation?

73. How are ions separated by adsorption chromatography and precipitation chromatography? What is the principle of ion-exchange chromatography? How is it used in quantitative analysis?

CHAPTER III

EXAMPLES OF GRAVIMETRIC DETERMINATIONS

36. Determination of Water of Crystallization in Barium Chloride

Water of crystallization is the water forming part of the crystal structure of certain substances, known as crystalline hydrates. The contents of such water in these hydrates correspond to definite chemical formulas, such as $BaCl_2 \cdot 2H_2O$; $CuSO_4 \cdot 5H_2O$; $Na_2SO_4 \cdot 10H_2O$; $Na_2SO_4 \cdot 7H_2O$, etc. Accordingly, water of crystallization is sometimes called stoichiometric water*.

When a crystalline hydrate is kept in a closed vessel which contains no water vapour, it partially decomposes to form the anhydrous substance and H_2O vapour. However, this continues only until the water-vapour pressure in the vessel has reached a value which is constant for the given hydrate at that temperature; this is known as the vapour pressure of the hydrate. A dynamic equilibrium is then established, for example:

$$BaCl_2 \cdot 2H_2O \rightleftarrows BaCl_2 + 2H_2O$$

$$CuSO_4 \cdot 5H_2O \rightleftarrows CuSO_4 + 5H_2O$$

etc.

Different hydrates have very different vapour pressures at a given temperature. For example, at 30°C it is 27 mm Hg for Glauber's salt $Na_2SO_4 \cdot 10H_2O$, 12.5 mm for copper sulphate $CuSO_4 \cdot 5H_2O$, and only 5 mm for barium chloride $BaCl_2 \cdot 2H_2O$. Such differences account for the differences in the behaviour of crystalline hydrates when exposed to air. If the vapour pressure of a hydrate is greater than the partial pressure of water vapour in the air, the crystals *effloresce*, i.e., they gradually lose water of crystallization at room

---

* It should be noted that the so-called *water of constitution* is also stoichiometric. As distinct from water of crystallization, water of constitution is not present as H_2O molecules but is formed from the H and O atoms present in a substance when it is decomposed by heat, for example:

$$2Fe(OH)_3 = Fe_2O_3 + 3H_2O$$

$$H_2SO_4 = SO_3 + H_2O$$

temperature. For example, Glauber's salt, washing soda, and similar substances effloresce when exposed to air. In contrast, crystalline hydrates with low vapour pressures do not effloresce, and some even absorb water vapour from the air. For example, the hydrate $CaCl_2 \cdot 2H_2O$ is converted into the more highly hydrated form $CaCl_2 \cdot 6H_2O$. The fact that $CaCl_2 \cdot 2H_2O$ absorbs water vapour is the reason for its use in desiccators and for drying gases.

When heated, crystalline hydrates decompose with liberation of water. This is the basis for the method of determining water of crystallization in most crystalline hydrates by volatilization. In the present example a weighed sample of $BaCl_2 \cdot 2H_2O$, contained in a weighing bottle (Fig. 3), is heated at 120-125°C in a drying oven (Fig. 21) until its weight ceases to change (i.e., it is dried to constant weight).

When the weight has become constant evidently all the water of crystallization has been removed. Its weight is equal to the weight loss of the sample.

The recrystallized chemically pure salt should be taken for this determination, so that the result can be checked against the formula of barium chloride.

Procedure. *Taking the Sample.* Wash a weighing bottle thoroughly (see Sec. 12), dry it in the drying oven and cool for 20 minutes, with the lid off, in a desiccator near the balance.*

Then weigh the bottle together with its lid accurately on an analytical balance, observing all the rules. Now put about 1.5 g of freshly recrystallized $BaCl_2 \cdot 2H_2O$ in the bottle, cover with the lid, and weigh accurately again.**

Drying. Put the lid edgewise (on a slant) on the weighing bottle, and place the latter on a shelf (not the floor) of the drying oven. A piece of paper with your name should be put under the bottle. Keep the bottle in the oven at about 125°C for approximately 2 hours.

During this time you can determine, for example, Ba^{++} or Cl^- in $BaCl_2 \cdot 2H_2O$.

At the end of 2 hours transfer the bottle and lid to a desiccator by means of crucible tongs (Fig. 23). Leave the desiccator near the balance for 20 minutes, take out the bottle and cover it with the lid, and weigh. Replace the weighing bottle with the substance in the drying oven and keep it there (not forgetting to open the lid) for about an hour; then cool and weigh it again.

---

* The hot weighing bottle must not be closed, because it would be difficult or even impossible to open when cool. For more details see p. 22.

** It is more convenient first to weigh out the required amount approximately (1.4-1.5 g) on a technical balance, and then weigh this sample in the bottle on an analytical balance.

If the second weighing gives the same result as the first, or does not differ from it by more than 0.0002 g, it may be assumed that practically all the water of crystallization has been removed.

Otherwise, continue the repeated drying and weighing, until the weight becomes constant. *The results of all the repeated weighings must be recorded in the laboratory log-book, even if they are the same.* It must be remembered that your instructor considers that anything which is not recorded has not been done in practice, while constancy of weight is the most important condition for correct analytical results.

If the work has to be interrupted, leave the weighing bottle in the desiccator. This is convenient because the drying of the substance continues owing to absorption of water vapour by calcium chloride. Obviously, drying can only occur in a desiccator if the ground-glass joint of the lid is properly greased.

Calculation. Suppose that the following numerical data were obtained and recorded in the laboratory note book:

Weight of bottle with substance	9.5895 g
Weight of bottle	8.1320 g
Weight of $BaCl_2 \cdot 2H_2O$	1.4575 g

Weight of bottle with substance after drying

I	9.3758 g
II	9.3748 g
III	9.3749 g

Rejecting the first weighing (9.3758 g), we find the weight of water of crystallization in the sample:

$$\begin{array}{r} 9.5895 \\ -\ 9.3748 \\ \hline 0.2147\text{g} \end{array}$$

We now calculate the percentage of water of crystallization in $BaCl_2 \cdot 2H_2O$:

1.4575 g of substance contains 0.2147 g H_2O

100 g of substance contains y g H_2O

$$y = \frac{0.2147 \times 100}{1.4575}\ \%$$

The tables of four-figure logarithms and antilogarithms (Appendices IX and X) are used for the calculation:

$$\begin{array}{ll} \log 0.2147 = \bar{1}.3318 \\ \log 100 \quad\ = 2.0000 \\ \hline \text{Sum} & 1.3318 \\ \log 1.4575 & 0.1636 \\ \hline \end{array}$$

Difference $= \log y = 1.1682$ and $y = 14.73\%$

Checking the Precision of the Determination. As a check, compare the result with the theoretically calculated percentage content of H_2O in $BaCl_2 \cdot 2H_2O$. Since one gram-molecule (244.3 g) of $BaCl_2 \cdot 2H_2O$ contains two gram-molecules or 36.03 g of H_2O, we have the following proportion.*

244.3 g $BaCl_2 \cdot 2H_2O$ contains 36.03 g H_2O
100 g $BaCl_2 \cdot 2H_2O$ contains x g H_2O

$$x = \frac{36.03 \times 100}{244.3} = 14.75\%$$

The absolute error is $14.73\% - 14.75\% = -0.02\%$. The relative error is therefore

$$D_0 = \frac{(-0.02) \times 100}{14.75} \approx -0.14\%$$

This error is easily accounted for by weighing errors.

If this determination is properly carried out the absolute error should not exceed $\pm 0.05\%$. In other words, only results between 14.70 and 14.80% are acceptable.

37. Determination of Hygroscopic Water

Solid substances adsorb water vapour from the air on their surfaces. This adsorbed water is termed *hygroscopic*. In distinction from stoichiometric water, the content of hygroscopic water cannot be represented in the chemical formula.

Substances of very large surface area can adsorb considerable amounts of water while retaining the appearance of dry powders. Hygroscopic water is in dynamic equilibrium with water vapour in the air. It is therefore partially removed from a substance kept in a dry place.

More complete removal and quantitative determination of water can be achieved by a method similar to that used for determination of water of crystallization; the substance is dried to constant weight at 105-130°C.

The weighing bottle used for the determination is first dried at 105-130°C and weighed. An average sample of the powdered substance (about 2-5 g) is weighed out and dried at 105-130°C to constant weight. The amount of hygroscopic water removed is found from the weight loss. The result is expressed as a percentage of the sample weight.

---

* Remember that, as was explained on p. 58, all the numerical data for calculation should be taken to four significant figures. Therefore, the weight of water of crystallization in a gram-molecule of barium chloride is taken as 36.03 g and not 36 g.

This method does not always give a correct idea of the amount of hygroscopic water. The loss in weight during drying depends not only on removal of hygroscopic water, but also on loss of water of crystallization and other volatile constituents. Another frequent source of error in this method is oxidation of the substance by atmospheric oxygen on heating. The loss in weight is then less than should correspond to the true content of hygroscopic water. This happens in analysis of many organic substances such as flour, leather, etc.

As has already been stated, the amount of hygroscopic moisture in a substance is not constant but depends on temperature and atmospheric humidity. Variations in the content of hygroscopic water must evidently influence the percentage contents of all the other constituents of a substance. Therefore, analytical results for substances containing appreciable amounts of hygroscopic water are recalculated for the absolutely dry substance in order to eliminate variations of composition with moisture content.

For example, suppose that a substance contains $p\%$ of a certain element and $h\%$ of hygroscopic water. The amount of dry substance in 100 g of the material is obviously $(100-h)$ g; therefore, we can write:

$(100-h)$ g of dry substance contains p g of the element
100 g of dry substance contains x g of the element

$$x = p\,\frac{100}{100-h}\,\%$$

Therefore, to recalculate for the absolutely dry substance the percentage (p) of the element found experimentally must be multiplied by

$$\frac{100}{100-h}$$

38. Determination of Barium in Barium Chloride

The Ba^{++} ion forms a number of sparingly soluble salts, such as $BaCO_3$, BaC_2O_4, $BaHPO_4$, $BaCrO_4$, $BaSO_4$, etc. The least soluble of them is barium sulphate $BaSO_4$ ($SP = 1.1 \times 10^{-10}$), so that this compound is the most convenient precipitated form for barium determination. The composition of $BaSO_4$ is not changed by ignition, so that this compound is also the weighed form. The composition of $BaSO_4$ corresponds strictly to its formula and it is very stable chemically. However, $BaSO_4$ precipitates have a strong tendency to form very small crystals which sometimes pass through the filter pores and complicate the work. Therefore, special care must be taken in precipitation to make the conditions favourable for formation of fairly coarse-grained precipitates.

The most vital of these conditions is slow addition of the precipitant which is also essential in obtaining the purer $BaSO_4$ precipitate (Sec. 27).

To avoid errors due to coprecipitation of the precipitant itself, the latter should for preference be volatile (Sec. 17). Therefore, Ba^{++} is precipitated by the action of sulphuric acid rather than sulphates. The reaction is:

$$BaCl_2 + H_2SO_4 = \downarrow BaSO_4 + 2HCl$$

The free acid can be used as the precipitant in this case because $BaSO_4$, being a sparingly soluble salt of a strong acid, is practically insoluble in acids. However, it was pointed out in Sec. 20 that its solubility nevertheless increases somewhat in presence of H^+ ions.* It is known that in precipitation of crystalline substance this increase of solubility is an advantage, because the degree of supersaturation of the solution with respect to the precipitated substance is decreased and the crystals deposited are larger.

To intensify this favourable influence of H^+ ions, a small amount of HCl is added to the solution in precipitation of Ba^{++}.

Rise of the solution temperature has an effect similar to addition of HCl. Of course, the increased solubility of $BaSO_4$ due to addition of HCl or heating must be lowered again at the end of the precipitation by addition of a suitable excess of precipitant (Sec. 19).

Before starting the analysis, carefully read through all the instructions and find what vessels are required, and how many. The vessels must be washed thoroughly beforehand. The crucible in which the precipitate is to be ignited must be brought to constant weight during the preparatory stages of the analysis (p. 122).

Procedure. *Weighing and Dissolving the Sample.* Barium sulphate precipitates are crystalline; therefore, the precipitate should weigh about 0.5 g. In the reaction one gram-molecule (233.4 g) of $BaSO_4$ is formed from one gram-molecule (244.3 g) of $BaCl_2 \cdot 2H_2O$. As the molecular weights are nearly equal in this case, about 0.5 g of $BaCl_2 \cdot 2H_2O$ should be taken to obtain 0.5 g of $BaSO_4$.

Weigh a clean and dry watch glass on the analytical balance. Weigh out roughly the required amount (0.4-0.6 g) of $BaCl_2 \cdot 2H_2O$ onto it on a technical balance, and then weigh the glass and substance together accurately on the analytical balance. Subtract the weight of the watch glass from the accurate total weight and thus find the weight of $BaCl_2 \cdot 2H_2O$ taken.

Transfer the sample quantitatively into a 200-300 ml beaker with a lip, and dissolve it in water. To do this, tip the substance into the

---

* The solubility of barium sulphate in 1 *N* hydrochloric acid is 20 time its solubility in water.

beaker from the tilted watch glass, taking care not to have any blown away, and then rinse in the remaining particles with a jet of water from a wash bottle. Add enough water to make the total volume of liquid in the beaker 80-100 ml.

Precipitation. Add 3-5 ml of 2 *N* HCl to this solution, and heat it on a gauze nearly to boiling (but do not allow it to boil because drops of liquid may be lost with steam bubbles escaping from the beaker). At the same time, heat to boiling about 3-5 ml of 2 *N* H_2SO_4 diluted with 30 ml of distilled water in another beaker (or flask).* Then add the hot H_2SO_4 solution *very slowly drop by drop* to the hot $BaCl_2$ solution, stirring the latter with a glass rod. Avoid touching the bottom and sides of the beaker with the rod, as otherwise the precipitate will cling firmly to the glass. Remember that *the rod must not be taken out of the beaker* because particles of precipitate adhering to it would be lost.

As the precipitation proceeds, the H_2SO_4 can be added rather more rapidly. When nearly all the acid (apart from a few drops) has been added, cover the beaker with a piece of paper or cardboard to protect the contents from dust, with the rod still in the beaker, and leave until the next session to allow the precipitate to ripen.** As soon as the $BaSO_4$ has settled to the bottom of the beaker, check whether precipitation of Ba^{++} is complete. To do this, add the last few drops of H_2SO_4 carefully down the side of the beaker to the clear liquid above the precipitate and note whether any turbidity appears.

While the precipitate is ageing bring the crucible to constant weight.

Filtration; Washing the Precipitate. Take a piece of the densest ashless filter paper (blue band), 7 cm in diameter, and fit it well into a funnel. Put the funnel in a ring on the stand, and decant the liquid down a glass rod through the filter into another clean beaker underneath. Follow carefully all the instructions given on pp. 115 et seq. When no more liquid can be poured off the precipitate, check that the filtrate is free from all traces of turbidity, and then throw it away.***

Now wash the precipitate 3-4 times by decantation (p. 120) putting 20-30 ml of cold distilled water slightly acidified with hydrochlo-

---

* See pp. 70-71 for calculation of the amount of precipitant necessary.

** This can be accelerated if the beaker with the precipitate is put on a boiling water bath for 2-3 hours.

*** The easiest way of detecting turbidity is to place the filtrate on a sheet of black paper (or on a black painted bench) and to look at it from above while slightly agitating the contents of the beaker by smooth circular movements. This causes any precipitate which has passed through the filter to collect on the bottom of the beaker, where it can easily be seen. If the filtrate is found to be turbid, it must be passed repeatedly through the same filter until the filter pores are blocked with precipitate particles and the liquid becomes quite clear.

ric acid (5 ml of 2 *N* HCl to 100 ml of water) into the beaker each time, and pouring it off as completely as possible into the filter. After the last decantation transfer the precipitate quantitatively to the filter (p. 121) very carefully (this is the most critical point in the work) and wash it with cold distilled water to remove Cl^-. Continue the washing until a portion of the filtrate, collected in a test tube and acidified slightly with HNO_3, no longer becomes turbid on addition of $AgNO_3$ (formation of AgCl) or of $Hg_2(NO_3)_2$ (formation of Hg_2Cl_2).

Drying and Igniting the Precipitate. Partially dry the filter with the washed precipitate,* put it together with the precipitate into the weighed crucible, and ignite the precipitate. The technique of these operations is described in detail on pp. 122, et seq. Continue the ignition for 20-25 minutes after the contents of the crucible have become white and the carbon deposit on the sides has disappeared. Cool the crucible in a desiccator and weigh. Ignite the crucible again for 10-15 minutes, cool, weigh again, etc., to constant weight.

When a $BaSO_4$ precipitate is ignited it is partially reduced to BaS by carbon from the filter paper:

$$BaSO_4 + 2C = BaS + 2CO_2 \uparrow$$

Barium sulphide is subsequently oxidized by atmospheric oxygen to $BaSO_4$:

$$BaS + 2O_2 = BaSO_4$$

When the weight has become constant, this is a sign that the oxidation is complete and the precipitate no longer contains BaS.

Calculation. Suppose that the following numerical data were obtained and recorded in the laboratory log-book:

	g
Weight of glass with $BaCl_2 \cdot 2H_2O$	6.1988
Weight of glass	5.7116
Weight of $BaCl_2 \cdot 2H_2O$	0.4872
Weight of crucible with $BaSO_4$,	
1st weighing	11.6876
2nd weighing	11.6878
Weight of empty crucible,	
1st weighing	11.2233
2nd weighing	11.2232

Weight of $BaSO_4$:

$$\begin{array}{r} 11.6877 \text{ g} \\ -\ 11.2232 \text{ g} \\ \hline 0.4645 \text{ g} \end{array}$$

* It is best to leave the filter slightly damp.

By proportion:

233.4 g $BaSO_4$ contains 137.3 g Ba
0.4645 g $BaSO_4$ contains x g Ba

$$x = \frac{0.4645 \times 137.3}{233.4}$$

This weight of barium was contained in 0.4872 g of barium chloride. Therefore 1 g of the latter contains

$$\frac{0.4645 \times 137.3}{233.4 \times 0.4872}$$

and 100 g contains 100 times as much, or

$$y = \frac{0.4645 \times 137.3 \times 100}{233.4 \times 0.4872} = \% \text{ Ba in } BaCl_2 \cdot 2H_2O$$

Now calculate log y by logarithms (Appendix IX):

$$\begin{array}{rl} \log 0.4645 = & \bar{1}.6670 \\ \log 137.3 = & 2.1377 \\ \log 100 = & 2.0000 \\ \hline \text{Sum} & 3.8047 \end{array} \qquad \begin{array}{rl} \log 233.4 = & 2.3681 \\ \log 0.4872 = & \bar{1}.6877 \\ \hline \text{Sum} & 2.0558 \end{array}$$

$$\begin{array}{r} 3.8047 \\ -\,2.0558 \\ \hline \log y = 1.7489 \end{array}$$

Use the antilogarithm tables (Appendix X) to find the number corresponding to this logarithm (1.7489):

$$y = 56.10\%$$

Of course, the calculation could be done in another way, by using the table of conversion factors F, which contains the following data:

Determined	Found	Factor F*	log F**
Ba	$BaSO_4$	0.5883	76,960

* The conversion factor F (see Sec. 32) shows how many grams of the element (or compound) being determined correspond to 1 g of precipitate. In this case:

$$F = \frac{137.3}{233.4}$$

** The five-figure mantissae of log F are given in this column.

The calculation is then continued by Formula (2) in Sec. 32.

Checking the Determination. To check the determination, compare the percentage of barium found with the value corresponding to the formula $BaCl_2 \cdot 2H_2O$.

By proportion:

$$244.3 \text{ g } BaCl_2 \cdot 2H_2O \text{ contains } 137.3 \text{ g Ba}$$
$$100 \text{ g } BaCl_2 \cdot 2H_2O \text{ contains } x \text{ g Ba}$$
$$x = \frac{137.3 \times 100}{244.3} = 56.20\%$$

The absolute error in this case is:

$$56.10 - 56.20 = -0.10\%$$

Now find the relative error, which is:

$$D_0 = \frac{(-0.10) \times 100}{56.20} = -0.18\%$$

39. Determination of Sulphur in Sulphuric Acid Solution

A method similar to that described above is used for determining sulphur in sulphuric acid solutions, soluble sulphates, and any materials containing sulphur which can be oxidized to SO_4^{--}. These include various sulphide ores of iron, copper, arsenic, etc. Let us consider the simplest case, the determination of sulphur in sulphuric acid solution.

Procedure. Put the solution of H_2SO_4 to be analysed in a thoroughly washed beaker, dilute it to about 100 ml, add 5 ml of 2 *N* HCl, and heat nearly to boiling. Precipitate SO_4^{--} from the hot solution by addition of 4-5 ml of 2 *N* $BaCl_2$ solution previously diluted with 30-50 ml of water and also heated to boiling. The precipitation conditions and all subsequent procedures are the same as in Ba^{++} determination, the only difference being that the $BaCl_2$ solution, which is the precipitant, is added drop by drop to the H_2SO_4 solution. It is especially important in this case to add the precipitant slowly, as otherwise much $BaCl_2$ is taken down with the precipitate. As $BaCl_2$ is non-volatile, the result would then be too high.

Calculation. This is done by proportion:

$$233.4 \text{ g } BaSO_4 \text{ contains } 32.06 \text{ g S}$$
$$a \text{ g } BaSO_4 \text{ contains } x \text{ g S}$$
$$x = a \times \frac{32.06}{233.4} \text{ g}$$

where a is the weight of $BaSO_4$ precipitate and $\frac{32.06}{233.4}$ is the conversion factor F.

As the solution analysed contains an unknown weight of H_2SO_4, the percentage content of S cannot be calculated in this case. Neither is it possible to check the analysis by theoretical calculation; therefore, the determination should be carried out at least in duplicate.

40. Determination of Chlorine in Barium Chloride

The least soluble chloride is silver chloride, and this is the form in which chlorine is determined gravimetrically. As AgCl readily forms colloidal solutions, Cl^- is precipitated by the action of $AgNO_3$ on heating in presence of a coagulant (HNO_3), the precipitate being left to stand for several hours to complete the coagulation. The precipitate is washed with water containing HNO_3 for the same reason.

In daylight AgCl decomposes with formation of metallic silver; the precipitate becomes first violet and then black. A violet colour is not yet a sign that the precipitate is unsuitable for further work. Blackening indicates considerable decomposition of AgCl, and is inadmissible. Therefore, care must be taken that the precipitate is not exposed to direct sunlight and does not remain for a long time in diffused light. It is best to surround the beaker containing the precipitate for settling with black paper. Silver chloride also decomposes very easily when heated. Therefore, it must be ignited with great care. Ignition can be avoided by drying the precipitate to constant weight at 130°C. Obviously paper filters cannot be used in that case, and the precipitates are collected in glass filter crucibles.

Procedure. It is easy to calculate (do this) from the reaction equation that about 0.26 g of $BaCl_2 \cdot 2H_2O$ should be taken to give about 0.3 g of AgCl.

Dissolve the weighed sample in 70-80 ml of distilled water and heat nearly (but not quite) to boiling. In another vessel heat nearly to boiling a previously calculated volume* of 0.1 *M* $AgNO_3$ solution acidified with 1 ml of diluted (1 : 1) HNO_3. Previously confirm that the HNO_3 does not give a turbidity with $AgNO_3$, i.e., does not contain Cl^-. Add the $AgNO_3$ solution to the $BaCl_2$ solution, continuing gentle heating.

Pour the $AgNO_3$ solution down a glass rod, and then stir the contents of the beaker vigorously for several minutes without brushing the sides.

The acid solution, heating and stirring help coagulation of the precipitate particles which form large curdy flakes settling rapidly to the bottom of the beaker. When this has occurred, stop the heating and test for completeness of precipitation by adding a few drops of

---

* By the reaction equation, precipitation of 1 gram-molecule (244.3 g) of $BaCl_2 \cdot 2H_2O$ takes 2 gram-molecules of $AgNO_3$. As 1 litre of 0.1 *M* solution contains 0.1 gram-molecule of $AgNO_3$, 2 gram-molecules of the latter are contained in 20 litres or 20,000 ml of solution. Use these values for the calculation. Take 5-10 ml more than the calculated volume of $AgNO_3$ for the determination.

$AgNO_3$ solution to the clear liquid down the side of the beaker. If turbidity occurs, add a few more ml of $AgNO_3$ solution, stir the liquid thoroughly again with the glass rod, test for completeness of precipitation, etc. When the precipitation is complete cover the beaker (with the rod left in) and leave it in the bench cupboard until the next session. It is useful to wrap black paper around the beaker to protect it from light.

The subsequent procedure depends on the filtration method used.

Filtration Through a Paper Filter. The ashless filter paper should be less dense than that used for $BaSO_4$ (white band).

At the end of the filtration wash the precipitate by decantation 3-4 times with hot water acidified with HNO_3 (5 ml of 2 *N* solution to 100 ml of water). Then use a glass rod with a rubber tip* to transfer the precipitate quantitatively to the filter, and wash at first with water containing HNO_3 and then with pure water. Continue the washing until the precipitant ($AgNO_3$) has been completely removed, i.e., until a separate portion of the filtrate no longer becomes turbid on addition of HCl. Put the funnel with the washed precipitate in a drying oven and dry it at 100-105°C.

AgCl, in contrast to $BaSO_4$, must be dried completely, as the precipitate must subsequently be removed from the filter. Take care not to let the temperature in the drying oven rise above 105°C, as otherwise the paper chars, and disintegrates when taken out of the funnel.

While the precipitate is being washed and dried, ignite a crucible to constant weight. Since AgCl is easily reduced by carbon and products of incomplete combustion of the filter, the latter must not be ignited together with the precipitate as in determination of Ba^{++}; the filter is burnt separately. Take the completely dry filter paper and precipitate out of the funnel, and transfer the precipitate as completely as possible to a sheet of black glazed paper, squeezing the filter lightly with the fingers. This must be done very carefully, avoiding loss due to dusting of the precipitate; collect the precipitate at one spot with a soft brush and cover it with an inverted funnel or, better still, with a black paper cone.

Put the filter with its residual particles of precipitate into a crucible which has been heated to constant weight, and ash it as described on p. 124. The small amount of AgCl on the filter is then reduced to metallic silver, which must be converted back into AgCl. Allow the crucible to cool and treat the precipitate with 3-4 drops of concentrated nitric acid, with *gentle heating* (preferably on a boiling water bath). The silver dissolves and $AgNO_3$ is formed.

---

* In this case pieces of ashless filter paper must not be used for transferring the precipitate.

Put one drop of concentrated HCl in the crucible and continue to heat it *very gently* until the contents are quite dry.* Allow the crucible to cool, wipe its outside with filter paper, and stand it on another sheet of glazed paper. Pour the AgCl precipitate which had been previously separated into the crucible, brushing the last few particles in with a small brush. Then put the crucible in a triangle and ring on the stand, and *heat it very gently and cautiously, holding the burner in the hand all the time, until the precipitate begins to melt* (AgCl *decomposes on stronger heating*). Cool the crucible in a desiccator and weigh it.

Filtration Through a Glass Filter Crucible. This determination is much simpler if a glass filter crucible is used instead of paper for filtration. Before starting the filtration take a No. 4 glass filter crucible and insert it in a rubber ring into the neck of a suction flask (see Fig. 19).

Wash the filter crucible thoroughly, with gentle suction, first with hot dilute HNO_3 (5 ml of 2 *N* solution to 100 ml of water) and then with hot water, and dry it at 130°C to constant weight.

Replace the filter crucible in the neck of the flask and start the filtration. As usual, decant the liquid down a glass rod into the filter crucible, which must not be more than $^3/_4$ full. At the end of the filtration wash the precipitate several times by decantation with hot water containing HNO_3. Transfer the precipitate quantitatively into the filter crucible by means of a rubber-tipped glass rod, and wash it thoroughly first with water acidified with HNO_3 and then with pure water.

At the end of the washing first release the vacuum by opening the tap of the flask *4*, shut off the water-jet pump, close the water tap, take out the filter crucible, and dry it again at 130°C to constant weight. Find the weight of AgCl from the difference between the weights of the empty crucible and the crucible with AgCl. The advantage of this method is obvious. Reduction of AgCl by carbon of the filter and decomposition during ignition are avoided.

Calculation. Knowing that one gram-molecule of AgCl contains one gram-atom of Cl, calculate the weight of the latter in the AgCl found, and express it as a percentage of the weight of $BaCl_2 \cdot 2H_2O$ taken. Compare the result with the theoretical chlorine content of barium chloride calculated from the formula $BaCl_2 \cdot 2H_2O$. Also find the relative error.

The sum of the results obtained in determinations of water of crystallization, barium and chlorine in $BaCl_2 \cdot 2H_2O$ should evidently

* Remember that with careless heating the precipitate can easily be spattered out of the crucible, so that the analysis must be started again. The safest way is to heat the *crucible* on a water bath.

be 100%. In reality it always differs somewhat from 100% because of inevitable analytical errors. With accurate work the difference usually does not exceed some tenths of 1%.

Silver is also determined in solutions of its salts or in alloys by precipitation as AgCl. In the case of an alloy, a weighed sample is dissolved in HNO_3, Ag^+ is precipitated with HCl, and the analysis is continued as described above. If excess of precipitant (HCl) is used, the soluble $[AgCl_2]^-$ complex may be formed.

41. Determination of Iron in Ferric Chloride Solution (III)

For gravimetric determination of Fe in solutions of ferric salts* iron is precipitated as $Fe(OH)_3$ by the action of NH_4OH:

$$FeCl_3 + 3NH_4OH = \downarrow Fe(OH)_3 + 3NH_4Cl$$

Ignition converts $Fe(OH)_3$ into anhydrous ferric oxide:

$$2Fe(OH)_3 = Fe_2O_3 + 3H_2O$$

which is weighed.

Ferric hydroxide is a typical amorphous precipitate which readily forms colloidal solutions. To avoid this, the precipitation must be effected in hot solution in presence of a coagulating electrolyte. It should be remembered that when solutions of ferric salts are heated they are strongly hydrolyzed, forming first basic iron salts and then $Fe(OH)_3$; for example:

$$FeCl_3 + 2H_2O \rightleftarrows Fe(OH)_2Cl + 2HCl$$

$$Fe(OH)_2Cl + H_2O \rightleftarrows Fe(OH)_3 + HCl$$

The slimy precipitate so formed sticks firmly to the bottom and sides of the beaker and is very difficult to filter off and wash. Its formation must therefore be prevented; this is done by acidifying the solution before it is heated. The above equations show that acid is formed as the result of hydrolysis. Therefore, an increase of the H^+ ion concentration in solution should suppress hydrolysis and prevent formation of the precipitate.

Subsequently the acid is neutralized with NH_4OH; the ammonium salt formed acts as a coagulating electrolyte in the precipitation.

It was said earlier (p. 101) that amorphous substances such as $Fe(OH)_3$ should preferably be precipitated from concentrated solutions. They are then less bulky, adsorb smaller amounts of impurities, and are easier to wash. Special care must be taken to wash out

* This determination is instructional in character, and provides a good example of the formation of amorphous precipitates. In practice, volumetric methods are used for determination of iron (Secs. 88, 89 and 94) as they are more precise and rapid.

all Cl^- ions, because they may form volatile ferric chloride $FeCl_3$ during the ignition so that some of the iron would be lost.

At the temperature of the ordinary gas burner flame Fe_2O_3 is not reduced by carbon from the filter paper, and therefore the precipitate is not removed from the filter for ignition. However, excessively strong or long heating should be avoided, as it leads to partial reduction of Fe_2O_3 to ferrosoferric oxide Fe_3O_4 by the reaction

$$6Fe_2O_3 = 4Fe_3O_4 + O_2 \uparrow$$

Procedure. Acidify the solution (containing not more than 0.1 g of iron) with 3-5 ml of 2 N HNO_3 solution and, without diluting with water, heat carefully over a small burner flame without allowing the liquid to boil. Add 10% ammonia solution to the hot solution until it smells faintly but distinctly of ammonia,* stir the contents of the beaker thoroughly with the glass rod, and add about 100 ml of hot distilled water to diminish adsorption. Stir the liquid well once again and allow the precipitate to settle for 5 minutes. Then check for complete precipitation by careful addition of 1-2 drops of NH_4OH and filter at once (the alkaline liquid must not be left for any length of time in the beaker, as alkalies extract silica from the glass and this increases the weight of the precipitate).

A filter paper of medium density (white band), 9 cm in diameter, should be used for the filtration. Decant the liquid from the precipitate through the filter, and then wash the precipitate several times by decantation with hot 2% NH_4NO_3 solution. Then transfer the precipitate quantitatively to the filter; particles adhering to the beaker and rod should be removed with pieces of ashless paper.

Continue to wash the precipitate on the filter until Cl^- ions have been completely removed, i.e., until a portion of the filtrate, acidified with HNO_3, no longer gives turbidity with $AgNO_3$ [or with $Hg_2(NO_3)_2$]. The precipitation, filtration and washing must all be completed during the same session.

Partly dry the washed precipitate and while it is still damp transfer it on the filter into a crucible which had been ignited to constant weight. Carefully dry the filter and char it over a small flame so that it does not catch fire. Then ash the paper and, gradually increasing the heat, ignite the crucible and precipitate to constant weight.

Calculation. Having found the weight of the precipitate, calculate its iron content. This is done by proportion:

$$M_{Fe_2O_3} - 2A_{Fe}$$

$$a - x$$

* In adding the ammonia, make sure that the smell comes from the solution and not from the glass rod or the sides of the beaker.

where a is the weight of the precipitate; $M_{Fe_2O_3}$ and A_{Fe} are the corresponding molecular and atomic weights.

Hence:

$$x = a\frac{2A_{Fe}}{M_{Fe_2O_3}} = aF$$

where

$$F = \frac{2 \times 55.85}{159.7} = 0.6994$$

As in the determination of S in H_2SO_4 solutions, the determination should be done in duplicate at least to confirm its accuracy.

A similar method is used for determination of iron in various materials. For example, in analysis of iron wire a weighed sample* (about 0.1 g) is dissolved with heating in 10-15 ml of 2 N HNO_3. The $Fe(NO_3)_3$ solution is analysed as described above. When the amount of iron in the Fe_2O_3 precipitate has been found, it is expressed as a percentage of the weight of the wire taken.

42. Determination of Aluminium in Alum

Aluminium (Al^{+++}) can be determined in the same way as Fe^{+++}, by precipitation with ammonia and subsequent conversion of the $Al(OH)_3$ precipitate into Al_2O_3 by ignition. However, this widely used method involves considerable complications in practice. Firstly, $Al(OH)_3$ is an amphoteric hydroxide and is appreciably soluble in excess NH_4OH. Therefore, for complete precipitation of Al^{+++} the solution pH must be adjusted very precisely.** Secondly, it is rather difficult to filter off the precipitate and to wash out adsorbed impurities. The weighed form (Al_2O_3) is very hygroscopic and special precautions must be taken when the ignited precipitate is cooled and weighed. Finally, ammonia precipitates a number of other cations in addition to Al^{+++}; many cations (such as Co^{++} Cu^{++}, Ni^{++}, Zn^{++}, etc.) which are not precipitated by ammonia by themselves are coprecipitated with aluminium hydroxide and are retained so strongly that a completely pure precipitate is not obtained even after reprecipitation.

Despite all these disadvantages, this method has been the most usual until recently. The most usual modern method is by precipitation of Al^{+++} with an organic reagent, 8-hydroxyquinoline (as was noted in Sec. 35).

---

* Before the sample is weighed the wire must be cleaned with emery paper to remove rust and then rubbed with a piece of filter paper.

** The solution must be exactly neutral (pH = 7); this can be done by performing the precipitation in presence of phenol red indicator, which has an orange colour at this pH.

The composition of 8-hydroxyquinoline corresponds to the formula

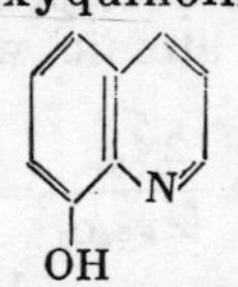

The following reaction takes place when Al^{+++} is precipitated with hydroxyquinoline:

$$Al^{+++} + 3H(C_9H_6NO) = \downarrow Al(C_9H_6NO)_3 + 3H^+$$

The precipitate is a chelate compound, in which one aluminium atom replaces hydrogen atoms of the hydroxyl groups in three hydroxyquinoline molecules, and also forms coordination bonds with nitrogen atoms:

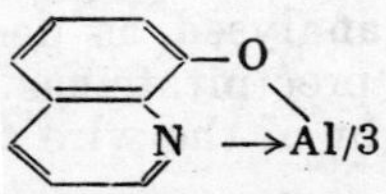

Since the reaction releases H^+ ions into solution, the degree of precipitation depends on the pH. Practically complete precipitation is achieved at pH = 4-10 (p. 142). It is performed in practice at pH of about 5, attained by addition of ammonium or sodium acetate to the acid solution.

The aluminium complex of hydroxyquinoline is a crystalline precipitate, unlike $Al(OH)_3$; it is easy to filter off and to wash. Ignition converts it into Al_2O_3. However, it is preferable to dry the precipitate to constant weight instead of igniting it, as the weighed form $Al(C_9H_6NO)_3$ is not hygroscopic and contains a much lower percentage* of aluminium than Al_2O_3 does. Obviously in this case the precipitate must be collected in a glass filter crucible (or a Gooch crucible) and not in a paper filter.

It was said in Sec. 35 that hydroxyquinoline is one of the most important organic reagents used in quantitative analysis. It was first recommended for determination of magnesium by R. Berg in 1923, but since then it has come to be widely used for determination of various other elements.

Procedure. Weigh out a sample of alum $KAl(SO_4)_2 \cdot 12H_2O$; the amount of Al in it should not exceed 0.05 g. Dissolve it in 100-150 ml of water, *slightly* acidify the solution with 2 *N* H_2SO_4 or HCl, add 30 ml of the precipitant (solution of 8-hydroxyquinoline in acetic acid**) and heat almost to boiling. Then transfer the beaker to a boiling water bath.

* This is an advantage because experimental errors have less effect on the final result than they would if Al_2O_3 is used as the weighed form (see Sec. 17).

** 3 g of 8-hydroxyquinoline is dissolved in the smallest possible amount of glacial acetic acid. The solution is diluted with water to 100 ml and ammo-

To precipitate $Al(C_9H_6NO)_3$ it is necessary to remove the H^+ ions introduced with the reagent* and formed during the reaction. To do this, add 2 *N* CH_3COONH_4 or CH_3COONa drop by drop to the solution until persistent turbidity appears. Interrupt the addition of 8-hydroxyquinoline for a few minutes in order to give the initially amorphous precipitate of the aluminium complex time to pass into the crystalline form. The rest of the solution (50 ml if the Al^{+++} content is about 0.05 g) may then be added.

The solution over the precipitate should be yellow (or orange-yellow), indicating an excess of 8-hydroxyquinoline. Let the solution with the precipitate stand for 10-15 minutes on the water bath, and then filter through a glass filter crucible, which must previously have been washed and dried to constant weight at 130°C. The filtration technique is described in Sec. 40.

Note. Sometimes the filtrate becomes turbid, either because of separation of 8-hydroxyquinoline on cooling, or because of continuing precipitation of $Al(C_9H_6NO)_3$, not completed at the proper time. Heat the solution to find the cause of the turbidity. It the turbidity disappears (indicating excess of reagent) it may be ignored. Otherwise the beaker with its contents must be kept for some time on the water bath, and the liquid must then be filtered again through the same crucible.

Wash the precipitated complex first with a small amount of hot water** and then with cold water; continue the washing until the filtrate is quite colourless.

Dry the crucible with the washed precipitate at 130°C (not higher, because partial decomposition may occur) to constant weight.

Calculation. Having found the weight of the $Al(C_9H_6NO)_3$ precipitate, calculate its aluminium content and express it as a percentage of the alum sample taken. Compare the result with the theoretical content of aluminium in alum, calculated from the formula $KAl(SO_4)_2 \cdot 12H_2O$.

43. Determination of Calcium in Calcium Carbonate

The substance to be analysed ($CaCO_3$) is insoluble in water. Before analysis a weighed sample must be dissolved in acid; for example:

$$CaCO_3 + 2HCl = CaCl_2 + H_2O + \uparrow CO_2$$

For quantitative determination Ca^{++} is precipitated in the form of calcium oxalate $CaC_2O_4 \cdot H_2O$ (salt of oxalic acid $H_2C_2O_4$).

---

nia is added drop by drop to the first appearance of turbidity which is then cleared by a few drops of CH_3OOH.

** The solubility of the precipitate in hot water is quite considerable. Therefore, hot water can be used for washing only as long as a sufficient excess of 8-hydroxyquinoline is present.

A solution of $(NH_4)_2C_2O_4$ is used; this reacts with $CaCl_2$ as follows:

$$CaCl_2 + (NH_4)_2C_2O_4 + H_2O = \downarrow CaC_2O_4 \cdot H_2O + 2NH_4Cl$$

The tendency of $CaC_2O_4 \cdot H_2O$ to form a microcrystalline precipitate which can pass through the filter greatly complicates the work. Therefore, it is very important in this case to observe the most important condition for formation of sufficiently coarse-grained precipitates; namely, to precipitate from a slightly supersaturated solution.

This is achieved by precipitation of CaC_2O_4 from an acid rather than a neutral solution (Sec. 25).

Let us consider what occurs in greater detail. Oxalic acid dissociates as follows:

$$H_2C_2O_4 \rightleftarrows H^+ + HC_2O_4^- \text{ (first stage)}$$

$$HC_2O_4^- \rightleftarrows H^+ + C_2O_4^{--} \text{ (second stage)}$$

The respective dissociation constants are:

$$K_1 = \frac{[H^+][HC_2O_4^-]}{[H_2C_2O_4]} = 5.9 \times 10^{-2}$$

$$K_2 = \frac{[H^+][C_2O_4^{--}]}{[HC_2O_4^-]} = 6.4 \times 10^{-5}$$

The $C_2O_4^{--}$ ions required appear as the result of the second dissociation stage; the value of the corresponding constant (K_2) shows that this dissociation is relatively slight. It follows that if the solution is acidified most of the $C_2O_4^{--}$ ions introduced in the form of $(NH_4)_2C_2O_4$ are combined as $HC_2O_4^-$ anions and then as free $H_2C_2O_4$:

$$C_2O_4^{--} + H^+ = HC_2O_4^-$$

$$HC_2O_4^- + H^+ = H_2C_2O_4$$

Their concentration therefore decreases progressively with the amount of H^+ ions introduced into the solution. At a high enough solution acidity the $C_2O_4^{--}$ concentration falls so much that the solubility product of CaC_2O_4

$$SP_{CaC_2O_4} = [Ca^{++}][C_2O_4^{--}] = 2.6 \times 10^{-9}$$

is not reached and no precipitate is formed.

However, if NH_4OH is added drop by drop to this acid solution, the H^+ ion concentration gradually falls while the $C_2O_4^{--}$ ion concentration rises.

Eventually, the product of concentrations $[Ca^{++}]\,[C_2O_4^{--}]$ becomes greater than the solubility product of the precipitate and the latter begins to form. Because the ammonia is added drop by drop the $C_2O_4^{--}$ ion concentration rises very slowly and gradually.

Therefore, the precipitation proceeds all the time from a solution very slightly supersaturated with CaC_2O_4, and the crystals are able to grow sufficiently.

The precipitation of Ca^{++} ions becomes increasingly complete with decrease of the H^+ ions concentration in solution.

Calculations (pp. 86-87) show that the precipitation is practically complete at $pH \geqslant 3.3$.

Any further addition of NH_4OH is pointless. To detect the point when the solution pH becomes 4 the precipitation should be performed in presence of methyl orange indicator, which changes its colour from pink to yellow at approximately this pH.

The CaC_2O_4 precipitate is appreciably soluble in water, and washing it with pure water would result in noticeable loss. Therefore, $C_2O_4^{--}$ ions must be introduced into the washing liquid to lower the solubility of the precipitate.

Removal of Cl^- ions by washing prevents losses due to formation of volatile $CaCl_2$ during ignition of the precipitate.

The usual weighed form in this determination is calcium oxide CaO, formed from $CaC_2O_4 \cdot H_2O$ at 900-1200°C by the reaction:

$$CaC_2O_4 \cdot H_2O \rightleftarrows CaO + \uparrow CO_2 + \uparrow CO + \uparrow H_2O$$

The disadvantage of CaO as the weighed form is that it is hygroscopic and adsorbs CO_2 from the air, so that suitable precautions must be taken in weighing. Moreover, the percentage content of Ca in CaO (and therefore the conversion factor) is high, which is also a disadvantage (p. 127).

Because of these disadvantages of CaO as the weighed form, it is sometimes preferred to convert $CaC_2O_4 \cdot H_2O$ into $CaCO_3$ by ignition at about 500°C or into $CaSO_4$ by treatment with H_2SO_4 solution, with subsequent removal of excess acid by careful evaporation and ignition of the dry residue.

Procedure. Weigh out a sample of chemically pure $CaCO_3$, calculated to contain about 0.1 g of Ca, into a 300 ml beaker with a lip. Put 5-10 ml of distilled water into the beaker and cover it with a watch glass to catch drops of liquid splashed out with the gas given off when the substance dissolves. Raise the watch glass very slightly and pour HCl (1 : 1) solution drop by drop carefully down the side of the beaker. After addition of each drop gently swirl the contents of the beaker by a smooth circular movement.

When all the substance has dissolved, rinse the sprayed liquid from the watch glass into the beaker with a jet of water from the wash bottle. Dilute the solution with water to about 100 ml and add 5 ml of HCl (1 : 1) solution, 35 ml of 0.5 N $(NH_4)_2C_2O_4$ solution, and 1-3 drops of methyl orange indicator. Heat the liquid to 70-80°C and add 5% NH_4OH solution slowly, drop by drop (1-2 drops per second) with continuous stirring. Continue the addition until the pink colour disappears,* and then allow the precipitate to settle completely (it is best to leave it overnight).

Decant the clear liquid through a dense filter paper (blue band) 7 cm in diameter and wash the precipitate three times by decantation with 0.5 *N* $(NH_4)_2C_2O_4$ solution diluted five- or six-fold with water. Then transfer the precipitate quantitatively to the filter and wash it until almost free of Cl^- ions (i.e., to the point when about 5 ml of the filtrate, acidified with 2 *N* HNO_3 solution to prevent precipitation of $Ag_2C_2O_4$, no longer gives turbidity with $AgNO_3$ solution**). Dry the washed precipitate in the drying oven.

While the precipitate is drying, prepare the crucible.

To avoid adsorption of water vapour and CO_2 from the air by the ignited CaO either it must be weighed very rapidly with the required weights and rider (in repeated weighings) previously put on the balance, or the crucible must be weighed in an air-tight stoppered bottle. In the latter case, of course, the same bottle must be used for weighing the empty crucible when it is being heated to constant weight.***

Transfer the dried precipitate on the filter into the crucible, put the latter in a triangle supported by a ring on the stand, and char the filter over a small burner flame. Then *carefully* ignite the crucible with the precipitate for some time, raising the temperature very slowly so as to avoid spattering of the precipitate by excessively rapid evolution of gases (CO_2 and CO) and water vapour.

The heating must then be intensified. After the carbon has burnt away transfer the crucible with the precipitate to a muffle (or crucible) furnace and heat it there for about an hour. Then cool the crucible in a desiccator and weigh as described above.

Continue the repeated heatings (about half an hour each) until the weight becomes constant; this takes some time, because calcium oxalate is a very difficult precipitate to decompose.

Calculation. Find the amount of Ca in the $CaCO_3$ sample in the usual way from the weight and formula of the precipitate (CaO) and express the result as a percentage. Compare your result with the theoretical percentage content of Ca in the compound with the formula $CaCO_3$.

---

* The solution turns yellow, but against the background of the white precipitate this is usually seen as decolorization of the pink solution.

** A slight opalescence is permissible in this test.

*** When weighing the crucible in a weighing bottle, avoid heating the air contained in the bottle (otherwise the weight of the bottle alters). Therefore, when putting the bottle on the balance pan, it should be touched only with the tips of the fingers for a short time. It is best to handle the bottle with crucible tongs tipped with pieces of rubber tubing.

44. Determination of Carbon Dioxide in Calcium Carbonate

The CO_2 contents of carbonates are determined by the volatilization method, a weighed sample being treated in a special apparatus with dilute HCl.

In the case of $CaCO_3$ the reaction is:

$$CaCO_3 + 2HCl = CaCl_2 + H_2O + CO_2 \uparrow$$

The amount of CO_2 given off is found (a) from the loss in weight of the apparatus containing the weighed sample (indirect method); (b) from the increase in weight of an absorbent, such as soda lime

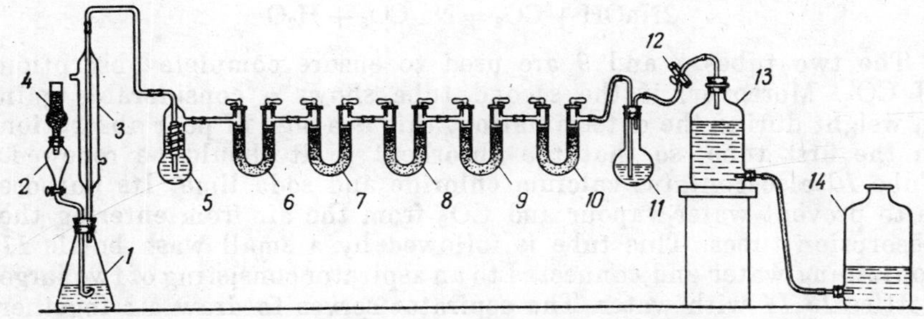

Fig. 28. Apparatus for CO_2 determination:
1—conical flask; *2*—dropping funnel; *3*—condenser; *4*—absorption tube; *5*, *11*—wash bottles; *6*, *7*, *8*, *9*, *10*—U-tubes; *12*—clip; *13*, *14*—aspirator bottles

(a mixture of NaOH with CaO), due to absorption of the liberated CO_2 (direct method). As we have already considered indirect methods for determination of volatile components in determination of water of crystallization and of hygroscopic water, only the direct method is described here.

In this method a weighed sample of the carbonate is treated with hydrochloric acid in the conical flask *1* (Fig. 28). Plugged in the neck of this flask is a bung through which are inserted a dropping funnel *2* fitted with a long tube with its tip bent upwards (so that the liberated CO_2 does not enter the tube) and a reflux condenser *3* which condenses most of the steam formed when the liquid in the flask is boiled. The top of the dropping funnel is closed by a bung through which is inserted an absorption tube *4* containing soda lime or ascarite* (soda asbestos) to remove CO_2 from the air drawn

* Ascarite is a mixture of asbestos with NaOH; it is made by impregnation of fibrous asbestos with highly concentrated NaOH solution and drying at 150-180°C. It should be ground down to pieces about the size of a wheat grain. Ascarite (or soda lime) is contained in the tube *4* between two layers of cotton wool.

through the apparatus. The top of the condenser is connected to an absorption system consisting of a wash bottle *5* with concentrated H_2SO_4 to absorb most of the water vapour leaving the condenser; a U-tube *6* containing pieces of pumice impregnated with anhydrous copper sulphate* for absorption of HCl (and any H_2S which may be evolved); a U-tube *7* with granulated calcium chloride** to retain the last traces of water vapour; and the U-tubes *8* and *9* for absorption of CO_2. Each of these U-tubes is two-thirds filled with soda lime or ascarite, the rest of the space being filled with granulated calcium chloride. The purpose of the latter is to retain the water vapour formed in the absorption of CO_2:

$$2NaOH + CO_2 = Na_2CO_3 + H_2O$$

The two tubes *8* and *9* are used to ensure complete absorption of CO_2. Moreover, if the second tube shows a considerable gain in weight during the determination, this is a sign of poor absorption in the first tube, so that the absorbent in it should be renewed. Tube *10* also contains calcium chloride and soda lime. Its purpose is to prevent water vapour and CO_2 from the air from entering the absorption tubes. This tube is followed by a small wash bottle *11* containing water and connected to an aspirator consisting of two large bottles *13*,*14* with water. The aspirator serves to draw air together with the CO_2 formed by the reaction through the whole system of absorbers. The rate of suction is regulated by the screw clip *12*. The separate absorbers are suspended by means of wire from a horizontal iron rod clamped in a stand.

Before the determination the apparatus must be tested for air-tightness. The top of the tube *4* is firmly closed with a rubber bung and the clip *12* is slightly opened so that 2-3 bubbles of air pass through the wash bottle *11* per second. If the apparatus is air-tight the bubbling soon stops.

Procedure. After preparing the apparatus as described above weigh out about 1 g of chemically pure $CaCO_3$ (or the mineral calcite) on a watch glass and transfer it quantitatively to the flask *1*.

---

* This is prepared by impregnation of pumice, crushed to about the size of a wheat grain, with saturated $CuSO_4$ solution and drying at 150-180°C. The material should be kept in a tightly closed vessel.

** Commercial calcium chloride is usually contaminated with lime, $Ca(OH)_2$. The latter absorbs CO_2 and is therefore inadmissible. Therefore, after the tubes have been filled with calcium chloride carbon dioxide is passed through them to convert $Ca(OH)_2$ into $CaCO_3$. Excess CO_2 is then removed by a current of dry air. Other absorbents are also used for absorption of water vapour, such as phosphoric anhydride P_2O_5, anhydrous magnesium perchlorate $Mg(ClO_4)_2$ ("anhydrone") or its hydrated form $Mg(ClO_4)_2 \cdot 3H_2O$ ("dehydrite"), etc.

Add enough water to cover the upturned tip of the funnel tube and attach the flask to the apparatus.

Now close the taps of the absorption tubes *8* and *9* and take them out of the system. Connect tube *7* directly to tube *10* and draw air through the whole system by means of the aspirator. This air is free from CO_2 which is removed in tube *4* filled with soda lime (or ascarite). The purpose of this operation is to remove CO_2 from the apparatus; it should be carried out fairly slowly* and should continue for 15-20 minutes. During this time weigh the absorption tubes *8* and *9* on the analytical balance. Before the weighing wipe the tubes thoroughly with a dry cloth and open their taps for an instant (to equalize the pressure). When air has been drawn through the system for a sufficient time put the weighed tubes *8* and *9* back in their places in the system. The side of each tube containing soda lime (or ascarite) should be towards the flask. Do not forget to open the tube taps.

Now take the calcium chloride tube *4* out of the funnel *2* and pour 50 ml of dilute (1:1) HCl solution into the funnel. Put the tube *4* back into the funnel and add acid from the funnel into the flask very slowly (drop by drop); CO_2 starts to come off at once. *Regulate the addition of* HCl *so that not more than 3-4 gas bubbles pass through the wash bottles (5 and 11) per second*, otherwise some CO_2 may escape absorption.

After all the acid has been added and evolution of CO_2 has slowed down, turn on the water in the condenser *3* and start to heat the flask very slowly, regulating the heating in accordance with the rate of bubbling through the absorbers. Eventually bring the liquid in the flask to the boil and draw a slow stream (2-3 bubbles per second) of air free from CO_2 through the solution for about 20 minutes by means of the aspirator. Then weigh the absorption tubes *8* and *9* again after they have been left for 20 minutes near the balance,** proceeding as in the first weighing.

With correct working the second tube should show very little increase in weight.

Calculation. Add the weight increases of both tubes together to find the weight of CO_2 given off; express it as a percentage of the sample taken. If chemically pure $CaCO_3$ was used for the analysis, compare your result with the percentage calculated from the formula and find the percentage error.

---

* Not more than 3-4 bubbles per second should pass through the wash bottle *11*.

** The tubes become appreciably warm during the absorption of CO_2.

45. Determination of Magnesium in Magnesium Sulphate

For quantitative determination, magnesium is precipitated either as the double phosphate of magnesium and ammonium, $MgNH_4PO_4 \cdot 6H_2O$, or as the hydroxyquinoline complex $Mg(C_9H_6NO)_2 \cdot 2H_2O$. We shall consider only the first of these methods. In this method the PO_4^{---} ions required to precipitate Mg^{++} are added in the form of Na_2HPO_4, and NH_4^+ ions are introduced with NH_4OH. The reaction can be represented by the equation:

$$MgSO_4 + Na_2HPO_4 + NH_4OH = \downarrow MgNH_4PO_4 + Na_2SO_4 + H_2O$$

When ignited, the precipitate loses ammonia and water and is converted into magnesium pyrophosphate $Mg_2P_2O_7$, which is the weighed form:

$$2MgNH_4PO_4 = Mg_2P_2O_7 + \uparrow 2NH_3 + \uparrow H_2O$$

It is known that ammonia is partially dissociated in aqueous solutions:

$$NH_4OH \rightleftarrows NH_4^+ + OH^-$$

Its dissociation constant is small, namely:

$$K = \frac{[NH_4^+][OH^-]}{[NH_4OH]} = 1.79 \times 10^{-5} \qquad (1)$$

Nevertheless, the OH^- ion concentration due to the ammonia is sufficient for the ionic product $[Mg^{++}]\,[OH^-]^2$ to exceed the solubility product of $Mg(OH)_2$, which is 5×10^{-12} (at 25°C). It follows that $Mg(OH)_2$ may be precipitated together with the required compound ($MgNH_4PO_4$), which would make the result wrong. To avoid this, NH_4Cl is added during the precipitation; this salt, having a common ion with NH_4OH, strongly suppresses dissociation of the latter. We see in Equation (1) that, since K is constant, the large increase of the NH_4^+ ion concentration due to the presence of NH_4Cl, and therefore the increase of the numerator, must lead to a corresponding increase of the denominator, i.e., of the concentration of undissociated NH_4OH molecules. In other words, NH_4^+ ions of the salt combine with OH^- ions of the ammonia solution, and the OH^- ion concentration falls so much that the ionic product $[Mg^{++}]\,[OH^-]^2$ becomes less than the solubility product of $Mg(OH)_2$, so that magnesium hydroxide is not precipitated.

However, a large excess of NH_4Cl should be avoided, as it favours the formation of the double salt $Mg(NH_4)_4(PO_4)_2$; this is undesirable because it yields P_2O_5 as well as $Mg_2P_2O_7$ when ignited.*

To obtain good crystalline $MgNH_4PO_4$ precipitates, they are precipitated from hydrochloric acid solutions containing Na_2HPO_4 and NH_4Cl by slow addition of dilute ammonia solution. The HCl is neutralized first, and the $MgNH_4PO_4$ precipitate is then formed. Different authors recommend different temperatures for the precipitation. The method described below is that of N. Tananayev; here the precipitation is performed at 40-45°C.

The $MgNH_4PO_4$ precipitate is appreciably soluble in water. From the equation

$$[Mg^{++}][NH_4^+][PO_4^{---}] = 2.5 \times 10^{-13}$$

we have

$$[Mg^{++}] = [NH_4^+] = [PO_4^{---}] = \sqrt[3]{2.5 \times 10^{-13}} = 6.3 \times 10^{-5}\,M$$

Therefore, 1 litre of solution contains $6.3 \times 10^{-5} \times 137 = 0.0086$ g of $MgNH_4PO_4$ in the form of ions.

In reality this rather high solubility is raised still further because of extensive hydrolysis of $MgNH_4PO_4$ with the formation of the more soluble acid salt:

$$MgNH_4PO_4 + H_2O \rightleftarrows MgHPO_4 + NH_4OH$$

The following calculation shows the extent of the $MgNH_4PO_4$ hydrolysis. Phosphoric acid dissociates in three stages; the dissociation constants are:

$$K_1 = \frac{[H^+][H_2PO_4^-]}{[H_3PO_4]} = 7.5 \times 10^{-3} \quad K_2 = \frac{[H^+][HPO_4^{--}]}{[H_2PO_4^-]} = 6.2 \times 10^{-8}$$

and

$$K_3 = \frac{[H^+][PO_4^{---}]}{[HPO_4^{--}]} = 2.2 \times 10^{-13}$$

Suppose that the solution pH is 7, i.e., that $[H^+] = 10^{-7}$ g-ion/litre. Then from the equation for K_3 we have:

$$\frac{[PO_4^{---}]}{[HPO_4^{--}]} = \frac{K_3}{[H^+]} = \frac{2.2 \times 10^{-13}}{10^{-7}} = 2.2 \times 10^{-6}$$

This result shows that even in a strictly neutral medium the PO_4^{---} ion concentration is only 0.000002 of the HPO_4^{--} concentration. It is easy to find (do this) from the equation for K_2 that nearly one half of all the HPO_4^{--} ions formed

---

* When ignited, $Mg(NH_4)_4(PO_4)_2$ is first converted into magnesium metaphosphate:

$$Mg(NH_4)_4(PO_4)_2 = Mg(PO_3)_2 + \uparrow 4NH_3 + \uparrow 2H_2O$$

On further heating the metaphosphate forms magnesium pyrophosphate and phosphoric anhydride:

$$2Mg(PO_3)_2 = Mg_2P_2O_7 + P_2O_5$$

are subsequently converted into $H_2PO_4^-$ ions:

$$HPO_4^{--} + H_2O \rightleftarrows H_2PO_4^- + OH^- \text{ (second hydrolysis stage)}$$

A similar calculation for pH = 12 shows that the HPO_4^{--} concentration is only 5 times the PO_4^{---} concentration, and not 500,000 times as at pH = 7.

This calculation shows that even in neutral solution nearly all the $MgNH_4PO_4$ is converted into $MgHPO_4$ and $Mg(H_2PO_4)_2$ as the result of hydrolysis, so that the solubility should increase considerably. However, the same calculation shows that hydrolysis is very much suppressed by increase of the solution pH. Therefore, at the end of the precipitation an excess of ammonia solution is added; this acts not only by its OH^- ions but also by NH_4^+ ions, common with the precipitate. With the same object of suppressing hydrolysis and decreasing solubility, dilute NH_4OH solution and not pure water is used to wash $MgNH_4PO_4$.

The tendency of $MgNH_4PO_4$ to form supersaturated solutions must be taken into account; accordingly, the precipitate must not be filtered off for at least 2-3 hours after formation.

Ignition of $MgNH_4PO_4$ precipitates involves certain difficulties. The reason is that this is a fairly fusible salt. When it melts it covers unburnt carbon particles and thus protects them from the air, so that complete combustion of the carbon becomes impossible. To avoid this, the filter should be ashed at the lowest temperature possible. It is easier to burn out the carbon if most of the precipitate is first removed from the filter, as is done in the determination of Cl^- in the form of AgCl. Alternatively, if the precipitate is dark because of the presence of unburnt carbon, it can be treated with a few drops of HNO_3. The excess nitric acid is removed by careful evaporation and the precipitate is then ignited. It must be remembered that *great care is needed* in both these methods. Careless work may result in large losses.

Procedure. Put an accurately weighed sample of about 0.7-0.9 g of crystalline magnesium sulphate $MgSO_4 \cdot 7H_2O$ into a 200-300 ml beaker and dissolve it in 50-60 ml of water. Acidify the solution with 5 ml of 2 *N* HCl, and add 15-20 ml of previously filtered 7% Na_2HPO_4 solution and 10 ml of 2 *N* NH_4Cl solution.* Heat the solution to 40-45°C and add 2.5% ammonia solution rapidly drop by drop,** stirring the liquid continuously with a glass rod. When the precipitate which forms begins to disappear rather slowly on stirring, slow down the ammonia addition to about 4-5 drops per

---

* If a precipitate forms when the solutions are mixed, it must be dissolved by addition of 2 *N* hydrochloric acid.

** This is most conveniently done from a burette or a dropping funnel with a tap.

minute. Continue the addition until the solution smells of ammonia. Stir the contents of the beaker vigorously all the time, taking care not to touch the bottom or sides of the beaker with the rod (the precipitate sticks to the glass at points of contact).

When the solution is quite cool add a further 25-30 ml of 10% ammonia solution to suppress hydrolysis and decrease solubility of $MgNH_4PO_4$, and leave for 2-3 hours. Then filter through a medium paper (white band) 9 cm in diameter. After all the liquid has been decanted from the precipitate wash the latter three times by decantation and then transfer it quantitatively to the filter, removing particles sticking to the glass with a rubber-tipped glass rod, and wash it with 2.5% ammonia solution, in which the precipitate is less soluble than in pure water (see above). The washing can be stopped when a portion of the filtrate, acidified with HNO_3,* does not give turbidity with $AgNO_3$ or $Hg_2(NO_3)_2$ (if all Cl^- ions have been removed we can be certain that all other extraneous substances such as Na_2HPO_4 have been washed out too).

When the washing is ended, it is useful to fill the filter with a mixture of 4 ml of 33% NH_4NO_3 and 1 ml of 1% NH_4OH to make subsequent ashing easier. When the liquid has drained out completely put the filter in its funnel into a drying oven and dry it thoroughly at 100°C. Then ash the filter separately from the precipitate as described for the determination of Cl^- (p. 162). Remember that *the ashing must be performed very carefully at the lowest possible temperature*, otherwise the precipitate on the filter would melt and make complete combustion of the carbon impossible.

When the filter has been ashed, transfer the separated precipitate quantitatively into the crucible and start ignition. As was said earlier, the precipitate loses water and ammonia and is converted into magnesium pyrophosphate $Mg_2P_2O_7$. The liberation of the gases should be as slow as possible to prevent loss of the precipitate; accordingly, the crucible must be heated very cautiously at the start. When evolution of ammonia has ceased the heating should be intensified. After half an hour of heating over the full flame transfer the crucible into a muffle furnace and continue heating it to constant weight.

Note. As was said earlier (124) it is possible to perform the ignition without removing the precipitate from the filter. In this case, however, if the precipitate is more or less dark owing to the presence of unburnt carbon, it should be treated in the crucible with a few drops of concentrated HNO_3. The excess acid is then removed by evaporation *to dryness on a water bath* (not on a gauze, because this inevitably leads to serious losses). When the precipitate is quite dry it is ignited. The ignition must again be started *very cautiously*, with the crucible high

* AgCl cannot be precipitated in an ammoniacal solution unless the latter is acidified, as it is soluble in ammonia.

above the flame. The heating is intensified very slowly, otherwise the gaseous nitrogen dioxide NO_2 liberated in the reaction would cause spattering of precipitate.

This procedure can also be used if the precipitate has been ignited separately from the filter but is nevertheless very dark (a faint colour may be ignored, as it has hardly any effect on the result).

Calculation. The result is calculated by proportion:

$$Mg_2P_2O_7 - 2Mg$$
$$a - x$$
$$x = a\frac{2Mg}{Mg_2P_2O_7} = a \times 0.2183 \text{ g Mg}$$

where a is the weight in grams of the $Mg_2P_2O_7$ precipitate.

The percentage of magnesium in the sample is calculated from the weight found. If chemically pure magnesium sulphate was taken for analysis, the accuracy of the result is checked against the formula $MgSO_4 \cdot 7H_2O$. Otherwise duplicate determinations are necessary.

46. Determination of Phosphate in Sodium Phosphate

The phosphate contents of soluble salts of phosphoric acid, such as $Na_2HPO_4 \cdot 12H_2O$, etc., are determined by a method quite analogous to that described in the preceding section. The only difference is that the reagent used is not sodium phosphate but a specially prepared mixture of $MgCl_2$, NH_4Cl, and HCl, known as "magnesia mixture".*

Procedure. Weigh out accurately about 0.8 g of $Na_2HPO_4 \cdot 12H_2O$, dissolve it in 50-60 ml of water, and add 5 ml of 2 *N* NH_4Cl solution and 15 ml of magnesia mixture. Now precipitate $MgNH_4PO_4$ by addition of ammonia; this (like all the subsequent operations) is done exactly as in the determination of magnesium (see Sec. 45). The only difference is that, to avoid precipitation of $Mg(OH)_2$, 10% ammonia solution must be added at the end of precipitation by small portions to the stirred solution and not all at once.

Calculation. Phosphate contents are usually expressed as percentages of P_2O_5. It is evident that one gram-molecule of $Mg_2P_2O_7$ (222.6 g) corresponds to one gram-molecule 141.9 g of P_2O_5. From this, calculate the weight of P_2O_5 in the $Mg_2P_2O_7$ precipitate and express the result as a percentage of the weight of $Na_2HPO_4 \cdot 12H_2O$ taken. As this salt effloresces rapidly in air, duplicate determinations are necessary to confirm the precision of the analysis.

* To prepare magnesia mixture, dissolve 55 g of $MgCl_2 \cdot 6H_2O$ and 105 g of NH_4Cl in water and make the volume up to 1 litre with water slightly acidified with HCl.

47. Determination of Calcium and Magnesium When Present Together

For quantitative determination of Mg^{++} it is precipitated as $MgNH_4PO_4$ in presence of ammonia. Under these conditions Ca^{++} also forms a sparingly soluble salt, $Ca_3(PO_4)_2$. Therefore, if the cations Ca^{++} and Mg^{++} are present together in a solution, which often happens in analysis of various natural materials or industrial products, Ca^{++} must first be precipitated as oxalate and thus separated from Mg^{++} before the latter can be determined.

For separation of Ca^{++} from Mg^{++} excess $(NH_4)_2C_2O_4$ is added. This precipitates Ca^{++} completely but does not precipitate Mg^{++}, which forms a complex with $C_2O_4^{--}$.

In reality, however, appreciable amounts of magnesium enter the precipitate because of coprecipitation and especially of post-precipitation (see p. 112). Therefore, the magnesium content found by analysis is too low, and the calcium content too high. This error is avoided by reprecipitation of CaC_2O_4 (p. 113). For the same reason the first precipitation of Ca^{++} is carried out in a fairly dilute solution.

After separation of the precipitate all the Mg^{++} of the original solution is contained in the filtrates and washings from both precipitations of Ca^{++}. It cannot be precipitated directly from such a dilute solution. Moreover, very large amounts of ammonium salts are added during the precipitation of Ca^{++}. In presence of a large excess of ammonium salts a precipitate with the composition of $Mg(NH_4)_4(PO_4)_2$ (see p. 176) may be formed instead of $MgNH_4PO_4$, giving rise to errors.

To avoid this error, ammonia salts must be removed by evaporation and calcination, or (which is simpler) $MgNH_4PO_4$ may be reprecipitated.

Procedure. *Determination of* Ca^{++}. To the solution under analysis, containing not more than 0.1 g Ca^{++} and 0.07 g Mg^{++}, add 5 ml of dilute (1 : 1) HCl solution and 50 ml of 0.5 *N* $(NH_4)_2C_2O_4$, and dilute with water to about 200 ml. Add 3-5 drops of methyl orange indicator, heat the solution to 70-80°C, and precipitate Ca^{++} by slow addition (1-2 drops per second) of dilute (2.5%) ammonia solution until the pink colour of the indicator disappears completely (the indicator turns yellow), stirring the solution vigorously all the time with a glass rod.

Leave the liquid to stand for $1^1/_2$-2 hours and then decant the clear liquid through a dense filter (blue band) and wash the precipitate 2-3 times by decantation, taking 20-25 ml of the washing solution* each time, and trying not to transfer any of the precipitate to the filter. Collect the washings together with the filtrate.

* This is prepared by 5-6-fold dilution of 0.5 *N* $(NH_4)_2C_2O_4$.

Dissolve the washed precipitate in HCl as follows. Put the beaker with the precipitate under the funnel with the filter paper and pour hot dilute HCl (10% hydrochloric acid diluted with twice its own volume of water) into the funnel. When the acid has drained through, wash the filter 3-4 times with hot water* and then add 20 ml of $(NH_4)_2C_2O_4$ solution to the acid liquid. If a precipitate is formed, dissolve it in HCl. Dilute the solution to 100 ml, heat it, and reprecipitate Ca^{++} with ammonia exactly as before.

The precipitate should be left to stand for $1^1/_2$-2 hours before filtration so that the precipitation should be complete. It should not be left for longer, otherwise an appreciable amount of magnesium would be coprecipitated. The filtration and all subsequent operations are then performed as described in Sec. 43.

Determination of Mg^{++}. Combine the filtrates from the two precipitations of calcium with the washings, and evaporate down to 100-120 ml. This should be done in a porcelain basin on the water bath (see Fig. 26), but not on any account on a gauze, as losses due to splashing would be inevitable. Add 2-3 drops of methyl orange indicator to the solution and then acidify with HCl until the indicator changes from yellow to red. Precipitate magnesium from this solution in the form of $MgNH_4PO_4$ as described in Sec. 45. Leave to stand for 2-4 hours, filter off the precipitate, and wash it 6-8 times with 2.5% NH_4OH solution by decantation, taking care not to transfer the precipitate to the filter. Then put the beaker with the washed precipitate under the filter funnel and dissolve the precipitate in dilute (1 : 1) hydrochloric acid. Add the acid drop by drop, wetting the filter uniformly. When the precipitate on the filter and in the beaker has dissolved, wash the filter 7-8 times with 1% hydrochloric acid and dilute the filtrate to about 100 ml. Add 3-5 ml of Na_2HPO_4 solution and repeat the precipitation of $MgNH_4PO_4$ by the action of NH_4OH as before. After 2-4 hours filter off the precipitate, wash it, and complete the determination as described in Sec. 45.

48. Determination of Nickel in Steel

As already noted (Sec. 35) nickel is precipitated with an organic reagent, dimethylglyoxime (L. Chugayev's reagent). The reaction results in the formation of a bright red crystalline precipitate of the nickel dimethylglyoxime internal complex ("dimethylglyoximate"). The reaction equation is given on p. 139.

* In order that this filter could be used for separation of the precipitate after reprecipitation of Ca^{++} it should be washed once with water containing a little ammonia and twice with pure water, and then kept under a piece of paper or a watch glass to protect it from dust.

The presence of H^+ ions, which combine with the anions formed from dimethylglyoxime, favours the reverse reaction whereby the precipitate is dissolved. Therefore, the completeness of precipitation depends very much on the solution pH. The precipitation is satisfactorily complete even in a weakly acid solution, for example, in presence of acetate buffer mixture ($CH_3COOH + CH_3COONa$), which maintains the pH at about 5. It is even better to complete the precipitation in presence of ammonia buffer solution ($NH_4OH + + NH_4Cl$) which gives pH ≈ 9. The precipitate is much more soluble both in strongly acidic and in strongly alkaline media; in the latter case probably owing to formation of disubstituted glyoximates.

The nickel dimethylglyoximate precipitate has very valuable analytical properties. Its solubility in water is very low ($SP = = 2.3 \times 10^{-25}$) and the Ni^{++} ion concentration is about $4 \times \times 10^{-9}$ g-ion/litre. This extremely low solubility is diminished still further by excess of precipitant. Further, the fact that the precipitate is pure is very valuable. Finally, the reaction is fairly specific. The only other cations to give insoluble precipitates with dimethylglyoxime are Pd and Pt, and these are rarely met in the normal course of analysis. All this makes dimethylglyoxime the most valuable precipitant for Ni^{++}.

When this reaction is used in analysis of materials containing iron, the latter must first be oxidized to Fe^{+++}; the reason is that Fe^{++} ions, which are usually formed when the samples are dissolved in acids, form a water-soluble red complex compound, and the solubility of the nickel dimethylglyoximate precipitate increases. As the precipitation is performed in presence of ammonia, Fe^{+++} ions, which give $Fe(OH)_3$ precipitates under these conditions, must also be absent. Therefore, Fe^{+++} ions are previously masked by addition of a sufficient quantity of tartaric or citric acid; this results in the formation of stable complexes of Fe^{+++} ions, not precipitated by alkalies.

The solubility of dimethylglyoxime in water is relatively low. It is therefore used in alcoholic or ammoniacal solution. In the former case it must be remembered that the precipitate is appreciably soluble in alcohol at concentrations above 50%. Therefore, the volume of the precipitant must be less than the volume of the aqueous solution being analysed.

The most convenient way of finishing the determination is to filter off the precipitate in a glass filter crucible and to dry it at 110-120°C to constant weight. The weighed form is then nickel dimethylglyoximate, which corresponds to the empirical formula $(C_4H_7N_2O_2)_2Ni$. Alternatively, the precipitate can be collected on a paper filter, washed, ignited, and weighed as NiO. However, this is less convenient because the conversion factor in this case is four times as large. Moreover, when the precipitate is ignited there is risk of loss owing to sublimation, which occurs at about 250°C. To avoid this, the precipitate must be ignited with good access of air to assist rapid combustion of the nickel dimethylglyoximate.

Procedure. Weigh out a sample of steel containing not more than 0.03 g of nickel. For example, if the nickel content is 2-3%, the sample should be about 1 g, and at higher nickel content it should be correspondingly less. Larger samples should not be taken because the precipitate is very bulky. Put the sample in a 300-400 ml beaker and dissolve it in 25-30 ml of dilute (1 : 1) HCl (in a fume cupboard), heating the beaker on a sand bath* or electric hot-plate, and covering it with a watch glass. Continue the heating until no more hydrogen bubbles are given off. Then oxidize Fe^{++} and carbides of nickel, iron, and other metals by careful addition of 3-5 ml of concentrated HNO_3. To do this, take the beaker off the sand bath or hot-plate, raise the watch glass slightly on one side, and pour in nitric acid in small portions down the side of the beaker. The first additions turn the liquid brown and brown nitrous fumes (NO_2) are abundantly evolved. When the HNO_3 has been added heat the solution again until the evolution of nitrous fumes ceases. Rinse any drops of solution off the watch glass into the beaker with a jet of water from a wash bottle, remove the watch glass, and dilute the solution to 120-150 ml with water. Add 5-7 g of solid tartaric acid (or 10-15 ml of a 50% solution) to complex the Fe^{+++} ions. After the tartaric acid has dissolved add ammonia to the solution until the smell persists. The solution must remain quite clear, as this shows that enough tartaric acid has been added. If the solution becomes turbid on addition of ammonia more tartaric acid must be added until it becomes clear again.

Now add dilute HCl to the ammoniacal solution to an acid reaction. If a small precipitate is found on the bottom of the beaker, collect it on a fast filter paper and wash it several times with hot water, combining the washings with the filtrate.**

Precipitate nickel from the solution as follows. Add 18-20 ml of 1% alcoholic dimethylglyoxime solution, heat to 80-90°C, and at once add NH_4OH solution drop by drop until the liquid smells of ammonia, stirring the liquid continuously with a glass rod. As in precipitation of CaC_2O_4 (p. 171), slow addition of ammonia gives a precipitate with larger crystals. The precipitate does not

* A sand bath is a metal vessel containing sand, heated by gas or electricity. The heating can be easily regulated by varying the thickness of the sand layer.

** The precipitate may contain carbon and silicic, tungstic and niobic acids.

always settle to the bottom of the beaker but may float on top. This does not affect the determination.

About one hour after the precipitation start the filtration. First, prepare (i.e., dry at 110-120°C and weigh) a No. 3 or No. 4 filter crucible. Insert it in the neck of a suction flask (see Fig. 19) and connect the flask to a water-jet pump. Before the filtration add a few drops of dimethylglyoxime solution to the clear liquid above the precipitate to confirm that the precipitation was complete. Now turn on the pump and filter. Transfer the precipitate to the crucible and wash it thoroughly until a portion of the washings acidified with HNO_3 gives a negative reaction for Cl^- ion. Dry the washed precipitate to constant weight at 110-120°C. Find the weight of nickel in the sample and its percentage content in the steel from the formula $(C_4H_7N_2O_2)_2Ni$ and the weight of the precipitate.

QUESTIONS AND PROBLEMS
(on Secs. 36-48)

1. In what cases do crystalline hydrates effloresce in air?
2. Why do crystalline hydrates decompose when heated, with formation of the corresponding anhydrous salts?
3. How is water of crystallization in crystalline hydrates determined? What does constancy of weight indicate in the determination?
4. What is hygroscopic water? How is it determined? What are the possible sources of error in determination of hygroscopic water in various substances?
5. A certain substance contains 15.00% of hygroscopic water. Its nitrogen content was found by analysis to be 4.25%. Calculate the nitrogen content of the absolutely dry substance.

Answer: 5.00%.

6. Why is Ba^{++} precipitated with H_2SO_4 and not with Na_2SO_4?
7. Explain the conditions for precipitation of Ba^{++}. Why is this precipitation performed in presence of HCl?
8. What happens to $BaSO_4$ during ashing of the filter and subsequent ignition of the precipitate?
9. For what purposes are (a) empty crucibles, (b) crucibles with precipitates, heated to constant weight?
10. What weight of H_2SO_4 is contained in 1 litre of sulphuric acid solution if 0.2126 g of $BaSO_4$ is formed from 50.00 ml of the solution by the action of $BaCl_2$ solution?

Answer: 1.787 g.

11. Why is the solution acidified, heated and stirred vigorously in precipitation of AgCl?
12. Explain why silver chloride eventually begins to pass through the filter and the filtrate becomes turbid after prolonged washing with pure water. Would this happen if AgCl was washed with HNO_3 solution?
13. Why must not AgCl be ignited with a paper filter? Why is it better to use a Sintered glass crucible in this case?
14. Will AgCl be precipitated if equal volumes of solutions made by dilution of 1 ml of 0.01 *M* $AgNO_3$ and KCl solutions to 1 litre each are mixed?

Answer: No precipitate.

15. Why is a solution of a ferric salt acidified before precipitation of iron with ammonia?

16. Why must adsorbed Cl^- ions be washed out completely from a $Fe(OH)_3$ precipitate? How is it confirmed that the washing is complete?

17. Why must not the precipitate in iron determination be ignited at too high a temperature?

18. What are the advantages of the hydroxyquinoline method over precipitation with ammonia for determination of aluminium?

19. In determination of metallic aluminium in bronze, the iron content is first found (by a volumetric method). Iron and aluminium are then precipitated with ammonia, the precipitate is ignited, and the total weight of $Fe_2O_3 + Al_2O_3$ is found. The aluminium content is then calculated as follows. The weight of iron is multiplied by 1.4297 and the result is subtracted from the total weight of $Fe_2O_3 + Al_2O_3$; the difference is multiplied by 0.5292. What is the significance of the factors 1.4297 and 0.5292 in this case?

20. Why is it preferable to precipitate Ca^{++} as oxalate from acid solution, gradually neutralizing the acid with ammonia?

21. The total weight of calcium in a determination is 0.1000 g and the error in weighing the precipitate is 0.0002 g. What is the percentage error if the weighed form is (a) CaO; (b) $CaC_2O_4 \cdot H_2O$?

Answer: (a) 0.14%; (b) 0.05%.

22. How is CO_2 in carbonates determined?

23. The following results were obtained in analysis of calcium carbonate: (a) 0.5493 g of $CaC_2O_4 \cdot H_2O$ from a sample weighing 0.3768 g; (b) 0.4013 g of CO_2 from a sample weighing 0.9160 g. By how much does the sum of the percentages of CaO and CO_2 differ from 100%?

Answer: By 0.25%.

24. Why is the precipitation of Mg^{++} as $MgNH_4PO_4$ performed in presence of NH_4Cl? Why should a large excess of the latter be avoided?

25. Why are $MgNH_4PO_4$ precipitates washed with dilute NH_4OH solution rather than with pure water? How is it confirmed that the washing is complete?

26. Why must the filter be ashed separately from a $MgNH_4PO_4$ precipitate? What chemical changes take place in the latter on ignition?

27. What is the percentage of $MgSO_4 \cdot 7H_2O$ in a crude product if a 0.4285 g sample gave 0.1920 g of $Mg_2P_2O_7$?

Answer: 99.22%.

28. The following formula is used for calculating the MgO content of cement:

$$\%MgO = \frac{a \times 36.21}{g}$$

Here a is the weight of the ignited $Mg_2P_2O_7$ precipitate; g is the weight of cement taken. How is the factor 36.21 calculated?

29. In determination of phosphorus in iron or steel the sample is dissolved in HNO_3, the phosphorus acid which is partially formed is oxidized to phosphoric, and phosphate is precipitated as $(NH_4)_3PO_4 \cdot 12MoO_3$. The precipitate is filtered off and dissolved in ammonia, and molybdic acid is precipitated as $PbMoO_4$, from the weight of which the phosphorus content is calculated. Calculate the conversion factor for this determination.

Answer: $F = 0.007015$.

30. Why is it necessary to reprecipitate $CaC_2O_4 \cdot H_2O$ in determination of Ca^{++} in presence of Mg^{++}? Why is the precipitate purer after the second precipitation?

31. Why must ammonia salts be removed from the solution obtained after separation of Ca^{++} before Mg^{++} can be precipitated?

32. What weight of a substance containing iron should be taken in order that the percentage of iron in it could be found by simple multiplication of the weight of the ignited Fe_2O_3 precipitate by 100?

Answer: The weight should be numerically equal to the conversion factor:

$$F = \frac{2Fe}{Fe_2O_3} = 0.6994$$

33. In a determination of MgO in a silicate, what weight of the silicate should be taken so that the percentage of MgO could be found by multiplying the weight of the ignited $Mg_2P_2O_7$ precipitate by 100?

Answer: 0.3621 g.

34. What properties of nickel dimethylglyoximate make it very valuable for quantitative determination of Ni^{++}?

35. Why does the solution pH influence the completeness of precipitation of Ni^{++} with dimethylglyoxime? What are the usual conditions for this precipitation?

36. Why does the presence of Fe^{++} ions interfere with determination of Ni^{++} by the dimethylglyoxime reaction? How are the Fe^{++} ions removed from solutions? Write the equation for this reaction.

37. Why is tartaric acid added before precipitation of nickel? How can you tell whether enough has been added?

38. Why is it preferable to collect a nickel dimethylglyoximate precipitate on a filter crucible and dry it to constant weight, rather than ignite it after filtration through a paper filter?

39. Percentage contents of nickel are calculated from the following formulas:

(a) in weighing as nickel dimethylglyoximate

$$\%\text{Ni} = \frac{a \times 20.32}{g}$$

(b) in weighing as NiO

$$\%\text{Ni} = \frac{a \times 78.58}{g}$$

where *a* is the weight of the precipitate and *g* is the weight of the sample taken. How are the factors 20.32 and 78.58 derived?

CHAPTER IV

VOLUMETRIC ANALYSIS

49. The Principle of Volumetric Analysis

Gravimetric analysis is the most precise chemical method of analysis. It also has a very wide range of applications, as every element (with isolated exceptions) forms insoluble compounds in the form of which it can be determined quantitatively by the gravimetric method.

However, the very serious disadvantage of gravimetric analysis is that the determinations are lengthy. At best, the results take several hours to obtain; more often the analysis is completed only on the following day.

Very often such slow analysis does not satisfy practical requirements. For example, in chemical control of a particular industrial process (such as blast-furnace or open-hearth smelting, etc.) the analytical results are required in good time so that the course of the process can be adjusted and faulty production prevented. Such timely analysis makes it possible to conduct the process in the best way and to obtain a high-quality product. Conversely, even the most careful analysis is useless if its results are provided too late.

Volumetric analysis has an enormous advantage over gravimetric with regard to speed. The determinations are more rapid because, instead of weighing the reaction product, the volume of a reagent solution required for the reaction is measured; the concentration (known as the *titre*) of this solution is accurately known.

The titre of a solution is usually taken to mean the number of grams of substance per 1 ml of solution. For example, the expression "the titre of the H_2SO_4 solution is 0.0049 g/ml" means that each millilitre of this sulphuric acid solution contains 0.0049 g H_2SO_4. The titre is denoted by the letter T together with the formula of the substance in question. Thus, in the present instance:

$$T_{H_2SO_4} = 0.0049 \text{ g/ml}$$

A solution of which the titre is accurately known is described as a *standard solution*.

In volumetric analysis a standard solution of the reagent is put in a measuring vessel known as a burette (see Fig. 30) and is then gradually added to the solution to be analysed* until it is found by a suitable method that the amount of reagent which has been added is equivalent to the amount of substance being determined. This operation is known as *titration*.

The volume of the reagent solution taken for the titration is read off the burette and multiplied by the known titre. This gives the amount of reagent in grams expended in the reaction. It is then easy to use the reaction equation for calculating the amount of substance in the unknown solution; if the volume of the latter is known, its titre can also be found.**

Comparing volumetric and gravimetric analyses, we see that instead of the lengthy and tedious operations: precipitation (and subsequent ripening of the precipitate), filtration, washing, ignition of the empty crucible and the crucible with the precipitate, etc., in volumetric analysis there is only one operation, that of titration, which usually takes only a few minutes with practice.

Volumetric determinations are usually somewhat less precise than gravimetric, because weighing on an analytical balance is rather more precise than volume determination with a burette. However, with proper working the difference is so small that it can be disregarded in most cases. Therefore, the more rapid volumetric methods are used whenever possible.

However, a particular reaction must satisfy a number of requirements if it is to serve as the basis for titration.

50. Requirements for Reactions Used in Volumetric Analysis

One of the most important differences between volumetric and gravimetric analysis is that *in titration the reagent is used not in excess, but in a quantity which exactly corresponds to the reaction equation and is chemically equivalent to the substance being determined.* It is on equivalence that calculation of the analytical results is based.

It is therefore obvious that it is necessary in titration *to determine the equivalence point* with sufficient accuracy.

In some cases this is possible because a coloured reagent changes colour during the reaction. For example, if a solution of $FeSO_4$ acidified with sulphuric acid is titrated with $KMnO_4$ solution the

---

* Sometimes the procedure is reversed, and the unknown solution is added from a burette to the standard solution in a flask.

** Other and more convenient methods for calculating the results of volumetric determinations are given in Sec. 56.

following reaction takes place:

$$10FeSO_4 + 2KMnO_4 + 8H_2SO_4 = 5Fe_2(SO_4)_3 + 2MnSO_4 + K_2SO_4 + 8H_2O$$

The colour of each drop of $KMnO_4$ disappears almost instantaneously when it is added. This is because Fe^{++} ions reduce the intensely coloured MnO_4^- ions to the almost colourless Mn^{++} ions. However, as soon as all the $FeSO_4$ has been oxidized to $Fe_2(SO_4)_3$ one more drop of $KMnO_4$ colours the solution a pale pink; this means that the equivalence point has been passed and the titration must be stopped. Thus the titration is ended not strictly at the equivalence point, but is slightly "overshot"; i.e., a slight excess of $KMnO_4$ is introduced with the last drop of standard solution. This gives rise to a slight *titration error*. As the standard $KMnO_4$ solution is very dilute and the excess is not more than one drop, this error may be ignored.

In titration of chlorides with $AgNO_3$ solution

$$NaCl + AgNO_3 = \downarrow AgCl + NaNO_3$$

addition of standard $AgNO_3$ solution can be continued until no more AgCl precipitate* is formed. However, it is easier to fix the equivalence point if a few drops of K_2CrO_4 solution are added to the NaCl solution. We know that Ag^+ ions precipitate both Cl^- and CrO_4^{--} ions. However, the solubility of AgCl (1.2×10^{-5} mole/litre) is considerably lower than the solubility of Ag_2CrO_4 (6.5×10^{-5} mole/litre), so that the solubility product of AgCl is reached first, and this compound is deposited in the form of a white precipitate. It is only when practically all the Cl^- ions have been precipitated that the solubility product of silver chromate is reached, and the latter appears as a brick-red precipitate. The instant at which precipitation of Ag_2CrO_4 begins an addition of one excess drop of $AgNO_3$ solution is very easy to establish, because the pure white precipitate turns reddish brown.

Substances which, like K_2CrO_4, undergo some easily detected change (such as change of colour, precipitation, etc.) during titration and which thereby indicate the equivalence point are called *indicators*. They include litmus, phenolphthalein, and methyl orange, which are used in neutralization reactions.

Indicators, for certain oxidation-reduction and precipitation reactions are also known. Various indicators and the mechanism of their action are discussed in the different sections on volumetric analysis. Here we must merely point out that suitable indicators

---

* Under suitable conditions the AgCl precipitate coagulates rapidly and the solution becomes clear at the equivalence point. This is a very precise method but is less convenient in practice than the method with the use of K_2CrO_4 which is described here.

are known for far from every reaction. On the other hand, even when indicators exist they cannot always be used. Highly coloured or turbid solutions usually cannot be titrated in presence of indicators, because colour changes are difficult to distinguish in such cases.

In such cases the equivalence point can sometimes be determined from changes in certain physical properties of the solution during titration. Electrovolumetric methods of analysis are based on this principle. These include conductometric titration, in which the equivalence point is found from the electrical conductance of the solution, and potentiometric titration, based on measurements of oxidation potentials.

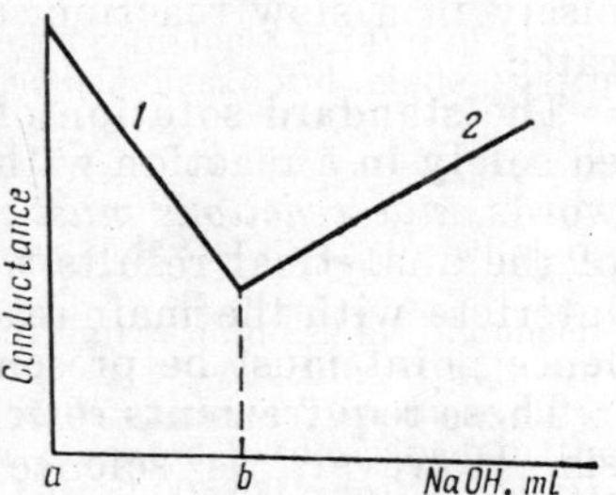

Fig. 29. Changes in the conductance during titration of HCl solution with NaOH solution

As an example of electrovolumetric methods, let us consider conductometric titration of a strong acid with a strong alkali; for instance

$$HCl + NaOH = NaCl + H_2O$$

In this titration the H^+ ions of hydrochloric acid gradually combine with OH^- ions of the alkali to form undissociated water molecules. The Na^+ ions of the alkali gradually accumulate in the solution, thus replacing the H^+ ions. But, since the mobility of the latter in electrolysis is considerably higher than the mobility of Na^+ ions, this replacement lowers the conductance of the solution.* At the equivalence point all the H^+ ions of hydrochloric acid are replaced by Na^+ ions and the conductance of the solution is at a minimum. On addition of excess alkali the conductance increases again owing to accumulation of Na^+ and OH^- ions in the solution. If the conductance of the solution is measured several times during the titration, before and after excess alkali has beed added, and the results are plotted on a graph, the two straight lines *1* and *2* (Fig. 29) intersect at the equivalence point. If we drop a perpendicular from this point to the abscissa axis, the intercept *ab* gives the volume of NaOH solution required to neutralize the HCl.

It is clear from what has been said above that *an essential condition for volumetric analysis is the possibility of determining the equivalence point by one method or another* (this is by no means always possible).

A second essential condition for the use of reaction in volumetric analysis is that it should *proceed quantitatively*, *with an equilibrium constant of the appropriate magnitude*. This constant should be large or, in other words, the equilibrium constant of the reverse reaction

* It will be remembered that electric charges in solutions are carried by ions, and therefore the more ions in a solution and the greater their mobility the higher is the conductance of the solution.

should be small; otherwise accurate titration becomes impossible. For example, accurate determination of weak acids by titration with solutions of strong bases is possible only if the reverse reaction (hydrolysis of the salt formed) is slight. This is the case only when the acid is not too weak (its dissociation constant should be greater than 1×10^{-7}). Similar considerations apply to other volumetric methods.

Only *rapid reactions* can be used in titration. It would be very difficult or even impossible to determine the equivalence point precisely in a slow reaction; the solution would inevitably be overtitrated.

The standard solution of reagent which is added must be expended solely in a reaction with the substance being determined. In other words, *side reactions must not occur in titration*, as exact calculation of the analytical results would be impossible. No substances which interfere with the main reaction or with determination of the equivalence point must be present in solution.

These requirements restrict the applicability of volumetric analysis. However, as science progresses, the scope of this method is broadening owing to the utilization of new reactions, discoveries of new indicators, etc.

51. Classification of Methods of Volumetric Analysis

The reactions used in volumetric analysis belong to various types. Accordingly, volumetric determinations can be subdivided into the following principal methods: neutralization, oxidation-reduction, precipitation, and complex-formation methods.

Neutralization. This comprises volumetric determinations based on reactions of acids with alkalies, i.e., on neutralization:

$$H^+ + OH^- \rightleftarrows H_2O$$

The neutralization method is used for determining the amount of acid (alkalimetry) or alkali (acidimetry) in a given solution, and for solving a number of other problems involving neutralization in one way or another.*

Oxidation-Reduction Methods (Oxidimetry). The commonest of these are:

---

* The terms "acidimetry" and "alkalimetry" are derived from the words *acid* and *alkali*. In determination of an acid the solution is titrated with an alkali solution the volume of which is measured by means of a burette. This accounts for the name *alkalimetry*. The name of the method for determining the amount of alkali, *acidimetry*, is derived analogously. However, this terminology is not universally accepted; some writers (for example, Treadwell) call determination of acids acidimetry, and determination of alkalies, alkalimetry.

permanganatometry, based on reactions of oxidation with potassium permanganate ($KMnO_4$);

iodometry, based on oxidation by the action of free iodine or reduction by I^- ions;

chromatometry, in which oxidation by the action of potassium dichromate $K_2Cr_2O_7$ is used;

bromatometry, involving oxidation with potassium bromate $KBrO_3$.

Other oxidation-reduction methods include *cerimetry* (oxidation by Ce^{++++} ions), *vanadatometry* (oxidation by VO_3^- ions), *titanometry* (reduction by Ti^{+++} ions), etc.

Methods Involving Precipitation and Complex Formation. These are volumetric determinations based on precipitation of various ions in the form of insoluble compounds, or on formation of weakly dissociated complexes.

Whichever method is used for a particular determination, it always involves:

(a) precise measurement of the volumes of the reacting solutions;
(b) the use of a "standard solution" for the titration;
(c) calculation of the analytical result.

Accordingly, before discussing the various methods of volumetric analysis, let us consider volume measurements, calculation of concentrations and preparation of standard solutions, and calculations used in volumetric determinations.

52. Volume Measurement

The primary unit of capacity in the metric system is the *litre*, which is the volume of 1 kg of water at the temperature of maximum density (3.98°C) and under normal atmospheric pressure. One thousandth part of a litre is called a *millilitre*. This does not quite coincide with a cubic centimetre, which is one thousandth of a cubic decimetre, because the mass of water in the latter is 1,000.028 g and not 1,000 g.

Burettes, pipettes, and measuring flasks are used for accurate volume measurements in quantitative analysis.

Burettes. The burette is used for titration, and consists of a cylindrical tube with a constricted end to which a narrow glass tube is attached by means of rubber tubing (Fig. 30; *2*, *3*).

On the free part of the rubber tube there is a spring clip (Fig. 30; *2*); when this is pressed with two fingers liquid is released from the burette. Sometimes a little glass ball inserted in the rubber tube (Fig. 30; *3*) is used instead of a spring clip. If the rubber is pressed gently over the glass ball, narrow channels are formed between the rubber and the ball, and the liquid can flow out of the burette.

Burettes with glass taps (Fig. 30; *1*) are used for solutions of substances (such as iodine) which attack rubber.

The burette is graduated in millilitres (usually 25 or 50) and tenths of millilitres, the zero being at the top.

Before a burette is filled with the solution the volume of which is to be measured, it (like any other measuring vessel) must be thoroughly washed. Special care must be taken not to leave the slightest trace of grease on the inside walls of the burette because greasy glass is not wetted by water and when the liquid runs out of the burette drops remain on the sides, making the measurement inaccurate. Burettes and other measuring vessels are washed as described in Sec. 12. When the burette is being washed the finger should not be put over the top, because otherwise grease will again enter the burette. The burette must be washed until the liquid flows uniformly off the sides *without leaving any drops.*

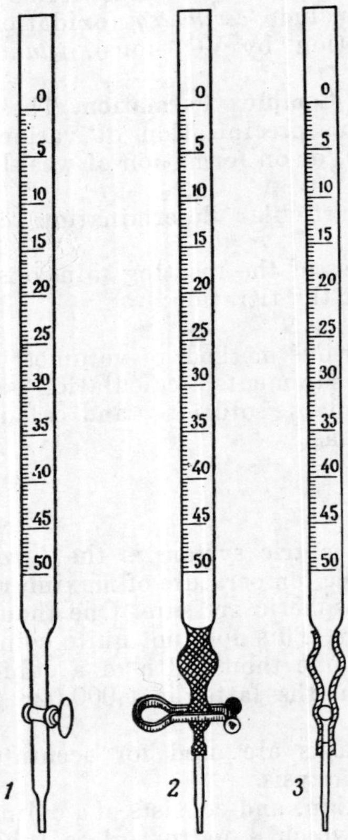

Fig. 30. Burettes

When the burette has been washed, there is no need to wait for it to dry. Instead, it is rinsed out twice with small amounts of the solution which is to be measured. The burette is filled through a funnel inserted in the top; the funnel must then be taken out.*

Care must be taken that no air bubbles remain in the narrow bottom tip of the burette. To remove this air, the spring clip is opened and the liquid is allowed to run out rapidly into a beaker or flask. If the burette has a glass tap, it is usually impossible to displace air in this way. In such cases the tip of the burette is placed in the same solution as is in the burette, the tap is opened, and a small amount of liquid is sucked in through the top. The burette is then filled in the usual way.

To keep burettes clean they are filled to the top with water and covered with glass hoods or clean test tubes to keep out dust.

* If the funnel is not taken out, drops of liquid remaining in it may drain down during the titration, making the measurement inaccurate.

If the same standard solution is used for a large number of analyses, the filling procedure described above is inconvenient and tedious. In such cases the burette is usually connected (as shown in Fig. 31) directly to a bottle containing a supply of standard solution.

When the system shown in Fig. 31*a*, is used, the bottle with standard solution stands on a shelf at a height such that the liquid

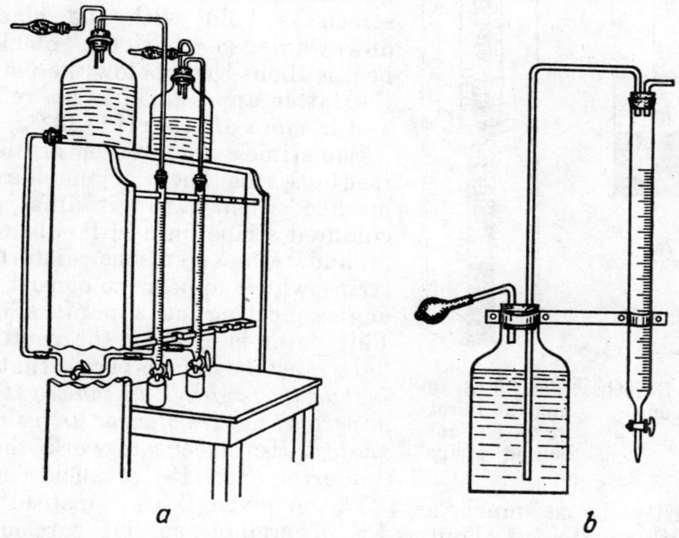

Fig. 31. Burettes connected to bottles containing standard solution

level in the burette is always below the liquid level in the bottle. The burette is then filled when the tap in the burette side-tube is opened. Conversely, in the system shown in Fig. 31*b*, the solution is forced into the burette by air pressure created by a squeezed rubber bulb. A similar device is shown in Fig. 55.

The liquid surface in the burette is seen as a wide concave band (meniscus). The reading is taken *from the division corresponding to the lower edge of the meniscus, with the eye on the same level as the latter*.

The burette divisions correspond to millilitres and tenths of millilitres. Further, if the lower edge of the meniscus cuts across a scale division, hundredths of a millilitre are estimated by eye. A magnifying glass is useful for this. Therefore, the precision of a burette reading is about 0.02-0.03 ml. In accordance with the rule given in Sec. 15, such readings should be recorded to two decimal places (for example, 24.00 and not 24.0 or 24).

To make the meniscus more distinct and to ensure that it always looks the same, it is convenient to place a screen behind the burette. This is made from a small (about 5 × 5 cm) piece of cardboard, covered with white paper, with the lower half blackened with Indian ink. If this screen is held with the black half downwards so that the black area begins about 1 mm below the meniscus, the latter appears dark by reflection and is more distinct (Fig. 32).

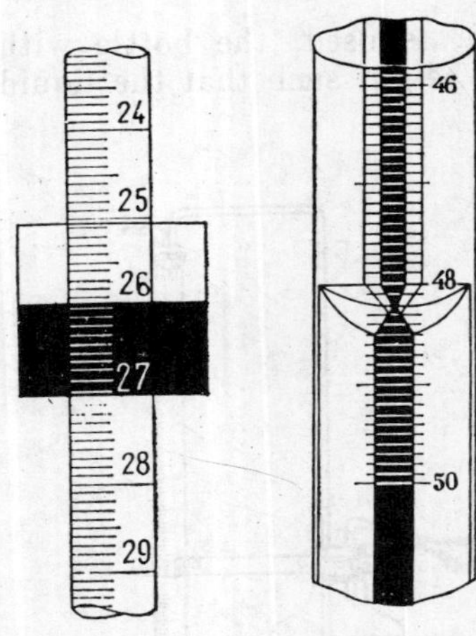

Fig. 32. Burette screen

Fig. 33. Reading a burette with a coloured stripe

Sometimes, for greater precision of readings, the back of the burette is marked with a longitudinal narrow coloured stripe on a milk-white background. The meniscus distorts this stripe which appears to consist of two angles meeting at a point (Fig. 33). This point is used for the readings.

It must be remembered that *errors in burette readings are among the most important sources of error in volumetric analysis.* In inaccurate work the relative error (Sec. 13) of such a reading can easily be as much as 0.3% or even 0.5%, instead of the permissible value of about 0.1%. Therefore, special care must be taken in this very important operation.

Always make quite sure that, when a reading is taken, *the eye is on the level of the lower edge of the meniscus.* It is easy to show that the readings vary appreciably with the position of the observer's eye (Fig. 34). The following procedure can be used for finding the proper eye level. A small mirror is put behind the burette and the eye level is adjusted so that the division nearest the bottom edge of the meniscus coincides with its own reflection in the mirror.

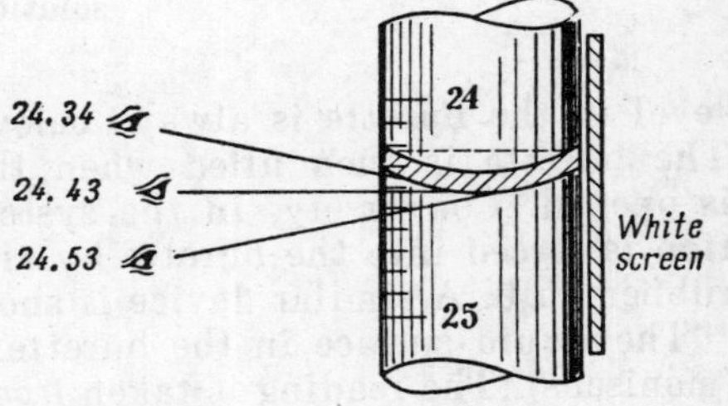

Fig. 34. Burette readings with the eye in different positions

The liquid must not be run too rapidly out of the burette, otherwise it does not have time to drain down the sides and the volume measurement becomes inaccurate. For the same reason at least 30 seconds must be allowed to elapse at the end of the titration before the reading is taken.

Before each titration the liquid level in the burette must always be adjusted to the zero mark, i.e., the same part of the burette must be used each time. It is easy to see that this is the best way to compensate graduation errors in the burette.

It must also be remembered that for accurate titration results the volume of solution used in a titration should not exceed the volume of the burette, but at the same time it should not be too small (not less than 10 ml). In the former case the burette would have to be filled twice, which would double the number of readings to be taken and would lower the accuracy considerably. In the second case the inevitable errors in readings would be an excessively high proportion of the total volume. For example, a reading error of 0.02 ml is 0.1% if the total solution volume is 20 ml, whereas with a total volume of 2 ml it is as much as 1%. The usual aim in titration is to choose the volume and concentration of the solution to be titrated so that it would take about 20-30 ml of the titrating solution

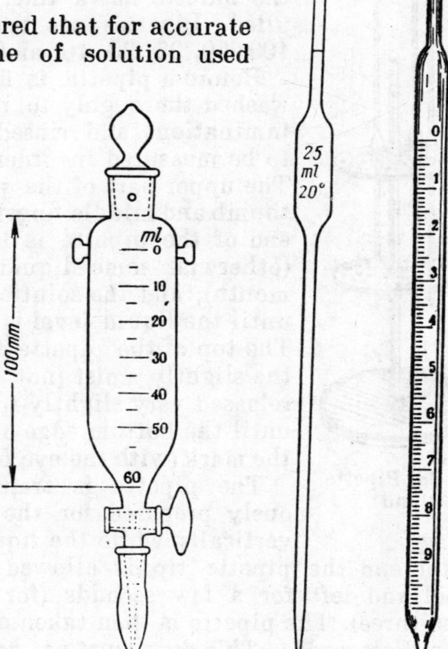

Fig. 35. Weighing burette Fig. 36. Pipette Fig. 37. Graduated pipette

In addition to the ordinary burettes described above, *weighing burettes* (Fig. 35) are sometimes used. With these burettes instead of finding the volume of a solution used in a titration its weight is found from the weight of the burette before and after the titration. Of course, the results are more accurate than with the use of ordinary burettes. For example, it is impossible to measure a volume of 30 ml with a precision of 0.01 ml by means of an ordinary burette, but with a weighing burette it is quite easy. Accordingly the precision of volume measurements with a weighing burette is about 0.01%, whereas the precision of an ordinary burette is 0.1%. However, work with weighing burettes takes more time, and they are used only when a particularly high degree of precision is required.

Pipettes. Pipettes are commonly used for accurate measurements of definite solution volumes; they are long narrow tubes with a bulb in the middle (Fig. 36). The upper narrow part of the burette has a line, up to which the burette is filled. Pipettes are usually made in capacities of 100, 50, 25, 20, 10, and 5 ml.

Before a pipette is filled with the solution it is washed thoroughly to remove grease and other contaminations and rinsed out twice with the solution to be measured in order to remove drops of water. The upper part of the pipette is then held by the thumb and middle finger of the right hand, the lower end of the pipette is lowered *deep* into the liquid (otherwise some liquid may be sucked into the mouth), and the solution is sucked into the pipette until the liquid level is about 2 cm above the mark. The top of the pipette is then quickly closed with the slightly moist (not wet) index finger, which is released very slightly to allow the liquid to run out until the bottom edge of the meniscus just touches the mark (with the eye held at the level of the mark).

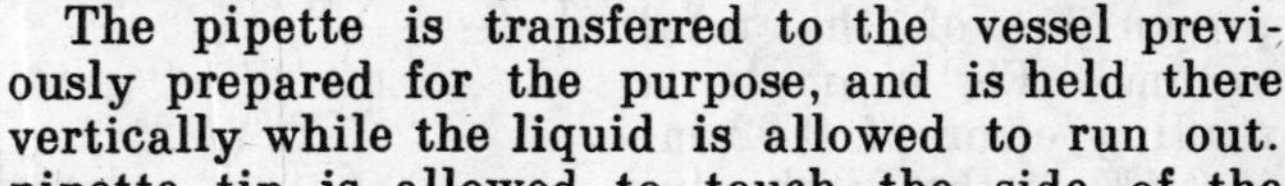

Fig. 38. Pipette stand

The pipette is transferred to the vessel previously prepared for the purpose, and is held there vertically while the liquid is allowed to run out. At the end the pipette tip is allowed to touch the side of the vessel and left for a few seconds (for example, while one counts up to three). The pipette is then taken out, the drop remaining in it being disregarded. *This drop must not be blown out.* It is in any case impossible to remove all the remaining liquid from the pipette, but it is important that the amount remaining should always be the same. This aim is achieved if the same method for emptying the pipette, as described above, is always used. Obviously such constant conditions cannot be obtained if the last drop is blown out, because the blowing force would vary.

Besides ordinary pipettes, the so-called graduated pipettes (Fig. 37) are sometimes used; they resemble burettes in shape and are similarly graduated.

At the end of the work pipettes are washed, placed in a special stand (Fig. 38), and covered with inverted test tubes or plugged with cotton wool to keep out dust.

Measuring Flasks. Measuring flasks (Fig. 39) are used for diluting solutions to a definite volume, parts being subsequently with-

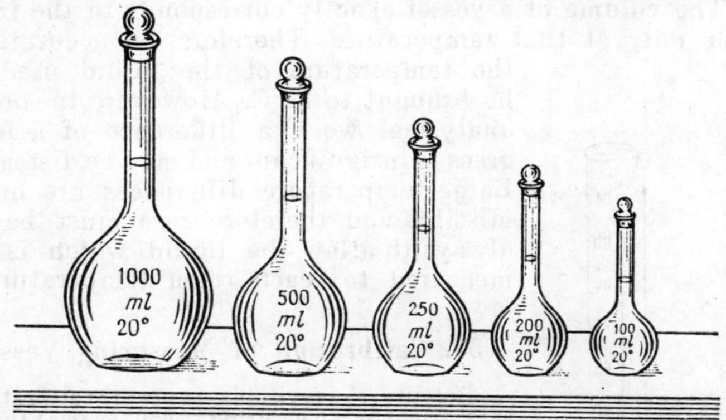

Fig. 39. Measuring flasks

drawn for titration by means of pipettes, and for preparation of standard solutions. Therefore, in distinction from burettes and pipettes, measuring flasks are usually designed to hold, but not to deliver, definite volumes of liquid.*

A measuring flask is a flask with a long narrow neck. A mark is made all round the neck to indicate the level to which the flask should be filled.

A measuring flask, like any other measuring vessel, must be washed thoroughly before use. Since measuring flasks are intended for dilution of definite quantities of solution, they cannot be rinsed out with these solutions as is done in the case of pipettes or burettes.

A measuring flask is filled first through a funnel inserted in the neck, and at the end from a dropping pipette (Fig. 40). The liquid is added from the latter drop by drop until the bottom of the meniscus touches the mark. The eye should be held at the level of the mark, so that the front side of the mark (facing the observer) hides the back.

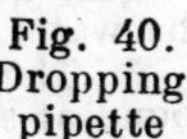

Fig. 40. Dropping pipette

Measuring Cylinders (Fig. 41) are unsuitable for volume measurement with the precision needed in volumetric analysis. Therefore, they are used only for measuring out various auxiliary reagents, the volumes of which are not needed for calculation of the results.

---

* Measuring flasks designed to deliver definite volumes of liquids also exist, but they are rarely used in practice.

Every measuring vessel is calibrated at a definite temperature (usually indicated on the vessel). The standard temperature is taken as 20°C. The volume of a vessel exactly corresponds to the indicated volume only at that temperature. Therefore, in accurate work the temperature of the liquid used must be brought to 20°C. However, in ordinary analytical work a difference of a few degrees is insignificant and may be disregarded. Large temperature differences are not permissible and therefore care must be taken always to allow the liquid which is to be measured to reach room temperature.

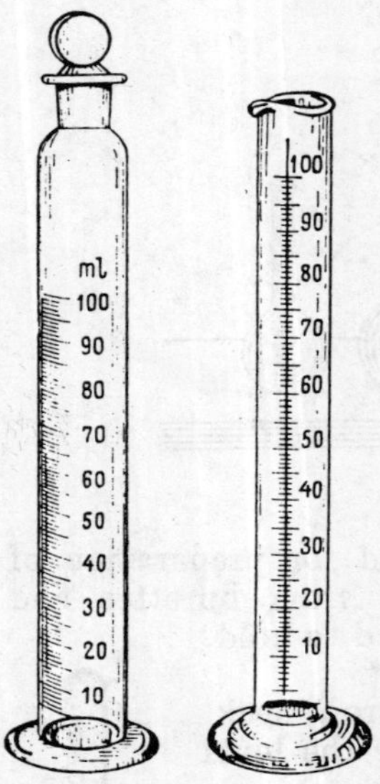

Fig. 41. Measuring cylinders

53. Calibration of Measuring Vessels

Because of inevitable errors in calibration, the capacity of any measuring vessel, even at the standard temperature, is not exactly equal to its marked (nominal) capacity, but deviates in one direction or the other. For example, in accordance with the official standard, the error for a measuring flask should not exceed $\frac{0.13}{\sqrt{V}}$, and of a pipette, $\frac{0.5}{\sqrt{V}}$ where V is the nominal capacity.

In fact, when these vessels are calibrated at the works even larger errors, far in excess of the permitted limit, may sometimes pass unnoticed. Therefore, although under certain conditions (see p. 205). it is possible to obtain correct analytical results with incorrectly calibrated measuring vessels, nevertheless the analyst must check the capacities of the vessels which he intends to use, in order to eliminate any incidental errors.

In calibration and checking, the capacity of a measuring vessel is estimated from the weight of water it holds (or delivers). This involves a number of corrections:

1. For determination of the volume of water from its weight, the water must be at the temperature of maximum density (3.98°C). Water at some other temperature is used in calibration. Therefore, a correction (which we denote by A) must be applied for the change in the density of water with temperature.

2. The volume of the water is considerably greater than the volume of the weights used. By the principle of Archimedes the latter lose less in weight than the water. Therefore, another correction (B) is applied for weighing in air*.

3. The capacity of the vessel at 20° C must be known, but in practice it is found at some other temperature. It is therefore necessary to apply a correction (C) for the change in the capacity of the vessel with temperature**.

---

* The calculation of the correction is discussed in Sec. 9.

** This correction is found from the formula:

$$V_{20} = V_t + 0.000025 V_t (20 - t)$$

where V_{20} and V_t are the capacities of the vessel at 20°C and $t°$, and 0.000025 is the coefficient of expansion of glass.

All these corrections have been calculated once and for all. They are summarized in Table IV.

Table IV

Calibration of Measuring Vessels

Temperature °C	Correction A g	Correction B g	Correction C g	Sum of corrections A+B+C	1,000—(A+B+C)
15	0.87	1.07	0.13	2.07	997.93
16	1.03	1.07	0.10	2.20	997.80
17	1.20	1.07	0.08	2.35	997.65
18	1.38	1.06	0.05	2.49	997.51
19	1.57	1.06	0.03	2.66	997.34
20	1.77	1.05	0.00	2.82	997.18
21	1.98	1.05	—0.03	3.00	997.00
22	2.20	1.05	—0.05	3.20	996.80
23	2.43	1.04	—0.08	3.39	996.61
24	2.67	1.04	—0.10	3.61	996.39
25	2.92	1.03	—0.13	3.82	996.18
26	3.18	1.03	—0.15	4.06	995.94
27	3.45	1.03	—0.18	4.30	995.70
28	3.73	1.02	—0.20	4.55	995.45
29	4.02	1.02	—0.23	4.81	995.19
30	4.32	1.01	—0.25	5.08	994.92

We now consider more fully the methods used for calibrating different types of measuring vessels.

Calibration of Measuring Flasks. Suppose that it is required to check the capacity of a measuring flask with a nominal capacity of 250 ml. The flask is thoroughly washed and dried, and put on the left-hand pan of a technical balance. Weights corresponding to the nominal capacity of the flask (250 g) are put on the same pan. The balance is then exactly counterpoised by a suitable load (lead shot, weights from another set, etc.). When this has been achieved, the balance is arrested and the weights and flask are removed from the left-hand pan while the counterpoise is left untouched. The flask is filled to the mark with distilled water, wiped on the outside with a cloth, and water wetting the inside of the top of the neck (above the mark) is wiped off with a piece of filter paper rolled in a tube. The flask is then replaced on the left-hand pan and small weights are put on the left- or right-hand pan of the balance, dependent on which is the lighter, until the weights and the flask balance.*

Suppose that 0.45 g is put on the left-hand pan. This means that the water in the flask weighs 0.45 g less than the weights originally on this pan. Therefore, the weight of the water is 250—0.45 = 249.55 g.

It is easy to calculate what this weight should be under the same conditions if the capacity of the flask at 20°C was exactly 250 ml.

* Weighing by substitution (Sec. 8) is used here in order to eliminate the error caused by inequality of the length of the balance arms.

Suppose that the temperature of the water filling the flask is 24°C. In the last column of Table IV the number corresponding to this temperature is 996.39. This represents the weight at 24°C, weighed in air, of the water contained in any glass vessel the capacity of which is exactly 1 litre at 20°C.

For a volume of 250 ml this gives $\frac{996.39}{4} = 249.10$ g. The weight actually found (249.55 g) is greater than this by 0.45 g.

This evidently means that the capacity of the flask is greater than 250 ml by 0.45 ml, i.e., it is 250.45 ml.*

Calibration of Pipettes. The temperature of some distilled water is measured, and the water is sucked into the pipette up to the mark. It is then discharged into a weighed weighing bottle. *Exactly the same procedure is used here as in subsequent work with the pipette*: all the rules in Sec. 52 are observed; in particular the last drop of liquid remaining in the pipette must on no account be blown out. The weighing bottle is then closed and weighed. The empty bottle and the bottle with water is weighed on an analytical balance to the nearest 0.001 g.

The experiment is performed at least three times and the average result is taken. The capacity of the pipette is calculated exactly as described for measuring flasks.

Calibration of Burettes. The capacity of a burette is checked either by a series of weighings of the amounts of water delivered by it between various divisions, or by means of a special pipette attached to the burette.

The first method is similar to the calibration of pipettes described above. Water is run out of the burette between 0-5 ml, 0-10 ml, etc., up to 0-50 ml into a previously weighed weighing bottle, which is weighed each time to the nearest 0.001 g. The volumes are calculated in the usual way from the weights and temperature of the water, and a correction table is prepared. This is used in work with the burette.

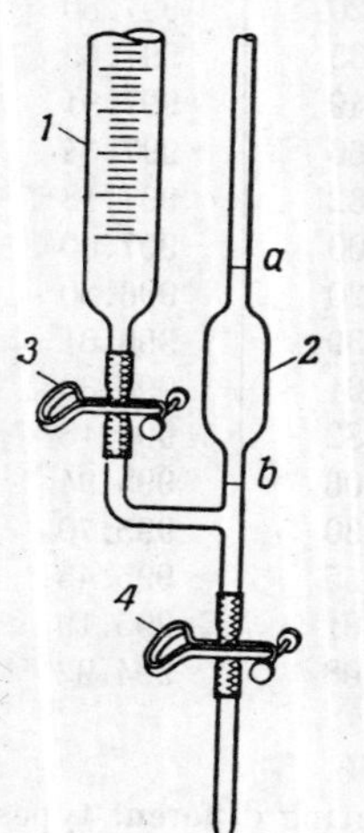

Fig. 42. Pipette for calibrating burettes:
1—burette; *2*—pipette; *3*, *4*—clips

For the second method a special pipette *2* (Fig. 42) is attached to the burette *1*. This pipette is previously calibrated accurately by weighing the water delivered by it between the marks *a* and *b*. This weighing is done on an analytical balance to the nearest 0.001 g and is repeated at least three times.

When the exact capacity of the pipette has been found, the water level in it is adjusted to mark *b*, while the level in the burette is set exactly at the zero mark. The clip *3* is then opened and the pipette is filled with water to mark *a*. The burette reading is noted down and water is let out of the pipette down to mark *b*, by means of the clip *4*, into a beaker or flask. The operation is repeated until the bottom of the burette scale is reached.

The burette readings are compared with the corresponding volumes (found by multiplying the volume of the pipette by the number of fillings) and a table of corrections is prepared. This is illustrated by Table V.

The burette readings in this table are rounded off and the table of corrections is compiled (Table VI).

---

* This calculation can be done in another way, by dividing the weight of water found experimentally (i.e., 249.55 g) by the weight of water corresponding to 1 ml under the given conditions. This weight is 0.001 of 996.39 g, i.e., 0.99639 g.

Table VI is used in work with this burette. It is also possible to use a calibration graph plotted from the values found.

Table V

Burette Calibration

Pipette fillings	Volumes, ml		Difference V_2-V_1
	Measured by burette, V_1	Measured by pipette, V_2	
1	2.02	1.99 *	−0.03
2	4.00	3.98	−0.02
3	5.99	5.97	−0.02
4	7.97	7.96	−0.01
5	9.94	9.95	+0.01
			etc.

* Here 1.99 ml is the pipette volume (V_2) found by calibration. All the other numbers in this column are found by multiplying this volume by the number of pipette fillings. Thus 9.95=1.99×5, etc.

Table VI

Table of Burette Corrections

Burette readings ml	Corrections ml
2	−0.03
4	−0.02
6	−0.02
8	−0.01
10	+0.01
	etc.

54. Preparation of Standard Solutions

Standard solutions are solutions of accurately known concentration. There are two methods for preparing standard solutions.

1. A quantity of the required substance is weighed out accurately on an analytical balance, dissolved in a measuring flask, and the volume is made up to the mark with water. If the weight of dissolved substance (g) and the volume of solution (V) are known, it is easy to calculate the titre of the solution. This is evidently

$$T = \frac{g}{V} \text{ g/ml}$$

Standard solutions prepared in this way are known as *primary standards*.

Obviously, this method of preparing standard solutions is very often not applicable. It cannot be used for preparing standard solutions of such substances as HCl, NaOH, etc. In fact, the exact concentration of an aqueous HCl solution is never known. Therefore, even if an axact weight of such a solution is taken, it is impossible to calculate the weight of hydrogen chloride it contains. The same applies to NaOH, which readily absorbs CO_2 and water vapour from the air, with a change of weight. Therefore, the amount of NaOH in a weighed sample is not known exactly either.

These examples show that the method described above can be used for preparation of standard solutions only of substances which satisfy the following conditions.

The substance must be chemically pure, i.e., it must not contain impurities in amounts which could affect analytical precision (not over 0.05-0.1%).

The composition of the substance must correspond exactly to its formula. For example, the water content of a crystalline hydrate must be exactly as indicated by the formula.

The substance must be stable on keeping, both in the solid state and in solution, as otherwise its composition would cease to correspond to its formula.

The gram-equivalent of the substance should be as large as possible, so that the precision in determining the normality of the solution is high.*

Substances satisfying these conditions are known as *primary*, as all other substances are standardized against them.

2. If the substance does not satisfy all the above conditions, a solution of approximately the required normality is first prepared. At the same time a standard solution of some suitable primary substance is prepared as described above. One of these solutions is then titrated with the other, and the exact concentration (titre) of the approximate solution is calculated, the concentration of the primary standard solution being known.

For example, the titre of a NaOH solution can be found by titrating a solution of oxalic acid with it. Oxalic acid is a crystalline substance which can be obtained chemically pure by recrystallization so that it exactly corresponds to its formula $H_2C_2O_4 \cdot 2H_2O$. The titre of the oxalic acid solution can therefore be found by dividing the exact weight of oxalic acid taken by the solution volume.

A standard solution the titre of which is found by titration (as in the case of NaOH) or by gravimetric analysis of the solution is described as *standardized*.

The great importance of primary substances in volumetric analysis is evident from all this. The better they satisfy the above conditions, the more accurately can the titres of the "working" solutions used in analysis be found, and the less will the analytical errors be.

It should be noted that working solutions are not always standardized against primary standards. For example, the titre of a NaOH solution can also be found by titration with HCl solution which has been standardized against a suitable primary standard. This method is convenient in that fewer primary standards are needed

* See Sec. 55 for explanations of gram-equivalent and normality.

and therefore the time required for their purification is saved. However, it is less accurate because the errors in determinations of the separate titres are cumulative.

Solutions are sometimes standardized by gravimetric analysis. For example, the titre of an HCl solution can be found from the weight of the AgCl precipitate formed by the action of $AgNO_3$ solution on a known weight of the HCl solution. Similarly, to find the titre of an H_2SO_4 solution we can add $BaCl_2$ solution to a definite volume of it and weigh the $BaSO_4$ precipitate formed, etc.

Finally, in analysis of natural substances or industrial products, the so-called *standard samples* are often used instead of primary standards. A standard sample is a sample of the material to be analysed, with an exactly known content of the element which is to be determined. For example, in determination of manganese in steel the sodium arsenite (Na_3AsO_3) solution used for the purpose is standardized against a known weight of a standard steel sample with an exactly known manganese content. Sodium thiosulphate ($Na_2S_2O_3$) solutions used for determination of copper in bronzes are standardized against standard bronze samples with exactly known copper contents, etc.

The use of standard samples is convenient because all the analytical operations prior to titration and all the impurities present in solution are the same in standardization as in the analysis. Therefore, they do not influence the analytical results and the precision is higher.

The use of standard samples for standardization of solutions illustrates the importance of one of the basic rules of volumetric analysis, which may be stated as follows: *as far as possible the conditions for standardization of working solutions should be the same as the conditions in analysis.*

If this is the case, all systematic errors (p. 48) are exactly the same in both cases and do not affect the results. For example, quite correct analytical results can be obtained with the use of an incorrectly calibrated pipette or measuring flask, if the same vessels were used for standardization of the working solution. It is therefore possible to work even without checking the measuring vessels. However, if the pipette or measuring flask should be broken the analyst must restandardize the solution. It is as a protection against such accidents that the measuring vessels are checked.

In practice, the commercially available Fixanal reagents are often used for preparation of standard solutions. These are accurately weighed amounts of various solids or exactly measured volumes of standard solutions, sealed in glass bulbs, each to give 1 litre of exactly 0.1 *N* solution. To prepare a standard solution from Fixanal, the contents of the bulb are transferred quantitatively into a 1 litre measuring flask, the substance is dissolved, and the solution is made up to the mark with water. The method used for transferring the substance from the bulb into the measuring flask is shown in Fig. 43. A funnel with a vertical projection for breaking the thin glass bottom of the bulb is inserted in the neck of the measuring flask. To remove the substance completely from the bulb, the latter is punctured in a cavity near its top by means of a pointed glass rod. The bulb is rinsed out thoroughly through the hole so made by a jet of water from a wash bottle. The funnel is then rinsed and removed, and the liquid in the flask is made up to the mark with water.

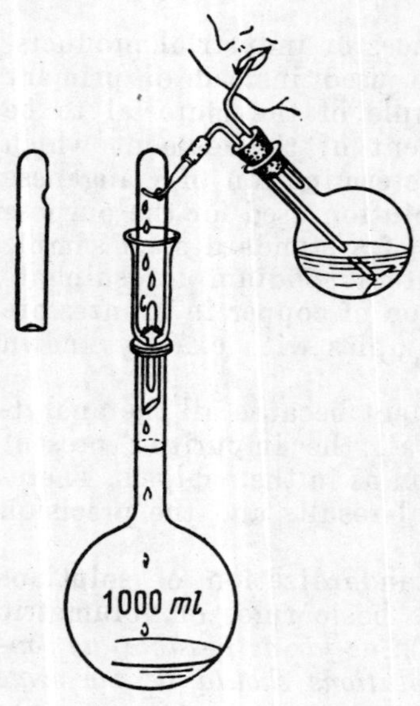

Fig. 43. Preparation of a standard solution from Fixanal

Titration can be performed by two different methods, both in standardization and in analysis.

1. A weighed sample of substance (either standard or for analysis) is dissolved in a measuring flask, diluted with water to the mark, and the solution is thoroughly mixed. Separate portions of the solution, each containing a definite or *aliquot* part of the sample, are withdrawn by means of a pipette and titrated. This is known as the *pipetting method.*

2. Separate samples of substance are weighed out, each is dissolved in any suitable volume of water, and the whole solutions are titrated. This is the *method of separate samples.*

It is easy to see that the method of separate samples, in which volumes are measured only once (with the burette), should give more accurate results than the pipetting method, where volumes are measured three times (with the measuring flask, pipette, and burette).* The chief advantage of the pipetting method is that it is easier to determine the equivalence point, because *equal* volumes of the solution are titrated each time. Moreover, it takes less time because it involves fewer weighings.

---

* However, this is true only if the samples weighed out are not too small, as otherwise the relative error in weighing can be very high.

55. Normality of Solutions. Gram-Equivalent

The concentrations of standard solutions in volumetric analysis are often expressed in terms of titre, which is the number of grams of substance contained in 1 ml of solution. It is even more convenient to express them in terms of normality.

The normality of a solution is the number of gram-equivalents of dissolved substance per litre of solution.

It is clear from this definition that the concept of normality is closely related to the concept of gram-equivalent, which is one of the most important concepts in volumetric analysis. We shall therefore consider it more fully.

The gram-equivalent of a substance is the number of grams of this substance chemically equivalent to one gram-atom (*or gram-ion*) *of hydrogen in a given reaction.*

To find the gram-equivalent we must write down the reaction equation and calculate how many grams of the substance correspond to one gram-atom or gram-ion of hydrogen in the reaction.

For example, in the equations

$$HCl + KOH = KCl + H_2O$$
$$CH_3COOH + NaOH = CH_3COONa + H_2O$$

the gram-equivalent is one gram-molecule (36.46 g) of HCl and one gram-molecule (60.05 g) of CH_3COOH, because these are the weights of the respective acids which yield one gram-ion of hydrogen, reacting with the hydroxyl ions of the alkali in the reactions. We also find that in the reactions

$$H_2SO_4 + 2NaOH = Na_2SO_4 + 2H_2O$$
$$H_3PO_4 + 3NaOH = Na_3PO_4 + 3H_2O$$

the gram-molecule of H_2SO_4 and H_3PO_4 correspond to two (H_2SO_4) and three (H_3PO_4) gram-ions of hydrogen respectively. Therefore, the gram-equivalent of H_2SO_4 is $^1/_2$ of the gram-molecule (49.04 g), and that of H_3PO_4 is $^1/_3$ of the gram-molecule (32.66 g).

It is known that molecules of di- and polybasic acids may react so that not all of the ionizable hydrogen atoms are involved. Evidently in such cases the values of their gram-equivalents are different.

For example, since each H_3PO_4 molecule yields only two hydrogen ions in the reaction

$$H_3PO_4 + 2NaOH = Na_2HPO_4 + 2H_2O$$

its gram-equivalent in this reaction is not $^1/_3$ but $^1/_2$ of the gram-molecule (49.00 g). Similarly, in the reaction

$$H_3PO_4 + NaOH = NaH_2PO_4 + H_2O$$

it is equal to the gram-molecule of H_3PO_4 (97.99 g).

Thus, in contrast to the gram-molecule, the gram-equivalent is not constant but depends on the reaction in which a given substance takes part. Therefore, in the above difinition of gram-equivalent special attention must be paid to the words *in a given reaction.*

Since one gram-ion of OH^- reacts with one gram-ion of H^+ and is therefore equivalent to the latter, gram-equivalents of bases are found similarly, except that their gram-molecular weights must be divided by the number of OH^- ions taking part in the reaction. For example, the gram-equivalents of the bases in the reactions

$$KOH + CH_3COOH = CH_3COOK + H_2O$$
$$3Ba(OH)_2 + 2H_3PO_4 = Ba_3(PO_4)_2 + 6H_2O$$
$$2Al(OH)_3 + 3H_2SO_4 = Al_2(SO_4)_3 + 6H_2O$$
$$Ca(OH)_2 + HCl = CaOHCl + H_2O$$

are, respectively, one gram-molecule of KOH, $^1/_2$ gram-molecule of $Ba(OH)_2$, $^1/_3$ of a gram-molecule of $Al(OH)_3$, and one gram-molecule of $Ca(OH)_2$.

We now turn to methods for calculating gram-equivalents of oxidizing and reducing agents, which we meet in oxidimetry. According to the modern theory introduced by L. Pisarzhevsky, an oxidation-reduction reaction consists in redistribution of electrons between the substances taking part in the reaction. The atom (or ions) of the reducing agent are oxidized, i.e., lose some of their valence electrons, while the atoms (or ions) of the oxidizing agents are reduced, i.e., accept these electrons.

For example, in the reaction

$$10FeSO_4 + 2KMnO_4 + 8H_2SO_4 = 5Fe_2(SO_4)_3 + 2MnSO_4 + K_2SO_4 + 8H_2O$$

the reducing agent is $FeSO_4$ or, more precisely, the Fe^{++} ion, which loses an electron and is oxidized to an Fe^{+++} ion:

$$Fe^{++} - 1e = Fe^{+++}$$

The oxidizing agent is $KMnO_4$, or, more precisely, its constituent MnO_4^- ion, which is reduced to Mn^{++} as follows*:

$$MnO_4^- + 8H^+ + 5e = Mn^{++} + 4H_2O$$

* The fact that the valence of manganese is decreased in the reaction from +7 (in $KMnO_4$) to +2 (in $MnSO_4$) also shows that the $KMnO_4$ molecule does in fact gain five electrons in the reaction; the decrease of the positive valence by one unit is evidently caused by addition of one electron.

Since the electrons do not remain free, the atoms of the oxidizing agent must together receive the exact number of electrons lost by the atoms of the reducing agent. This condition determines the coefficients in oxidation-reduction reaction equations and the weight proportions in these reactions. It is therefore clear that calculations of the gram-equivalents of oxidizing and reducing agents must also be based on the number of electrons gained or lost by one molecule of substance in a given reaction.

It was stated above that in the oxidation of $FeSO_4$ (in acid solution) the $KMnO_4$ molecule gains five electrons, which is as many as would be gained by five H^+ ions. Therefore, in this reaction one gram-ion of hydrogen is equivalent to $^1/_5$ of a gram-molecule of $KMnO_4$ (i.e., 31.61 g). This is the oxidation gram-equivalent of the substance in question.

Therefore, *to find the oxidation gram-equivalent the gram-molecular weight of an oxidizing agent must be divided by the number of electrons gained by one molecule of it in the given reaction.* Gram-equivalents of reducing agents are found similarly, except that the electrons gained and not lost by the molecule are considered. For example, the reduction gram-equivalent of $FeSO_4$ in the reaction under consideration is equal to its gram-molecule, because the $FeSO_4$ molecule contains one Fe^{++} ion which loses one electron.

Similarly we find that in the reaction

$$Cr_2(SO_4)_3 + 2KMnO_4 + 8KOH = \\ = \downarrow 2MnO(OH)_2 + 2K_2CrO_4 + 3K_2SO_4 + 2H_2O$$

the reduction gram-equivalent of $Cr_2(SO_4)_3$ is $^1/_6$ of the gram-molecule, since each chromium atom increases its valence from $+3$ to $+6$, i.e., loses three electrons, and since the $Cr_2(SO_4)_3$ molecule contains 2 chromium atoms, the $Cr_2(SO_4)_3$ molecule as a whole loses 6 electrons. As regards $KMnO_4$, its oxidation gram-equivalent in this reaction is no longer $^1/_5$ but $^1/_3$ of the gram-molecule, since manganese decreases its valence from $+7$ to $+4$, i.e., gains three electrons. It follows that in oxidation-reduction reactions too the value of the gram-equivalent of a substance depends on the reaction in which it takes part.

It is also necessary to distinguish the oxidation or reduction gram-equivalents of substances from their gram-equivalents in exchange reactions. For example, it was shown above that the reduction gram-equivalent of $FeSO_4$ is equal to its gram-molecule: but in the exchange reactions

$$FeSO_4 + 2NaOH = \downarrow Fe(OH)_2 + Na_2SO_4$$

or

$$FeSO_4 + BaCl_2 = FeCl_2 + \downarrow BaSO_4$$

the gram-equivalent of $FeSO_4$ is $^1/_2$ of a gram-molecule (see below).

The milligram-equivalent is also often used in analytical chemistry. *The milligram-equivalent* (mg-eq) is one thousandth of a gram-equivalent (g-eq: 1,000), and represents *the equivalent weight of a substance expressed in milligrams.* For example, 1 g-eq of HCl is 36.46 g, and 1 mg-eq of HCl is 36.46 mg. Similarly, the gram-equivalents of H_2SO_4 and NaOH are 49.04 g and 40.00 g of the respective substances, while the respective milligram-equivalents are the same numbers of milligrams.

It follows from the concept of the chemical equivalent that gram-equivalents or milligram-equivalents are exactly the weight proportions in which substances interact. For example, neutralization of 1 g-eq of any acid takes 1 g-eq of any alkali. Likewise, in terms of milligram-equivalents, alkali will neutralize 1 mg-eq of any acid; the precipitation of 15 mg-eq of $AgNO_3$ takes exactly as many milligram-equivalents of any soluble chloride, etc.

It is evident that, since a titration is ended at the equivalence point, the numbers of gram-equivalents (or milligram-equivalents) of the titrating and the titrated substance must be equal to each other. This is the basis on which the results of volumetric determinations are calculated if solution concentrations are expressed as normalities (see Sec. 56).

A solution containing 1 g-eq of substance per litre is said to be normal (or uninormal). For example, a normal solution of sulphuric acid contains 98.08 : 2 = 49.04 g H_2SO_4 per litre, a normal permanganate solution contains 158.04 : 5 = 31.61 g $KMnO_4$ per litre, etc. It is obvious that 1 mg-eq (which is 0.001 g-eq) of one of these substances is contained in 1 ml of a normal solution. Therefore, *the normality of a solution is the number of gram-equivalents of substance per litre or the number of milligram-equivalents per millilitre.*

Normal solutions are not very suitable for volumetric analysis, as they are too concentrated. In titration with such a solution the last drop would contain a considerable amount of the substance, and the so-called *drop error* would be large.

This also applies to solutions of half this strength, seminormal solutions (0.5 *N*). Solutions of one-tenth or even one-fiftieth of the normal strength, known as decinormal (0.1 *N*) and bicentinormal (0.02 *N*), are used much more often. The former contain 0.1 and the latter 0.02 g-eq of the corresponding substance per litre (or the same number of milligram-equivalents per millilitre).

The advantage of using exactly 0.1 *N*, exactly 0.02 *N*, etc., solutions is that *equal volumes of solutions of the same normality are consumed in a reaction.* For example, titration of 25.00 ml of 0.1 *N* solution of any alkali takes exactly the same volume of 0.1 N solution of any acid, etc.

The reason for this is easy to see. One ml of a 0.1 N solution of any substance contains 0.1 mg-eq and 25 ml contains $0.1 \times 25 = 2.5$ mg-eq. Since in a titration equal numbers of milligram-equivalents of the two reacting substances are used up in the reaction, equal volumes of 0.1 N solutions must be needed for the reaction between them. The same is true whenever solutions of equal normality are taken for a reaction.

If the solutions are of different normalities, then the volume of the solution of the higher normality required for the titration will be proportionately smaller. For example, 20 ml of 0.1 N, or 10 ml of 0.2 N, or 5 ml of 0.4 N alkali solution, etc., would be required for neutralization of 20 ml of 0.1 N acid solution. It follows that *the volume of solution taken in a titration is inversely proportional to its normality*. If we represent the volume and normality of one solution in a titration by V_1 and N_1, and those of the other by V_2 and N_2, we can write:

$$\frac{V_1}{V_2}=\frac{N_2}{N_1} \text{ or } N_1V_1=N_2V_2$$

In other words, *the product of the volume of a solution used in a titration and its normality is a constant value for both reacting substances*. This is clear from the fact that the products N_1V_1 and N_2V_2 are the number of milligram-equivalents of the two substances used in the titration. Therefore, the two products must be equal to each other.

Despite the convenience of using solutions of definite normality, the so-called *empirical* solutions are also often used in practice. The concentration of an empirical solution does not depend in some simple manner on the gram-equivalent but is determined by various practical considerations.

For example, if a particular standard solution is used for repeated determinations of some element, it is convenient to choose its concentration so that 1 ml of it corresponds exactly to 0.01 g or 0.001 g, etc., of the substance to be determined.* It is then possible to find the weight of the substance in grams directly from the volume of solution taken for the titration, without calculations of any kind.

It is even more convenient to choose the concentration of the working solution so that the volume taken for the reaction (with

* Concentrations of empirical solutions are usually expressed in terms of "titre for the substance determined". This method of expressing concentrations and the calculations which it involves are discussed in Sec. 56.

a given weight of the substance being analysed) gives the percentage content of the substance or element required in the sample. Clearly the use of empirical solutions in repeated analyses offers great advantages, and such solutions are therefore often used in industrial laboratories.

56. Calculation of the Results of Volumetric Determinations

We now consider how the results of volumetric determinations are calculated with different ways of expressing the concentrations of the working solutions. We start with the commonest method, based on the use of solutions of definite normalities.

Calculations with Concentrations Expressed in Terms of Normality. The calculation procedure depends on whether the pipetting method or the method of separate samples (p. 206) is used in the determination.

Calculations with the Pipetting Method. Suppose that we wish to find the weight of $Ba(OH)_2$ present in a sample dissolved in water in a measuring flask 250.0 ml in capacity, made up to the mark with water, if 20.00 ml of this solution took 22.40 ml of 0.09884 N HCl solution.

It was stated earlier that the product of the volume and the normality should be the same for both solutions used in the titration. Therefore, denoting the normality of the $Ba(OH)_2$ solution by N, we can write:

$$20.00 \times N = 22.40 \times 0.09884$$

and hence

$$N = \frac{22.40 \times 0.09884}{20.00} = 0.1108$$

If the $Ba(OH)_2$ solution was required merely for titration of some other solutions, this result would be sufficient to indicate its concentration and no other calculations would be necessary.

However, in the present instance we have to find the amount of $Ba(OH)_2$ in 250.0 ml of the solution. To do this, we can calculate the titre of the $Ba(OH)_2$ solution from its normality and then multiply the result by 250.

Since the gram-equivalent of $Ba(OH)_2$ is $M : 2$ or 85.68 g, 1 litre of 0.1108 N solution contains 0.1108×85.68 g $Ba(OH)_2$. Therefore, the titre of the $Ba(OH)_2$ solution is

$$T_{Ba(OH)_2} = \frac{0.1108 \times 85.69}{1,000} = 0.009491 \text{ g/ml}$$

250.0 ml of this solution contains

$$Q = VT = 250.0 \times 0.009491 = 2.373 \text{ g } Ba(OH)_2$$

It is not necessary to calculate the titre in this case; we can at once find the weight of $Ba(OH)_2$ in 250 ml (i.e., in 0.25 litre) of solution as follows:

$$Q = 0.1108 \times 85.68 \times 0.2500 = 2.373 \text{ g}$$

Such calculations must be performed to the necessary degree of precision. Since volume measurements with a burette are performed to hundredths of a millilitre and the results have four significant figures (for example, 18.76 ml, or 24.60 ml, etc.), the normalities, titres, amounts of substance being determined, etc., must also be calculated to four significant figures.

In the above example it would not be permissible to round off the normality (0.1108) to 0.111, or the titre (0.009491) to 0.0095, as the precision would be lowered. Neither would there be any sense in writing 2.3735 instead of 2.373 in the final result, because in that case not one but the last two figures (35) would be uncertain (see Sec. 15).

Calculations with the Method of Separate Samples. 1. It is required to find the normality and titre of a NaOH solution if 24.60 ml of it is used in titration of 0.1590 g of chemically pure oxalic acid $H_2C_2O_4 \cdot 2H_2O$ (dissolved in an arbitrary volume of water).

It is obvious that we cannot use the equation $N_1V_1 = N_2V_2$ for solving this problem, because we know the volume of only one of the solutions (NaOH), while in the case of oxalic acid we know the weight, and not the normality of the solution. In any titration the numbers of gram-equivalents of the reacting substances are equal to one another; we therefore have to find the numbers of gram-equivalents of NaOH and $H_2C_2O_4 \cdot 2H_2O$ and equate them. This gives an equation from which the required normality of the NaOH solution can easily be found.

In the reaction oxalic acid is converted into the neutral salt $Na_2C_2O_4$, i.e., it behaves as a dibasic acid. Therefore, the gram-equivalent of oxalic acid is half of its gram-molecule, or 63.03 g. The sample of oxalic acid taken contains $\frac{0.1590}{63.03}$ g-eq.

On the other hand, if the normality of the NaOH solution is N, this means that 1 litre of it contains N g-eq, and 1 ml contains $\frac{N}{1,000}$ g-eq NaOH.

Therefore, the 24.60 ml of the caustic soda solution taken in the titration contains

$$\frac{24.60 \times N}{1,000} \text{ g-eq NaOH}$$

We form the equation:

$$\text{number of g-eq NaOH} = \text{number of g-eq } H_2C_2O \text{ } 2H_2O$$

i.e.,

$$\frac{24.60 \times N}{1,000} = \frac{0.1590}{63.03}$$

Solving it, we have

$$N = \frac{0.1590 \times 1,000}{24.60 \times 63.03} = 0.1026$$

The concentration of the NaOH solution is therefore 0.1026 N. From this it is easy to find the titre of the NaOH which is

$$T_{NaOH} = \frac{0.1026 \times 40.00}{1,000} = 0.004104 \text{ g/ml}$$

2. Find the amount of acetic acid in a solution if 20.50 ml of 0.1145 N NaOH solution was required to neutralize it.

Reasoning as before, we find that

$$\frac{20.50 \times 0.1145}{1,000} \text{ g-eq NaOH}$$

was used in the titration.

The number of gram-equivalents of acetic acid was equal to this. Since the gram-equivalent of acetic acid is 60.05 g, we have

$$Q_{CH_3COOH} = \frac{20.50 \times 0.1145 \times 60.05}{1,000} = 0.1410 \text{ g}$$

In calculations of analytical results it is sometimes more convenient to convert the volume of a solution taken into the equivalent volume of a 1 N solution of the same substance. For this calculation *the volume of the solution must be multiplied by its normality.*

For example, if 20.00 ml of 0.25 N HCl solution was taken for titration of a certain alkali solution, this is equivalent to the use of $20.00 \times 0.25 = 5$ ml of a hydrochloric acid of four times that concentration (i.e., 1 N HCl).

Calculations with Concentrations Expressed in Terms of the Solution Titre. One example of calculation of analytical results when the concentrations are expressed in terms of titre has already been given (p. 15). Let us consider another example of this type.

It is required to find the number of grams of H_2SO_4 contained in 500 ml of a solution if 25.00 ml of the solution took 22.80 ml of a NaOH solution the titre of which was 0.004257 g/ml.

The amount of NaOH used in the reaction is

$$Q_{NaOH} = T_{NaOH} V_{NaOH} = 0.004257 \times 22.80 \text{ g}$$

Since 1 g-eq (40.00 g) of NaOH reacts with 1 g-eq (49.04 g) of H_2SO_4, we can write

$$\begin{array}{l} 49.04 \text{ g } H_2SO_4 \text{ corresponds to } 40.00 \text{ g NaOH} \\ x \text{ g } H_2SO_4 \text{ corresponds to } 0.004257 \times 22.80 \text{ g NaOH} \end{array}$$

$$x = \frac{49.04 \times 0.004257 \times 22.80}{40.00} = 0.1190 \text{ g}$$

Further,

$$T_{H_2SO_4} = \frac{0.1190}{25.00} = 0.004758 \text{ g/ml}$$

and

$$Q_{H_2SO_4} = T_{H_2SO_4} \times 500.0 = 0.004758 \times 500.0 = 2.380 \text{ g}$$

This is a less convenient method than the others, and is therefore hardly ever used now.

Calculations with Concentrations Expressed in Terms of Titre for the Substance Determined. In repeated analyses it is very convenient to express concentrations of working solutions in terms of the so-called *titre for the substance determined* rather than normality or titre, because the calculations are thereby considerably simplified.

For example, the titre of an $AgNO_3$ solution used for repeated determinations of Cl^- is usually given for chlorine; i.e., the number of grams of Cl^- equivalent to 1 ml of the $AgNO_3$ solution is indicated.

The titre for the substance determined is very easy to find from the known normality. In the present example, if the normality of the $AgNO_3$ solution is, say, 0.1100, then 1 ml of this solution contains $\frac{0.1100}{1,000}$ g-eq $AgNO_3$ and reacts with the same number of gram-equivalents of Cl^-. Since the gram-equivalent of Cl^- is 35.45 g, the titre of the $AgNO_3$ solution for chlorine is

$$T_{AgNO_3/Cl^-} = \frac{0.1100 \times 35.45}{1,000} = 0.003899 \text{ g/ml}$$

For example, if in the determination of Cl^- in some substance 20.00 ml of this $AgNO_3$ solution was used for titration, then the solution which was titrated contained

$$x = T_{AgNO_3/Cl^-} V_{AgNO_3} = 0.003899 \times 20.00 = 0.07798 \text{ g } Cl^-$$

The convenience of this method is obvious for repeated analyses; the titre of the working solution for the substance determined having once been found, the amount of the substance in a sample is found simply by multiplying the titre by the volume of solution used. Therefore, this method is used very widely in laboratories which have to deal with repeated determinations of the same element in a large number of samples. On the other hand, if the determinations are not of the multiple type and a particular standard solution is used for determining not always one but different elements, it is more convenient to calculate results from the normality.

Let us consider several more examples of calculations with the concentrations expressed in terms of titre for the substance determined.

1. The titre of a $K_2Cr_2O_7$ solution is 0.005000 g/ml. Find the titre of this solution for iron, $T_{K_2Cr_2O_7/Fe}$.

The titres of a solution expressed in grams of different substances are obviously in the same ratio as the gram-equivalents of these substances. Therefore, we can write

$$\frac{T_{K_2Cr_2O_7/Fe}}{T_{K_2Cr_2O_7}}=\frac{\text{g-eq}_{Fe}}{\text{g-eq}_{K_2Cr_2O_7}}$$

But the electron-ion equations for the oxidizing and reducing agent in the reaction

$$Fe^{++}-1e=Fe^{+++}$$

$$Cr_2O_7^{--}+14H^{+}+6e=2Cr^{+++}+7H_2O$$

show* that $\text{g-eq}_{Fe}=A_{Fe}=55.85$ g, and $\text{g-eq}_{K_2Cr_2O_7}=\frac{M}{6}=49.03$ g. Consequently

$$T_{K_2Cr_2O_7/Fe}=T_{K_2Cr_2O_7}\cdot\frac{\text{g-eq}_{Fe}}{\text{g-eq}_{K_2Cr_2O_7}}=0.005000\cdot\frac{55.85}{49.03}=0.005696\text{ g Fe/ml}$$

2. Find the titre of a $KMnO_4$ solution for iron, given that 20.00 ml of this solution is required for titration of a solution containing 0.1170 g Fe^{++}.

If 20.00 ml of $KMnO_4$ solution reacts with 0.1170 g Fe^{++}, one millilitre of the same solution is equivalent to 1/20 of this weight of Fe^{++}. Therefore

$$T_{KMnO_4/Fe}=\frac{0.1170}{20.00}=0.005850\text{ g Fe/ml}$$

3. Find the amount of acetic acid in a solution if 20.50 ml of 0.1145 *N* NaOH solution was required to neutralize it (p. 214).

We first find the titre of the NaOH solution for acetic acid:

$$T_{NaOH/CH_3COOH}=\frac{0.1145\times 60.05}{1,000}$$

---

* *A* is the atomic weight.

This number of grams of CH_3COOH reacts with 1 ml of the NaOH solution; since 20.50 ml of NaOH solution was used, the weight of acetic acid is:

$$Q_{CH_3COOH} = \frac{0.1145 \times 60.05 \times 20.50}{1,000} = 0.1410 \text{ g}$$

Thus, in calculating analytical results by the method of separate samples we can find the amount of the element being determined in two ways. We either calculate the number of gram-equivalents of the solution taken for the titration and multiply it by the gram-equivalent of the substance being determined, or we convert the titre of the solution into its titre for the substance determined and multiply the result by the volume of solution used. Both methods are equally convenient and both yield the same expression for finding *Q*.

It follows from the above that the titre for the substance determined is to some extent analogous to the conversion factor in gravimetric analysis. Indeed, just as the conversion factor shows what amount of the substance (or element) being determined corresponds to 1 g of the weighed form, the titre for the substance determined shows what amount of the latter corresponds to 1 ml of the particular solution used. Just as the amount of substance or element being determined is found by multiplying the weight of the precipitate (weighed form) by the conversion factor, in volumetric analysis this amount is found by multiplying the volume of solution used by its titre for the substance determined.

57. Calculations in Preparation and Dilution of Solutions

In Sec. 56 we considered methods for calculating analytical results. In addition to such calculations, it is also necessary to perform various calculations when solutions are prepared or diluted, when it is necessary to convert their concentrations from one system into another, etc. We shall now consider these calculations in some detail.

The concentration of a solution is usually taken to mean the amount of substance dissolved in unit volume (or weight) of solution. The unit of volume is usually the litre, while the amount of dissolved substance is generally expressed in moles (gram-molecules) or in gram-equivalents. In the former case we have the molar concentration or *molarity* of the solution, and in the second, its *normality*. Conversion from one to the other is very simple; it is merely necessary to know what fraction of the molecular weight is the equivalent of the substance. Consider the following examples.

Example 1. Calculate the molarity of a 0.3 *N* $Al_2(SO_4)_3$ solution.

Solution. As was shown on p. 209, the gram-equivalent of $Al_2(SO_4)_3$ is 1/6 of a gram-molecule of it. Therefore, in order to find how many moles are present in 0.3 g-eq of this salt we must multiply 0.3 by 1/6. Therefore,

$$M = N \times 1/6 = 0.3 \times 1/6 = 0.05$$

i.e., the molarity of the solution is 0.05.

Example 2. Calculate the normality of a 0.2 *M* $Bi(NO_3)_3$ solution.

Solution. Since a gram-molecule of $Bi(NO_3)_3$ corresponds to 3 gram-molecules of HNO_3, i.e., to 3 g-ions of H^+, the gram-equivalent of this salt is equal to 1/3 of a gram-molecule. Therefore, a 1 *M* solution is 3 *N*, and a 0.2 *M* solution is $0.2 \times 3 = 0.6$ *N*.

Calculations relating to solution concentrations are somewhat complicated by the fact that, in addition to the methods for expressing concentrations already described, *percentage concentrations* are also often used in practice. It must be remembered that unless otherwise stated *the percentage concentration is the number of parts of solute by weight per 100 parts of solution by weight.* For example, the expression "3% NaCl solution" means that each 100 g of solution contains 3 g NaCl and 97 g water.

In converting percentage concentrations to molarities or normalities we must take into account the specific gravity (density) of the solution. It is known from physics that the weight (*P*) of a body, its density (*d*), and its volume (*V*) are connected as follows:

$$P = Vd \text{ or } V = \frac{P}{d}$$

Let us consider some numerical examples.

Example 3. Calculate the normality of a 20.0% sulphuric acid solution.

Solution. First find from tables (Appendix V) the specific gravity of 20.0% H_2SO_4 solution. It is (rounded off) 1.14. Then calculate the volume of 100 g of 20.0% H_2SO_4 solution:

$$V = \frac{P}{d} = \frac{100}{1.14} = 87.7 \text{ ml}$$

Now calculate the number of grams of H_2SO_4 in 1 litre of 20.0% sulphuric acid solution:

87.7 ml contains 20.0 g H_2SO_4

1,000 ml contains x g H_2SO_4

and hence

$$x = \frac{1{,}000 \times 20.0}{87.7} = 228 \text{ g}$$

We now have to find how many gram-equivalents this weight of H_2SO_4 corresponds to. Since the gram-equivalent of H_2SO_4 is half its gram-molecular weight, i.e., 49.04 g, we have

$$N = \frac{228}{49.04} = 4.65$$

Therefore, a 20.0% sulphuric acid solution is approximately 4.65 *N*. The molarity of the same solution is $4.65 : 2 = 2.32$.

Standard acid solutions, such as 0.1 *N* HCl or H_2SO_4 solutions, are prepared from the corresponding concentrated acid solutions. The volume of the concentrated solution which must be taken to give a required volume of the diluted solution is calculated from the density and the corresponding concentration of the concentrated solution. When the solution has been prepared it is standardized as described in Sec. 54. The calculations used in such cases are illustrated by the following example.

Example 4. Find how many mullilitres of concentrated sulphuric acid, sp. gr. 1.84, containing 96% H_2SO_4, must be taken for preparation of 5 litres of an approximately 0.1 *N* solution.

Solution. First calculate how many grams of anhydrous H_2SO_4 is required for the given volume of 0.1 *N* solution. Since the gram-equivalent of H_2SO_4 is *M* : 2, approximately 49 g, and 1 litre of 0.1 *N* solution contains 0.1 g-eq, the total amount of H_2SO_4 required is

$$x = 0.1 \times 49 \times 5 \approx 25 \text{ g}$$

Now find the weight of 96% sulphuric acid which contains this weight of anhydrous H_2SO_4:

100 g of 96% acid contains 96 g H_2SO_4

y g of 96% acid contains 25 g H_2SO_4

and hence

$$y = \frac{25 \times 100}{96} = 26 \text{ g}$$

We now convert the weight of 96% sulphuric acid into the corresponding volume:

$$V = \frac{26}{1.84} = 14 \text{ ml}$$

Therefore, to prepare 5 litres of approximately 0.1 *N* sulphuric acid solution we must measure out (in a small measuring cylinder) about 14 ml of concentrated H_2SO_4, sp. gr. 1.84, and dilute it with water (*the acid must be poured into water, not water into the acid*) to 5 litres.

Let us now consider some examples of calculations used when solutions are diluted from one normality to another or from one percentage concentration to another.

Example 5. Find the volume to which 50.0 ml of 2 *N* HCl must be diluted to convert it into 0.3 *N* solution*.

Solution. It was shown in Sec. 55 that the product of the volume of a solution and its normality gives the number of milligram-equivalents of the substance present in that volume of solution. If the solution is diluted its volume and normality change but the total number of milligram-equivalents of the dissolved

---

* In this and similar problems the concentrations (2 *N* and 0.3 *N*) are taken as exact. The answer must be found to a degree of precision sufficient for practical purposes (1 ml or 0.1 ml).

substance remains constant. It follows that, as in titration, the following equation is true in dilution:

$$N_1V_1 = N_2V_2$$

Applying this equation in the present case, we have

$$V \times 0.3 = 50.0 \times 2$$

and hence

$$V = \frac{50.0 \times 2}{0.3} = 333 \text{ ml}$$

Therefore, to convert a 2 N HCl solution into a 0.3 N solution 50.0 ml of the 2 N solution must be diluted with water to 333 ml.

Example 6. What volume of a 1 N solution contains the same amount of a given dissolved substance as 30 ml of a 0.2 N solution?

Solution. Since the amount of substance is the same in both solutions, the products of the solution volumes and normalities should be equal.

Therefore

$$V \times 1 = 30.0 \times 0.2, \quad \text{and } V = 6 \text{ ml}$$

To convert the volume of a solution of a given normality into the equivalent volume of a 1 N solution the volume must be multiplied by the normality.

Example 7. Calculate the proportions by weight and by volume in which a 54% solution of nitric acid (sp. gr. 1.33) must be mixed with a 14% solution of nitric acid (sp. gr. 1.08) to give a 20% solution.

Solution. Represent the weight of the first solution by x, and of the second by y. The total weight of the mixture will be $(x + y)$ g. Now calculate the number of grams of pure (anhydrous) HNO_3 contained in x g of 54% acid. 100 g of the latter contains 54 g, 1 g contains $\frac{54}{100}$ g, and x g contains $\frac{54x}{100}$ g HNO_3. Similarly, we find that y g of 14% acid contains $\frac{14y}{100}$ g HNO_3, and $(x + y)$ g of 20% solution (mixture) contains $\frac{(x+y)\,20}{100}$ g HNO_3. But the amount of HNO_3 is the same after as before mixing. Therefore, we have the equation

$$\frac{54x}{100} + \frac{14y}{100} = \frac{20\,(x+y)}{100}$$

or

$$54x + 14y = 20x + 20y$$

Rearranging this equation, we have

$$\frac{x}{y} = \frac{20-14}{54-20}$$

This result shows that to obtain a 20% solution of HNO_3 we must take 20—14=6 parts by weight of 54% acid to 54—20=34 parts by weight of 14% acid. The volume proportions can be easily found from these weight proportions. The volume of 6 g of 54% acid is $\frac{6}{1.33} = 4.5$ ml, and the volume of 34 g of 14% acid is $\frac{34}{1.08} = 31.5$ ml. Therefore, 4.5 ml of 54% HNO_3 must be added to each 31.5 ml of 14% HNO_3.

If the volume proportions of the solutions to be mixed are known, it is easy to calculate the volume of one of the solutions which must be mixed with a given volume of the other. For example, if we have 100 ml of 54% HNO_3 we must add $\frac{31.5 \times 100}{4.5} = 700$ ml of 14% HNO_3.

In practice, weight proportions of solutions to be mixed are calculated by means of the very convenient graphical device shown below:

$$\begin{matrix} 54 & & 6 \text{ (i.e., } 20-14) \\ & 20 & \\ 14 & & 34 \text{ (i.e., } 54-20) \end{matrix}$$

On the left we write, one above the other, the percentage concentrations of the two original solutions, and the final concentration of the mixture is written in the centre. On the right, at the opposite ends of the diagonals (i.e., crosswise) we write the differences between the final and each of the initial concentrations (or vice versa), the smaller quantity being subtracted from the larger. Each of the differences represents the weight of the solution the percentage concentration of which is written in the same horizontal line. Thus, in this instance the diagram shows that 6 parts by weight of 54% acid must be taken with 34 parts by weight of 14% acid.

The same device can be used in calculations relating to dilution of solutions with water. The percentage concentration of water is taken as zero. This is illustrated by the following examples.

Example 8. Calculate the weight of water to be added to 100 ml of 72% sulphuric acid (sp. gr. 1.63) to convert it into 26% acid.

Solution. We use the above graphical method to find the relative weights of 72% acid solution and water:

$$\begin{matrix} 72 & & 26 \\ & 26 & \\ 0 & & 46 \end{matrix}$$

Therefore, we must take 46 parts of water to 26 parts of 72% acid solution by weight. We now convert to volume proportions:

$$V_{H_2SO_4} : V_{H_2O} = \frac{26}{1.63} : \frac{46}{1} = 16 : 46$$

By proportion

To 16 ml H_2SO_4 we must add 46 ml H_2O
To 100 ml H_2SO_4 we must add x ml H_2O

and finally

$$x = \frac{46 \times 100}{16} \approx 290 \text{ ml}$$

Example 9. How much water must be added to 200 ml of hydrochloric acid of sp. gr. 1.18 to obtain an acid of sp. gr. 1.10?

Solution. This problem is quite analogous to the previous one. The only difference is that the percentage concentrations are not given but must be found from tables (Appendix V). We find from the table that acid of sp. gr. 1.18 contains 36% HCl, and acid of sp. gr. 1.10 contains 20% HCl.

We can therefore write

$$\begin{matrix} 36 & & 20 \\ & 20 & \\ 0 & & 16 \end{matrix}$$

Therefore, 16 g of water must be added to 20 g of HCl solution of sp gr. 1.18. Converting to volumes, we have $\frac{20}{1.18} = 17$ ml for HCl and 16 ml for water.

By proportion:

To 17 ml HCl we must add 16 ml H_2O
To 200 ml HCl we must add x ml H_2O

and finally

$$x = \frac{200 \times 16}{17} \approx 190 \text{ ml}$$

QUESTIONS AND PROBLEMS
(on Secs. 49-57)

1. What is the principle of volumetric analysis, and how does it differ from gravimetric analysis?
2. 250.0 ml of a NaOH solution contains 10.00 g NaOH. What is the titre of this solution?

Answer: $T_{NaOH} = 0.04000$ g/ml.

3. What is the equivalence point in titration, and how is it determined?
4. Free iodine oxidizes various substances; for example,

$$I_2 + Na_2SO_3 + H_2O = Na_2SO_4 + 2HI$$

Knowing that I_2 solutions are dark brown in colour while I^- ions are colour less, say how the equivalence point may be determined in titration of Na_2SO solution with iodine. Would it be possible to use starch solution as an indicato in order to obtain a higher degree of precision in this titration? What would be the colour change at the end of the titration in that case?

5. Explain the use of K_2CrO_4 as indicator in titration of NaCl solution with $AgNO_3$ solution.
6. What is the principle of conductometric titration of strong acids with strong bases?
7. Specify the conditions to which reactions used in titration must conform.
8. Give exact definitions of the units of volume used in volumetric analysis.
9. Explain why burettes and pipettes must be rinsed out before use with the solutions for which they are to be used. Can this be done with measuring flasks (designed to hold definite volumes of solution)?
10. Explain why the last drop of solution must not be blown out of a pipette.
11. A student took a burette reading with his eye below the level of the meniscus. How did this affect the volume measurement?
12. When the capacity of a 25 ml pipette was checked the weight of water delivered by it (average from three experiments) was 24.82 g. The temperature of the water was 15°C. Calculate the volume of water delivered by the pipette.

Answer: 24.87 ml.

13. The coefficient of expansion of glass is 0.000025. What is the decrease in the capacity of a 200 ml measuring flask calibrated at 20°C if it is used for measuring the volume of a liquid at 10°C?

Answer: 0.05 ml (or 0.025%).

14. What weight of water must be weighed out at 14°C with brass weights (sp. gr. of brass is 8.4) for calibration of a 100 ml measuring flask at 20°C? What is the percentage error if exactly 100 g of water is weighed out in the calibration?

Answer: 99.80 g; +0.2%.

15. In preparation of a standard sodium carbonate solution 1.3250 g of chemically pure Na_2CO_3 was dissolved in a measuring flask and made up to 250.0 ml with water. Calculate the titre of the solution.

Answer: $T_{Na_2CO_3} = 0.005300$ g/ml.

16. What substances are known as "primary standards" and to what requirements must they conform?

17. In preparation of a standard solution of sulphuric acid 2.9 ml of concentrated (approximately 96%) sulphuric acid of sp. gr. 1.84 was diluted with water to 1 litre. Can the *exact* titre of this solution be determined from these data?

18. In standardization of an H_2SO_4 solution prepared as described in the previous problem 25.00 ml of Na_2CO_3 solution of titre 0.005300 g/ml was titrated with the H_2SO_4 solution. The volume of the latter was 24.50 ml. Knowing that the reaction equation is

$$Na_2CO_3 + H_2SO_4 = Na_2SO_4 + H_2O + CO_2$$

calculate the titre of the H_2SO_4 solution.

Answer: $T_{H_2SO_4} = 0.005003$ g/ml.

19. What is the titre of an HCl solution if 0.2868 g AgCl was formed by addition of 20.00 ml of $AgNO_3$ solution to it?

Answer: $T_{HCl} = 0.003646$ g/ml.

20. What are standard samples? What is the advantage in determining titres of working solutions against standard samples?

21. Under what conditions would the use of wrongly calibrated measuring vessels not affect the accuracy of analytical results?

22. Describe volumetric determinations (a) by the pipetting method, (b) by the method of separate samples.

23. Define the terms *gram-equivalent*, *milligram-equivalent*, and *normality* of a solution.

24. Find the gram-equivalents of the acids, bases, and salts in the following reactions:

$$HBr + NH_4OH = NH_4Br + H_2O$$
$$H_2SO_4 + Ca(OH)_2 = CaSO_4 + 2H_2O$$
$$H_2SO_4 + NaCl = NaHSO_4 + HCl$$
$$Mg(OH)_2 + HCl = MgOHCl + H_2O$$
$$2Al(OH)_3 + 3H_2SO_4 = Al_2(SO_4)_3 + 6H_2O$$
$$K_2Cr_2O_7 + 2BaCl_2 + H_2O = 2BaCrO_4 + 2HCl + 2KCl$$

25. Calculate the titres of: (a) 1,000 N HBr, NH_4OH, and $BaCl_2$ solutions; (b) 0.1000 N $Ca(OH)_2$ and NaCl solutions; (c) 0.02000 N $K_2Cr_2O_7$ solution when the respective substances take part in the reactions listed in the preceding problem.

Answer: (a) 0.08092 g/ml, 0.03505 g/ml, 0.1041 g/ml; (b) 0.003705 g/ml, 0.005844 g/ml; (c) 0.001471 g/ml.

26. What are the gram-equivalents of the oxidizing and reducing agents in the following reactions:

$$2KMnO_4+5KNO_2+3H_2SO_4=2MnSO_4+K_2SO_4+5KNO_3+3H_2O$$

$$2CrCl_3+3Br_2+16KOH=2K_2CrO_4+6KCl+6KBr+8H_2O$$

$$K_2Cr_2O_7+3H_2S+4H_2SO_4=Cr_2(SO_4)_3+K_2SO_4+7H_2O+\downarrow 3S$$

$$KClO_3+6HCl+6FeCl_2=6FeCl_3+KCl+3H_2O$$

27. What does n represent in the formula for the gram-equivalent

$$\text{g-eq}=\frac{M}{n}$$

(a) in oxidation-reduction reactions; (b) in exchange reactions?

28. What are the normalities of solutions containing, per litre, (a) 4.0106 g HCl; (b) 4.8059 g H_2SO_4?

Answer: (a) 0.1100; (b) 0.09797.

29. Find the normality of an HCl solution if its titre is 0.003592 g/ml.

Answer: 0.09851.

30. What is the titre of a 0.1205 N H_2SO_4 solution?

Answer: 0.005909 g/ml.

31. What is the weight of KOH in 200 ml of a 0.09200 N solution?

Answer: 1.032 g.

32. What are the normality and titre of an HNO_3 solution if 20.00 ml of it takes 15 ml of 0.1200 N NaOH solution?

Answer: Normality, 0.09000; titre, 0.005671 g/ml.

33. Calculate the weight of H_2SO_4 in 5 litres of a solution if titration of 25.00 ml of this solution takes 22.50 ml of 0.09500 N KOH solution.

Answer: 20.97 g.

34. Now many gram-equivalents are contained in (a) 1.8909 g of chemically pure oxalic acid $H_2C_2O_4 \cdot 2H_2O$; (b) 20 ml of 0.12 N NaOH solution?

Answer: (a) 0.03000; (b) 0.0024.

35. How many milligram-equivalents are contained in (a) 0.4240 g of chemically pure Na_2CO_3; (b) 50 ml of 0.20 N H_2SO_4 solution?

Answer: (a) 8.0000; (b) 10.

36. What are the normality and titre of a KOH solution if 26.00 ml of it was required for titration of 0.1560 g of chemically pure (dibasic) succinic acid $H_2C_4H_4O_4$?

Answer: $N = 0.1016$; $T = 0.005700$ g/ml.

37. What is the percentage of $H_2C_2O_4 \cdot 2H_2O$ in a sample if 25.60 ml of 0.09000 N KOH solution was required for titration of 0.1500 g of the sample dissolved in an arbitrary volume of water?

Answer: 96.79%.

38. Explain the meaning of the expressions T_{HCl/Na_2CO_3} and $T_{Na_2CO_3/HCl}$. In grams of which substance is each of these titres given?

39. Titration of 0.0340 g $AgNO_3$ took 20.00 ml of an HCl solution. Calculate $T_{HCl/Ag}$.

Answer: 0.001077 g/ml Ag.

40. What is $T_{HCl/CaO}$ if 27.65 ml of this hydrochloric acid solution is required for titration of 0.1144 g Na_2CO_3 (see Problem 39)?

Answer: 0.002189 g CaO/ml.

41. In determinations of free P_2O_5 in superphosphate the H_3PO_4 present in an aqueous solution of the superphosphate is titrated with NaOH, NaH_2PO_4 being formed. What is T_{NaOH/P_2O_5} if 0.1035 g of $H_2C_2O_4$ takes 25.15 ml of the given NaOH solution?

Answer: 0.006486 g P_2O_5/ml.

42. What is the percentage of iron in an ore if titration of a $FeCl_2$ solution obtained from 0.2000 g of the ore takes 20.00 ml of a dichromate solution if titre $T_{K_2Cr_2O_7/Fe} = 0.006500$ g/ml?

Answer: 65.00%.

43. What are the titres of 0.09000 *N* sulphuric acid solution: (a) for $Ba(OH)_2$; (b) for NH_3; (c) for N?

Answer: (a) 0.007712 g/ml; (b) 0.001533 g/ml; (c) 0.001261 g/ml.

44. Calculate the weight of Na_2CO_3 in a solution which took 22.00 ml of 0.1200 *N* HCl solution for titration: (a) by calculation of the number of gram-equivalents of HCl used; (b) by calculation of T_{HCl/Na_2CO_3}:

$$\text{g-eq}_{Na_2CO_3} = \frac{M}{2} = \frac{106.0}{2} = 53.00$$

Answer: 0.1399 g

45. What weight of chemically pure Na_2CO_3 should be taken so that titration of its solution would take 20-30 ml of 0.1 *N* H_2SO_4 solution?

Answer: About 0.11-0.16 g.

46. How many millilitres of 0.0200 *N* $KMnO_4$ solution would be required for titration of 20.00 ml of 0.0300 *N* $FeSO_4$ solution?

Answer: 30.00 ml.

47. How many millilitres of 0.02000 *N* $KMnO_4$ solution would be required for titration of an $FeSO_4$ solution containing 0.0200 g of iron?

Answer: 17.9 ml.

48. It is required to prepare a solution each millilitre of which precipitates (in the presence of NH_4OH) 1.0 mg of Ca^{++} from solutions of calcium salts. What weight of chemically pure $H_2C_2O_4 \cdot 2H_2O$ should be taken, dissolved in water, and made up to 250.0 ml in a measuring flask for this purpose?

Answer: 0.7863 g.

49. What is the titre of a $K_2Cr_2O_7$ solution if 1.00 ml of it corresponds to exactly 0.5% of iron in titration of a $FeCl_2$ solution prepared from an ore sample weighing 0.2000 g?

Answer: $T_{K_2Cr_2O_7} = 0.000878$ g/ml.

50. Calculate the normality of a 40% $CaCl_2$ solution of sp. gr. 1.396.

Answer: Approximately 10 *N*.

51. Calculate the molar concentration of 10% NH_3 solution (sp. gr. 0.958).

Answer: Approximately 5.6 *M*.

52. How many millilitres of 2.00 *N* HNO_3 solution should be taken for preparation of 3 litres of 0.1000 *N* solution?

Answer: 150 ml.

53. What volume of 1 *N* HCl solution is equivalent to 23.8 ml of 0.20 *N* HCl solution?

Answer: 4.8 ml.

54. How many millilitres of 20% HCl solution of sp. gr 1.098 should be taken for preparation of 5 litres of 0.1 *N* solution?

Answer: 83 ml.

55. How many millilitres of 10% HCl solution (sp. gr. 1.047) should be added to 50 ml of 37.23% solution of sp. gr. 1.19 to give a 25% HCl solution?

Answer: 46 ml.

56. How much water must be added to 200 ml of 46% HNO_3 solution (sp.gr. 1.285) to convert it into 10% solution?

Answer: 925 ml.

57. How much water must be added to 1 litre of HNO_3 of sp. gr. 1.405 to obtain nitric acid of sp. gr. 1.193?

Answer: 1,581 ml.

CHAPTER V

THE NEUTRALIZATION METHOD

58. The Principle of the Neutralization Method

The neutralization method includes all volumetric determinations based on the neutralization reaction:

$$H^+ + OH^- \rightleftarrows H_2O$$

By this method a standard solution of an acid can be used for quantitative determination of alkalies (acidimetry), or a standard solution of an alkali can be used for quantitative determination of acids (alkalimetry).*

This method is used for various other volumetric determinations which involve neutralization in one way or another; for example, for determination of certain salts which, like Na_2CO_3 and $Na_2B_4O_7$ have a strongly alkaline reaction as the result of hydrolysis and which can therefore be titrated with acids; for determination of the hardness of water; for determination of ammonium salts; for determination of nitrogen in organic compounds, etc.

The main working solutions in the neutralization method are an acid solution (usually HCl or H_2SO_4) and an alkaline solution (usually NaOH or KOH).

These substances do not conform to the conditions for primary standards, and therefore standard solutions of them cannot be prepared from exact weights diluted to definite volumes; they must be standardized by titration (or gravimetrically).

The commonest primary standards for standardization of acids are borax $Na_2B_4O_7 \cdot 10H_2O$ or sodium carbonate Na_2CO_3. These substances can be obtained practically pure and strictly corresponding to their formulas by recrystallization. As stated, their solutions are strongly alkaline and can be titrated with acids.

Alkalies are generally standardized against oxalic acid $H_2C_2O_4 \times \times 2H_2O$ or succinic acid $H_2C_4H_4O_4$. Both these acids are crystalline solids. They are also obtained quite pure and correspond to their

---

* See footnote to p. 192.

formulas after recrystallization. Succinic acid is more convenient as a primary standard than oxalic acid, as it does not contain water of crystallization and there is no risk of efflorescence when it is kept.

We know from qualitative analysis* that any aqueous solution, regardless of its reaction, contains H^+ and OH^- ions as the result of dissociation of water. The product of the concentrations of these ions at a given temperature is (approximately) constant.** At 22°C in any aqueous solution

$$[H^+][OH^-] = K_{H_2O} = 10^{-14} \quad (1)$$

Table VII shows that the ionic product of water K_{H_2O} increases rapidly with temperature.

Table VII

Ionic Product of Water (K_{H_2O}) at Various Temperatures

Temperature °C	K_{H_2O}	$[H^+] = [OH^-]$	Temperature °C	K_{H_2O}	$[H^+] = [OH^-]$
0	0.13×10^{-14}	0.36×10^{-7}	40	3.80×10^{-14}	1.95×10^{-7}
10	0.36×10^{-14}	0.59×10^{-7}	50	5.60×10^{-14}	2.40×10^{-7}
20	0.86×10^{-14}	0.93×10^{-7}	60	12.6×10^{-14}	3.50×10^{-7}
22	1.00×10^{-14}	1.00×10^{-7}	80	34.0×10^{-14}	5.80×10^{-7}
30	1.89×10^{-14}	1.37×10^{-7}	100	74.0×10^{-14}	8.60×10^{-7}

By the theory of electrolytic dissociation, acidic properties of solutions depend on H^+ ions, and basic properties on OH^- ions. The concentrations of these ions should be equal in water and in all neutral aqueous solutions. Therefore, at 22°C these concentrations are:

$$[H^+] = [OH^-] = \sqrt{K_{H_2O}} = \sqrt{10^{-14}} = 10^{-7} \text{ g-ion/litre}$$

In acid solutions

$$[H^+] > [OH^-], \text{ i.e., } [H^+] > 10^{-7} \text{ and } [OH^-] < 10^{-7}$$

In alkaline solutions

$$[OH^-] > [H^+], \text{ i.e., } [OH^-] > 10^{-7} \text{ and } [H^+] < 10^{-7}$$

---

* V. Alexeyev, *Qualitative Analysis*, Sec. 39, Goskhimizdat, 1960; and V. Alexeyev, *Course of Qualitative Chemical Semimicroanalysis*, Sec. 19, Goskhimizdat, 1962.

** Strictly speaking, it is not the product of the concentrations but the product of the activities of the H^+ and OH^- ions which is constant, i.e.,

$$a_{H^+} \cdot a_{OH^-} = K_{H_2O}$$

Since the concentrations of H^+ and OH^- ions are in inverse proportion, as represented by Equation (1), it is possible to represent the reaction of any solution quantitatively by the concentration of one of these ions, as the concentration of the other is thereby fully determined. For example, if the H^+ ion concentration of a solution is 10^{-10} g-ion/litre, the OH^- ion concentration is

$$10^{-14} : 10^{-10} = 10^{-4}$$

and the solution has an alkaline reaction.

Instead of the actual concentrations of H^+ or OH^- ions it is more convenient to represent the reaction of a solution by their negative logarithms, known as the hydrogen and hydroxyl exponents, pH and pOH. Therefore*

$$\mathrm{pH} = -\log [H^+]; \ \mathrm{pOH} = -\log [OH^-]$$

If we take logarithms of Equation (1) and reverse the signs, we have

$$-\log [H^+] - \log [OH^-] = 14$$

or

$$\mathrm{pH} + \mathrm{pOH} = 14 \quad (2)$$

The relationship between the H^+ and OH^- ion concentrations, the pH and pOH values, and solution reactions is illustrated in Table VIII.

From Table VIII it follows that: (a) in neutral solutions the pH (and also pOH) is 7; (b) in acid solutions pH is less than 7 and diminishes with increasing acidity; (c) in alkaline solutions pH is greater than 7 and increases with increasing alkalinity; (d) a pH increase of one unit corresponds to a tenfold decrease of H^+ ion concentration.

If a solution of any acid is titrated with an alkaline solution, the OH^- ions of the latter combine with the H^+ ions of the acid and the concentration of the latter gradually decreases while the solution pH increases. At a certain definite pH value the equivalence point is reached and no more alkali should be added.

When a solution of an alkali is titrated with an acid solution the OH^- ions are removed by the H^+ ions, and the concentration of the

---

* In accordance with the footnote to p. 228, pH and pOH are defined more precisely as the negative logarithms of the activities of H^+ and OH^- ions, i.e.,

$$\mathrm{pH} = -\log a_{H^+} \text{ and } \mathrm{pOH} = -\log a_{OH^-}$$

Here we use concentrations of the ions instead of their activities, because this changes the pH values very little and the resulting inaccuracy does not invalidate any of the conclusions.

latter gradually increases while the solution pH decreases. At a certain definite pH value the equivalence point is reached and the titration must be ended at that point.

Table VIII

Relationship Between $[H^+]$, $[OH^-]$, pH, pOH, and Solution Reaction *

$[H^+]$	$[OH^-]$	pH	pOH	Reaction
1	10^{-14}	0	14	Acid ↑
10^{-1}	10^{-13}	1	13	
10^{-2}	10^{-12}	2	12	
10^{-3}	10^{-11}	3	11	
10^{-4}	10^{-10}	4	10	
10^{-5}	10^{-9}	5	9	
10^{-6}	10^{-8}	6	8	
10^{-7}	10^{-7}	7	7	Neutral
10^{-8}	10^{-6}	8	6	Alkaline ↓
10^{-9}	10^{-5}	9	5	
10^{-10}	10^{-4}	10	4	
10^{-11}	10^{-3}	11	3	
10^{-12}	10^{-2}	12	2	
10^{-13}	10^{-1}	13	1	
10^{-14}	1	14	0	

* Vertical arrows indicate the directions of acidity and alkalinity increase.

The pH value at the equivalence point depends on the nature and concentrations of the reacting substances (acid and base).*

For example, the titration of a strong acid with a strong alkali proceeds as follows:

$$HCl + NaOH = NaCl + H_2O$$

In this case when the equivalence point has been reached the amount of alkali added is equivalent to the amount of acid being titrated, i.e., at that point the solution contains only the salt (NaCl) formed in the reaction, without any excess of acid or alkali. Salts

* The method for calculating pH at the equivalence point will be described later.

of strong acids and strong bases are not hydrolyzed and therefore have a neutral reaction (pH = 7).

Therefore, in this instance the pH value at the equivalence point should be 7. The same is evidently true in titration of any other strong acid with any strong base, or in titration of a strong base with a solution of a strong acid.

However, if a weak acid such as acetic is used, the following reaction occurs in the titration:

$$CH_3COOH + NaOH \rightleftarrows CH_3COONa + H_2O$$

At the equivalence point the solution contains the salt CH_3COONa, which is hydrolyzed as follows:

$$CH_3COONa + H_2O \rightleftarrows CH_3COOH + NaOH$$

It is seen that *hydrolysis is a reaction which is the reverse of neutralization. In this case the reaction taking place during the titration is reversible and does not go to completion.* Some of the acid and alkali used remains in the solution in the free state. At the equivalence point the amounts of free CH_3COOH and NaOH are, of course, equivalent to each other. However, whereas acetic acid, present mainly in the form of undissociated CH_3COOH molecules, yields very few free H^+ ions into solution, caustic soda (which dissociates almost completely) gives rise to a much higher concentration of OH^- ions in solution.

Therefore, titration must be stopped at pH > 7, and not at pH = 7 as in titration of HCl.

The ionic equation for hydrolysis shows especially clearly that solutions of salts formed from weak acids and strong bases must have an alkaline reaction. For example, the equation for hydrolysis

$$CH_3COONa + H_2O \rightleftarrows CH_3COOH + NaOH$$

may be written in the following form:

$$Na^+ + CH_3COO^- + H_2O \rightleftarrows CH_3COOH + Na^+ + OH^-$$

Omitting the Na^+ ions, which remain unchanged, we finally have:

$$CH_3COO^- + H_2O \rightleftarrows CH_3COOH + OH^-$$

It is clear from this ionic equation that in this case hydrolysis is accompanied by an increase of OH^- ion content, and must therefore make the solution alkaline.

Similarly we find that when weak bases are titrated with strong acids, as, for example,

$$NH_4OH + HCl \rightleftarrows NH_4Cl + H_2O$$

the reaction of the solution at the equivalence point is determined by hydrolysis of NH_4Cl, which leads to an increase of H^+ ion content, as is evident from the ionic equation for the hydrolysis:

$$NH_4^+ + H_2O \rightleftarrows NH_4OH + H^+$$

Therefore, in this case the pH at the equivalence point must be less than 7.*

To summarize the above, *in different cases titration must be ended at different pH values, depending on the nature (and concentrations) of reacting acid and base.*

59. Indicators for the Neutralization Method

It is known that neutralization is not accompanied by visible changes such as alteration in the colour of the solution. Therefore, a suitable indicator must be added to the titrated solution in order to determine the equivalence point.

It was stated earlier that when the solution acquires a definite pH value this is a sign that the equivalence point has been reached. Therefore, substances which change colour in accordance with pH are used as neutralization indicators. They include litmus, methyl orange, phenolphthalein, and many other substances. The colour of each of these changes over a definite narrow range of pH, and this range depends only on the properties of the given indicator and is quite independent of the nature of the reacting acid and base. Because of this, the colour change of an indicator generally takes place not strictly at the equivalence point but with some deviation from it. This deviation leads to a certain error, known as the *indicator error* in titration. The magnitude of this error varies over a wide range, in accordance with the indicator used and with the kind of acid and alkali used in the reaction. If the indicator is chosen correctly the error does not exceed the usual limits of analytical error and may be disregarded. On the other hand, if an unsuitable indicator is used the error may be very considerable.

One of the most widely used indicators is methyl orange, which is yellow with alkalies and red with acids. However, if a 0.1 *N* acetic acid solution is titrated with 0.1 *N* NaOH solution in its presence the red colour of the indicator changes to orange** at the point when

---

* For fuller details of hydrolysis, see V. Alexeyev, *Qualitative Analysis*, Sec. 41, Goskhimizdat, 1960; or V. Alexeyev, *Course of Qualitative Chemical Semimicroanalysis*, Sec. 46, Goskhimizdat, 1962.

** Titration in presence of methyl orange is usually ended when the colour becomes orange, intermediate between red and yellow.

only 15% of the CH_3COOH has been neutralized. In this case the indicator error is enormous (85%).

It might seem at first sight that it is nevertheless possible to obtain the correct result. If it can be found exactly how much alkali is required for neutralization of 15% of the acid taken, it should be easy to calculate how much would be needed for 100%.

However, in reality the situation is much more complicated, because in this instance the indicator does not change colour sharply (i.e., by addition of one drop of alkali), but very slowly and gradually. When 25 ml of 0.1 *N* CH_3COOH solution is titrated with NaOH solution of the same concentration about 4 ml of the NaOH solution is required to change the red colour of the indicator to orange. This evidently makes titration of CH_3COOH in presence of methyl orange practically impossible, because the point at which the titration must be stopped cannot be determined exactly. On the other hand, if the same titration is performed with phenolphthalein as indicator one drop of alkali at the end of the titration produces a sharp colour change and the indicator error is only 0.02%, i.e., it is within the limits of experimental error.

This example shows *the great significance of the selection of a proper indicator in titration*. For a clear understanding of this fundamental problem in volumetric analysis we must consider the theory of indicators.

60. Theory of Indicators

Chemists have long been aware of the importance of indicators in volumetric analysis. However, until the end of the last century investigations of indicators were purely empirical in character and did not touch upon the principles of the physico-chemical processes which take place when an indicator changes colour. This was because of the lack of a general chemical theory which could be the basis of a theory of indicators and which could provide a common viewpoint for all the great variety of available experimental data.

The theory of electrolytic dissociation, put forward in 1887 by S. Arrhenius, proved to be suitable for the purpose. After only 7 years (in 1894) Ostwald was able to formulate the *ionic theory of indicators.*

By this theory, *neutralization indicators are weak organic acids or bases in which undissociated molecules differ in colour from their ions.*

For example, according to this theory litmus contains a certain acid (azolitmic), the undissociated molecules of which are red while its anions are blue. We shall denote any indicator acid by the symbol HInd, and its anions by Ind^-. The dissociation of litmus can then be represented as follows:

$$\text{HInd} \leftrightarrows \text{H}^+ + \text{Ind}^-$$

Red **Blue**

When litmus is dissolved in water its undissociated molecules, present together with its ions, confer an intermediate (violet) colour to the solution. If a drop of an acid such as HCl is added the above equilibrium is shifted to the left. In other words, the added H^+ ions combine with most of the Ind^- anions present in the solution to form undissociated HInd molecules, and the solution turns red.

On the other hand, if an alkali is added to litmus solution then the OH^- ions of the alkali combine with H^+ ions of the indicator to form undissociated H_2O molecules. As a result the dissociation equilibrium of the indicator is shifted to the right, leading to an increase in the amount of Ind^- anions, and the solution turns blue.

Both forms of litmus (HInd molecules and Ind^- ions) are coloured. It is an example of a *two-colour* indicator. There are also *one-colour* indicators; such an indicator has only one coloured form while the other is colourless. They include phenolphthalein, which is colourless in acid solutions and red in alkaline solutions. Since this indicator is a weak acid, so that its undissociated molecules should predominate in acid solutions and anions in alkaline solutions, the dissociation of phenolphthalein may be represented as follows on the basis of the theory:

$$\text{HInd} \rightleftarrows \text{H}^+ + \text{Ind}^-$$

Colourless **Red**

By analogy, the colour changes of other basic indicators can also be explained in the light of the ionic theory of indicators.

If the undissociated molecules of such an indicator are denoted by IndOH, and its cations by Ind^+, then its dissociation in solution may be represented as follows:

$$\text{IndOH} \rightleftarrows \text{Ind}^+ + \text{OH}^-$$

Addition of alkali to the solution shifts the dissociation equilibrium of the indicator to the left, and the solution acquires the colour of undissociated IndOH molecules. When acid is added (and OH^- ions thereby removed) it is shifted to the right, and the solution acquires the colour of Ind^+ cations.

Thus, the ionic theory of indicators explains very simply and clearly the changes in the colours of indicators when H^+ or OH^- ions are added to their solutions. Another important advantage of this theory is that it allows of quantitative interpretations.

However, recent experimental investigations by a number of scientists have shown that this theory is not quite correct. It was found that the colouring of organic compounds depends on the structure of their molecules, and a colour change can therefore occur only as the result of some intramolecular rearrangement which changes the structure of the indicator. These investigations have given rise to another theory of indicators, known as the *chromophore theory*.

The origin of this name is that the colour of organic compounds is attributed to the presence in their molecules of certain atomic groups (radicals) or groups of double bonds, known as *chromophores*.

The chromophores include the nitro group* $O{=}\overset{|}{N}{\rightarrow}$, which can be converted into the $HO{-}\overset{\|}{N}{\rightarrow}$ group, and the azo group $-N{=}N-$, which under certain conditions is transformed into the $=N{-}NH-$ group. The quinoid group is another very important chromophore.

The quinoid group is formed from the benzenoid group as follows:

Benzene nucleus Quinoid group

and, by the chromophore theory, it is very often responsible for colour changes of indicators. In addition to the groups mentioned above, the chromophores include arrangements of several carbonyl groups $>C{=}O$ or double bonds close to each other, etc.

The colour of organic compounds is also influenced by the presence of another type of groups, known as *auxochromes*. In distinction from chromophores, auxochromes cannot by themselves confer colour to a compound but when present together with chromophores they augment the action of the latter and deepen the colour produced by them. The most important auxochromes are the $-OH$ and $-NH_2$ groups, and also groups formed by replacement of hydrogen atoms in $-NH_2$ by various radicals; for example, $-OCH_3$, $-N(CH_3)_2$, $-N(C_2H_5)_2$, etc.

By the chromophore theory the colour change of an indicator is the consequence of an isomeric change, i.e., an intramolecular regrouping which changes the structure of the indicator.** If this regrouping results in the formation (or disappearance) of groups

---

* Arrows (→) in the formulas of organic compounds indicate semipolar (coordination) bonds. For details consult an organic chemistry textbook.

** It will be remembered that isomers is the name given in organic chemistry to compounds of the same composition but of different structure, and therefore differing in properties.

which influence the colour (chromophores, auxochromes), the colour also changes. It should be noted that the interconversion of isomeric forms is a reversible process in indicators. This reversible isomerism is known as *tautomerism*, and the corresponding isomers, as *tautomers*. By the chromophore theory any neutralization indicator contains different tautomeric forms, differing from each other in colour and in equilibrium with each other.

This theory can be illustrated by the example of paranitrophenol indicator, which has a much simpler structure than other common indicators. In this case the following tautomeric change occurs*:

O ← N=O ← ⇄ O ← N—OH

O |H| ⇄ O

Colourless Yellow

The above scheme shows that this change essentially consists in the conversion of the benzene nucleus into the quinoid nucleus. Formation of the quinoid nucleus is the cause of the colour change of paranitrophenol when the solution is made alkaline. When it is acidified the equilibrium between the two tautomeric forms is shifted in the opposite direction and the indicator changes from yellow to colourless.

The colour changes of other indicators are explained similarly by the chromophore theory.**

It may appear that the ionic and the chromophore theories give quite different pictures of the processes taking place in indicators, and at first sight seem incompatible. However, they are not mutually exclusive; on the contrary, they augment each other very well.

It may be regarded as conclusively established that colour changes of indicators are associated with changes in their structure. Why do changes in structure take place when acids or alkalies are added to the solutions? An answer to this question must be sought in the ionic theory of indicators. In full agreement with this theory, one

* The arrowed dotted line in the first formula shows that the tautomeric change is the consequence of transfer (migration) of the hydrogen atom from the hydroxyl group to one of the oxygens in the nitro group. As a result the single bonds between the O and N atoms and the benzene rings become double bonds. This, in its turn, causes a redistribution of double bonds within the benzene nucleus.

** Fuller details are given in the descriptions of the most important indicators.

(and sometimes both) of the tautomeric forms of a neutralization indicator is either a weak acid, or a weak base, or an amphoteric substance. In the case of paranitrophenol the yellow tautomer is an acid. This becomes evident if we notice that the —OH group in the molecule of this tautomer is a part of the $O \leftarrow \overset{\overset{O}{\|}}{N} - OH$ group, i.e., it is linked to an oxidized nitrogen atom, as in molecules of nitric $(O - \overset{\|}{N} - OH)$ or nitrous $(O = N - OH)$ acids.

The structural analogy should correspond to an analogy in properties, such that all three compounds have acidic properties, i.e., are able to split off hydrogen from the hydroxyl groups in the form of H^+ ions when in aqueous solutions.

Therefore, in a solution of paranitrophenol there should be two equilibria; equilibrium (I) between the two tautomers, and the dissociation equilibrium (II):

$$\underset{\substack{\text{Colourless} \\ \text{(A)}}}{O \leftarrow N{=}O\text{-}C_6H_4\text{-}OH} \;\underset{\rightarrow}{\overset{\text{(I)}}{\leftarrow}}\; \underset{\substack{\text{Yellow} \\ \text{(B)}}}{O \leftarrow N(-OH){=}C_6H_4{=}O} \;\underset{\leftarrow}{\overset{\text{(II)}}{\rightarrow}}\; H^+ + \underset{\substack{\text{Yellow} \\ \text{(C)}}}{O \leftarrow N(-O^-){=}C_6H_4{=}O}$$

The existence of these equilibria makes it quite easy to understand the connection between the solution reaction and the colour of a given indicator. Suppose, for example, that we have a yellow solution of paranitrophenol. Nearly all of the indicator is present in solution in the form of anions (C) which are in equilibrium with a small amount of undissociated molecules of tautomer (B), and the latter are in equilibrium with the tautomer (A). If any acid is added to the solution, equilibrium (II) is shifted to the left. In other words, most of the indicator anions combine with H^+ ions of the acid to form undissociated molecules of tautomer (B). This conversion is not in itself accompanied by a colour change, because these ions and molecules are of exactly the same structure and therefore of the same colour.

However, the resultant increase in the concentration of tautomer (B) must also cause a shift in the equilibrium (I) between the two tautomeric forms of the indicator. The yellow form (B) is converted into the colourless form (A), and the solution becomes colourless.

Conversely, addition of any alkali to a colourless solution of paranitrophenol results in removal of its H^+ ions and a shift of equilibrium (I) and then of equilibrium (II) to the right. As a result, molecules of form (A) almost disappear from the solution while the concentration of anions (C) increases and the solution turns yellow.

It is thus clear that as science developed the two theories merged in a single *ionic-chromophore theory of indicators.*

It should be borne in mind that, whereas the dissociation equilibrium of an indicator is established almost instantaneously, a tautomeric change takes time. Therefore, the colour changes of indicators are not always rapid enough. This is one of the most convincing proofs of the existence of tautomeric changes in colour changes of indicators, and it is quite inexplicable in the light of the ionic theory of indicators. Obviously only indicators which change colour rapidly enough can be used in volumetric analysis.

It must be pointed out that the problem of the relationship between the colour and structure of organic compounds has not been finally solved.* Other theories, such as the coordination-ionic and the quinophenolate theories, have also been put forward.

In conclusion we consider some of the indicators most commonly used in analytical practice.

Phenolphthalein is an acidic indicator. One of the three benzene nuclei in the phenolphthalein molecule undergoes quinoid rearrangement and the following equilibrium is established in solution:

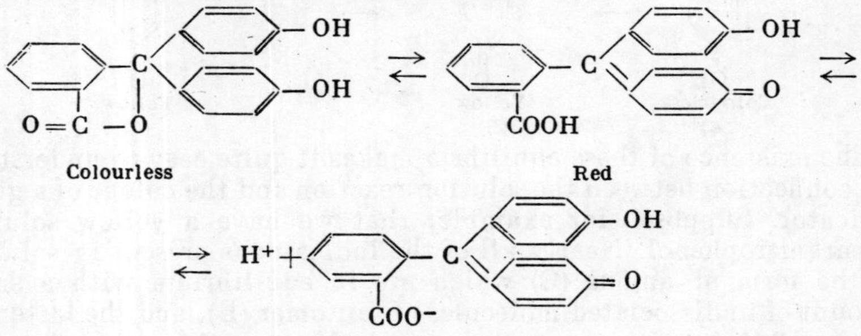

— OH
C
— OH
O = C — O
$\rightleftarrows$
— C
— OH
= O
COOH
$\rightleftarrows$

Colourless Red

$\rightleftarrows$ H^+ +
— C
— OH
= O
COO^-

Red

When OH^- ions are introduced into the solution the equilibrium shifts to the right. This results in a change of colour.

Phenolphthalein is used as 0.1% and 1% solutions in 50% alcohol.

Litmus is the colouring matter from a species of lichen (*Lacca musci*). Its active principle is azolitmic acid, of which 4-5% is present in litmus. Its structure is unknown.

---

* The formulas given for the indicators do not represent their true chemical structure and properties quite accurately. For example, in accordance with modern data a quinoid structure cannot be ascribed to only one of the nuclei in the indicator molecule, and the structure of the nitro group does not correspond to a simple formula with quinquivalent nitrogen. These matters are discussed more fully in the course of organic chemistry.

For preparation of litmus solution the commercial product is first treated several times with 80% alcohol on heating to extract all coloured impurities, and the residue is boiled with water. The aqueous extract is used as the indicator.

Methyl orange is classed as a basic indicator. More correctly it is amphoteric, as its molecules contain both acidic radicals SO_3H and basic groups $N(CH_3)_2$. Dissociation of methyl orange molecules gives rise to amphoteric ions bearing positive and negative charges simultaneously:

$$(H_3C)_2\overset{+}{N}{=}C_6H_4{=}N{-}NH{-}C_6H_4{-}SO_3^-$$

When the solution is acidified the concentration of these ions increases and the solution becomes red. When alkali is added these amphoteric ions react with OH^- ions; this reaction is accompanied by a change in the structure of the indicator and a colour change from red to yellow:

$$(H_3C)_2\overset{+}{N}{=}C_6H_4{=}N{-}NH{-}C_6H_4{-}SO_3^- + OH^- \rightleftarrows$$

Red

$$\rightleftarrows (H_3C)_2N{-}C_6H_4{-}N{=}N{-}C_6H_4{-}SO_3^- + H_2O$$

Yellow

Methyl orange is used as an 0.1% aqueous solution.

Methyl red is also a basic indicator. Its change of colour occurs in a way similar to methyl orange according to the scheme

$$(H_3C)_2\overset{+}{N}{=}C_6H_4{=}N{-}NH{-}C_6H_4(COO^-) + OH^- \rightleftarrows$$

Red

$$\rightleftarrows (H_3C)_2N{-}C_6H_4{-}N{=}N{-}C_6H_4(COO^-) + H_2O$$

Yellow

Generally a 0.2% solution in 60% alcohol is used.

61. Indicator Range

Neutralization indicators change colour on introduction of H^+ or OH^- ions into their solutions. However, introduction of these ions obviously alters the solution pH. Therefore, we can say that *the colour of an indicator depends on* pH and therefore such indicators can be described as pH *indicators.*

The relationship between the colour of a particular pH indicator and the solution pH can be established with the aid of the ionic-chromophore theory of indicators. By this theory the following system of interrelated equilibria exists in a solution of an acidic indicator:

$$HInd^0 \overset{(I)}{\rightleftarrows} HInd \overset{(II)}{\rightleftarrows} H^+ + Ind^-$$

Here $HInd^0$ represents one and HInd the other tautomeric form, and Ind^- represents the anions formed from the latter. Since the indicator is present almost entirely in the form of $HInd^0$ molecules in strongly acidic solutions and in the form of Ind^- anions in strongly alkaline solutions, we can call the former the acidic and the latter the alkaline form of the indicator.* We can apply the law of mass action to each of the above equilibria (I) and (II). We then have:

(a) for equilibrium (I)

$$\frac{[HInd]}{[HInd^0]} = K_{taut.}$$

(b) for equilibrium (II)

$$\frac{[H^+][Ind^-]}{[HInd]} = K_{diss.}$$

Multiplying these equations together term by term we have:

$$\frac{[H^+][Ind^-][HInd]}{[HInd][HInd^0]} = K_{diss.} K_{taut.}$$

Cancelling [HInd] from the fraction and denoting the product of the two constants by K we have

$$\frac{[H^+][Ind^-]}{[HInd^0]} = K$$

or

$$\frac{[H^+] \cdot C_{alk.\,f.}}{C_{acid.\,f.}} = K \qquad (1)$$

The constant K is known as *the apparent dissociation constant of the indicator.***

---

* Clearly, in the case of basic indicators where the solution equilibria can be represented as

$$IndOH^0 \rightleftarrows IndOH \rightleftarrows Ind^+ + OH^-$$

the acidic form consists of Ind^+ cations, and the alkaline form of $IndOH^0$ molecules.

** Evidently the same equation could be derived from the ionic theory of indicators, the only difference being that K would then be the true and not the apparent dissociation constant of the indicator.

Solving Equation (1) for $[H^+]$, we have

$$[H^+] = K \frac{C_{acid.\,f.}}{C_{alk.\,f.}}$$

and hence

$$-\log [H^+] = -\log K - \log \frac{C_{acid.\,f.}}{C_{alk.\,f.}}$$

and finally

$$pH = pK - \log \frac{C_{acid.\,f.}}{C_{alk.\,f.}} \qquad (2)$$

Here $pK = -\log K$ is the so-called *indicator exponent.*

Equation (2), which is the fundamental equation in the theory of indicators, represents the relationship between the colour of an indicator and the solution pH.

When several drops of an indicator are added to a solution of a definite pH value, the $\frac{C_{acid.\,f.}}{C_{alk.\,f.}}$ ratio corresponding to this pH should become established. However, these two forms of the indicator differ in colour, and therefore the colour shade of the indicator in the solution depends on the value of this ratio.

Since the indicator exponent pK is constant for any given indicator (at constant temperature), it follows from Equation (2) that any change of solution pH must alter the $\frac{C_{acid.\,f.}}{C_{alk.\,f.}}$ ratio. However, far from every change of this ratio is perceived as a colour change. The ability of the human eye to perceive colours is limited, and usually the eye fails to detect the presence of one of the coloured forms of an indicator together with the other if the concentration of the former is one-tenth of the concentration of the latter. Accordingly, *the colour of any indicator changes, not with any change of* pH, *but only within a certain* pH *range which is known as the useful range of that indicator*. This is illustrated more clearly by Table IX.

The data in Table IX apply to the case where the acidic form of the indicator, i.e., the undissociated $HInd^0$ molecules, is red (as in litmus), while the alkaline form (Ind^- cations) is blue. Let us first assume that the concentrations of the two forms in a given solution are equal, each being 50% of the total indicator concentration. The colour of the solution is then evidently violet. At what pH does this colour appear? This is easy to calculate from the equation

$$pH = pK - \log \frac{C_{acid.\,f.}}{C_{alk.\,f.}}$$

Substituting the appropriate values of $C_{acid.\,f.}$ and $C_{alk.\,f.}$ into this equation we have:

$$pH = pK - \log \frac{50}{50} = pK - \log 1 = pK$$

Table IX

Colour Changes of an Indicator with Changes of Solution pH

				pK − 1			pK			pK + 1				
$C_{acid.f.}$ *	99.99	99.9	99	91	70	60	50	40	30	9	1	0.1	0.01	etc.
$C_{alk.f.}$ *	0.01	0.1	1	9	30	40	50	60	70	91	99	99.9	99.99	etc.
Colour		Red		Redder ←			Violet			→ Bluer		Blue		
				Useful Range										

* The concentrations $C_{acid.f.}$ and $C_{alk.f.}$ are given as percentages of the total indicator concentration.

Thus, the intermediate violet colour appears at the point when the solution pH is equal to the indicator exponent pK. For example. if K for the indicator is 2.5×10^{-6}, this occurs* at

$$pH = pK = -\log 2.5 \times 10^{-6} = -(0.4 - 6) = 5.6$$

Now suppose that the solution pH is gradually lowered by addition of some acid. The equilibrium between the two forms of the indicator is then progressively shifted towards an increase of $C_{acid.\ f.}$ with a corresponding decrease of $C_{alk.\ f.}$.

While $C_{acid.\ f.}$ passes from 50 to 91% and $C_{alk.\ f.}$ from 50 to 9% the solution becomes progressively redder. At the point when the ratio $\frac{C_{acid.\ f.}}{C_{alk.\ f.}}$ becomes $\frac{91}{9} \approx 10$, the eye ceases to perceive the blue colour of the Ind^- ions altogether and the solution appears red (without the slightest sign of a violet tinge).

This colour appears at $pH = pK - \log \frac{91}{9} = pK - \log 10 = pK - 1$ (i.e., at pH = 4.6 in this example).

If the addition of acid is continued, no further colour change perceptible to the eye is produced despite the continuing increase of $C_{acid.\ f.}$ and decrease of $C_{alk.\ f.}$. In fact, the blue alkaline form of the indicator can no longer be detected when its concentration is 0.1 of $C_{acid.\ f.}$ (i.e., at pH = pK − 1). Therefore, now (at $pH < pK - 1$), at an even lower concentration of the alkaline form, its presence in solution cannot possibly affect the colour.

* These values refer to the indicator lacmoid, which owes its name to the similarity of its colour changes to those of litmus.

Quite analogous effects are observed when alkali is added to a violet solution of the indicator. The equilibrium between the two forms of the indicator is then shifted towards an increase of $C_{\text{alk. f.}}$ and a decrease of $C_{\text{acid. f.}}$. Until the former reaches 91% and the latter 9%, i.e., until the ratio $\frac{C_{\text{acid. f.}}}{C_{\text{alk. f.}}}$ becomes 0.1, the solution will be getting progressively more blue, the colour reaching its maximum at

$$\text{pH} = \text{p}K - \log 0.1 = \text{p}K + 1$$

(i.e., at pH = 6.6 in this example).

No matter how much more alkali is added to the solution after this, its colour remains exactly the same (blue) as at pH = pK + 1.

Therefore, *the useful range of an indicator usually extends by one unit of* pH *on each side of the* pK *of that particular indicator*, i.e.,

$$\text{pH range} = \text{p}K \pm 1 \tag{3}$$

For example, the dissociation constant of phenolphthalein is 10^{-9} and its useful range should therefore be between pH = 8 and pH = 10; this is found to be the case. Up to pH = 8 the colour of the acidic form of the indicator is observed, i.e., the solution is colourless, while from pH = 10 onwards the colour of the alkaline form (red) is seen. In the range from pH = 8 to pH = 10 the colourless solution gradually turns bright red.

Similarly, for the indicator phenol red ($K = 6.3 \times 10^{-8}$) pK = $= -\log 6.3 \times 10^{-8} = -(0.8-8) = 7.2$. Therefore according to Equation (3), its range should be between pH = 6.2 and pH = 8.2. In reality it is somewhat narrower (6.4 to 8.0), because the eye is less sensitive to the colours of this indicator. In this case the eye ceases to perceive one of the forms of this indicator at the point when the concentration of one form is 6.3 and not 10 times the concentration of the other. Therefore, the range is pH $= 7.2 \pm \log 6.3 = 7.2 \pm 0.8$, i.e., 6.4 to 8.0.

In the case of methyl orange the eye ceases to perceive one of the coloured forms when its concentration is only $^1/_4$ that of the other. Therefore, the useful range of this indicator is considerably narrower than that of the other indicators, being between 3.1 and 4.4. At pH = 3.1 or less the eye sees the colour of the acidic form of the indicator (red), and at pH = 4.4 it sees the colour of the alkaline form (yellow). Within this pH range the colour of methyl orange gradually passes from red to yellow, so that a definite tinge corresponds to each pH value in this range.

Many pH indicators are known, and their apparent dissociation constants vary considerably. Because of this, the ranges of different indicators cover almost the entire pH scale from pH = 0 to pH = 12

Table X

Ranges of the Most Important pH Indicators

Indicator	Solvent	Concentration %	Nature of indicator	Colour: Acid form	Colour: Alkaline form	pH range
Alizarin yellow	Water	0.1	Acid	Yellow	Violet	10.1-12.0
Thymolphthalein	90% alcohol	0.1	Acid	Colourless	Blue	9.3-10.5
Phenolphthalein	60% alcohol	0.1 & 1.0	Acid	Colourless	Red	8.0-10.0
Cresol purple	20% alcohol	0.05	Acid	Yellow	Purple	7.4-9.0
Neutral red	60% alcohol	0.1	Basic	Red	Yellow-brown	6.8-8.0
Phenol red	20% alcohol *	0.1	Acid	Yellow	Red	6.4-8.0
Bromthymol blue	20% alcohol **	0.05	Acid	Yellow	Blue	6.0-7.6
Litmus (azolitmin)	Water	1.0	Acid	Red	Blue	5.0-8.0
Methyl red	60% alcohol	0.1 & 0.2	Basic	Red	Yellow	4.2-6.2
Methyl orange	Water	0.1	Basic	Red	Yellow	3.1-4.4
Bromphenol blue	Water	0.1	Acid	Yellow	Blue	3.0-4.6
Tropeoline 00	Water	0.01, 0.1 & 1.0	Basic	Red	Yellow	1.4-3.2
Crystal violet	Water	—		Green	Violet	0.0-2.0

* Or water with 5.7 ml of 0.05 *N* NaOH per 100 mg of indicator.
** Or water with 3.2 ml of 0.05 *N* NaOH per 100 mg of indicator.

and over. This is illustrated by Table X and Fig. 44, where the ranges of the most important pH indicators are represented by shaded squares. The figure also shows (by initials) the colours of the acidic (left) and alkaline (right) forms of the indicators.

Of all the intermediate colours of an indicator the one of greatest interest is the one at which the titration is ended. For example, if 0.1 *N* NaOH solution (the pH of which is about 13) is titrated with hydrochloric acid in presence of methyl orange, the colour of the latter remains pure yellow all the time, despite the continuously decreasing pH, up to the point at which the solution pH reaches 4.4. Beyond this point the colour of the indicator begins to change.

However, this change becomes quite distinct only at pH = 4.0, when the colour of the solution becomes an easily distinguishable pinkish orange. Titration in presence of methyl orange is continued until this colour is reached at pH = 4.0.

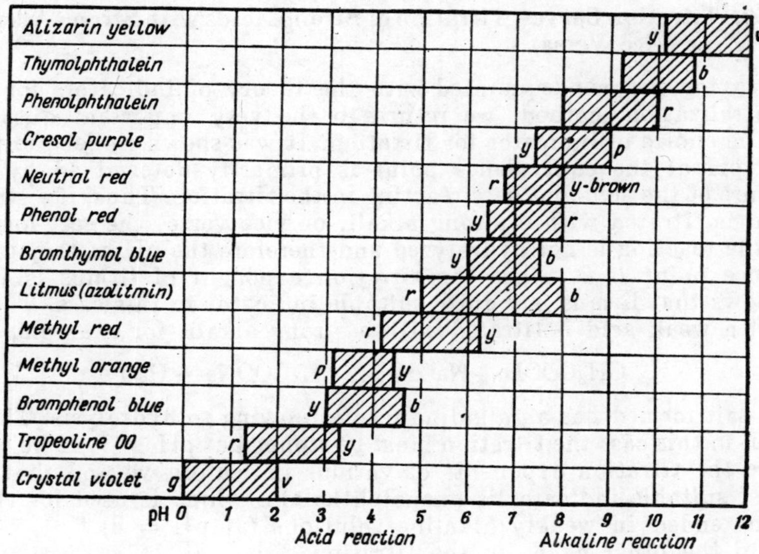

Fig. 44. Ranges and colours of the most important pH indicators

The pH *at which titration in presence of a given indicator is ended is sometimes known as its titration exponent, denoted by* pT. Therefore, the titration exponent of methyl orange is pT = 4.0

The pT values for four of the best-known indicators are given below:

Methyl orange	pT = 4.0
Methyl red	pT = 5.5
Litmus	pT = 7.0
Phenolphthalein *	pT = 9.0

As the pT value corresponds to one of the intermediate colours of the indicator, it lies within its useful range. Therefore, when the

* It should be noted that the pT of phenolphthalein and other one-colour indicators depends on their concentration in solution. For example, if 2-3 drops of 0.1% phenolphthalein solution are used per 50 ml of solution the pale pink colour at which the titration is ended appears at pH = 9. On the other hand, if the same number of drops of 1% phenolphthalein solution is used a quite distinct pink colour appears at pH = 8. Therefore, in this case pT of phenolphthalein is 8.

pT is not given it may be assumed to lie in the middle of the useful range, i.e., it can be taken as approximately equal to the indicator exponent pK.

62. Titration Curves. Titration of Strong Acids with Strong Alkalies (or Vice Versa)

Having become acquainted with the theory of indicators for the neutralization method, we return to the very important question of the choice of indicator for titration. It was shown in Sec. 58 that the pH at the equivalence point is primarily determined by the nature of the acid and base reacting in the titration. Thus, if a strong acid is titrated with a strong alkali, or vice versa, the salt formed in the reaction is not hydrolyzed and therefore the pH at the equivalence point is 7. Since the titration exponent of litmus is 7, it follows that litmus is a quite suitable indicator in this case.

If a weak acid is titrated with a strong alkali, for example,

$$CH_3COOH + NaOH \rightleftarrows CH_3COONa + H_2O$$

the salt formed has an alkaline reaction owing to hydrolysis. Therefore, in this case the titration must be stopped at pH > 7. If we compare the titration exponents of various indicators we find that the most suitable indicator is phenolphthalein, which is used for titrations ended in weakly alkaline solutions (at pH $= 9$).*

On the other hand, in the titration

$$NH_4OH + HCl \rightleftarrows NH_4Cl + H_2O$$

the salt formed has an acid reaction owing to hydrolysis, and therefore more suitable indicators are methyl orange (pT $= 4$) and methyl red (pT $= 5.5$), which are used for titrations ended in acid solutions.

It is very useful to take these considerations into account when an indicator is chosen in order to avoid serious errors. However, it is easy to see that they alone are not a sufficient guide in the choice of an indicator. It is impossible to predict the precision of the titration, whereas an error of 2% is just as inadmissible as one of 20%.

On the other hand, such qualitative considerations cannot answer the question of the extent to which we may deviate from the

---

* Note that the pT of phenolphthalein and of other single-colour indicators depends on their concentration in the titrate. For example, if 2-3 drops of an 0.1 per cent phenolphthalein solution is added to 50 ml of titrate the pale pink colour masking the end point appears at pH 9. But if the same amount of a 1 per cent phenolphthalein solution is used, a fairly pronounced pinkish colour will appear at pH 8. Therefore, in this case the pT of phenolphthalein is 8.

equivalence point in any given instance. For example, titration of a strong acid with a strong alkali (or vice versa) must be ended at pH = 7. However, is it permissible to use methyl orange and end the titration at pH = 4, or to use phenolphthalein and to end it at pH = 9? It might seem that such large deviations from the equivalence point should give rise to large indicator errors (p. 232), and yet this is found not to be the case in practice. In this instance all four of the commonest indicators give results which virtually coincide, and all can be used successfully in the titration.

Therefore, a qualitative approach is insufficient in the choice of an indicator; the problem must be solved quantitatively. Two quantitative methods are available for this purpose:

(a) plotting of "titration curves",

(b) calculation of the indicator error in titration.

Let us first consider titration curves. Suppose, for example, that 100 ml of 0.1 *N* HCl solution is titrated with 0.1 *N* NaOH solution. Let us calculate the solution pH at different stages of the titration. In calculating the pH values of solutions of strong acids or alkalies the concentration of H^+ (or OH^-) ions may be taken as equal to the total concentration of acid (or alkali), because, in the modern view, such acids and alkalies are almost completely dissociated in solution. To simplify the calculations we assume that the total volume of the solution remains unchanged during the titration. In reality its volume is doubled at the end of the titration. Evidently the error if the pH is calculated without the change of volume taken into account is log 2, or about 0.3. This error does not affect the general conclusions and can therefore be disregarded.

Before the start of the titration we have a 0.1 *N* solution of HCl, the pH of which is 1. Now suppose that 90 ml of 0.1 *N* NaOH solution is added to 100 ml of 0.1 *N* HCl solution. Then 90% of the total amount of acid is neutralized. The amount of free acid left is one-tenth of the amount present before the start of the titration. Since volume changes are disregarded, we can assume that the concentration of free acid (C_{acid}) becomes one-tenth of its initial value, or 0.01 mole/litre. Therefore, the pH of the solution at this point is approximately 2.*

When 99 ml of NaOH has been added, the concentration of free HCl is decreased tenfold again, down to 0.001 mole/litre, and the pH of the solution rises to about 3. Similarly we find that on addition of 99.9 ml of NaOH C_{acid} falls to 0.0001 mole/litre, and the pH rises to approximately 4.

---

* If the volume change is taken into account C_{acid} is $\frac{0.1 \times 10}{190} = 5.3 \cdot 10^{-3}$, and hence the pH = $-(0.72 - 3) = 2.28$

If exactly 100 ml of a NaOH solution is added to 100 ml of the HCl solution of the same normality, the amount of alkali added is exactly equivalent to the amount of acid present, i.e., the equivalence point is reached. At this point the solution contains only the salt NaCl formed in the reaction. Since this salt is not hydrolyzed the solution pH is 7. This is the point at which the titration must be ended. However, in order to have an idea of the course of pH variations in titration of an alkali with acid, we continue the calculation up to 100% excess of NaOH.

Table XI

pH Variation in Titration of 100 ml of 0.1 *N* HCl with 0.1 *N* NaOH (or Vice Versa)

NaOH added ml	c_{acid} *M*	$c_{alk.}$ *M*	$[H^+]$	$[OH^-]$	pH
—	0.1	—	10^{-1}	10^{-13}	1
90	0.01	—	10^{-2}	10^{-12}	2
99	0.001	—	10^{-3}	10^{-11}	3
99.9	0.0001	—	10^{-4}	10^{-10}	4
100 equiv. pt.	—	—	10^{-7}	10^{-7}	**7**
100.1	—	0.0001	10^{-10}	10^{-4}	10
101.0	—	0.001	10^{-11}	10^{-3}	11
110	—	0.01	10^{-12}	10^{-2}	12
200	—	0.1	10^{-13}	10^{-1}	13

Suppose that the amount of alkali added is 0.1 ml too much, i.e., 100.1 ml. Since the NaOH concentration is the same as that of the HCl, this excess (0.1 ml) of alkali must give rise to an OH^- ion concentration equal to the H^+ ion concentration produced by 0.1 ml excess HCl.

Therefore, $[OH^-]$ at this point is approximately 10^{-4}, $[H^+] = 10^{-10}$, and pH $= 10$.

Similarly we find that with 1 ml excess alkali $[OH^-] = 10^{-3}$, $[H^+] = 10^{-11}$ and pH $= 11$, etc.

These results are summarized in Table XI and are plotted in the form of a curve in Fig. 45.

Such curves, representing the variations of pH *in titration, are known as titration curves.*

To plot a titration curve, the amounts of excess acid or alkali present in solution (in percentages)* are taken along the abscissa

---

* If 100 ml of solution is titrated, each millilitre of excess acid (or alkali) in solution of course corresponds to 1%.

axis, while the ordinates represent the corresponding pH values. If we follow the curve from left to right, we have the pH variation when the acid is titrated with the alkali. Conversely, the pH variation when the alkali is titrated with the acid is represented by the curve taken from right to left. The amounts of excess acid and alkali in the graph are limited to 10% in order that the figure should not be too large.

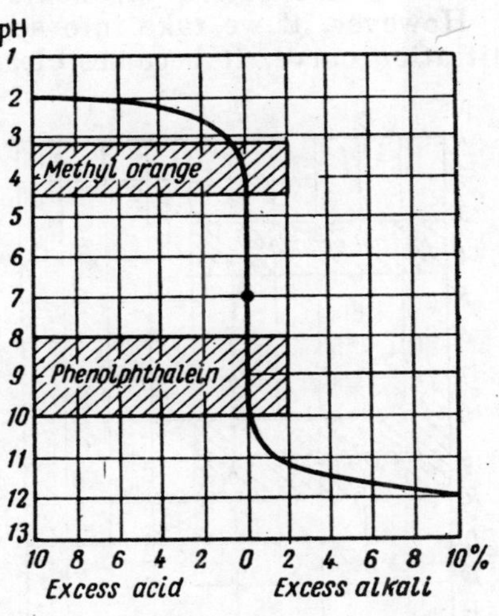

Fig. 45. Titration curve of 0.1 *N* HCl with 0.1 *N* NaOH (or vice versa)

If we examine the titration curve of 0.1 *N* hydrochloric acid solution with 0.1 *N* caustic soda solution we see that the equivalence point (indicated by a black dot in the graph) coincides in this case with the point of neutrality (pH = 7).

Further, we note *the extremely abrupt change of* pH *at the end of the titration.* Whereas addition of nearly all (99.9 ml) the alkali changes the pH by only 3 units (from 1 to 4), in the transition from 0.1 ml excess acid to 0.1 ml excess alkali (i.e., from 99.9 ml to 100.1 ml of added alkali) the pH changes by 6 units (from 4 to 10). If, as is usually the case in practice, 25 ml and not 100 ml of solution is titrated, this pH change, which corresponds to a millionfold decrease of the H^+ ion concentration, is produced by addition not of 0.2 ml but $\frac{0.2}{4} = 0.05$ ml of NaOH solution. This amount represents only 1-2 drops.

It is easy to see that this abrupt pH change at the end point is very advantageous.

Indeed, it follows from the equation

$$\mathrm{pH} = \mathrm{p}K - \log \frac{C_{\text{acid. f.}}}{C_{\text{alk. f.}}}$$

that the break of pH produced by addition of the last 1-2 drops of solution must correspond to an abrupt change of the $\frac{C_{\text{acid.f.}}}{C_{\text{alk.f.}}}$ ratio, and hence to a sharp change in the colour of the indicator. If there was no abrupt pH change on the titration curve the colour change would be slow and gradual and it would not be possible to determine the end point. Accurate titration would then be impossible

What conclusions can be drawn from these characteristics of the titration curve with regard to the problem of choice of an indicator?

It might seem at first sight that it is essential to use an indicator which changes colour at pH = 7, i.e., exactly at the equivalence point of this titration; for example, litmus or bromthymol blue, which have titration exponents of about 7.

However, if we take into account the abrupt pH change on the titration curve, it becomes clear that an indicator such as methyl orange can be used with equal success, although the end point with this indicator is at pH = 4 and not at pH = 7. It is evident from Table XI that the pH reaches 4 when 99.9 ml of NaOH solution has been added. Therefore, the indicator error in titration in this case is 0.1 ml per 100 ml, and only 0.025 in titration of 25 ml; i.e., it is not more than one drop in volume.

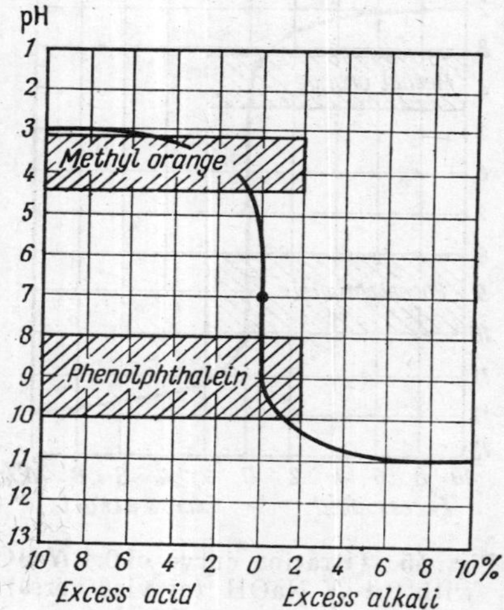

Fig. 46. Titration curve of 0.01 *N* HCl with 0.01 *N* NaOH (or vice versa)

Similarly, if phenolphthalein was used the amount added in excess would be less than 0.025 ml per 25 ml (or 0.1 ml per 100 ml). With this excess of alkali the solution pH would be 10, whereas the end point with this indicator is at pH = 9.

From all this it is easy to derive the basic rule for choice of an indicator: *the indicator used in any given titration must have a titration exponent within the range of the abrupt* pH *change on the titration curve.*

For example, in titration of 0.1 *N* solutions of strong acids with strong bases (or vice versa) all indicators from methyl orange (pT = 4.0) to thymolphthalein (pT = 10)* would give practically identical results.

On the other hand, if an indicator such as tropeoline 00 is used (pT ≈ 2), it follows from Table XI that in titration of HCl the amount of alkali added would be about 10 ml too small, which is, of course, quite inadmissible.

---

* It will be shown later that this is true only if the alkali solution is free from carbonates (see p. 278).

An even more important fact is that at pH = 2 the titration curve is almost horizontal. Therefore, tropeoline 00 would be unsuitable also because its colour would change very slowly and gradually, and not on addition of one drop of NaOH. Neither would alizarin yellow (pT $\approx$ 11) be suitable, as the amount of NaOH added would be about 1 ml too much, and the colour change would again not be sharp.

So far we have considered titration of 0.1 *N* solutions. If 0.01 *N* solutions are used we can plot the titration curve shown in Fig. 46 from data calculated as described above.

This curve shows that the region of abrupt pH change is narrower here; it is between pH 5 and 9.

Therefore, methyl orange (pT = 4) and thymolphthalein (pT = = 10) cannot be used in this case. On the other hand, methyl red, litmus, phenolphthalein, and similar indicators would be suitable.

63. Titration of Weak Acids with Strong Alkalies (or Vice Versa)

We now turn to titration of weak acids with strong alkalies. Suppose, for example, that 100 ml of 0.1 *N* CH_3COOH solution is titrated with 0.1 *N* NaOH solution. In this case, when calculating the pH, we cannot assume that the H^+ ion concentration is equal to the total acid concentration, because most of the acid is present in the form of undissociated molecules and only a small proportion is dissociated with formation of H^+ ions.

Therefore, in such cases the pH calculation is based on the equation for the dissociation constant of the weak acid, i.e.,

$$\frac{[H^+][CH_3COO^-]}{[CH_3COOH]} = K_{acid} = 1.86 \times 10^{-5} \tag{1}$$

Initially the acetic acid in solution is partially dissociated in accordance with the equation

$$CH_3COOH \rightleftarrows H^+ + CH_3COO^-$$

which shows that for each H^+ ion formed one CH_3COO^- ion is present in solution. Therefore, their concentrations are equal, i.e.,

$$[CH_3COO^-] = [H^+]$$

Since the degree of dissociation of acetic acid is very low, we may assume that

$$[CH_3COOH] \approx C_{acid}$$

where C_{acid} is the total acetic acid concentration, 0.1 *M* in this instance.

We then have from Equation (1):

$$[H^+]^2 = K_{acid}C_{acid}$$

and

$$[H^+] = \sqrt{K_{acid}C_{acid}} \tag{2}$$

To convert $[H^+]$ to pH we take logarithms of Equation (2) and reverse the signs. We then have:

$$-\log[H^+] = -\frac{1}{2}\log K_{acid} - \frac{1}{2}\log C_{acid}$$

or

$$pH = \frac{1}{2}pK_{acid} - \frac{1}{2}\log C_{acid} \tag{3}$$

Here $pK_{acid} = -\log K_{acid}$ is the dissociation exponent of the acid, which we met earlier (p. 241). In the present instance it is*

$$pK_{acid} = -\log 1.86 \times 10^{-5} = -(0.27 - 5) = 4.73$$

Hence from Equation (3) we have

$$pH = \frac{1}{2} \times 4.73 - \frac{1}{2}\log 0.1 = 2.37 + 0.5 = 2.87$$

This is the pH of 0.1 *N* acetic acid solution corresponding to the initial point of the titration curve which we are considering.

Note. The pH could also be calculated in another way, by first determining the H^+ ion concentration from Equation (2) and then converting it to pH. We then have:

$$[H^+] = \sqrt{1.86 \times 10^{-4} \times 0.1} = \sqrt{1.86 \times 10^{-6}} = 1.34 \times 10^{-3} \text{ g-ion/litre}$$

and hence

$$pH = -\log[H^+] = -\log 1.34 \times 10^{-3} = -(0.13 - 3) = 2.87$$

However, Equation (3) is more convenient to use because p*K* is calculated only once and can then be used for finding a number of points on the given titration curve, whereas if we use the equations for $[H^+]$ we have to use logarithms each time. Moreover, instead of calculating p*K* we can take its values from tables (Appendix II).

We now turn to derivation of formulas for calculating intermediate points on the titration curve. These points correspond to instants at which only a certain proportion of the total amount of acid has been titrated, i.e., converted into salt. Therefore, at these points the solution contains free weak acid (CH_3COOH) and its salt

* Since the precision in experimental determinations of pH does not exceed 0.01, the logarithms are rounded off to the nearest 0.01 in calculations of pH and p*K*.

(CH_3COONa). To calculate the pH of such solutions we solve for $[H^+]$ the equation for the dissociation constant of acetic acid. We then have:

$$[H^+] = K_{acid} \frac{[CH_3COOH]}{[CH_3COO^-]}$$

But CH_3COOH is a weak acid and is present almost entirely in the form of undissociated CH_3COOH molecules. Therefore, the concentration of the latter can be assumed, without appreciable error, to be the same as the total acid concentration in solution, i.e.:

$$[CH_3COOH] \approx C_{acid}$$

On the other hand, as the salt CH_3COONa is completely dissociated while acetic acid is dissociated very slightly, nearly all the CH_3COO^- anions present in the solution are formed by dissociation of the salt, each dissociated salt molecule giving one CH_3COO^- anion. It follows that the concentration of the anions may be taken as equal to the total salt concentration, i.e.,

$$[CH_3COO^-] \approx C_{salt}$$

Accordingly, we have from the equation given earlier

$$[H^+] = K_{acid} \frac{C_{acid}}{C_{salt}}$$

Taking logarithms and reversing signs, we have:

$$-\log [H^+] = -\log K_{acid} - \log \frac{C_{acid}}{C_{salt}}$$

and hence

$$pH = pK_{acid} - \log \frac{C_{acid}}{C_{salt}} \qquad (4)$$

This equation* is used for calculating the intermediate points on the titration curve. Let us perform two such calculations. First we calculate the solution pH when 50% of the acetic acid has been titrated (i.e., when half the amount of alkali required by the reaction equation has been added, 50 ml of alkali to 100 ml of acid). The titrated part of the acid has been converted into its salt. Therefore, the ratio $C_{acid} : C_{salt}$ is equal to the ratio of the number of millilitres of remaining acid to the number of millilitres of acid which has been titrated (or the number of millilitres of added alkali, which is equal to it). Therefore, at this point

$$pH = pK_{acid} - \log \frac{50}{50} = 4.73$$

---

* Equation (4) is evidently quite analogous to the equation derived for indicators (Equation 2, p. 241). Indeed, $C_{acid.\ f.}$ and $C_{alk.\ f.}$ are nothing more than the concentrations of the free indicator acid and its salt.

Thus, *at the point when exactly one half of the weak acid has been titrated the solution* pH *is equal to* pK_{acid}.

The region of the abrupt change (break) on the titration curve is of special practical interest. This region is the pH range from the point at which 0.1 ml of free acetic acid remained to the point at which 0.1 ml excess alkali had been added. Therefore, at the start of the break

$$pH = 4.73 - \log\frac{0.1}{99.9} = 4.73 - (-3) = 7.73$$

We now pass to the derivation of the equation for calculating pH at the equivalence point. The solution contains the salt CH_3COONa which is partially hydrolyzed (see p. 231):

$$CH_3COO^- + H_2O \rightleftarrows CH_3COOH + OH^-$$

Applying the law of mass action to this reversible reaction, we write:

$$\frac{[CH_3COOH][OH^-]}{[CH_3COO^-][H_2O]} = K$$

Taking $[H_2O]$ to the right-hand side of the equation and noting that the concentration of water (which is present as solvent in enormous excess) may be regarded as almost constant and not changed appreciably with any shifts of the hydrolysis equilibrium, we have

$$\frac{[CH_3COOH][OH^-]}{[CH_3COO^-]} = K \cdot [H_2O] = K_h \quad (5)$$

Here the product $K \cdot [H_2O]$ is also constant; it is known as the *hydrolysis constant* and is denoted by K_h. Its numerical value is easily found from the ionic product of water K_{H_2O} and the dissociation constant K_{acid} of acetic acid. From the expression for K_{H_2O} we have

$$[OH^-] = \frac{K_{H_2O}}{[H^+]} = \frac{10^{-14}}{[H^+]} \text{ (at 22° C)}$$

Substituting this value for $[OH^-]$ into Equation (5), we have

$$\frac{[CH_3COOH] \times 10^{-14}}{[CH_3COO^-][H^+]} = K_h$$

However, the fraction $\frac{[CH_3COOH]}{[CH_3COO^-][H^+]}$ is the reciprocal of K_{acid} and is equal to $1/K_{acid}$.

Therefore, we may write:

$$K_h = \frac{10^{-14}}{K_{acid}}$$

and

$$\frac{[CH_3COOH][OH^-]}{[CH_3COO^-]} = \frac{10^{-14}}{K_{acid}} \tag{6}$$

By the ionic equation for the reaction, one $[CH_3COOH]$ molecule is formed in solution for each H^+ ion, and hence $[CH_3COOH] = [OH^-]$.

At the same time, as the dissociation of CH_3COOH yields very few CH_3COO^- ions, we may assume that $[CH_3COO^-] \approx C_{salt}$. We therefore have from Equation (6):

$$\frac{[OH^-]^2}{C_{salt}} = \frac{10^{-14}}{K_{acid}}$$

and

$$[OH^-] = \sqrt{\frac{10^{-14} \times C_{salt}}{K_{acid}}} \tag{7}$$

Taking logarithms and reversing signs, we have

$$-\log [OH^-] = 7 + \frac{1}{2}\log K_{acid} - \frac{1}{2}\log C_{salt}$$

and

$$pOH = 7 - \frac{1}{2}\,pK_{acid} - \frac{1}{2}\log C_{salt}$$

But $pH = 14 - pOH$. We thus finally find the formula for calculating the pH at the equivalence point in this titration:

$$pH = 7 + \frac{1}{2}\,pK_{acid} + \frac{1}{2}\log C_{salt} \tag{8}$$

Let us use this formula for calculating the pH at the equivalence point in the titration of 0.1 N CH_3COOH with 0.1 N NaOH (or vice versa). Since the volume change in titration is disregarded (p. 247), we assume C_{salt} to be equal to the initial concentration of the acid, or 0.1 M. Therefore, we have

$$pH = 7 + \frac{4.73}{2} + \frac{1}{2}\log 0.1 = 7 + 2.37 - 0.5 = 8.87$$

We now calculate pH at the points in the titration when excess NaOH has been added. The NaOH is present in solution together with the salt CH_3COONa formed in the reaction; solutions of this salt have an alkaline reaction and should therefore augment the action of the NaOH, i.e., raise the pH due to the latter. In reality the increase is so small that it can be disregarded.* In other words, we may assume that the pH is determined entirely by the free NaOH

* The reason is that the presence of the strong alkali NaOH has a very strong suppressing effect of hydrolysis of the CH_3COONa. However, this is so only if the acid being titrated is not too weak. Otherwise hydrolysis of the salt cannot be disregarded and the pH must be calculated from other and more complicated equations which are not considered in this book

present in solution. Since it is a strong alkali, the OH^- ion concentration may be assumed equal to the total NaOH concentration. At the end of the break the excess of NaOH is 0.1 ml of 0.1 *N* solution in a volume of 100 ml.* This corresponds to 1 ml of 0.1 *N* solution per litre and this contains $\frac{0.1}{1,000}$ or 10^{-4} g-ion OH^-. Therefore, the OH^- ion concentration is 10^{-4} g-ion/litre, and the H^+ ion concentration is $10^{-14} : 10^{-4} = 10^{-10}$ g-ion/litre and the solution pH is 10. Thus, we have the same pH value as in the titration of 0.1 *N* HCl solution. All the subsequent points on the titration curve will similarly coincide with the curve considered earlier (Fig. 45).

The calculated pH values are given in Table XII.

Table XII

pH Variations in Titration of 100 ml of 0.1 *N* CH_3COOH Solution with 0.1 *N* NaOH (or Vice Versa)

NaOH added ml	Excess, ml		$\frac{C_{acid}}{C_{salt}}$	Calculations	pH
	acid	alkali			
0	100.0	—	—	$pH = \frac{4.73}{2} - 1/2 \log 0.1$	2.87
2.0	98.0	—	98/2	$pH = 4.73 - \log 98 + \log 2$	3.04 *
15.0	85.0	—	85/15	$pH = 4.73 - \log 85 + \log 15$	3.98
31.0	69.0	—	69/31	$pH = 4.73 - \log 69 + \log 31$	4.38
50.0	50.0	—	50/50	$pH = 4.73 - \log 50 + \log 50$	4.73
90.0	10.0	—	10/90	$pH = 4.73 - \log 10 + \log 90$	5.68
99.0	1.0	—	1/99	$pH = 4.73 - \log 1 + \log 99$	6.73
99.9	0.1	—	0.1/99.9	$pH = 4.73 - \log 0.1 + \log 99.9$	7.73
100 (equiv. pt.)	—	—	—	$pH = 7 + \frac{4.73}{2} + \frac{1}{2} \log 0.1$	8.87
100.1	—	0.1	—	$[OH^-] = 10^{-4}$; $[H^+] = 10^{-10}$	10
101.0	—	1.0	—	$[OH^-] = 10^{-3}$; $[H^+] = 10^{-11}$	11
110.0	—	10.0	—	$[OH^-] = 10^{-2}$; $[H^+] = 10^{-12}$	12
200.0	—	100.0	—	$[OH^-] = 10^{-1}$; $[H^+] = 10^{-13}$	13

* The pH values with 2, 15 and 31 ml NaOH were calculated for comparison with the indicator range of methyl orange; these data may be omitted when the titration curves are plotted.

* Since the volume change in titration is disregarded.

We plot the titration curve from these data in the usual way (Fig. 47).

Comparing this curve with the titration curve for 0.1 *N* HCl solution we see that: (a) the equivalence point no longer coincides, as it does in the case of HCl with the neutral point but is in the alkaline range, at pH = 8.87; (b) the break of pH in the titration curve is less than in titration of HCl; the break extends from pH = = 7.73 (with 0.1 ml excess acid) to pH = 10 (with 0.1 ml excess

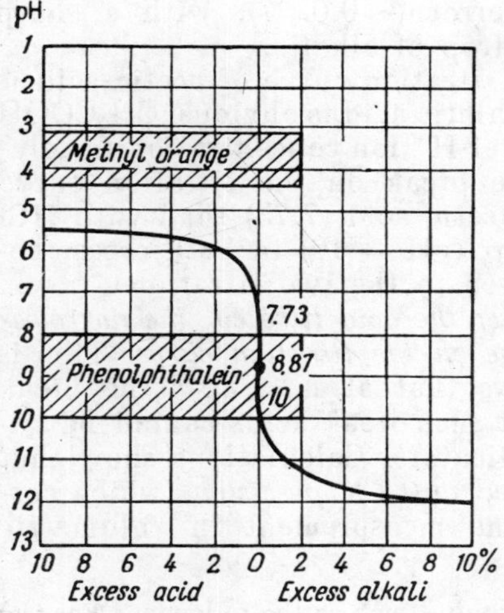

Fig. 47. Titration curve of 0.1 *N* CH_3COOH with 0.1 *N* NaOH (or vice versa)

Fig. 48. Relationship between the dissociation constant of the acid titrated and the range of the break on the titration curve

alkali); (c) it follows that in titration of acetic acid only phenolphthalein can be used out of the four commonest indicators. The colour change of methyl orange, corresponding to pH = 4, appears at the instant when only about 15% of the total amount of CH_3COOH has been titrated (see Table XII). Therefore, the indicator error in this case is about 85%. Even more important is the slowness of the colour change of the indicator near the equivalence point. To pass through the whole range of intermediate colours of this indicator, from pure red corresponding to pH ≈ 3.1 (with addition of 2 ml NaOH solution) to pure yellow, corresponding to pH ≈ 4.4 (with addition of 31 ml NaOH solution), we must add 29 ml of 0.1 *N* NaOH per 100 ml of the CH_3COOH solution. With 25 ml of the latter this corresponds to about 7.25 ml of the alkali solution. It is obvious that because of this very slow change in the colour of the indicator it is impossible to titrate acetic acid in its presence.

Methyl red, with pT $\approx$ 5.5, is likewise unsuitable in this case. Even litmus, with pT $\approx$ 7, gives an indicator error of about 0.5% in titration of acetic acid, and its colour change is not sharp enough either.

Only phenolphthalein, the titration exponent of which lies in the pH break region (pT = 9) and is very close to the equivalence point (pH = 8.87), gives a very small error ($\sim$0.02%), with a sharp colour change on addition of one drop of alkali.

The reason why the break in the titration curve of acetic acid is narrower than in the curve of hydrochloric acid is obvious: CH_3COOH being a weak acid, gives a much lower H^+ ion concentration in solution than does HCl. Therefore, the break on the titration curve should begin at a higher pH with acetic acid (7.73) than with HCl (pH = 4). It ends at the same point (pH = 10) in both cases, because the same alkali solution is used in the two titrations.

It follows from this that *the weaker the acid titrated, the narrower is the range of the abrupt* pH *change on the titration curve*. This is illustrated by Fig. 48, which shows that at $K = 10^{-9}$ the break vanishes completely. It follows that such weak acids cannot be titrated in presence of any of the indicators. Calculations show that *only acids of $K \geqslant 10^{-7}$ can be titrated to 0.1% precision* (which corresponds to the precision of volume measurement in volumetric analysis).

This conclusion may be reached by reasoning such as the following. For the precision of the titration to be 0.1%, not more than 0.1% of the unchanged initial substances must be present in solution in equilibrium with the reaction products at the equivalence point. For example, in titration of 0.1 *N* solution of a weak acid (designated as HA) with NaOH solution not more than 0.1% of the free acid HA and OH^- ions must remain, as the result of hydrolysis, at the equivalence point. In other words, their maximum permissible concentration at the equivalence point is

$$[HA] = [OH^-] = \frac{0.1 \times 0.1}{100} = 10^{-4}\ M$$

The concentration of the salt NaA formed in the reaction (and therefore of A^- anions) must be 0.1 (if we disregard the change in the solution volume during the titration).

Substituting these concentrations into the equation for the hydrolysis constant of the salt NaA:

$$\frac{[HA][OH^-]}{[A^-]} = \frac{K_{H_2O}}{K_{HA}}$$

we have

$$\frac{10^{-4} \times 10^{-4}}{10^{-1}} = \frac{10^{-8}}{K_{HA}}$$

and hence

$$K_{HA} = \frac{10^{-14} \times 10^{-1}}{10^{-8}} = 10^{-7}$$

Therefore, if K_{HA} is equal to or greater than 10^{-7} the acid can be titrated with satisfactory precision. On the other hand, an acid with $pK < 10^{-7}$ cannot be titrated satisfactorily.

It follows from the foregoing that at $K = 10^{-7}$ the OH^- ion concentration at the equivalence point is 10^{-4}. This means that at that point $[H^+] = 10^{-10}$ and pH = 10.*

It follows that in titrations of weak acids which are feasible in practice the pH at the equivalence point cannot exceed 10. Therefore, only indicators with pT not greater than 10 are used in titrations.

It should be noted that the strength of a weak acid can sometimes be increased considerably by introduction of a substance which forms a complex acid with it. For example, boric acid H_3BO_3, which is one of the weakest inorganic acids ($K = 5.7 \times 10^{-10}$), cannot be directly titrated in presence of any indicator. The two most suitable indicators with regard to the pT value, thymolphthalein (pT = 10) and phenolphthalein (pT = 9), give indicator errors of 15% and 37% respectively. However, if mannitol, glucose, or glycerol, which form much more strongly dissociated complex acids with boric acid, are added to the latter, it can be titrated in presence of phenolphthalein.**

64. Titration of Weak Bases with Strong Acids (or Vice Versa)

Suppose, for example, that 100 ml of 0.1 *N* NH_4OH solution ($K = 1.8 \times 10^{-5}$, $pK = 4.75$) is titrated with 0.1 *N* HCl. At the initial stage of the titration we have a 0.1 *N* solution of the weak base NH_4OH, the pH of which is found from the equation:

$$\frac{[NH_4^+][OH^-]}{[NH_4OH]} = K_{base} = 1.8 \times 10^{-5}$$

Since $[NH_4^+] = [OH^-]$ and $[NH_4OH] \approx C_{base}$, we can write:

$$[OH^-] = \sqrt{K_{base} C_{base}}$$

and

$$pOH = \frac{1}{2} pK_{base} - \frac{1}{2} \log C_{base} \qquad (1)$$

Hence:

$$pH = 14 - pOH = 14 - \frac{1}{2} pK_{base} + \frac{1}{2} \log C_{base} \qquad (2)$$

It is evident that Equation (1), obtained during derivation of Equation (2), is quite analogous to the equation derived earlier for

---

* This can also be confirmed by the use of Equation (8) (p. 255) for calculation of pH at the equivalence point:

$$pH = 7 + \frac{1}{2} pK + \frac{1}{2} \log C_{salt} = 7 + \frac{7}{2} - 0.5 = 10$$

** Strictly speaking, the complex acids formed are titrated, and not H_3BO_3

solutions of weak acids

$$pH = \frac{1}{2} pK_{acid} - \frac{1}{2} \log C_{acid}$$

the only difference being that it gives pOH instead of pH.

The same applies to calculations of the intermediate titration points and of the equivalence point. The appropriate equations are derived exactly as shown above (those who wish can derive them independently).

For the intermediate points in the titration, when the solution contains the salt NH_4Cl formed in the reaction together with residual free base (NH_4OH), we can write:

$$pOH = pK_{base} - \log \frac{C_{base}}{C_{salt}}$$

and

$$pH = 14 - pK_{base} + \log \frac{C_{base}}{C_{salt}} \quad (3)$$

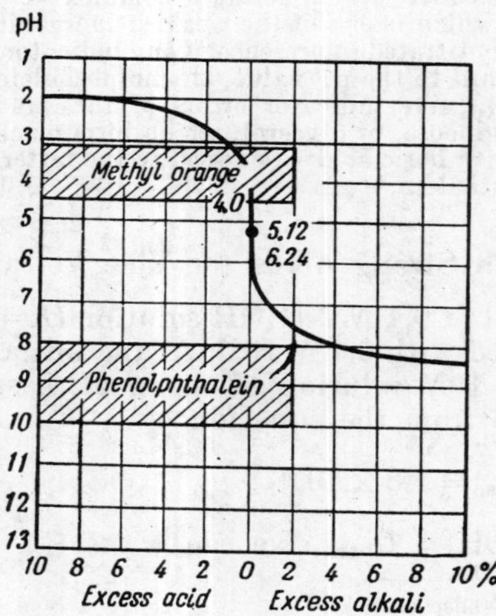

Fig. 49. Titration curve of 0.1 *N* NH_4OH with 0.1 *N* HCl (or vice versa)

At the equivalence point, when the solution contains the salt hydrolyzed in accordance with the equation

$$NH_4^+ + H_2O \rightleftarrows NH_4OH + H^+$$

the equation for the hydrolysis constant

$$\frac{[NH_4OH][H^+]}{[NH_4^+]} = \frac{10^{-14}}{K_{base}}$$

gives:

$$pH = 7 - \frac{1}{2} pK_{base} - \frac{1}{2} \log C_{salt} \quad (4)$$

It must be noted that this equation differs from that derived earlier for the pH of solutions of salts of weak acids and strong bases in one respect only: previously the terms $\frac{1}{2}$ pK and $\frac{1}{2}$ log C_{salt} were added to 7, since the pH had to be greater than 7. In the present instance it is less than 7, and these terms must therefore be subtracted from 7.

The pH at points corresponding to additions of excess HCl is calculated from the total HCl concentration in solution by the method already described above.

Calculated data for the titration curve are given in Table XIII, and the curve itself is plotted in Fig. 49.

Table XIII shows that: (a) the equivalence point lies in the acid range (pH = 5.12); (b) the region of abrupt pH change extends from pH = 6.24 to pH = 4.00, which is over only 2.24 pH units, whereas in titration of 0.1 *N* caustic soda with 0.1 *N* hydrochloric acid it extended over a range of 6 pH units.

Table XIII

pH Variation in Titration of 100 ml of 0.1 *N* NH_4OH Solution with 0.1 *N* HCl (or Vice Versa)

HCl added, ml	Excess, ml		$\frac{C_{base}}{C_{salt}}$	Calculations	pH
	NH_4OH	HCl			
0	100	—	—	$pH = 14 - \frac{4.75}{2} - 1/2 \log 0.1$	11.13
65	35	—	35/65	$pH = 14 - 4.75 + \log 35 - \log 65$	9.02
90	10	—	10/90	$pH = 14 - 4.75 + \log 10 - \log 90$	8.30
99	1	—	1/99	$pH = 14 - 4.75 + \log 1 - \log 99$	7.25
99.9	0.1	—	0.1/99.9	$pH = 14 - 4.75 + \log 0.1 - \log 99.9$	6.24
100 (equiv. pt.)	—	—	—	$pH = 7 - \frac{4.75}{2} - 1/2 \log 0.1$	5.12
100.1	—	0.1	—	$[H^+] = 10^{-4}$	4.0
101.0	—	1.0	—	$[H^+] = 10^{-3}$	3.0
110.0	—	10.0	—	$[H^+] = 10^{-2}$	2.0
200.0	—	100.0	—	$[H^+] = 10^{-1}$	1.0

Therefore, we can say that *the weaker the base which is titrated the narrower is the range of abrupt* pH *change on the titration curve and the more restricted is the choice of indicators which can be used in the titration*. Very weak bases with $K < 10^{-7}$, like very weak acids, cannot be titrated with accuracy because of the absence of an abrupt pH change.*

* It was shown on p. 259 that in titration of weak acids the pH at the equivalence point cannot be higher than 10 for the titration to be practically possible. Just in the same way it can be shown that in titration of weak acids the pH at the equivalence point cannot be less than 4. Therefore, only indicators with values of pT or p*K* (since the two are similar) between 4 and 10 can be used in acid-base titrations. The indicators listed in Table X (p. 244) from methyl orange (pT = 4) to thymolphthalein (pT = 10) conform to this condition.

All indicators with pT between 6.25 and 4.0 are suitable for the titration in question. In particular, methyl orange (pT = 4.0) and methyl red (pT = 5.5) would serve very well, but phenolphthalein (pT = 9) cannot be used.

Indeed it is clear from Table XIII that the titration exponent of phenolphthalein (pT = 9) is reached when only about 65% of the NH_4OH has been neutralized. As the curve is nearly flat over this region, the colour change of phenolphthalein is slow and gradual, so that NH_4OH cannot be titrated in its presence.

65. Titration of Weak Acids with Weak Bases (or Vice Versa)

In titration of weak acids with weak bases (or vice versa) the acid portion of the titration curve corresponds to titration of a weak acid with a strong base. The alkaline portion of the same curve is the same as the curve for titration of a weak base with a strong acid. The pH at the equivalence point is found from the equation of the hydrolysis constant of the salt as follows.

Suppose that acetic acid is titrated with NH_4OH solution. The salt formed is hydrolyzed in accordance with the equation

$$CH_3COONH_4 + H_2O \rightleftarrows NH_4OH + CH_3COOH$$

or

$$NH_4^+ + CH_3COO^- + H_2O \rightleftarrows NH_4OH + CH_3COOH$$

and hence

$$K_h = \frac{[NH_4OH][CH_3COOH]}{[NH_4^+][CH_3COO^-]} \tag{1}$$

Replacing the concentrations of NH_4OH and CH_3COOH in this equation by the values found from the equations for the corresponding dissociation constants, we have:

$$K_h = \frac{[NH_4^+][OH^-][H^+][CH_3COO^-]}{K_{base}K_{acid}[NH_4^+][CH_3COO^-]} = \frac{[OH^-][H^+]}{K_{base}K_{acid}} = \frac{10^{-14}}{K_{base}K_{acid}} \tag{2}$$

Substituting the value found for K_h into Equation (1) and noting that in accordance with the hydrolysis equation

$$[NH_4^+] = [CH_3COO^-] = C_{salt} \text{ and } [NH_4OH] = [CH_3COOH]$$

we have:

$$\frac{[CH_3COOH]^2}{C_{salt}^2} = \frac{10^{-14}}{K_{base}K_{acid}}$$

Putting the value of $[CH_3COOH]$ from the equation for the dissociation constant of acetic acid:

$$[CH_3COOH] = \frac{[H^+][CH_3COO^-]}{K_{acid}} = \frac{[H^+]\,C_{salt}}{K_{acid}}$$

We have:

$$\frac{[H^+]C_{salt}}{K_{acid}}\sqrt{\frac{10^{-14}\times C^2_{salt}}{K_{base}K_{acid}}}$$

and hence

$$[H^+]=\sqrt{\frac{10^{-14}\times K_{acid}}{K_{base}}}$$

Taking logarithms and reversing signs, we finally have:

$$pH=7+\frac{1}{2}pK_{acid}-\frac{1}{2}pK_{base} \qquad (3)$$

In the present instance, since $pK_{acid}=4.73$ and $pK_{base}=4.75$

$$pH=7+2.37-2.38=6.99$$

Regardless of the salt concentration, the solution pH at the equivalence point is almost 7, i.e., it coincides with the point of neutrality. However, this is true only if $pK_{acid} = pK_{base}$, i.e., if the reacting acid and base are of equal strength. If the acid is stronger (if $pK_{acid} < pK_{base}$) then the pH of the salt solution is less than 7 and so the solution has an acid reaction. Otherwise $pH > 7$, and the salt solution has an alkaline reaction.

Since this case is of no practical interest, we give only the titration curve (Fig. 50), without the relevant calculations.

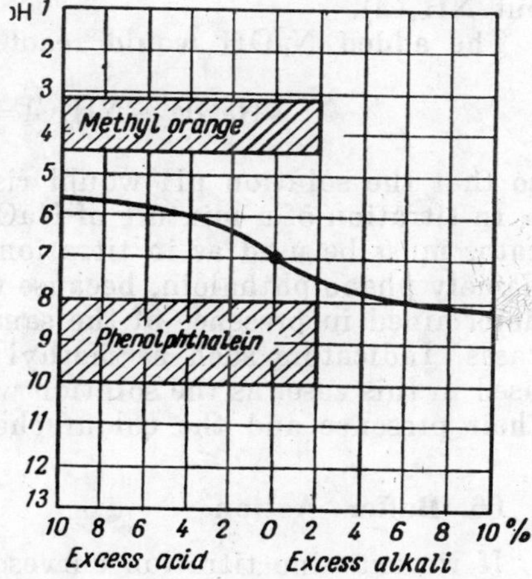

Fig. 50. Titration curve of 0.1 N CH_3COOH with 0.1 N NH_4OH (or vice versa)

Figure 50 shows that there is no pH break at all in this case. This means that the titration cannot be performed accurately with any of the known indicators. Hence it follows that *in titrations by the neutralization method at least one of the reacting substances must be a strong electrolyte.*

The working solutions for the neutralization method must always be solutions of strong alkalies or acids in order that weak as well as strong acids or bases can be titrated.

It should be remembered that the pH break on the titration curve also disappears if a very weak acid or base is titrated or if very dilute solutions are used. Calculations show that to ensure a degree of precision of about 0.1% the values of K_{acid} or K_{base} must not be less than 10^{-7}, and the solution concentrations must not be below 0.0001 N.

In conclusion, let us consider that case when a solution to be titrated contains, in addition to an acid or base, certain extraneous substances which influence the pH at the equivalence point. Suppose, for example, that a solution containing NH_4Cl together with HCl is titrated with caustic soda. Which indicator should be used in this titration? To answer this question, we note that at the equivalence point the solution contains, in addition to NaCl, NH_4Cl which gives it an acid reaction. Therefore, the equivalence point is no longer at pH = 7 but at pH < 7, as in titration of HCl with ammonia solution. Accordingly, the same indicator (methyl orange or methyl red) as in the latter case should be used. If phenolphthalein was used instead, the end point would be at pH = 9. To bring the solution pH to this value it would be necessary to add a large excess of NaOH, and not one drop as in the titration of pure HCl (without NH_4Cl).

The added NaOH would react with NH_4Cl:

$$NaOH + NH_4Cl = NH_4OH + NaCl$$

so that the solution pH would rise very slowly.

In titration of a mixture of NaOH and CH_3COONa the same indicator must be used as in titration of acetic acid with caustic soda, namely phenolphthalein, because the pH at the equivalence point is determined in presence of the same substance, CH_3COONa, in both cases. Indicators such as methyl orange or methyl red cannot be used in this case, as the solution would be very much overtitrated in their presence and the colour change would not be sharp enough.

66. Buffer Action

If we examine titration curves we see that they have regions of two types. In the region of abrupt pH change the curves are almost vertical, so that additions of extremely small amounts of acid or alkali produce very large changes of solution pH. On the other hand, in other regions the curves are flat and almost horizontal. This means that at the corresponding titration stages the solution pH is changed very little by addition of acid or alkali. Such solutions are said to have *buffer action* or are known as *buffer solutions*.

The term "buffer" is applied to such solutions because, just as buffers of railway carriages resist shocks, buffer solutions resist the action of various factors which alter pH. If a buffer is introduced into a reacting system, the solution pH remains almost constant despite the formation of an acid or a base in the reaction.

To illustrate this we may refer to the reaction whereby Zn^{++} is separated from the other Group III cations by precipitation with hydrogen sulphide. It is found in practice that ZnS is completely precipitated even at pH = 2, whereas CoS, NiS, and other Group III sulphides are not precipitated under such conditions. Therefore, if we first neutralize the solution, add a sufficient quantity of a buffer mixture of pH = 2, and then pass H_2S through the solution, Zn^{++} is completely precipitated despite the fact that an acid is formed in the reaction; for example:

$$ZnCl_2 + H_2S = \downarrow ZnS + 2HCl$$

All other Group III cations remain in solution. A suitable buffer for this separation is a mixture of free formic acid HCOOH with a salt of the same acid—ammonium or sodium formate; this mixture is known as formate buffer mixture.

The buffer action of such a mixture is quite easy to understand. The strong acid formed in the reaction reacts with the formate and produces an equivalent amount of the relatively weak formic acid:

$$HCOONH_4 + HCl = NH_4Cl + HCOOH$$

or

$$HCOO^- + H^+ = HCOOH$$

In other words, nearly all the H^+ ions introduced into the solution combine with the $HCOO^-$ (formate ions) and do not remain free, and the solution pH therefore changes very little.

The same thing happens if an alkali is introduced into a solution containing formate buffer. The OH^- ions of the alkali do not remain free but combine at once with the H^+ ions of formic acid:

$$OH^- + HCOOH = H_2O + HCOO^-$$

Therefore, here again the solution pH remains almost unchanged.

The titration curves of weak acids also show that mixtures of weak acids and their salts should have buffer action. For example, the flat portion of the curve representing titration of acetic acid with caustic soda (Fig. 47) on the acid side corresponds to the stages when only part of the CH_3COOH has been titrated (i.e., converted into its salt), while the rest remains free. Therefore, the mixture of CH_3COOH and CH_3COONa is a buffer in presence of which the pH changes very slowly on addition of acid or alkali (this is known as the acetate buffer).

The pH of this buffer can be easily calculated for any free acid and salt concentrations from the well-known equation

$$pH = pK - \log \frac{C_{acid}}{C_{salt}}$$

For example, if the solution contains 0.1 mole each of acetic acid and its salt, then

$$pH = 4.73 - \log \frac{0.1}{0.1} = 4.73$$

If 0.01 mole of any strong acid is added to 1 litre of this solution, 0.01 mole of the salt (CH_3COONa) is converted into the equivalent amount of free acid (CH_3COOH). Therefore, the solution pH becomes

$$pH = 4.73 - \log \frac{0.11}{0.09} = 4.64$$

Similarly, if we add 0.01 mole of alkali to 1 litre of the solution we have

$$pH = 4.73 - \log \frac{0.09}{0.11} = 4.82$$

Therefore, in either case the pH alters by only 0.09.

On the other hand, if the same amount of acid or alkali is added to 1 litre of pure water, the pH alters by 5 units (falls from 7 to 2 or rises from 7 to 12). It is evident that the pH of a buffer mixture remains unchanged on dilution, as C_{acid} and C_{salt} alter in the same ratio.

The curve for titration of NH_4OH solution with hydrochloric acid (Fig. 49) shows that mixtures of weak bases and their salts ($NH_4OH + NH_4Cl$ in this instance) should have buffer action, because here again the region of the titration curve corresponding to the presence of these substances in solution is flat. The pH of such mixtures is calculated from the formula:

$$pH = 14 - pK_{base} + \log \frac{C_{base}}{C_{salt}}$$

A mixture of equivalent amounts of NH_4OH and NH_4Cl gives a pH value of $14 - pK_{base} = 14 - 4.75 = 9.25$.

It will be remembered that this buffer mixture is constantly used in qualitative analysis; for example, in separation of Group II and Group I cations, or in separation of Group III cations from Group II and I cations. In both cases the presence of ammonia buffer prevents precipitation of magnesium hydroxide (or basic carbonate), the solubility product of which is not reached at $pH \approx 9$.

Mixtures of acid salts of different basicities, such as NaH_2PO_4 + + Na_2HPO_4, should also have buffer action; here the first salt acts as a weak acid and the second as its salt.

Finally, curves representing titration of strong acids with strong alkalies or vice versa (see Figs. 45 and 46) show that strong acids and strong alkalies also have buffer action if their concentrations are high enough, because here again the corresponding regions of the titration curves are very flat. Of course, the mechanism of the buffer action here is very different from that in the cases considered earlier. The reason is, if the concentration of acid (or alkali) is fairly high, the amount of it which must be added to the solution to produce any appreciable pH change is rather large. Additions of small amounts of acid or alkali would have hardly any effect on the pH.

For example, if 0.01 mole of HCl is added to 1 litre of 0.1 *N* HCl solution (the pH of which is 1), the H^+ ion concentration rises to 0.11 g-ion/litre and the pH falls to 0.96, or by only 0.04. Similarly, on addition of 0.01 mole of NaOH the H^+ ion concentration falls to 0.09, so that the pH rises to 1.05. When small amounts of acids or alkalies are added to fairly concentrated solutions of strong alkalies the pH changes are also slight. On the other hand, very dilute solutions of strong acids and alkalies, salt solutions, and pure water do not have buffer action. For example, if 0.01 mole of NaOH is added to 1 litre of a solution containing 10^{-4} *M* HCl all the acid is converted into its salt and an excess of alkali equal to $0.01-0.0001=$ $= 0.0099$ *M* is left. The OH^- ion concentration in the resultant solution is $[OH^-] = 9.9 \times 10^{-3}$, pOH = 2, and pH = 12. Therefore, addition of 0.01 mole of NaOH changes the pH from 4 to 12.

In the light of all that has been said about buffer action, we can formulate the rule for choice of indicators in titration in another way: *the indicator chosen for any particular reaction should change colour at a point when the solution being titrated does not exert a buffer effect*, because only then is the colour change sharp enough.

Buffer mixtures are wide[illegible] us[illegible] in analytical practice both in qualitative and quantitati[illegible]s when it is necessary to maintain the solution pH at a [illegible]level in a particular analytical operation. They are also [illegible] experimental determinations of pH (Sec. 127).

67. Indicator Error in Tit[illegible]

In addition to plotting of titration c[illegible]es, there is another method for choosing an indicator (p. 247), which involves [illegible]lculation of the indicator error. It will be remembered that *the indicator error* [illegible] *the error caused by the difference between the titration exponent of a given in[illegible]ator and the* pH *at the equivalence point.* Because of this difference a solution is [illegible]sually either somewhat overtitrated or undertitrated. As a result, the solution contains an excess of free acid or free alkali at the end of the titration.

If this excess acid is a strong acid and is therefore present in the form of free H^+ ions, the error is described as the "hydrogen" or "H^+ error". If on the contrary, the acid is weak and is present almost entirely in the form of undissociated molecules (HA), the "acid error" or "HA error" is decisive. Similarly, if the excess alkali is strong it gives rise to the "hydroxyl error" or "OH^- error"; if it is weak, the "alkali error" or "MeOH error" has to be taken into account. Let us now consider methods for calculating the magnitude of all these four types of indicator errors.

Hydrogen Error. Suppose that the titration exponent of the indicator is pT, the normality of the strong acid being titrated is N, its volume is V_1 ml, and the total solution volume at the end of the titration is V_2 ml.

We reason as follows: each millilitre of N solution contains $\frac{N}{1{,}000}$ gram-equivalents of acid. Therefore, the total amount of acid taken for the titration is $\frac{NV_1}{1{,}000}$ gram-equivalents, containing the same number of gram-ions of H^+. Let us now calculate how many gram-ions of H^+ remain at the end of the titration. The titration is ended when the pH is equal to the pT of the indicator used; for example, at pH $= 4$ with methyl orange or at pH$=9$ with phenolphthalein, etc. However, since pH $= -\log[H^+]$, these pH values correspond to H^+ ion concentrations $[H^+] = 10^{-4}$; $[H^+] = 10^{-9}$ g-ion/litre, etc. It follows that in the general case the concentration of the residual H^+ ions is $[H^+] = 10^{-pT}$ g-ion/litre. The V_2 ml of solution at the end of the titration contains $\frac{10^{-pT} \times V_2}{1{,}000}$ gram-ions of H^+.

This amount represents the hydrogen error. To express it as a percentage of the amount of H^+ ions taken, we have by proportion:

$$\frac{NV_1}{1{,}000} - 100\%$$

$$\frac{10^{-pT} \times V_2}{1{,}000} - x\%$$

Hence the H^+ error is

$$x = \frac{10^{-pT} \times V_2}{NV_1} \times 100\% \qquad (1)$$

Hydroxyl Error. Suppose that V_1 ml of a strong alkali of normality N is titrated with a strong acid, and that the volume of the solution at the end of the titration is V_2 ml.

Reasoning as before, we find that the total amount of OH^- ions taken for the titration is $\frac{NV_1}{1{,}000}$ g-ions. The titration is ended when the pH is equal to the pT of the indicator, i.e., at pOH $= 14 -$ pT. Therefore, at the end of the titration $[OH^-] = 10^{-(14-pT)}$ and V_2 ml of the solution contains $\frac{10^{-(14-pT)} \times V_2}{1{,}000}$ gram-ions of OH^- (the OH^- error). As before, we express the OH^- error as a percentage:

$$\frac{NV_1}{1{,}000} - 100\%$$

$$\frac{10^{-(14-pT)} \times V_2}{1{,}000} - x\%$$

Therefore, the OH^- error is

$$x = \frac{10^{-(14-pT)} \times V_2}{NV_1} \times 100\% \qquad (2)$$

Acid Error. To calculate the acid error, i.e., the error due to the presence of undissociated molecules of a weak acid (HA) in solution at the end of the titration, we first write the equation for the dissociation constant of the acid:

$$\frac{[H^+][A^-]}{[HA]} = K$$

Rearranging this equation, we have:

$$\frac{[HA]}{[A^-]} = \frac{[H^+]}{K}$$

As HA is a weak acid, [HA] is practically equal to the total concentration of free acid in the solution, and $[A^-]$, to the concentration of the salt. However, each gram-molecule of the salt is formed by neutralization of one gram-molecule of acid. Therefore, the ratio $[HA] : [A^-]$ may be regarded as the ratio of the concentrations of the residual and neutralized acid and taken as a measure of the acid error in the titration. Noting further that $[H^+] = 10^{-pT}$ and $K = 10^{-pK}$, we have from the above equation:

$$\text{HA error} = \frac{\text{acid not neutralized}}{\text{acid neutralized}} = \frac{10^{-pT}}{10^{-pK}}$$

Finally

$$\text{HA error} = 10^{pK-pT} \qquad (3)$$

If the indicator error in a titration is not to exceed 0.1%, i.e., if the amount of residual acid is not to exceed 0.001 of the amount of acid neutralized, the following conditions must be satisfied:

$$10^{pK-pT} \leqslant 10^{-3}$$

or

$$pT \geqslant pK + 3$$

This means that *when the use of a particular indicator gives rise to an acid error in titration, this indicator is suitable only if the indicator exponent* pT *is at least 3 units greater* than the acid exponent p*K*.

For example, it can be said in advance that acetic acid ($pK = 4.73$) can be titrated accurately only in presence of indicators with $pT \gg 7.73$. This means that methyl orange ($pT=4$), methyl red ($pT=5.5$), and even litmus ($pT=7$) are unsuitable here. On the other hand, phenolphthalein ($pT = 9$) should be suitable if the OH^- error is not too large.

Alkali Error. Reasoning as before, we can write:

$$\frac{[Me^+][OH^-]}{[MeOH]} = K; \qquad \frac{[MeOH]}{[Me^+]} = \frac{[OH^-]}{K}$$

but

$$\frac{[MeOH]}{[Me^+]} = \frac{\text{alkali not neutralized}}{\text{alkali neutralized}} = \text{MeOH error}$$

On the other hand, pH at the end of the titration is equal to pT, and pOH = 14 — pT. Therefore:

$$\text{MeOH error} = \frac{10^{-(14-\text{pT})}}{10^{-\text{p}K}} = 10^{\text{p}K+\text{pT}-14} \quad (4)$$

With the same reasoning as in the preceding case we find that the titration may be sufficiently precise if the MeOH error is equal to or less than 10^{-3}; i.e., provided that

$$\text{p}K + \text{pT} - 14 \leqslant -3$$

or

$$\text{pT} \leqslant 11 - \text{p}K$$

For example, in titration of NH_4OH (pK = 4.75) indicators with pT $\leqslant$ 6.25 may be used. Therefore, neither phenolphthalein (pT = 9) nor litmus (pT = 7) is suitable. On the other hand, methyl red (pT = 5.5) and methyl orange (pT = 4) should be quite suitable if the H^+ error does not exceed the permissible limit.

We now consider a few examples of the use of these formulas for choice of indicators.

Example 1. What is the indicator error in titration of 0.1 *N* HCl with 0.1 *N* NaOH in presence of methyl orange?

Solution. We first decide which of the errors must be taken into account in this case. Here the equivalence point is at pH = 7, while the end point with methyl orange is at pH = 4. Therefore, the solution contains some excess HCl at the end of the titration. Since it is a strong acid, it gives rise to an H^+ error.

As both solutions are of the same normality, equal volumes are used in the titration. This means that the volume of the solution is doubled during the titration, i.e., $V_2 = 2V_1$. From Equation (1) we have

$$H^+ \text{ error} = -\frac{10^{-4} \times 2V_1}{10^{-1} \times V_1} \times 100 = -0.2\%$$

The minus sign here means that the HCl solution is undertitrated. Since 0.2% is not beyond the usual limits of experimental error we conclude that methyl orange can be used in this case.

Example 2. Solve the same problem for titration in the presence of phenolphthalein.

Solution. The end point in titration in the presence of phenolphthalein is at pH = 9, so that the solution is somewhat overtitrated. As the alkali is strong, it gives rise to an OH^- error. Therefore

$$OH^- \text{ error} = +\frac{10^{-(14-9)} \times 2V_1}{10^{-1} \times V_1} \times 100 = +0.02\%$$

It follows that phenolphthalein is quite suitable for this titration.

Example 3. Can 0.01 *N* hydrochloric acid be titrated with caustic soda in presence of methyl orange?

Solution. Here the error is evidently of the same type as in Example 1. Therefore

$$H^+ \text{ error} = -\frac{10^{-4} \times 2V_1}{10^{-2} \times V_1} \times 100 = -2\%$$

This error is too large. Therefore, methyl orange cannot be used in this titration. However, with phenolphthalein the OH^- error is +0.2%, and this indicator is therefore quite suitable here.

Example 4. Calculate the titration error in titration of 0.1 *N* acetic acid with 0.1 *N* caustic soda in the presence of methyl orange indicator.

Solution. To determine the type of error, we find the solution pH at the equivalence point *:

$$pH = 7 + \frac{4.73}{2} + {}^1/_2 \log 0.05 = 8.72$$

As the end point in titration with methyl orange is at pH = 4, the solution contains excess CH_3COOH at the end of the titration. This is a weak acid, so that it gives rise to an HA error. We can therefore write:

$$\text{HA error} = 10^{pK - pT} = 10^{4.73-4} = 10^{0.73}$$

Hence log HA error is 0.73 and the HA error is approximately 5.4.

This means that the amounts of residual and neutralized acetic acid are in the ratio of 5.4 to 1. In other words, out of 6.4 parts of the CH_3COOH initially taken 5.4 parts remain not neutralized. From this it is easy to calculate the HA error as a percentage:

$$6.4 - 100\%$$

$$5.4 - x\%$$

$$x = \text{HA error} = -\frac{5.4 \times 100}{6.4} \approx -84\%$$

The conclusion is that acetic acid cannot be titrated in the presence of methyl orange.

It will be remembered that the same conclusion was reached previously without calculation, by the use of the expression $pT \gg pK + 3$ (p. 269).

Example 5. Solve the same problem for titration of CH_3COOH in the presence of phenolphthalein.

Solution. Since the pH at the equivalence point is 8.72 and pT of phenolphthalein is 9.0, CH_3COOH is somewhat overtitrated in the presence of this indicator. As a strong alkali is used in the titration, an OH^- error is to be expected here:

$$OH^- \text{ error} = +\frac{10^{14-9} \times 2V_1}{10^{-1} \times V_1} \times 100 = +0.02\%$$

As in titration of HCl, this indicator is suitable.

Example 6. What is the indicator error in titration of 0.1 *N* NH_4OH with 0.1 *N* HCl in the presence of the following indicators: (a) phenolphthalein; (b) methyl orange?

Solution. (a) The pH at the equivalence point is

$$pH = 7 - \frac{4.75}{2} - {}^1/_2 \log 0.05 = 5.28$$

The end point in titration with phenolphthalein is at pH = 9; at the end of the titration the solution contains a certain excess of NH_4OH. Therefore, an MeOH error is to be expected here:

$$\text{MeOH error} = 10^{4.75+9-14} = 10^{-0.25}$$

---

* In this calculation we take into account the doubling of the solution volume in the titration. Therefore, C_{salt} is taken as 0.05 *N*. It will be remembered that *pK* of acetic acid is 4.73 (p. 269).

Hence $\log(\text{MeOH error}) = -0.25 = \bar{1}.75$; MeOH error $= 0.56$.

Therefore, out of 1.56 parts by weight of the NH_4OH initially taken 0.56 part remains not neutralized. By proportion:

$$1.56 - 100\%$$

$$0.56 - x\%$$

$$x = \text{MeOH error} = -\frac{0.56 \times 100}{1.56} \approx -36\%$$

The conclusion is that the indicator is unsuitable.

The same conclusion was reached from the expression $pT \ll 11 - pK$ (p. 270).

(b) In titration of NH_4OH in presence of methyl orange the end point is at pH = 4.0 instead of 5.28. We therefore expect an H^+ error:

$$H^+ \text{ error} = +\frac{10^{-4} \times 2V_1}{10^{-1} \times V_1} \times 100 = +0.2\%$$

Therefore, the indicator is suitable.

It was shown above how the suitability of any specified indicator can be determined by calculation of the indicator error in titration. If no indicator is specified, then one is chosen such that its titration exponent is as close as possible to the pH at the equivalence point (which can be found from known formulas), and the indicator error is calculated for this indicator.

68. Titration of Dibasic and Polybasic Acids

In accordance with the stepwise dissociation of di- and polybasic acids, their neutralization is also stepwise. For example, the following reactions take place in titration of orthophosphoric acid with caustic soda:

$$H_3PO_4 + NaOH = NaH_2PO_4 + H_2O$$

$$NaH_2PO_4 + NaOH = Na_2HPO_4 + H_2O$$

$$Na_2HPO_4 + NaOH = Na_3PO_4 + H_2O$$

Accordingly, the H_3PO_4 titration curve, shown in Fig. 51, has not one but three equivalence points.*

The first of these corresponds to formation of the monosubstituted acid salt (NaH_2PO_4), the second, to the disubstituted acid salt (Na_2HPO_4), and the third, to the trisubstituted salt (Na_3PO_4). The first equivalence point is reached after one mole of NaOH has been added per mole of H_3PO_4, the second after addition of two moles of NaOH, and the third after addition of three moles. For example, if 30 ml of 0.1 *M* H_3PO_4 solution is titrated, the first equivalence point is reached after addition of 10 ml, the second, of 20 ml, and the third, of 30 ml of 0.1 *M* NaOH solution.

---

* In Fig. 51 the abscissa axis shows the number of moles of NaOH per mole of H_3PO_4.

The position of the first equivalence point is found from the equation

$$pH_I = \frac{pK_1 + pK_2}{2} \quad (1)$$

The acid salt NaH_2PO_4 formed at the first equivalence point gives rise to $H_2PO_4^-$ ions, and these in their turn dissociate according to the equation

$$H_2PO_4^- \rightleftarrows H^+ + HPO_4^{--}$$

Here the concentrations of H^+ and HPO_4^- ions are not equal because some of the H^+ ions combine with $H_2PO_4^-$ ions to give undissociated H_3PO_4 molecules.

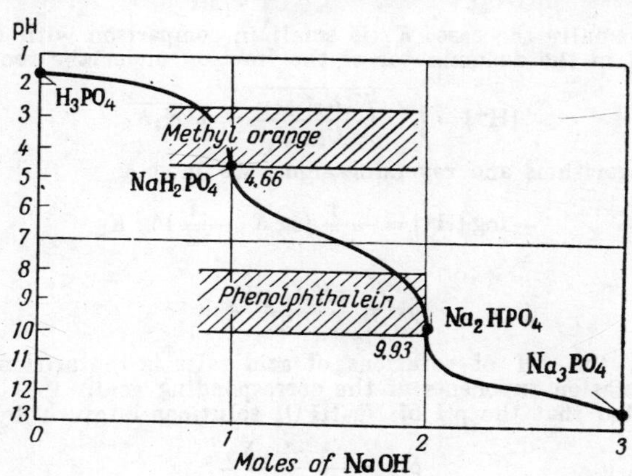

Fig. 51. Titration curve of 0.1 *M* H_3PO_4 solution with 0.1 *N* NaOH

The amount of H^+ ions involved in this process is evidently equal to the number of undissociated H_3PO_4 molecules in solution. We can therefore write:

$$[H^+] + [H_3PO_4] = [HPO_4^{--}] \quad (2)$$

In addition, we can write the equations for K_1 and K_2

$$\frac{[H^+][H_2PO_4^-]}{[H_3PO_4]} = K_1 \quad (3)$$

$$\frac{[H^+][HPO_4^{--}]}{[H_2PO_4^-]} = K_2 \quad (4)$$

We find $[HPO_4^{--}]$ and $[H_3PO_4]$ from Equations (3) and (4) and substitute their values into Equation (2). This gives

$$[H^+] + \frac{[H^+][H_2PO_4^-]}{K_1} = \frac{K_2[H_2PO_4^-]}{[H^+]}$$

or

$$K_1[H^+]^2 + [H_2PO_4^-][H^+]^2 = K_1K_2[H_2PO_4^-]$$

and hence

$$[H^+]=\sqrt{\frac{K_1K_2[H_2PO_4^-]}{K_1+[H_2PO_4^-]}}$$

Since NaH_2PO_4 is a strong electrolyte and each molecule dissociates to yield one $H_2PO_4^-$ ion, we can assume, disregarding the second and third hydrolysis stages, that

$$[H_2PO_4^-]\approx C_{salt}$$

Consequently

$$[H^+]=\sqrt{\frac{K_1K_2C_{salt}}{K_1+C_{salt}}} \tag{5}$$

If, as is usually the case, K_1 is small in comparison with C_{salt}, it may be disregarded in the denominator of the fraction under the root sign. Then

$$[H^+]=\sqrt{\frac{K_1K_2C_{salt}}{C_{salt}}}=\sqrt{K_1K_2}$$

Taking logarithms and reversing signs, we have

$$-\log[H^+]=-\frac{1}{2}\log K_1-\frac{1}{2}\log K_2$$

or

$$pH=\frac{pK_1+pK_2}{2} \tag{6}$$

Therefore, the pH of solutions of acid salts is the arithmetic mean of the two dissociation exponents of the corresponding acid.

We also find that the pH of Na_2HPO_4 solutions is given by

$$pH=\frac{pK_2+pK_3}{2} \tag{7}$$

In pH calculations in such cases the following processes must be taken into account: (a) dissociation of HPO_4^{--} ions; (b) combination of the latter with H^+ ions to form $H_3PO_4^-$; these processes have the constants:

$$\frac{[H^+][PO_4^{---}]}{[HPO_4^{--}]}=K_3 \text{ and } \frac{[H^+][HPO_4^{--}]}{[H_2PO_4^-]}=K_2$$

The numerical values of the dissociation constants of phosphori acid and the corresponding values of pK are

$$K_1=7.51\times10^{-3}; \qquad pK_1=-\log 7.51\times10^{-3}=2.12$$

$$K_2=6.23\times10^{-8}: \qquad pK_2=-\log 6.23\times10^{-8}=7.21$$

$$K_3=2.2\times10^{-13}; \qquad pK_3=-\log 2.2\times10^{-13}=12.67$$

Therefore, at the first equivalence point

$$pH_I=\frac{2.12+7.21}{2}=4.66$$

And at the second equivalence point

$$pH_{II}=\frac{pK_2+pK_3}{2}=\frac{7.21+12.67}{2}=9.94$$

The pH at the third equivalence point can be calculated from the formula for pH of salts of weak acids and strong bases:

$$pH_{III} = 7 + {}^1/_2 pK + {}^1/_2 \log C_{salt}$$

Although this formula was derived for salts of monobasic acids (Sec. 63), it can be used in the present instance with an accuracy adequate for practical purposes Hydrolysis of Na_3PO_4 is confined mainly to the first stage, corresponding to the equation

$$PO_4^{---} + H_2O \rightleftarrows HPO_4^{--} + OH^-$$

The hydrolysis in the subsequent stages is so slight that it may be disregarded.

Taking this into account and noting that the first hydrolysis stage of Na_3PO_4 depends on K_3, we have:

$$pH \approx 7 + \frac{12.67}{2} + {}^1/_2 \log 0.1 \approx 12.8$$

Therefore, the first equivalence point (pH = 4.6) is close to the range of methyl orange (pH = 3.1-4.4), and the second (pH = 9.93) is in the phenolphthalein range (pH = 8.0-10.0).

However, we know that the suit bility of a particular indicator in titration depends not only on the position of the equivalence point but also on the abruptness of pH change on the titration curve, without which the colour change would not be distinct.

Investigations of this problem have shown that a break sharp enough for precise titration appears on titration curves of di- and polybasic acids only if the ratio of their dissociation constants at the different stages is high enough (at least 10^4). In the present instance these ratios are: for the first equivalence point

$$\frac{K_1}{K_2} = \frac{7.51 \times 10^{-3}}{6.23 \times 10^{-8}} \approx 1.2 \times 10^5$$

for the second equivalence point

$$\frac{K_2}{K_3} = \frac{6.23 \times 10^{-8}}{2.2 \times 10^{-13}} \approx 3 \times 10^5$$

Therefore, pH breaks large enough to allow accurate titration of H_3PO_4 should occur at both equivalence points.

It is clear from all that has been said that in presence of methyl orange indicator H_3PO_4 is titrated as a monobasic acid, i.e.,

$$H_3PO_4 + NaOH = NaH_2PO_4 + H_2O$$

In this case the gram-equivalent of H_3PO_4 is one gram-molecule.

In contrast to this, in presence of phenolphthalein (or, more precisely, of thymolphthalein) phosphoric acid is titrated in accordance with the equation

$$H_3PO_4 + 2NaON = Na_2HPO_4 + 2H_2O$$

i.e., it behaves as a dibasic acid. There the gram-equivalent of H_3PO_4 is a half of the gram-molecule.

Direct titration of orthophosphoric acid as a tribasic acid:

$$H_3PO_4 + 3NaOH = Na_3PO_4 + 3H_2O$$

is impossible with any indicator, because the corresponding dissociation constant of orthophosphoric acid is very small ($K_3 = 2.2 \times \times 10^{-13}$). It is known (p. 258) that even at $K = 10^{-9}$ there is no break at all on the titration curve.

However, such titration may be performed indirectly. The H_3PO_4 is replaced by an equivalent amount of HCl by the action of $CaCl_2$, and the hydrochloric acid is titrated:

$$2H_3PO_4 + 3CaCl_2 = \downarrow Ca_3(PO_4)_2 + 6HCl$$

$$6HCl + 6NaOH = 6NaCl + 6H_2O$$

These equations show that the reaction between H_3PO_4 and $CaCl_2$ gives the insoluble salt $Ca_3(PO_4)_2$ and hydrochloric acid (in an equivalent amount), and the latter is titrated with alkali. In this case the gram-equivalent of H_3PO_4 is $^1/_3$ of a gram-molecule.

Now consider the titration of carbonic acid. It is neutralized as follows:

$$H_2CO_3 + NaOH = NaHCO_3 + H_2O$$

$$NaHCO_3 + NaOH = Na_2CO_3 + H_2O$$

Accordingly, the titration curve (Fig. 52) has two equivalence points.* One corresponds to formation of $NaHCO_3$ and the other, of Na_2CO_3.

For carbonic acid:

$$K_1 = 4.31 \times 10^{-7};$$

$$pK_1 = -\log 4.31 \times 10^{-7} = 6.37$$

$$K_2 = 5.61 \times 10^{-11};$$

$$pK_2 = -\log 5.61 \times 10^{-11} = 10.25$$

and the pH values at the two equivalence points are

$$pH_I = \frac{pK_1 + pK_2}{2} = \frac{6.37 + 10.25}{2} = 8.31$$

---

* In Fig. 52 the abscissa axis shows the number of moles of NaOH per mole of H_2CO_3.

and

$$pH_{II} = 7 + {}^1/_2 pK_2 + {}^1/_2 \log C_{salt} = 7 + \frac{10.25}{2} + {}^1/_2 \log 0.1 \approx 11.6$$

Since the first equivalence point is within the phenolphthalein range, carbonic acid is titrated as a monobasic acid in its presence. However, the pH break is not sharp enough, as the ratio $K_1 : K_2$ is somewhat less than 10^4 (actually 0.8×10^4). Therefore, the titration is not very precise.

Direct titration of carbonic acid as a dibasic acid is clearly impossible because of the very low value of K_2 and the consequent absence of a pH break on the titration curve.*

The reverse process to that considered above, namely titration of Na_2CO_3 solution with HCl solution, is of considerable practical importance. The following reactions take place:

$$Na_2CO_3 + HCl = NaHCO_3 + NaCl$$

$$NaHCO_3 + HCl = H_2CO_3 + NaCl$$

The equations show that Na_2CO_3 is first converted into $NaHCO_3$; the solution pH changes from 11.6 to 8.31 in the process (see Fig. 52).

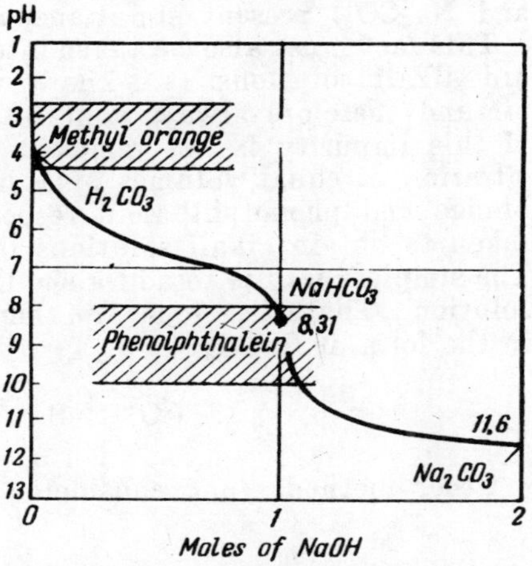

Fig. 52. Titration curve of H_2CO_3 solution with NaOH solution.

If phenolphthalein is added to the Na_2CO_3 solution before the start of the titration, a bright red colour is produced.

At the equivalence point corresponding to formation of $NaHCO_3$ the solution becomes colourless (at pH $\approx$ 8).

However, if methyl orange is now added to the solution its colour becomes yellow. It will remain yellow on further addition of HCl up to the point when all the $NaHCO_3$ is converted into free H_2CO_3, a saturated solution of which has pH of about 4.0, which is the same as the titration exponent of this indicator.

If Na_2CO_3 is titrated in presence of methyl orange from the start, two moles of HCl would be taken per mole of Na_2CO_3, in accordance with the equation

$$Na_2CO_3 + 2HCl = H_2CO_3 + 2NaCl$$

---

* Such titrations can be performed by indirect methods only.

In presence of phenolphthalein the amount of acid required for the titration would be a half of this, or 1 mole:

$$Na_2CO_3 + HCl = NaHCO_3 + NaCl$$

Therefore, we can say that in presence of phenolphthalein only a half of the Na_2CO_3 present is titrated, whereas in presence of methyl orange this salt is completely titrated.

The difference in the titration of Na_2CO_3 in presence of methyl orange and phenolphthalein respectively can be used for determination of caustic alkalies and alkali carbonates (for example, NaOH and Na_2CO_3) present simultaneously in solution (Sec. 72).

This fact must also be taken into account in preparation of standard alkali solutions. It is known that alkalies absorb CO_2 from the air and therefore always contain some carbonate as an impurity. If this impurity is not removed different results are obtained in titration of equal volumes of a strong acid in presence of methyl orange and phenolphthalein respectively. Steps must therefore be taken to obtain alkali solutions free from the carbonate impurity. The simplest way is to add a small amount of $BaCl_2$ solution to the solution. The CO_3^{--} ions are then precipitated almost completely in the form of $BaCO_3$:

$$CO_3^{--} + Ba^{++} = \downarrow BaCO_3$$

Other methods (not considered here) are also available.

69. Titration of Salt Solutions

The neutralization method can be used for titration not only of acid and alkali solutions, but also of certain salts, such as Na_2CO_3 and $NaHCO_3$. Similarly, it might be possible to titrate NaH_2PO_4 with caustic soda as far as Na_2HPO_4 (in presence of phenolphthalein), and Na_2HPO_4 with hydrochloric acid as far as NaH_2PO_4 (in presence of methyl orange). However, it is far from always possible to titrate salt solutions, which are alkaline or acid because of hydrolysis, in this way. To understand the reasons for this let us consider the general aspects of titration of salt solutions.

It is easy to see that if a solution of a salt of the type NaA, formed from a strong base (NaOH) and a weak acid (HA), is titrated with a solution of a strong acid the solution pH must change exactly as it does in the titration of weak bases.

To show this, let us calculate and plot the titration curve for such a case.

At the start of the titration we have a solution of the salt NaA, the pH of which is found from the formula

$$\mathrm{pH} = 7 + \frac{1}{2}\,\mathrm{p}K_{\mathrm{HA}} + \frac{1}{2}\log C_{\mathrm{NaA}}$$

derived in Sec. 62.

At the intermediate stages of the titration the solution contains the free weak acid HA, formed by the reaction

$$\mathrm{NaA} + \mathrm{HCl} = \mathrm{HA} + \mathrm{NaCl}$$

together with residual unconverted salt NaA. The pH of such mixtures can be calculated from the formula (see Sec. 62):

$$\mathrm{pH} = \mathrm{p}K - \log\frac{C_{\mathrm{HA}}}{C_{\mathrm{NaA}}}$$

At the equivalence point all the salt taken is converted into the free acid HA, the pH of which can be calculated from the formula (see Sec. 62).

$$\mathrm{pH} = \frac{1}{2}\,\mathrm{p}K_{\mathrm{HA}} - \frac{1}{2}\log C_{\mathrm{HA}}$$

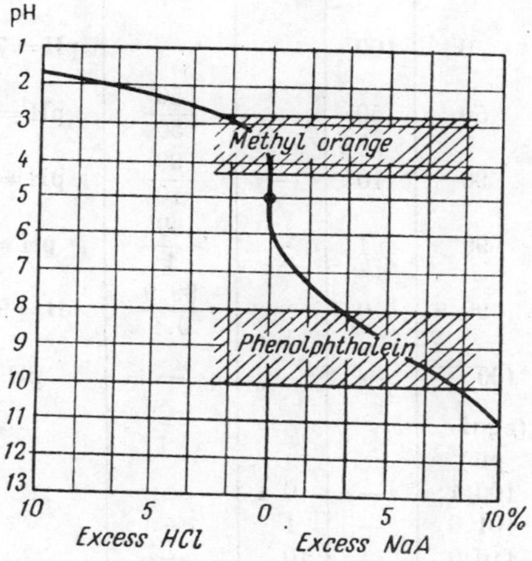

Finally, when the titrating acid is present in excess the solution pH is calculated in the usual way, from the total HCl concentration in solution.*

Fig. 53. Titration of a salt NaA of a weak acid HA ($K_{\mathrm{AH}} = 10^{-9}$) with 0.1 *N* HCl solution

Table XIV contains calculated data for a titration curve of a salt of the NaA type for the case when $K_{\mathrm{HA}} = 10^{-9}$, i.e., $\mathrm{p}K_{\mathrm{HA}} = 9$, and the curve itself is plotted in Fig. 53.

It is clear from an examination of this curve that it is quite similar to the titration curves of weak bases with strong acids. Indeed: (a) as in the titration of weak bases, the equivalence point here lies in the acid region (at pH = 5.0); (b) the pH changes sharply near the equivalence point (from pH = 6 to pH = 4) so that accurate titration is possible; (c) accordingly, this salt (like weak bases) can be titrated in presence of methyl orange and methyl red indicators, but not in presence of phenolphthalein.

---

* The presence of the free acid HA, the dissociation of which is slight and is, moreover, suppressed by the presence of the strong acid, has virtually no effect on the solution pH and may be disregarded.

Table XIV

Variations of pH in Titration of 100 ml of 0.1 *N* Solution of Salt NaA of a Weak Acid HA (p*K* = 9) with 0.1 *N* HCl Solution

HCl added, ml	Excess, ml		$\frac{C_{HA}}{C_{NaA}}$	Calculations	pH	pH in titration of weak base MeOH of pK=5*
	NaA	HCl				
0	100	—	—	$pH = 7 + \frac{9}{2} + 1/2 \log 0.1$	11.0	11.0
50	50	—	$\frac{50}{50}$	$pH = 9 - \log 50 + \log 50$	9.0	9.0
90	10	—	$\frac{90}{10}$	$pH = 9 - \log 90 + \log 10$	8.05	8.05
99	1	—	$\frac{99}{1}$	$pH = 9 - \log 99 + \log 1$	7.0	7.0
99.9	0.1	—	$\frac{99.9}{0.1}$	$pH = 9 - \log 99.9 + \log 0.1$	6.0	6.0
100 (equiv. pt.)	—	—	—	$pH = \frac{9}{2} - 1/2 \log 0.1$	5.0	5.0
100.1	—	0.1	—	$[H^+] = 10^{-4}$	4.0	4.0
101.0	—	1	—	$[H^+] = 10^{-3}$	3.0	3.0
110.0	—	10	—	$[H^+] = 10^{-2}$	2.0	2.0
200	—	100	—	$[H^+] = 10^{-1}$	1.0	1.0

* The values in this column were calculated as described on p. 255. Volume changes were disregarded in the calculations.

The last column of Table XIV, which gives the pH values for the corresponding points of the curve representing titration of a weak base MeOH of pK = 5 (i.e., 14—9) shows that the titration curves in the two cases are not merely analogous but identical.

Titration of a salt formed from a strong base and a weak acid of dissociation exponent pK *is the same thing as titration of a solution of a weak base of dissociation exponent 14*—pK, *of the same concentration*: the two titration curves are absolutely identical.

The identity of the titration curves is explained as follows. We know tha salts of weak acids (HA) and strong bases form alkaline solutions owing to hydrol ysis of the salts, the extent of which increases with increasing hydrolysis constant. Therefore, the pH of a solution of a salt of type NaA should be determined by the negative logarithm of the hydrolysis constant $K_{h.}$, just as the pH of a solution of a weak base is determined by pK of the base. However,

$$pK_{h.} = -\log K_{h.} = -\log \frac{10^{-14}}{K_{HA}} = 14 - pK_{HA} \quad (1)$$

Because of the above-mentioned role of the value of pK_h and by virtue of the relationship (1) between this value and pK_{HA} of the weak acid HA formed by hydrolysis, if we replace pK_{base} in the formulas used for calculating the titration curves of weak bases by $14 - pK_{HA}$ we obtain formulas which are used for calculating the titration curves of salts of the NaA type with strong acids. For example, if in the formula

$$pH = 14 - \frac{1}{2}\,pK_{base} + \frac{1}{2}\log C_{base} \quad (2)$$

we perform this replacement and also replace C_{base} by C_{salt}, we obtain the formula

$$pH = 7 + \frac{1}{2}\,pK_{HA} + \frac{1}{2}\log C_{salt} \quad (3)$$

These formulas are used for calculation of the initial points on the titration curves of a weak base (2) and a salt NaA (3) with a strong acid. These points should therefore coincide. It is easy to show that the same applies to all other points on both titration curves.

The following important conclusion follows from the identity of the titration curves: *titration of a salt of a weak acid, of the* NaA *type, with strong acids is possible only if the weak acid* HA *has a fairly low dissociation constant* (i.e., fairly high pK). In fact, it was stated earlier that if $pK_{HA} = 9$, i.e., $K_{HA} = 10^{-9}$, the corresponding salt can be accurately titrated like a base of $pK = 5$.

However, if $pK_{HA} = 5$, the titration curve with a strong acid for such a salt would be identical to the titration curve of a base of $pK = 9$, i.e., $K = 10^{-9}$. On titration curves of such weak bases there is no sharp pH change, and therefore they cannot be accurately titrated (p. 263).

For example, salts such as CH_3COONa or HCOONa, etc., cannot be titrated, because the dissociation constants of the corresponding acids (acetic, formic) are relatively large (1.8×10^{-5} and 2×10^{-4}). On the other hand, salts such as KCN ($K_{HCN} = 7 \times 10^{-10}$ and $pK = 9.15$) can be titrated with strong acids.*

The same is true of salts of di- and polybasic acids. For example, salts such as Na_2CO_3 or $Na_2B_4O_7$, being salts of very weak acids, can be effectively titrated with strong acids. On the other hand, salts such as $Na_2C_2O_4$ and $Na_2C_4H_4O_6$, derived from the much stronger oxalic and tartaric acids, cannot be titrated with acids.

* It was noted earlier that only weak acids and bases with $pK \geqslant 7$ can be titrated to a precision of 0.1%. Evidently salts of weak acids can be titrated with the same precision only provided that the pK of the corresponding acid is equal to or greater than 7.

It should be noted, however, that even such salts as CH_3COONa, etc., can be titrated if they are dissolved in alcohol (C_2H_5OH) or acetone (CH_3COCH_3), as in these solvents the acids formed by the reactions dissociate much less than in water (i.e., have much lower dissociation constants than in aqueous solutions). Nearly all salts of organic acids can be titrated in a mixture consisting of 70% alcohol or acetone and 30% water.

Exactly analogous considerations apply in the titration of salts of weak bases and strong acids. For example, titration of a solution of NH_4Cl with NaOH solution is equivalent to titration of a weak acid HA with $pK_{HA} = 14 - pK_{NH_4OH} = 14 - 4.75 = 9.25$.

This value of pK_{HA} corresponds to dissociation constant $K_{HA} = 10^{-9.25} = 5.6 \times 10^{-10}$, and with this value of K there is no pH break on the titration curve. Therefore, an NH_4Cl solution cannot be titrated directly with NaOH in presence of any indicator. However, this salt can be determined volumetrically by indirect methods. One such method is as follows. A solution of NH_4Cl is heated with an exactly measured volume of standard NaOH solution taken in known excess. The heating is continued until the ammonia formed in the reaction

$$NH_4Cl + NaOH = NaCl + H_2O + NH_3 \uparrow$$

is completely removed.

The residual NaOH is titrated with HCl solution. The amounts of NaOH taken initially, remaining unchanged, and neutralized by the HCl are known; the number of millilitres of NaOH solution used in the reaction with NH_4Cl is found by difference. From this the amount of salt can be easily calculated (Sec. 77).

This procedure, known as *back-titration* (or residual titration) is very often used in volumetric analysis and extends its range considerably. In particular, it is used for determinations of various salts by the neutralization method. For example, in order to determine a calcium salt in a given solution, we can add to it a known excess of standard Na_2CO_3 solution and then titrate the residual Na_2CO_3 with HCl solution in presence of phenolphthalein. The amount of Na_2CO_3 required for the reaction with Ca^{++} is found from the difference between the total amount taken and the amount neutralized by HCl. From this it is easy to calculate the amount of the original salt.

Back-titration is a method of great practical importance. For example, it is used for determinations of the permanent hardness of water (see Sec. 74), phosphorus in fertilizers and ferrous alloys, tungsten and chromium in ferrous alloys, nitrogen in organic substances, etc.

Calculation methods in back-titration will be considered in detail later.

70. Effects of Various Factors on Indicator Changes

In conclusion, let us consider the effects of various factors on indicator changes.

One such factor is temperature. It is known that the dissociation constants of electrolytes vary with temperature. The colour range of an indicator depends on K. Therefore, the range of an indicator should also change with temperature. Table XV compares the ranges of the most usual indicators at 18 and 100°C.

Table XV

Effect of Temperature on Indicator Range

Indicator	pH range		Indicator	pH range	
	at 18°C	at 100°C		at 18°C	at 100°C
Methyl orange	3.1-3.4	2.5-3.7	Phenolphthalein	8-10	8.1-9.0
Methyl red	4.2-6.3	4.0-6.0	Thymolphthalein	9.3-10.5	8.7-9.5
Phenol red	6.8-8.4	7.3-8.3	Nitramine	11.0- -12.5	9.0-10.5

In addition, the colour intensity and sharpness of the colour change may also alter with temperature, and as a result some indicators may become quite unsuitable.

Another factor is the presence of non-electrolytes such as alcohol, acetone, etc., in solution; these may sometimes take part in titration as solvents. Being non-ionizing (or weakly ionizing) solvents, such substances depress the dissociation of the acids and bases which are being titrated and weaken their influence on indicators. Of course, the indicator ranges also alter.

The presence of proteins, colloids, and neutral salts in solution also generally influences indicator ranges. Although only indicators which give small "protein" and "salt" errors are used in titrations, nevertheless at high protein or salt concentrations in solution these errors may become considerable.

In order to exclude the effects of all these factors on the final analytical result, whenever a titration has to be carried out with heating or in presence of non-electrolytes, large amounts of salts, etc., *the solution used must always be standardized under the same conditions.* This is, in general, one of the most important rules in volumetric analysis.

Let us now consider the very important question of the amount of indicator which should be added in titration. Beginners often take too much, thinking that the more indicator is taken the easier it is to detect the colour change. In reality the reverse is true. Although the colour of the solution is brighter if more indicator is used, the colour change is more difficult to detect, because it occurs more gradually. To understand the cause of this, let us consider as an example the colour change of any indicator when OH^- ions are introduced into a solution containing it. We know that this change is caused by conversion of molecules of one tautomeric form of the indicator ($HInd^0$) into another (HInd) and then into (Ind^-) anions as follows:

$$HInd^0 \rightleftarrows HInd \rightleftarrows H^+ + Ind^-$$

If a small amount of indicator is taken then the concentration of $HInd^0$ molecules in solution is low. Therefore, when only a single drop of alkali is added they are nearly all converted into Ind^- anions and the colour change is sharp. With a large amount of indicator evidently a correspondingly larger amount of alkali is needed to produce an equally strong colour change. This is what occurs in titration. Under given conditions the less indicator is taken the sharper is the colour change, and vice versa.

It follows from all this that *a large amount of indicator should not be used in titration*. It is nearly always sufficient to add 1-2 drops per 25 ml of solution to be titrated.*

The degree of precision with which the equivalence point is determined depends not only on the nature and the amount of indicator but also on the *titration sequence*. Suppose, for example, that alkali is being added from a burette to an acid. In this case in presence of methyl orange indicator the end point should be accompanied by a change of colour from pink to yellow on addition of one drop of alkali. This colour change is usually difficult to detect and cannot be determined very accurately. It is much easier to detect the reverse change, from yellow to pink. Therefore, titrations in presence of methyl orange are usually performed by addition of acid to alkali.

In presence of phenolphthalein, when alkali is added to acid an easily detectable colour change takes place (from colourless to pink). However, the reverse change can also be observed quite accurately Therefore, in this case the titration sequence is not so important as with methyl orange.

It should be noted that different titration sequences involve titration to different shades of colour and therefore to different pH values. For example, in titrations of alkali with acid in presence of

* In titrations in presence of indicators such as phenolphthalein, which are very sensitive to weak acids, a larger amount (8-10 drops) of indicator is sometimes taken in order to decrease the effect of absorption of CO_2 from the air by the solution.

methyl orange the end point is at pH =4.0. If acid is titrated with alkali (i.e., if the solution becomes yellow at the end point), the end point is at pH = 4.4. Similarly, in titrations in presence of phenolphthalein the end point is at pH = 9 when acid is titrated with alkali (to a faint pink colour), and at pH = 8 (until colourless) when alkali is titrated with acid. If the break on the titration curve is fairly sharp and both pH values are within its limits this is of no practical significance; otherwise it may be very important.

In order to detect the colour change at the end point more easily, especially with methyl orange, the following procedure is convenient. Distilled water of roughly the same volume as the solution at the end of the titration is put in a beaker or flask. The same number of drops of methyl orange as are taken in the titration is added, followed by 1-2 drops of acid from the burette, so that a weak but distinct pink colour appears. The colour of the titrated solution should then be taken to the same shade.

In this way it is possible not only to determine the end point more reliably and accurately, but also to apply a correction for the amount of excess acid required to produce an appreciable colour change in titrations with methyl orange.

For example, if 24.30 ml of HCl solution is taken for titration of an alkali solution, and 2 drops of acid were used in preparation of the comparison solution, it follows that the amount taken in the titration was 2 drops more than is required to neutralize the alkali. If the volume of a single drop is, say, 0.03 ml* then the actual amount of acid taken for neutralization is 24.30 — 0.06 = 24.24 ml.

It is obvious, of course, that such corrections should be applied if the determination and the standardization of the solution used were carried out under different conditions. If the conditions were the same, then the errors in both cases are equal and compensate each other, so that the result is not affected.

Sometimes, in addition to (or instead of) such a comparison solution another one is used, without acid and therefore of pure yellow colour. If both these comparison solutions are placed by the side of the titrated solution and the colours are compared continuously, the end point can be detected even more accurately.

The so-called *mixed indicators* are used in order to obtain sharper colour changes and to coordinate them with narrower ranges of pH. They are usually mixtures of indicators with indifferent dyes. The colour of the dye should be complementary to the colour of the indicator at the pH equal to the titration exponent of the indicator. It follows that when this pH is reached the solution becomes colourless.

---

* The drop volume depends on the diameter of the burette orifice and must be measured. To do this, 50 or 100 drops of liquid are discharged from the burette, the volume is read off, and divided by the number of drops.

Sometimes suitable mixtures of two different indicators are used for this purpose.

Let us consider the indicator consisting of a solution of 1 g of methyl orange and 2.5 g of indigo carmine per litre of water. Indigo carmine is a blue dye the colour of which does not change during titra-

Table XVI

Mixed Indicators

Composition of indicator solution	A : B *	Colour: Acid form	Colour: Basic form	pT	Notes
A. Methyl orange (0.1% in water) B. Indigo carmine (0.25% in water)	1 : 1	Violet	Green	4.1	Very convenient for titrations by artificial light
A. Bromcresol blue (0.2% in alcohol) B. Methyl red (0.2% in alcohol)	3 : 1	Red	Green	5.1	Very sharp colour change
A. Neutral red (0.1% in water) B. Methylene blue (0.1% in water)	1 : 1	Blue-violet	Green	7.0	Should be kept in a dark bottle
A. Phenolphthalein (0.1% in 50% alcohol) B. α-Naphtholphthalein (0.1% in 50% alcohol)	3 : 1	Pale pink	Violet	8.9	Pale green at pH = 8.6
A. Thymol blue (0.1% in 30% alcohol) B. Phenolphthalein (0.1% in 50% alcohol)	1 : 3	Yellow	Violet	9.0	Green at pH = 9.0

* Volume proportions in which solutions A and B are mixed before use.

tion. Therefore, its colour is merely added optically to the colours given by the methyl orange.

In alkaline solution (more accurately, at pH $\geqslant$ 4.4) this indicator is green (combination of yellow and blue) In acid solution (at pH $\leqslant$ 3.1) it should be violet (combination of pink and blue). At the pH corresponding to the pT of the indicator (i.e., 4) the colour components are pinkish orange and blue, which are complementary colours, and the solution is therefore pale grey, almost colourless. The instant when the green or violet solution becomes colourless in presence of this mixed indicator is much easier to detect than the appearance of the intermediate pinkish orange colour of methyl orange itself.

Many mixed indicators are now available. Some of them are detailed in Table XVI.

Mixed indicators can be used for detecting pH changes of the order of 0.1-0.15. Such indicators are therefore very convenient if the pH change on the titration curve is not large. Sometimes titration is even possible with these indicators when there is no sharp pH change at all. For example, it has been found that a solution of NH_4OH can be titrated with acetic acid in presence of a mixed indicator consisting of neutral red and methylene blue (Table XVI). It is known (p. 263) that this titration is impossible in presence of single indicators.

QUESTIONS AND PROBLEMS.
(on Secs. 58-70)

1. What are the pH values of solutions containing: (a) 2×10^{-4} g-ion H^+ per litre; (b) 0.008 g-ion OH^- per litre?

Answer: (a) 3.7; (b) 11.9.

2. Two solutions have pH values of: (a) 2.63; (b) 12.45. What are the H^+ and OH^- ion concentrations in these solutions?

Answer:

$$[H^+] = 2.34 \times 10^{-3}; \quad [OH^-] = 4.27 \times 10^{-12}$$
$$[H^+] = 3.54 \times 10^{-13}; \quad [OH^-] = 2.82 \times 10^{-2}$$

3. What are the pH values of: (a) 0.015 *N* HCl; (b) 0.005 *N* KOH?

Answer: (a) 1.82; (b) 11.70.

4. What are the degree of dissociation of 0.1 *N* acetic acid solution and the dissociation constant of acetic acid if the pH of the 0.1 *N* solution is 2.87?

Answer: $\alpha = 1.35\%$; $K = 1.82 \times 10^{-5}$

5. Calculate the pH of 0.01 *N* formic acid solution, given that $K_{HCOOH} = 2 \times 10^{-4}$.

Answer: pH = 2.85.

6. Calculate the pH of 0.01 *N* NH_4OH solution, given that $K_{NH_4OH} = 1.8 \times 10^{-5}$.

Answer: pH = 10.63

7. Calculate the pH of a mixture containing 0.01 *M* CH_3COOH and 0.1 *M* CH_3COONa.

Answer: pH = 5.73.

8. Calculate the pH of a mixture containing 0.2 *M* NH_4OH and 0.02 *M* NH_4Cl.

Answer: pH = 10.25.

9. Calculate the hydrolysis constant and pH of 0.01 *N* NH_4Cl solution at 22° C.

Answer: $K_{h.} = 5.6 \times 10^{-10}$; pH = 5.63.

10. Calculate the pH of buffer mixtures containing: (a) 0.01 *M* CH_3COOH and 0.01 *M* CH_3COOK; (b) 0.01 *M* CH_3COOH and 0.05 *M* CH_3COOK; (c) 0.5 *M* CH_3COOH and 0.01 *M* CH_3COOK.

Answer: (a) 4.73; (b) 5.43; (c) 3.03.

11. A solution contains NaOH in 10^{-5} *N* concentration. How is its pH changed by addition of 0.001 mole of (a) NaOH; (b) HCl to 1 litre of the solution?

Answer: (a) increased by ~ 2; (b) decreased by ~ 6.

12. A solution contains 0.056 *M* NH_4OH and 0.1 *M* NH_4Cl. Calculate its pH and find how this value is changed by addition of 0.001 mole of (a) NaOH; (b) HCl to 1 litre of the solution. (Compare the answer with the preceding problem.).

Answer: pH = 9.00; (a) increased by 0.01; (b) decreased by 0.01.

13. Calculate the concentration ratio [HCOOH]: [HCOONa] required to give a solution of pH = 2, given that $K_{HCOOH} = 2 \times 10^{-4}$.

Answer: 50 : 1.

14. In what cases is the equivalence point at pH = 7; at pH > 7; at pH < < 7?

15. The indicator bromthymol blue is a weak acid; it is yellow in strongly acid and blue in strongly alkaline solutions. Explain the change of colour with pH in the light of the ionic theory of indicators.

16. Briefly state the chromophore theory of indicators. What are chromophores and auxochromes?

17. Write the structural formulas of both tautomeric forms of the indicator paranitrophenol. Explain the mechanism of its colour change on the basis of the ionic chromophore theory of indicators.

18. The indicator alizarin yellow is an acid of apparent dissociation constant $K = 10^{-11}$. Its acid and alkaline forms are yellow and blue respectively. Explain how the range of this indicator arises and find its position on the pH scale.

19. Taking the preceding answer into account, state the colour of alizarin yellow at the following pH values: 2; 7; 10; 11; 12; 14. In which of these cases are the colours exactly the same in appearance?

20. The pH values of two solutions are 8.5 and 11.0 respectively. Will they give different colours with litmus (pH range 5-8) and with phenolphthalein (pH range 8-10)?

21. The dissociation constant (apparent) of bromthymol blue is 1.6×10^{-7}. The presence of one of the coloured forms of this indicator can no longer be detected when its concentration becomes 1/6 of the concentration of the other. Calculate the range of this indicator.

Answer: Approximately 6.0-7.6.

22. What is the titration exponent of an indicator? Give the titration exponents of four of the most important indicators. What (approximately) are the titration exponents of bromthymol blue (Problem 21) and alizarin yellow (Problem 18)?

23. Describe how, without calculation, it is possible to decide approximately which indicator is the most suitable for a given titration. Explain why a qualitative approach to this problem is not sufficient.

24. 30 ml of 0.1 *N* NaOH solution is added to 20 ml of 0.1 *N* HCl. Find the pH of the resultant solution.*

Answer: pH = 12.30.

25. To 25 ml of 0.1 *N* HCl solution is added (a) 24.95 ml; (b) 25.05 ml of 0.1 *N* NaOH solution. Find the pH of the resultant solution in each case.

Answer: (a) 4; (b) 10.

26. Calculate and plot the titration curve for titration of 0.02 *N* KOH with 0.02 *N* HNO_3 (disregarding volume changes). What is the pT range of indicators suitable for this titration? Which of the four most common indicators can be used in this case?

Answer: From pT = 4.7 to pT = 9.3.

27. Calculate and plot the titration curve for titration of 0.1 *N* formic acid (HCOOH) with 0.1 *N* KOH. Which of the usual indicators are suitable in this case? Can the indicators bromphenol blue (pH range 3.0-4.6) or neutral red (pH range 6.8-8.0) be used?

28. 24 ml of 0.2 *N* NaOH is added to 25 ml of 0.2 *N* CH_3COOH. What is the pH of the resultant solution?

Answer: pH = 6.11.

29. 25.1 ml of 0.2 *N* NaOH is added to 25 ml of 0.2 *N* CH_3COOH. Calculate the pH of the resultant solution (taking the volume change into account).

Answer: 10.6.

30. Find (disregarding volume changes) the region of pH break and the equivalence point on the titration curve of 0.5 *N* NH_4OH with 0.5 *N* HNO_3. Which of the usual indicators may be used?

Answer: Region of pH break from 6.25 to 3.30; equivalence point 4.78.

31. What is the pH at the equivalence point in titration of 0.1 *N* NH_4OH with 0.1 *N* HCOOH?

Answer: pH = 6.50.

32. What is the indicator error in titration? List the types of such errors.

33. What are the indicator errors in the following titrations: (a) 0.1 *N* HCl with 0.1 *N* NaOH in the presence of methyl red (pT = 5.5); (b) 0.1 *N* NaOH with 0.1 *N* HCl in presence of nitramine (pT $\approx$ 12)?

Answer: (a) —0.0064%; (b) +20%.

34. What are the indicator errors in the following titrations: (a) 0.1 *N* HCOOH with 0.1 *N* NaOH in the presence of thymolphthalein (pT = 10); (b) 0.1 *N* NH_4OH with 0.1 *N* HNO_3 in the presence of methyl red (pT = 5.5)?

Answer: (a) +0.2%; (b) —0.018%.

---

* Take the volume change into account.

35. Calculate the indicator error in titration of 0.1 *N* NaOH with 0.1 *N* HCOOH in the presence of neutral red (pT = 7).

Answer: −0.056%.

36. The dissociation constants of a tribasic acid H_3A are: $K_1 = 1 \times 10^{-2}$, $K_2 = 1 \times 10^{-6}$, and $K_3 = 1 \times 10^{-12}$. Calculate the pH values at the first and second equivalence points in titration of this acid with a strong alkali (NaOH). What indicators should be used in titration of this acid to the mono- and disubstituted salt? Is direct titration as far as the neutral salt possible? What is the pH at the third equivalence point (with $C_{salt} = 0.1$ *M*)?

Answer: The pH values at the equivalence points are: $pH_I = 4.0$; $pH_{II} = 9.0$; $pH_{III} = 12.5$.

37. How are K_2CO_3 and $KHCO_3$ titrated in the presence of methyl orange and phenolphthalein respectively? How can the carbonate and bicarbonate contents be determined if they are present simultaneously?

38. Explain why carbonate should be removed in the preparation of a standard alkali solution. Is this necessary if only strong acids are to be titrated with the alkali solution?

39. What factors influence indicator ranges? How can their influence on analytical results be excluded?

40. Why is it wrong to take too much indicator in a titration?

41. What is the significance of a particular titration sequence? What are comparison solutions and how are they used?

42. How are mixed indicators prepared? What are their advantages?

43. Calculate and plot the curve for titration of 0.1 *N* KCN with 0.1 *N* HCl. What indicators can be used in this titration?

44. The dissociation constant of a base MeOH is 1×10^{-10}. Calculate and plot the curve for titration of its salt MeCl with 0.1 *N* NaOH solution and compare this curve with the titration curve of a 0.1 *N* solution of a weak acid HA with a dissociation constant of 1×10^{-4}. What indicators can be used for this titration?

45. In what cases can salts of (a) weak acids, (b) weak bases be titrated with sufficient accuracy?

46. How should CH_3COOK be titrated with H_2SO_4 solution to give accurate results?

47. How should boric acid be titrated with caustic alkali to give sufficiently accurate results?

48. What are the pT ranges of indicators used in the neutralization method? Explain this.

CHAPTER VI

EXAMPLES OF DETERMINATIONS BY THE NEUTRALIZATION METHOD

71. Preparation of Standard HCl Solution

Laboratory solutions of HCl are usually standardized (see Sec. 58) against borax or sodium carbonate. Borax is the more convenient, as it is easily obtained in a chemically pure state, corresponding to the formula $Na_2B_4O_7 \cdot 10H_2O$, by recrystallization at 60°C. It satisfies the other requirements for primary standards: it is quite stable and it has a high gram-equivalent (190.7 g). In contrast, sodium carbonate is more difficult to purify and its gram-equivalent is considerably smaller (52.99 g). Moreover, anhydrous Na_2CO_3 is hygroscopic, so that it must be heated before use to remove water. We shall therefore use borax as the primary standard.

When dissolved in water, borax undergoes hydrolysis:

$$Na_2B_4O_7 + 7H_2O \rightleftarrows 2NaOH + 4H_3BO_3$$

The resultant orthoboric acid is one of the weakest acids while NaOH is a strong base; the solution is therefore strongly alkaline and (as was explained in Sec. 70) can be titrated with acids. We can easily derive the reaction equation by assuming that the alkali formed by hydrolysis is consumed in the reaction with HCl:

$$2NaOH + 2HCl = 2NaCl + 2H_2O$$

Adding the two equations, we obtain the aggregate equation for the reaction:

$$Na_2B_4O_7 + 2HCl + 5H_2O = 2NaCl + 4H_3BO_3$$

This equation shows that the solution at the equivalence point contains a mixture of NaCl with free boric acid, H_3BO_3. The solution pH is evidently determined by the presence of H_3BO_3. Disregarding the volume change in titration, and taking pK of boric acid as 9.24, we have:

$$pH = {}^1/_2\, pK_{acid} + {}^1/_2 \log C_{acid} \doteq \frac{9.24}{2} + 0.5 = 5.1$$

Therefore, the most suitable indicator for the titration is methyl red with pT = 5.5. Borax can also be titrated in presence of methyl orange, as its titration exponent (pT = 4), is not outside the limits of the break on the titration curve (pT = 4.0-6.2). On the other hand, phenolphthalein (pT = 9) or litmus (pT = 7) cannot be used.

Preparation of Borax Solution. Use a 250 ml or 200 ml measuring flask for preparation of a standard borax solution.

First calculate how much borax should be taken. A gram-molecule (381.4 g) of $Na_2B_4O_7 \cdot 10H_2O$ reacts with two gram-molecules of HCl, i.e., with two gram-ions of hydrogen. Its gram-equivalent is therefore $\frac{381.4}{2} = 190.7$ g. Therefore, 19.07 g is required for 1 litre of 0.1 *N* solution, and $\frac{19.07}{4} = 4.7875$ g for 250 ml.

It is not necessary to weigh out exactly the calculated amount—this is of no advantage, and takes longer. Weigh out 4-5 g of borax on a technical balance, put it in a weighing bottle (or on a watch glass), and weigh the bottle with the borax accurately on an analytical balance. Then tip the borax out carefully through a *dry* funnel* into a thoroughly washed measuring flask. Then weigh the bottle with any remaining grains of borax accurately again and by difference find the weight of borax transferred to the flask. Wash all the borax carefully out of the funnel into the flask in a stream of hot water (borax is not readily soluble in cold water) from a wash bottle.

Add more hot water to the flask until it is two-thirds full, remove the funnel, and smoothly swirl the contents of the flask until all the borax dissolves. Then cool the solution to room temperature and make up to the mark with distilled water. At the end add the water drop by drop, keeping the eye level with the mark until the bottom of the meniscus touches the mark. Then cork the flask and mix the contents thoroughly by repeatedly inverting and shaking the flask. Now calculate the titre and normality of the borax solution. To find the titre, divide the weight of borax taken by the volume of the solution.**

For example, if 4.6812 g of borax was taken, then

$$T = \frac{4.6812}{250.0} = 0.01873 \text{ g/ml}$$

* The substance sticks to a wet funnel and clogs its tube. It is best to use special funnels for powders, with wide and short tubes (or ordinary funnels with cut-off tubes).

** Of course, if in the calibration of the measuring flask (Sec. 53) it was found that its capacity was not exactly 250.0 ml, the actual volume found experimentally should be used in the calculation. The same applies to the volume of the pipette (see p. 202).

To convert the titre to normality, multiply it by 1,000 (to convert to litres) and divide by the gram-equivalent:

$$N = \frac{0.01873 \times 1{,}000}{190.7} = 0.09819$$

Preparation of HCl Solution. One litre of 0.1 N hydrochloric acid contains 3.646 g (in round numbers, 3.6 g) of HCl. First calculate the volume of concentrated hydrochloric acid (sp. gr. 1.19) which contains this amount of HCl. Use Appendix V, which gives a table of specific gravities of strong acids and alkalies, for the calculation. The table shows that hydrochloric acid of sp. gr. 1.19 contains approximately 38% HCl.

By proportion:

100 g of HCl solution contains 38 g HCl

x g of HCl solution contains 3.6 g HCl

$$x = \frac{100 \times 3.6}{38} = 9.6 \text{ g}$$

To convert this weight of acid to volume it must be divided by the specific gravity of the acid (1.19). We then have

$$V = \frac{9.6}{1.19} \approx 8.1 \text{ ml}$$

Measure out the calculated volume (8-9 ml) of concentrated HCl roughly in a small measuring cylinder and dilute it to 1 litre with distilled water with the aid of a large measuring cylinder. Mix the solution thoroughly.

Titration. Having prepared the solutions, start the titration. First read all that was said above concerning the use of burettes and pipettes for volume measurements (Sec. 53). Wash the burette thoroughly and finally rinse it out twice with small portions of the prepared HCl solution in order to remove remaining water. Then fill the burette almost to the top with the HCl solution, put a flask or beaker under it and open the tap slightly so as to fill the tip of the burette without leaving any air bubbles in it.

Now take a clean conical flask and a thoroughly washed pipette; rinse the pipette out twice with the standard borax solution and then transfer 25.00 ml of this solution into the conical flask.

In using the pipette, obey the rule given on p. 198: *do not blow out* the last drop remaining in the pipette but remove it, if possible, by touching the side of the flask with the tip.

Having measured out the borax solution, add one or, at most, two drops of methyl orange solution.

Prepare a comparison solution in a similar flask. For this, measure out 50 ml of distilled water with a measuring cylinder, add 1-2 drops of methyl orange and then one drop of acid from the burette so that the liquid turns slightly pink.* Then adjust the level of the HCl solution in the burette to the zero mark.

Place the flask with borax solution on a sheet of white paper under the burette and gradually add HCl from the burette, continuously agitating the liquid by a smooth circular movement of the flask. It is necessary to detect the point at which addition of *one drop of hydrochloric acid* changes the original pure yellow colour of the solution to slightly pinkish, exactly the same as that of the comparison solution.

It is difficult to detect this point exactly in the first titration. Therefore, first determine the volume of acid needed approximately, say to the nearest 1 ml. For example, suppose that in the first titration it was found that with 23.00 ml HCl the solution was still yellow, and with 24.00 ml it was bright pink. In this case, in repeating the titration with a fresh portion of borax solution, it is safe to add 23.00 ml of acid.** Beyond this add the HCl solution drop by drop.

If you are in doubt whether the colour of the solution has changed, take the burette reading (see below) and then add another drop of HCl solution. If a colour change had taken place, the added drop is too much and makes the solution very distinctly pink. Of course, this excess drop must be disregarded.

Having obtained a colour change by the addition of one drop of hydrochloric acid, read the burette and write down the reading.

If the bottom of the meniscus is not exactly on a scale division, try to estimate hundredths of a millilitre by eye.

In every reading care must be taken to have the eye level with the meniscus.

The precise titration must be performed at least three times, with a fresh portion of solution each time and with the acid level in the burette adjusted to zero. With accurate work the differences between the readings amount to only a few hundredths of a millilitre. In any case, they should not exceed 0.1 ml. If the deviations are larger, repeat the titrations until you have three concordant results and take the average. *All readings must be recorded in the laboratory log-book*, even if they are the same.

---

* It is also possible to prepare the comparison solution without HCl. This has a pure yellow colour, which readily shows colour changes of the titrated solution by comparison. It is better still to have both comparison solutions.

** Of course, before a fresh portion of borax is pipetted out the liquid must be poured out of the flask and the flask itself must be rinsed out thoroughly first with tap and then with distilled water. The acid level in the burette must again be adjusted to zero.

Calculating the Tirte of Hydrochloric Acid Solution. Consider the following example. Suppose that 23.40; 23.20; 23.28; and 23.20 ml of HCl solution was taken in four titrations of 25.00 ml lots of borax solution of normality 0.09504. Rejecting the very high reading (23.40), we find the average:

$$V_{HCl} = \frac{23.20 + 23.28 + 23.20}{3} = 23.23 \text{ ml}$$

where V_{HCl} is the average of the readings.

Denoting the normality of the HCl solution by N and using the rule derived above (p. 211), according to which the products of the volumes and normalities of the reacting solutions are equal, we can write:

$$23.23 \times N = 25.00 \times 0.09504$$

and hence

$$N = \frac{25.00 \times 0.09504}{23.23} = 0.1023$$

The value of N so found completely characterizes the concentration of the HCl solution and is sufficient for analytical calculations. Therefore, no other calculations are needed at this stage. If the titre of the HCl solution is also required, the normality must be multiplied by the gram-equivalent of HCl (36.46 g) and divided by 1,000:

$$T_{HCl} = \frac{0.1023 \times 36.46}{1{,}000} = 0.003729 \text{ g/ml}$$

All these calculations should be done with the aid of four-figure logarithms and antilogarithms to the same precision as the analysis itself (to four significant figures). On the other hand, the calculations of the weight of borax to be taken and of the volume of concentrated HCl used for preparing the solution are approximate and the quantities involved in them should be rounded off.

72. Determination of Alkali in a Solution

When a standard HCl solution has been prepared it can be used for determining the contents of various alkalies in solutions. For such a determination, put the solution of alkali in a measuring flask, dilute it with distilled water exactly to the mark, mix thoroughly, and titrate several separate portions (25.00 ml each) with the standard HCl in presence of methyl orange, proceeding exactly as in the standardization of the HCl.*

* In taking the portions of solution for titration remember to rinse out the pipette with the alkali solution to be titrated.

Take the average of three concordant results (agreeing to within 0.1 ml) and calculate the normality and titre of the unknown solution and the total amount of alkali in the measuring flask.*

The contents of such salts as Na_2CO_3, K_2CO_3, and $Na_2B_4O_7$, solutions of which are distinctly alkaline and can be titrated in presence of methyl orange (Sec. 69), in solutions can be determined in exactly the same manner. The only difference is that the gram-equivalent of the particular salt must be used in calculations of the titre.

73. Determination of NaOH and Na_2CO_3 in the Same Solution

It is known that alkalies absorb CO_2 from the air and are converted into carbonates:

$$2NaOH + CO_2 = Na_2CO_3 + H_2O$$

Therefore, a solution of caustic soda always contains some Na_2CO_3. In some cases it may be necessary to know the amounts of NaOH and Na_2CO_3 present in a solution. Therefore, as our second example of the determination of alkalies, we consider the determination of NaOH and Na_2CO_3 present in the same solution. There are two possible methods. One involves the determination of both equivalence points on the titration curve of Na_2CO_3 (Sec. 68); in the other method NaOH is determined after precipitation of CO_3^{--} ions by Ba^{++} ions.

Determination of Two Equivalence Points

It was shown in Sec. 68 that, because of the existence of two equivalence points on the titration curve of Na_2CO_3, titration of this salt in presence of phenolphthalein gives results different from those obtained by titration in presence of methyl orange. In presence of phenolphthalein the end point is the point at which all the Na_2CO_3 is converted into $NaHCO_3$:

$$Na_2CO_3 + HCl = NaHCO_3 + NaCl$$

When Na_2CO_3 is titrated in the presence of methyl orange the indicator turns pink only after all the salt has been converted into H_2CO_3:

$$Na_2CO_3 + 2HCl = H_2CO_3 + 2NaCl$$

Comparison of the two equations shows that when Na_2CO_3 is titrated in presence of phenolphthalein the amount of HCl required (1 molecule) is half the amount required in presence of methyl orange (2 molecules). Therefore, we can say that only half the Na_2CO_3

* The course of the calculations is described in detail in Sec. 56.

is titrated in presence of phenolphthalein, and all of it in presence of methyl orange. This is the principle of the determination.

Procedure. Put the mixture of NaOH and Na_2CO_3 in a 250 ml measuring flask, make up to the mark with distilled water* free from CO_2, and mix thoroughly. Pipette out 25.00 ml of this solution, and 8-10 drops of 0.1% phenolphthalein solution, and titrate with standard HCl solution until the colour disappears after addition of a single drop. Write down the burette reading.

Now add 1-2 drops of methyl orange to the titrated solution. The solution turns yellow. Continue the titration until the solution becomes a permanent pink and take the burette reading again. Repeat the precise titration once or twice more and take the average reading for each indicator.

Calculations. When the unknown solution is titrated in presence of phenolphthalein, all the NaOH and half the Na_2CO_3 are titrated. After addition of methyl orange the other half of the Na_2CO_3 is titrated (Fig. 54).

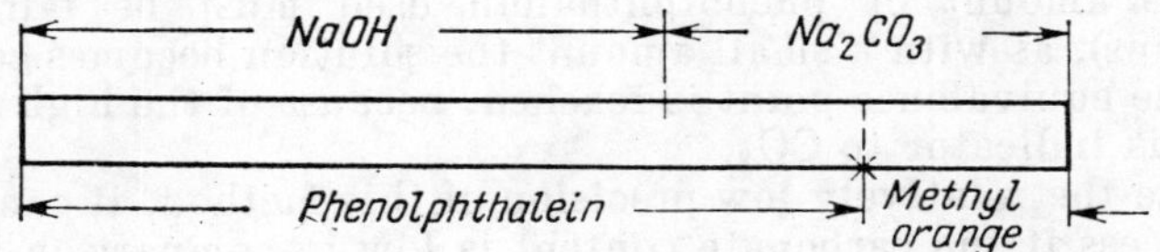

Fig. 54. Titration of a mixture of NaOH and Na_2CO_3 with HCl solution in presence of phenolphthalein and of methyl orange

Therefore, if the burette reading was 23.20 ml in the titration with phenolphthalein and 24.60 ml with methyl orange, the volume of HCl taken for titration of half the Na_2CO_3 was 24.60 — 23.20 = = 1.40 ml, and all of the Na_2CO_3 would take 2.80 ml. This means that the volume of HCl used for titration of the NaOH was 24.60 — — 2.80 = 21.80 ml.

Having thus found the volumes of HCl solution taken for neutralization of NaOH and Na_2CO_3 respectively, the normalities of the solution with respect to the two components are calculated in the usual way. Thus, the normality of the solution with respect to Na_2CO_3 is

$$N_{Na_2CO_3} = \frac{0.1023 \times 2.80}{25.00} = 0.01146$$

where 0.1023 is the normality of the HCl solution.

Hence the amount of Na_2CO_3 in 250 ml of solution is

$$Q_{Na_2CO_3} = 0.01146 \times 53.00 \times 0.25 = 0.1518 \text{ g}$$

* See footnote to p. 298.

The normality of the solution with respect to NaOH and the amount of NaOH in 250 ml of solution are found similarly.

It was stated in Sec. 68 that, since the ratio $K_1 : K_2$ of the dissociation constants of carbonic acid is less than 10^4, the pH break near the equivalence point, corresponding to formation of $NaHCO_3$, is not large enough. Therefore, the precision of this method is relatively low (not better than 1%). Another factor lowering the precision is absorption of CO_2 by the solution from the air (or water), so that part of the NaOH is converted into Na_2CO_3. Therefore the following precautions must be taken during the analysis:

(a) water free from CO_2* must be used for diluting the solution;

(b) the solution must be titrated immediately it has been measured out;

(c) at the end of the titration with phenolphthalein the acid must be added slowly to avoid formation of free H_2CO_3 instead of $NaHCO_3$;

(d) violent agitation of the solution must be avoided, as this helps absorption of CO_2 from the air;

(e) the amount of phenolphthalein used must be fairly large (8-10 drops), as with a small amount the solution becomes colourless before the equivalence point is reached, because of the high sensitivity of this indicator to CO_2.

Despite the relatively low precision of this method, it can be used with success if the carbonate content is low in comparison with the NaOH content.

Method Based on Precipitation of CO_3^{--} *Ions*

In this, more accurate, method two portions of the unknown solution are taken. One is titrated with HCl in the presence of methyl orange while $BaCl_2$ is first added to the other to precipitate CO_3^{--}. The $BaCO_3$ precipitate is not filtered off, and the solution is titrated in presence of phenolphthalein.** The first titration evidently gives the total volume (V_1) of hydrochloric acid required to neutralize the NaOH and Na_2CO_3 together, and the second gives the volume (V_2) required to neutralize the NaOH. The difference $(V_1 - V_2)$ is the volume of hydrochloric acid taken for neutralization of Na_2CO_3.

Procedure. Put the solution containing NaOH and Na_2CO_3 into a 250 ml measuring flask, dilute it to the mark with water free from CO_2, and mix thoroughly. Pipette out an aliquot portion***

* To remove CO_2, water is boiled and then cooled in a vessel protected from CO_2 by means of an absorption tube containing soda lime.

** If methyl orange is used as indicator instead of phenolphthalein, not only the NaOH but also the $BaCO_3$ reacts with the HCl, because in the presence of methyl orange the end point is in the acid range.

*** See p. 206.

(25.00 ml) of this solution, add 1-2 drops of methyl orange, and titrate with standard HCl solution. Repeat the precise titration 2-3 times and take the average reading.

Now pipette out 25.00 ml of the solution and add 8-10 ml of 1 *N* $BaCl_2$ solution and 8-10 drops of phenolphthalein. Without filtering off the precipitate ($BaCO_3$), titrate the solution with hydrochloric acid, stirring carefully, until the red colour has completely disappeared. Repeat the titration once or twice more and take the average of the concordant results.

Calculation. Suppose that in the titration with methyl orange an average of 24.42 ml of hydrochloric acid solution was used, and that 20.16 ml was taken in the titration with phenolphthalein (after precipitation of CO_3^{--} ions). The latter volume is the amount of HCl solution required to neutralize the NaOH. Therefore, the volume of HCl taken for neutralization of Na_2CO_3 was 24.42 — 20.16 = = 4.26 ml of HCl solution. Then, with the same reasoning as in the first method, we can calculate the amounts of NaOH and Na_2CO_3 in 250 ml of solution.

74. Determination of the Hardness of Water

The hardness of water depends on the presence of soluble calcium and magnesium salts.* A distinction is made between carbonate and permanent hardness in accordance with the nature of the salts present.

Carbonate hardness is due to the presence of calcium and magnesium bicarbonates, $Ca(HCO_3)_2$ and $Mg(HCO_3)_2$. When water containing these salts is boiled, they decompose with precipitation of the neutral salts and the hardness is removed; for example:

$$Ca(HCO_3)_2 = \downarrow CaCO_3 + H_2O + CO_2 \uparrow$$

Accordingly, carbonate hardness is also known as temporary hardness.** The precipitate formed when water is boiled is responsible for scale formation in boilers, kettles, etc.

Permanent hardness is due to the presence in the water of other soluble salts of calcium and magnesium (usually sulphates).

In contrast to carbonate hardness, permanent hardness cannot be removed by boiling. The sum of the permanent and carbonate hardness is the *total hardness* of water.

---

* In some cases hardness is also caused by the presence of iron salts.

** The terms "carbonate" and "temporary" hardness are not quite synonymous, because the decrease of hardness when water is boiled depends not only on decomposition of $Ca(HCO_3)_2$ and $Mg(HCO_3)_2$ but also on the decrease of $CaSO_4$ solubility with rise of temperature.

In the past, hardness was generally expressed in special units known as "degrees of hardness"*. This has now been replaced in the USSR by a standard whereby *the hardness is expressed in terms of the number of milligram-equivalents* (see p. 210) *of soluble calcium and magnesium salts per litre of water.*

Acidimetric determinations of carbonate and permanent hardness of water are considered separately below.

In addition to acidimetric methods for determination of water hardness, the complexometric method is now widely used; this is discussed in detail in Sec. 116.

Determination of Carbonate Hardness

A known volume of water is titrated with hydrochloric acid in presence of methyl orange, when the following reactions take place:

$$Ca(HCO_3)_2 + 2HCl = CaCl_2 + 2H_2O + 2CO_2 \uparrow$$

$$Mg(HCO_3)_2 + 2HCl = MgCl_2 + 2H_2O + 2CO_2 \uparrow$$

Procedure. Pipette out 100-200 ml of the water with a 50 or 100 ml pipette, add 2-3 drops of methyl orange, and titrate with standard HCl solution. Repeat the titration two or three times and take the average of the concordant results.

Calculation. Suppose that titration of 200 ml of water took, on the average, 10.13 ml of 0.1023 *N* HCl solution. This corresponds to $10.13 \times 5 = 50.65$ ml per litre of water. One litre of the HCl solution contains 0.1023 gram-equivalent of HCl, and 1 ml contains 0.1023 milligram-equivalent. Therefore, 0.1023×50.65 milligram-equivalents of HCl are required for titration of the $Ca(HCO_3)_2$ and $Mg(HCO_3)_2$ present in 1 litre of the water. This is therefore the total number of milligram-equivalents of these salts per litre of water.

The carbonate hardness of the water is therefore

$$x = 0.1023 \times 50.65 = 5.181 \text{ mg-eq/litre}$$

Determination of Permanent Hardness

This determination is based on precipitation of calcium and magnesium salts in the form of carbonates by the action of excess standard Na_2CO_3 solution. After separation of the precipitate the residual unchanged Na_2CO_3 is titrated with HCl solution in the presence

* The degree of hardness was the number of milligrams of CaO equivalent to the total amount of calcium and magnesium salts contained in 100 ml of water.

of methyl orange and the volume of Na_2CO_3 solution taken for precipitation of the calcium and magnesium salts is found by difference (the back-titration method; see p. 282). The hardness is easily calculated from the result.

After addition of Na_2CO_3 the solution is evaporated to dryness, when the acid salts $Ca(HCO_3)_2$ and $Mg(HCO_3)_2$ decompose completely to form insoluble carbonates. Therefore, this method gives not the total but only the permanent hardness of water.*

Procedure. Pipette out 100 ml of the water into a porcelain basin and add from a burette an exactly measured volume (10-25 ml) of approximately 0.1 *N* Na_2CO_3 solution. Evaporate the mixture to dryness on a water bath. Treat the dry residue with 15-20 ml of distilled water free from carbon dioxide** to extract residual (excess) Na_2CO_3.

Filter off the undissolved residue consisting of calcium and magnesium carbonate and wash the residue (and the basin) three or four times with the same water; collect the filtrate and washings in a conical flask for titration.

At the end of the washing add 1-2 drops of methyl orange to the solution and titrate it with hydrochloric acid.

Now determine the relationship between the equivalent volumes of Na_2CO_3 and HCl solutions. The simplest way to do this is to measure out with a burette into a flask the same volume of Na_2CO_3 solution as was used for the determination, and to titrate it (in duplicate or triplicate) with the HCl solution in the presence of 1-2 drops of methyl orange.

Calculation. Suppose that 20.00 ml of Na_2CO_3 solution was taken for the determination, and that the back-titration of the residual sodium carbonate after the reaction with calcium and magnesium salts took 16.48 ml of 0.1023 *N* HCl solution. Further, titration of 20.00 ml of the Na_2CO_3 solution took 19.16 ml of the standard HCl. It follows from these figures that the amount of calcium and magnesium salts, causing permanent hardness, in 100 ml of the water is equivalent to $19.16 - 16.48 = 2.68$ ml of 0.1023 *N* HCl solution. This corresponds to 26.8 ml of HCl solution per litre of water; hence, reasoning as before, we find the permanent hardness:

$$x = 0.1023 \times 26.8 = 2.7416 \text{ mg-eq/litre}$$

---

* If the water is first titrated with hydrochloric acid, so that bicarbonates are converted into chlorides, it is possible to determine total hardness by a method similar to that described here. Usually the total hardness is found as the sum of the carbonate and permanent hardness.

** Water containing CO_2 dissolves carbonates, for example:

$$CaCO_3 + H_2O + CO_2 = Ca(HCO_3)_2$$

See the footnote to p. 298 concerning the preparation of water free from CO_2.

75. Preparation of Standard NaOH Solution

So that we can determine the contents of various acids in solutions, we prepare another standard solution essential for the neutralization method, namely, a standard alkali solution such as NaOH.

Preparation of NaOH Solution. Caustic soda always contains an admixture of Na_2CO_3 owing to absorption of CO_2 from the air. We know (Sec. 68) that this is a very harmful impurity, because in its presence titration of the same acid solution in presence of methyl orange and of phenolphthalein gives different results.

The sodium carbonate must be removed*; the most convenient way to do this is to precipitate carbonate by addition of $BaCl_2$ solution:

$$Na_2CO_3 + BaCl_2 = \downarrow BaCO_3 + 2NaCl$$

To prepare the solution, put pieces of NaOH in a beaker and wash them 2-3 times with small portions of distilled water, pouring off the water each time and replacing it by a fresh portion. Most of the sodium carbonate on the surface of the NaOH dissolves. Now weigh out the required amount of NaOH as quickly as possible on a technical balance, transferring the washed pieces with forceps specially used for this purpose to a previously counterpoised watch glass or beaker (*not a piece of paper*). For preparation of a litre of 0.1 *N* solution 4 g NaOH should be weighed out. However, the NaOH contains water and Na_2CO_3, so that rather more, about 4.5 g, should be taken.

At the end of the weighing dissolve the NaOH in a litre of distilled water from a measuring cylinder.

To the solution add a few ml of 2 *N* $BaCl_2$ solution, allow the precipitate to settle thoroughly, check for complete precipitation,** and decant the clear liquid carefully by means of a siphon tube into another vessel.

Rather than adding $BaCl_2$ by guess, it is better to determine the Na_2CO_3 content of the prepared alkali solution (Sec. 73). Having found the normality of the Na_2CO_3 present, we can easily calculate the volume of 2 *N* $BaCl_2$ solution needed for the precipitation. Thus, if the normality of the Na_2CO_3 solution was found to be 0.01, we can write:

$$2 \times x = 1{,}000 \times 0.01$$

and hence $x = 5$ ml. As explained earlier, 1.5 times the calculated

* However, if it is proposed to use the solution exclusively for titrations in the presence of methyl orange (i.e., if weak acids are not to be determined), Na_2CO_3 does no harm and need not be removed.

** Add H_2SO_4 solution to 1-2 ml of the clear solution. If a precipitate (turbidity) of $BaSO_4$ is formed, this shows that there is an excess of Ba^{++} in the solution, which means that the CO_3^{--} ions have been completely precipitated.

amount of precipitant should be taken to ensure more complete precipitation.

The NaOH solution so prepared must be protected against absorption of CO_2 from the air. A special apparatus for titration, which can be easily assembled by the student himself, is shown in Fig. 55.

The necks of the bottle *1* and the burette *2* are plugged with bungs in which special absorption tubes with soda lime are inserted (Sec. 44). Soda lime absorbs CO_2 and prevents it from entering the NaOH solution.

When the tubes *3* are filled, the upper end of the narrow bottom tube is plugged with a piece of cotton wool, and the tube is then packed with pieces of soda lime (or Ascarite) the size of a pea. The soda lime is covered with a layer of cotton wool and a bung fitted with a narrow tube is inserted in the neck of the absorption tube.

To fill the burette, the clip *4* is opened and air is sucked by the mouth through the tube *5*. After the burette has been filled the clip is closed and the burette is then used in the ordinary way. A more complicated apparatus for titration with alkali solutions, generally used in laboratories, is shown in Fig. 31*a*.

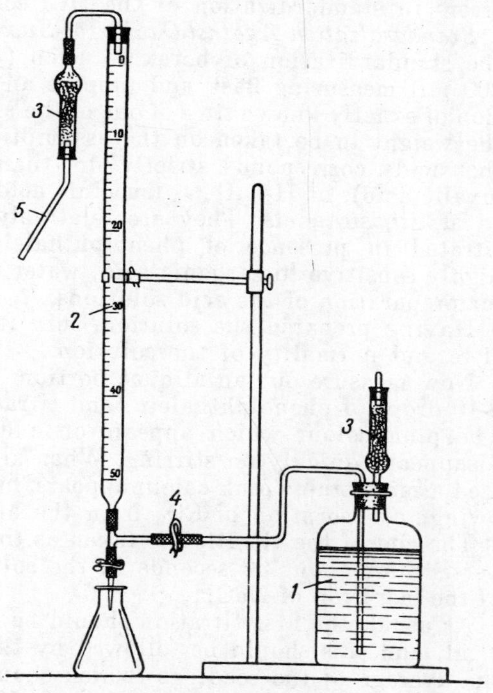

Fig. 55. Apparatus for titration with caustic alkalies:

1—bottle; *2*—burette; *3* — absorption tube; *4*—clip; *5*—glass tube

Standardization. The NaOH solution can be standardized either against a standard HCl solution or against a solution of a primary standard such as oxalic acid.

Standardization of NaOH *Solution Against* HCl. Measure out exactly 25.00 ml of the NaOH solution from the burette, add 1-2 drops of methyl orange, and titrate the solution in the usual way with standard HCl solution until one drop of the acid gives a pink colour.

Repeat the precise titration 2-3 times and calculate the normality of NaOH by the usual method from the normality of the HCl and the volumes of NaOH and HCl solutions used. Although this method is rapid and simple, it has the disadvantage that all the errors in standardization of the HCl solution influence the result.

Standardization Against Oxalic (or Succinic) Acid. Proceeding as in the standardization of borax solution (p. 292), take a 250 ml (or 200 ml) measuring flask and prepare an approximately 0.1 *N* solution of exactly known titre of one of the above-named salts. Calculate the weight to be taken on the assumption that the composition of the acids corresponds strictly to their formulas: $H_2C_2O_4 \cdot 2H_2O$ (oxalic acid), or $H_2C_4H_4O_4$ (succinic acid), and that both are titrated as dibasic acids. They are relatively weak acids, and must be titrated in presence of phenolphthalein. Since this indicator is highly sensitive to carbonic acid, water free from CO_2 must be used for preparation of the acid solutions.

Having prepared the solution, mix it thoroughly. Calculate the titre and normality of the solution.

Now measure out an aliquot portion (25.00 ml) into a flask, add 8-10 drops of phenolphthalein, and titrate with the NaOH solution. The pink colour which appears on addition of the alkali at first disappears quickly on stirring. When all the acid has been neutralized a more stable pink colour appears, but this also fades eventually owing to absorption of CO_2 from the air by the solution.

The end of the titration is taken as the point at which the colour persists for about 30 seconds in the solution stirred after addition of the last drop of NaOH.

As usual, the first titration should be approximate, to the nearest 1 ml, and this should be followed by three precise titrations. Take the average of the readings (which should not differ by more than 0.1 ml). Calculate the normality of the NaOH solution from the volumes of solutions taken in the titration and from the known normality of the oxalic (or succinic) acid solution.

This standardization method is free from the defect inherent in the first method: errors of the individual determinations are not additive. In this sence it is more reliable. With careful work the two methods should, nevertheless, give very close results. Any considerable deviations indicate an error of some sort.

76. Determinations of Acids

If a standard alkali solution is available, we can determine the contents of various acids in solutions. If the acid is strong, it is titrated in presence of methyl orange as described for the standardization of NaOH against HCl: the alkali solution is titrated with the acid solution until addition of one drop changes the colour of the indicator to pink. If the NaOH solution is free from Na_2CO_3 (Sec. 75) it can be equally well titrated in presence of phenolphthalein, but here alkali must be added to the acid.

In determinations of weak acids it is imperative to use phenolphthalein and not methyl orange (Sec. 63). The procedure is then the same as in standardization of NaOH against oxalic acid; the acid is titrated with the alkali until a pale pink colour is obtained which persists for 30 seconds.

Such acids as H_3PO_4 can be titrated with caustic alkali either in presence of methyl orange as far as NaH_2PO_4 or in presence of phenolphthalein (or, better, thymolphthalein), as far as Na_2HPO_4. In the first case the equivalent of H_3PO_4 is equal to M, and in the second, to $\frac{M}{2}$ (Sec. 68).

For determination of the percentage content of a concentrated acid, a sample is weighed out exactly on an analytical balance* to give an approximately 0.1 N solution when dissolved in a 250 ml measuring flask. *Concentrated acids should be weighed out in stoppered weighing bottles; great care must be taken.* The weighed sample is poured through a funnel into a measuring flask containing 50-100 ml of water; the weighing bottle and funnel are then rinsed out several times with water, the solution is made up to the mark and stirred thoroughly, and aliquot portions are titrated with alkali (or vice versa).

The normality of the diluted acid solution and the amount of acid present in the measuring flask are calculated from the titration results. The result is expressed as a percentage of the sample taken.

77. Determination of Ammonia in Ammonium Salts

The neutralization method can be used for determining ammonia in ammonium salts (Sec. 69). However, ammonium salts cannot be titrated directly with alkalies because of the absence of a break on the titration curve (p. 260); indirect titration methods must therefore be used. These are the back-titration and the substitution methods. Let us consider them individually.

The Back-Titration Method

This determination can be performed in various ways; the one considered here is the simplest although not the most accurate

* The required weight is calculated from the specific gravity of the acid, the reasoning being the same as in preparation of HCl solution. See also Sec. 57, Example 4 (p. 219).

Procedure. In contrast to the determinations already described, in which pipetting was used, the method of separate samples (p. 206) is used here. Weigh out about 0.15 g of NH_4Cl on an analytical balance into a titration flask and dissolve it in 50-60 ml of distilled water. Now add from a burette an exactly measured volume, known to be in excess, of standard NaOH solution (for example, 40.00 ml), and heat the liquid until the ammonia formed in the reaction

$$NH_4Cl + NaOH = NaCl + H_2O + NH_3 \uparrow$$

has been completely removed. The heating must be continued until a piece of filter paper moistened with $Hg_2(NO_3)_2$ solution no longer turns black in the vapour from the liquid.*

At this stage cool the solution and titrate the excess alkali with standard HCl solution in presence of methyl orange.

Calculation. Suppose that 40.00 ml of 0.09964 *N* NaOH solution was taken, and titration of the excess took 14.60 ml of 0.1023 *N* HCl. First we calculate the volume (V) of NaOH solution equivalent to the amount of HCl used in the titration.

From the equation

$$V \times 0.09964 = 14.60 \times 0.1023$$

we have

$$V = \frac{14.60 \times 0.1023}{0.09964} = 14.96 \text{ ml}$$

It follows that of the 40.00 ml NaOH taken, 40.00 — 14.96 = = 25.04 ml was used in the reaction with NH_4Cl. Since a litre of 0.09964 *N* NaOH contains 0.09964 gram-equivalent, 25.04 ml of this solution contains

$$\frac{0.09964 \times 25.04}{1{,}000} \text{ g-eq NaOH}$$

Since the substances react in equivalent amounts, this was also the amount of gram-equivalents of NH_4Cl in the sample weighed out. In the reaction loss of one NaOH molecule corresponds to formation of one NH_3 molecule; hence the gram-equivalent of NH_3 is M = 17.03 g. Therefore, the amount of NH_3 in the sample is

$$Q_{NH_3} = \frac{0.09964 \times 25.04 \times 17.03}{1{,}000} = 0.04248 \text{ g}$$

---

* The blackening of the paper is due to the reaction of $Hg_2(NO_3)_2$ with NH_3:

$$2Hg_2(NO_3)_2 + 4NH_3 + H_2O = \left[O\begin{matrix} Hg \\ Hg \end{matrix}NH_2 \right] NO_3 + 2Hg + 3NH_4NO_3$$

This amount of ammonia is now expressed as a percentage of the sample taken.

The precision of this method is relatively low, because NaOH reacts with glass when heated in glass vessels, so that a certain amount of alkali (not taken into account) is lost.

A more precise method is by distillation of the ammonia liberated in the reaction with alkali into a measured volume of standard HCl solution, which reacts with the NH_3:

$$HCl + NH_3 = NH_4Cl$$

The residual acid is then titrated with alkali in presence of methyl orange,* and the volume of HCl used in the reaction with NH_3 is found by difference as in the preceding method. The amount of NH_3 in the sample can then be calculated.

This method is used for determining nitrogen content in substances of plant and animal origin, and in organic substances in general. A weighed sample of the material is heated in concentrated H_2SO_4 (sp. gr. 1.84) in the presence of a catalyst (e.g., mercury). The organic substance is oxidized to CO_2 and H_2O and all its nitrogen is converted into $(NH_4)_2SO_4$. Excess concentrated alkali solution is added, the ammonia formed is distilled off, and determined in the usual way.

The Substitution Method

In the substitution method a substance (such as NH_4Cl) which cannot be directly titrated with a particular standard solution (NaOH) is replaced by an equivalent quantity of another substance (HCl) which can be so titrated. In the present instance this substitution is effected by addition of a solution of formaldehyde CH_2O (formalin) to the NH_4Cl solution, when the following reaction takes place:

$$4NH_4Cl + 6CH_2O = (CH_2)_6N_4 + 4HCl + 6H_2O$$

The compound $(CH_2)_6N_4$ formed in the reaction is known as urotropine (hexamethylenetetramine). The amount of HCl produced in the reaction is equivalent to the amount of NH_4Cl taken; therefore, after the HCl has been titrated with NaOH solution it is easy to calculate the amount of NH_4Cl and therefore of NH_3 in the sample. The method is fairly accurate and very convenient.

Procedure. Weigh out accurately about 0.15 g NH_4Cl, dissolve it in 25 ml of water, add 5 ml of 40% formalin (which must first be

* Phenolphthalein cannot be used, because the solution contains NH_4Cl which gives it an acid reaction at the equivalence point (Sec. 65).

made exactly neutral by addition of caustic soda*) and 2-5 drops of 1% phenolphthalein solution.**

Leave the mixture to stand for a few minutes and then titrate it with standard NaOH solution until addition of one drop produces a pink colour which persists for 30 seconds.

Calculation. The calculation is quite analogous to that used in the first method: the number of gram-equivalents of NaOH taken for the reaction is calculated from the volume and normality of the NaOH solution taken. This value is exactly equal to the number of gram-equivalents of HCl, and therefore of NH_4Cl and NH_3. This result is multiplied by the gram-equivalent of NH_3 (17.03 g) and the result is expressed as a percentage of the sample.

QUESTIONS AND PROBLEMS
(on Secs. 71-77)

1. What volume of HNO_3 of sp. gr. 1.4 should be taken to prepare 5 litres of 0.1 *N* solution?

***Answer*: About 34 ml.**

2. A 4 *N* solution of H_2SO_4 is available. How can a 0.1 *N* solution be made from it?

3. Why cannot the titre of an H_2SO_4 solution be calculated from the exact weight of a sample of concentrated acid?

4. Calculate the weight of Na_2CO_3 which should be taken for standardizing 0.1 *N* H_2SO_4 solution if a 200 ml measuring flask and a 50 ml pipette are available and if methyl orange is to be used in the titration.

***Answer*: About 0.53 g.**

5. Calculate the normality and titre of an H_2SO_4 solution if 24.00 ml of it is required for titration of 50.00 ml of a solution made by dissolving 0.5000 g Na_2CO_3 in a 200 ml measuring flask, with methyl orange as the indicator.

***Answer*: $N = 0.09826$; $T = 0.004819$ g/ml.**

6. Explain why burettes and pipettes must be rinsed out with the solutions with which they are to be filled. Is it permissible to rinse out the titration flask with the solution to be titrated?

7. Calculate the weight of succinic acid $H_2C_4H_4O_4$ which should be taken for standardization of 0.1 *N* KOH solution by the pipetting method if a 250 ml measuring flask and a 25 ml pipette are to be used. What indicator should be used?

***Answer*: About 1.5 g.**

---

* Formalin usually contains formic acid (HCOOH) as an impurity, and if it is not neutralized an incorrect result is obtained. For the neutralization, alkali is added in the presence of phenolphthalein to a faint pink colour.

** The reaction between formaldehyde and ammonium salts is reversible. To ensure that it goes practically to completion, the acid formed in the reacton should be fully neutralized; this is achieved by titration in the presence of phenolphthalein (the titration ends in a slightly alkaline solution at pH = 9). In titrations in the presence of such indicators as methyl orange or methyl red the end point is in the acid range and the reaction is not complete.

8. Find the normality and titre of a KOH solution if 25.20 ml of it was taken for titration of 0.1495 g of $H_2C_4H_4O_4$ dissolved in a random volume of water.

Answer: $N = 0.1005$; T = 0.005637 g/ml.

9. Calculate the percentage of HNO_3 in concentrated nitric acid if, after 9.7770 g of it had been diluted with water in a 1 litre measuring flask, 25.45 ml of the resultant solution was required for titration of 25.00 ml of 0.1040 *N* NaOH solution.

Answer: 65.85%.

10. Calculate the weight of H_3PO_4 in a given solution if titration of this solution in presence of phenolphthalein took 25.50 ml of 0.2000 *N* NaOH. In the calculation, first find the number of gram-equivalents of NaOH used.

Answer: 0.2499 g.

11. Calculate the weight of H_3PO_4 in a given solution if titration of this solution in the presence of methyl orange took 25.50 ml of 0.2000 *N* NaOH solution.
To solve this problem, first find T_{NaOH/H_3PO_4}.

Answer: 0.4998 g.

12. Find the weights of KOH and K_2CO_3 in a sample of technical caustic potash if the following burette readings were obtained when it was dissolved in an arbitrary volume of water and titrated with 0.09500 *N* HCl solution: in presence of phenolphthalein, 22.40 ml; in presence of methyl orange, 25.80 ml.

Answer: 0.0446 g K_2CO_3 and 0.1013 g KOH.

13. Titration of 25.00 ml of a solution containing a mixture of Na_2CO_3 and $NaHCO_3$ took 9.46 ml of 0.1200 *N* H_2SO_4 solution in presence of phenolphthalein, and 24.86 ml in presence of methyl orange. Find the weights of Na_2CO_3 and $NaHCO_3$ in 250 ml of this solution.

Answer: 1.203 g Na_2CO_3; 0.5989 g $NaHCO_3$.

14. State which of the compounds KOH, K_2CO_3, and $KHCO_3$ are present in a given solution if (a) equal volumes of HCl are required in titrations in presence of phenolphthalein and of methyl orange; (b) twice as much HCl is taken in the methyl orange titration as in the phenolphthalein titration; (c) the solution is not alkaline to phenolphthalein but can be titrated in the presence of methyl orange.

15. Explain the principle of back-titration.

16. Find the weight of $CaCO_3$ in a sample if, after it had been treated with 50.00 ml of 0.2000 *N* HCl solution, titration of the residual HCl took 10.00 ml of a NaOH solution. It is given that 24.00 ml of this NaOH solution is required for titration of 25.00 ml of the HCl solution.

Answer: 0.3962 g.

17. Calculate the carbonate hardness of water sample if 100 ml of it took 5.00 ml of 0.09000 *N* HCl solution.

Answer: 4.50 mg-eq/litre.

18. Calculate the degree of permanent hardness of a water sample, given that after 100 ml of it had been treated with 10.00 ml of 0.1100 *N* Na_2CO_3 solution and evaporated, back-titration of excess Na_2CO_3 took 6.20 ml of 0.1000 *N* HCl.

Answer: 4.80 mg-eq/litre.

19. A sample of metallic magnesium was dissolved in 50.00 ml of 0.5200 *N* HCl solution; back-titration of the residual HCl took 15.00 ml of 0.2000 *N* NaOH. Find the weight of magnesium metal.

Answer: 0.2795 g.

20. In a magnesium determination Mg^{++} was precipitated in the form of $MgNH_4PO_4$. The precipitate was filtered off, washed, and dissolved in 50.00 ml of an HCl solution. The following reaction took place:

$$MgNH_4PO_4 + 2HCl = MgCl_2 + NH_4H_2PO_4$$

The excess acid was titrated with 0.1010 *N* NaOH solution in the presence of methyl orange; the volume of NaOH taken was 15.5 ml. Find the weight of Mg^{++} if titration of 25.00 ml of the HCl solution took 22.50 ml of the alkali.

Answer: 0.0362 g.

21. For determination of NH_3 in technical $(NH_4)_2SO_4$, 1.6160 g of the latter was dissolved in a 250 ml measuring flask; 25.00 ml of the solution was boiled with concentrated NaOH solution and the ammonia was absorbed in standard H_2SO_4 solution. The excess sulfuric acid was titrated with NaOH solution. Calculate the percentage content of ammonia in the $(NH_4)_2SO_4$ given that 40.00 ml of 0.1020 *N* H_2SO_4 solution was taken for absorption of the NH_3, while the back-titration took 17.00 ml of 0.0960 *N* NaOH solution.

Answer: 25.79%.

22. The nitrogen in 0.8880 g of an organic substance was converted into $(NH_4)_2SO_4$ by the action of concentrated H_2SO_4; the ammonium sulphate was then boiled with concentrated alkali to liberate ammonia, which was absorbed in 50.0 ml of 0.1200 *N* H_2SO_4 solution. Titration of the excess H_2SO_4 took 12.00 ml of 0.09800 *N* NaOH. Calculate the percentage of nitrogen in the organic substance.

Answer: 7.61%.

23. For determination of tungsten content, a sample of steel weighing 1.0000 g was heated with HCl, and the tungsten present in the steel was then oxidized to tungstic acid, H_2WO_4, by boiling with HNO_3. The solution was diluted with water, the precipitated H_2WO_4 was filtered off, washed thoroughly, and dissolved in 40.00 ml of standard NaOH solution. Given that $T_{NaOH/W} = 0.001020$ g/ml, calculate the percentage of tungsten in the steel if back-titration of the excess NaOH in the presence of phenolphthalein took 18.00 ml of HNO_3 solution, one millilitre of which is equivalent to 1.02 ml of the NaOH solution.

Answer: 2.21%.

CHAPTER VII

OXIDATION-REDUCTION METHODS (OXIDIMETRY)

78. Oxidation Potentials and Reaction Direction

In contrast to neutralization and precipitation methods, in which the titration reaction consists in particular ions forming undissociated molecules of a weak electrolyte (water, weak acid) or a precipitate, oxidimetry involves oxidation-reduction reactions associated with transfer of electrons.* In a reaction of this type the *oxidizing agent gains electrons and is reduced, and the reducing agent loses electrons and is oxidized.* This exchange of electrons leads to changes in the valence of the corresponding atoms or ions; *the valence of an oxidized atom or ion is increased, and the valence of a reduced atom or ion is decreased.* For example, conversions of Fe^{++} into Fe^{+++}, Cl^- into Cl_2, and Cu into Cu^{++} are oxidations, because in all three cases the valence of the atom or ion increases (from $+2$ to $+3$, from -1 to 0, and from 0 to $+2$).

Oxidizing and reducing agents may differ among themselves in strength, i.e., in chemical activity. Strong oxidizing agents have a pronounced tendency to gain electrons. Therefore, they are able to remove electrons from many reducing agents, including those which are relatively weak, i.e., which yield electrons with difficulty. Conversely, weak oxidizing agents have a much less pronounced tendency to gain electrons. Therefore, they can only oxidize the strongest reducing agents (i.e., those which yield electrons readily). Obviously, the direction of an oxidation-reduction reaction can be predicted only if some quantitative characteristic of the relative force of the oxidizing and reducing agents involved is known. This characteristic is called the *redox potential.* We have already met the concept of oxidation potential in the course of qualitative analysis. It is of even greater significance in quantitative analysis. We must therefore consider it more fully here.

* Modern concepts of oxidation-reduction processes as processes of electron transfer were introduced by L. Pisarzhevsky during 1910-14.

If a metal is dipped into water or an aqueous solution cations from the crystal lattice of the metal may pass into the adjacent zone of the solution, setting up an excess of positive charges in the solution and of negative ones in the metal (double electric layer). Thus a certain difference of potentials appears between the metal and the solution.

The reverse process, namely, passage of cations from the solution to the metal, is also possible. In this case the solution acquires a negative charge (owing to the excess of anions in the vicinity of the metal), and the metal, a positive one; the net result is also a difference of potentials, but now it is of the opposite sign.

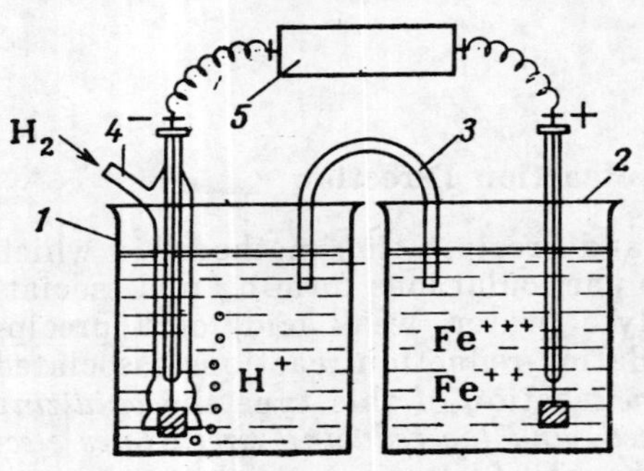

Fig. 56. Apparatus for determination of the standard oxidation potential of the system Fe^{+++}/Fe^{++}:
1, 2—glass vessels; *3*—electrolytic bridge; *4*—tube for hydrogen gas; *5*—potentiometer

It is very difficult to measure the difference of potentials between the metal and the solution, but, as we saw in the course of qualitative analysis, it is easy to measure the potential difference between two systems by connecting them up into a galvanic cell (see Fig. 56). Any galvanic element consists of two half-elements each of which is an oxidation-reduction couple, i.e., a system consisting of the oxidized and the reduced forms of the chemical element or ion in question.

The oxidation state of the element is higher in the oxidized form (Fe^{+++}; Cl_2, MnO_4^-) and lower in the reduced (Fe^{++}, Cl^-, Mn^{++}).* The oxidized form of each oxidation-reduction couple is an oxidant and its reduced form, a reductant. *The more powerful the oxidant of a pair, the weaker its reductant should be, and vice versa.* For instance, if Cl_2 is said to be a powerful oxidizing agent, this means that its atoms possess pronounced ability to accept electrons, i.e., to change into Cl^- ions. But this being the case, the Cl^- ions should keep a strong hold on these electrons, i.e., should be a very weak reducing agent. Likewise, since Sn^{++} ion is a rather strong reductant, i.e., yields its electrons readily to form Sn^{++++} ion, it follows that the latter is not very apt to accept electrons, i.e., is a weak oxidant, etc.

---

* It will be recalled that when comparing the valence of different elements and ions its sign should be taken into account. For example, the valence of chlorine in Cl_2 (0) is higher than that of the ions Cl^- (-1).

It should be noted that in practice one never has to do with an absolutely pure oxidizing agent or an absolutely pure reducing agent: their solutions always contain the products of their reduction or oxidation, respectively. For example, the reductant Fe^{++} always contains some Fe^{+++} formed from it and possessing oxidizing properties; the oxidants Cl_2, MnO_4^-, etc. always contain, though in insignificantly small quantities, admixtures of the reducing agents they form, viz., Cl^- ion, Mn^{++} ion and so on.

That is why it is more correct to speak of the redox potentials of *oxidation-reduction couples* such as Fe^{+++}/Fe^{++}, MnO_4^-/Mn^{++}, etc., rather than of the potentials of individual oxidants or reductants. When determining the oxidation potentials of various couples experimentally it must be taken into account that their values depend not only on the strengths of the oxidizing and reducing agents making up the couple, but also on the ratio of their concentrations. To obtain comparable results the concentrations must be made *the same*, equal to unity in the general case. The oxidation potentials obtained under such conditions are known as *standard* oxidation potentials and are denoted by E_0. To obtain comparable results when determining standard oxidation potentials different oxidation-reduction couples should always be paired with the same standard couple. The so-called *standard hydrogen electrode* is used for this purpose, this electrode being a $2H^+/H_2$ couple with the concentration (or rather the activity) of the H^+ ions equal to 1 g-ion per litre and at a hydrogen gas pressure of 1 atm. One of the designs of a standard hydrogen electrode is shown in Fig. 56 (left). Vessel *1* contains a H_2SO_4 solution of the required concentration, into which a platinum electrode coated with a layer of finely divided platinum ("platinum black") is dipped. Chemically pure hydrogen is passed into the solution through tube *4* and on coming in contact with the electrode is adsorbed by the finely divided platinum. As a result the electrode acts as if it were made of hydrogen.

The potential of the standard hydrogen electrode is conventionally taken as zero, just like the temperature of melting ice is conventionally taken as zero for measuring temperatures.

In determination of the standard oxidation potential of any particular system, such as Fe^{+++}/Fe^{++}, it is combined with a standard hydrogen electrode in the form of a cell, as shown in Fig. 56.

The vessel *2* is filled with a mixture of equal volumes of $FeCl_3$ and $FeCl_2$ solutions of the same molar concentration and a platinum electrode is immersed in it. The two electrodes are joined by a conductor, and the instrument *5* for e.m.f. measurement (potentiometer) is inserted in the circuit. The solutions are connected by an inverted U-tube *3* containing an electrolyte solution (KCl). Along this tube known as an "electrolytic bridge", the ions diffuse from one vessel to the other (thus closing the internal circuit).*

The resultant cell acts as follows. Its negative pole (cathode) is the standard hydrogen electrode, and the positive pole (anode) is the Fe^{+++}/Fe^{++} system. At the cathode H_2 molecules give electrons to the platinum, i.e., they are oxidized to H^+ ions:

$$H_2 - 2e = 2H^+$$

The liberated electrons travel through the conductor to the anode, where they are taken up by the Fe^{+++} ions, which are thereby reduced to Fe^{++} ions:

$$2Fe^{+++} + 2e = 2Fe^{++}$$

Adding these two equations, we have the general equation for the reaction taking place in the operation of the cell:

$$2Fe^{+++} + H_2 = 2Fe^{++} + 2H^+$$

The electromotive force (e.m.f.) of this cell is found to be 0.77 V. Since it represents the difference between the standard oxidation potentials of the two systems, we can write

$$\text{e.m.f.} = E_{0\ Fe^{+++}/Fe^{++}} - E_{0\ 2H^+/H_2} = 0.77\ \text{V}$$

However, $E_{0\ 2H^+/H_2}$ is taken as zero. Therefore

$$E_{0\ Fe^{+++}/Fe^{++}} = +0.77\ \text{V}$$

The plus sign shows that the system in question acts as the positive pole when combined with a standard hydrogen electrode. Conversely, if it should be a negative pole (giving electrons to H^+ ions and reducing them to H_2 during operation of the cell), its potential is regarded as negative.

The standard oxidation potential (+0.77 V) found for the system Fe^{+++}/Fe^{++} *is a measure of the power of* Fe^{+++} *ions to gain electrons from* H_2 *molecules, i.e., to oxidize them to* H^+ *ions.*

If a standard hydrogen electrode is combined with the $Cl_2/2Cl^-$ system instead of Fe^{+++}/Fe^{++}, the result is a cell the operation of which can be represented as follows:

$$H_2 - 2e = 2H^+ \text{ (at the cathode)}$$

$$\underline{Cl_2 + 2e = 2Cl^- \text{ (at the anode)}}$$

$$H_2 + Cl_2 = 2H^+ + 2Cl^-$$

---

* The tube *3* is filled with heated KCl solution containing gelatin or agar; when the solution cools it sets to a gel which retains it in the tube but does not prevent migration of ions through it.

The standard oxidation potential of the $Cl_2/2Cl^-$ system is considerably greater than that of the Fe^{+++}/Fe^{++} system; its value is $E_{0Cl_2/2Cl^-} = +1.36$ V. It follows that free Cl_2 has a much higher tendency than Fe^{+++} ions to gain electrons (i.e., it has much higher oxidation activity). Accordingly, Cl^- ions are a weaker reducing agent than Fe^{++} ions. It follows that *the higher the standard oxidation potential of a given system, the stronger the oxidizing power of its oxidized form and the weaker the reducing power of its reduced form.*

The standard oxidation potentials of various systems of importance in quantitative analysis are given in Appendix VI. The first and third columns of this table give the formulas of the individual components of the various systems; these components are arranged in increasing order of their corresponding standard oxidation potentials E_0 (fourth column). The second column gives the number of electrons (n) gained or lost when the reducing agent (first column) is converted into the corresponding oxidizing agent (third column) or vice versa.

Since the strengths of oxidizing agents increase and the strengths of reducing agents decrease with increasing oxidation potential, the strongest oxidizing agents are found at the end of the third column, and the strongest reducing agents, at the top of the first column of the table of oxidation potentials. For example, the strongest of all oxidizing agents is free fluorine, with the highest value of E_0 (+2.87 V). Other very strong oxidizing agents include permanganate ions MnO_4^- in acid solution ($E_0 = +1.51$ V); dichromate ions $Cr_2O_7^{--}$ in acid solution ($E_0 = +1.36$ V); free chlorine Cl_2 ($E_0 = +1.36$ V); free bromine Br_2 ($E_0 = +1.07$ V). Ferric ions Fe^{+++} ($E_0 = +0.77$ V), AsO_4^{---} ions ($E_0 = +0.57$ V), free iodine I_2 ($E_0 = +0.54$ V), Sn^{++++} ions ($E_0 = +0.15$ V) and H^+ ions ($E_0 = 0$ V) are weaker oxidizing agents, while Zn^{++} ions ($E_0 = -0.76$ V), Al^{+++} ($E_0 = -1.70$ V), etc., are very weak oxidizing agents.

The strongest reducing agents include the alkali and alkaline-earth metals and also Mg, Al, Zn, etc. Hydrogen arsenide AsH_3 is a very powerful reducing agent. Some very strong reducing ions are V^{++}, Ti^{+++}, S^{--}, and Sn^{++}; I^-, AsO_3^{---}, Fe^{++} and others are somewhat weaker in this respect. F^- ions are practically devoid of reducing properties, as there is no oxidizing agent which could gain electrons from them. It is known that electrons can be removed from F^- ions only by electrolysis.

If any two redox systems are combined, *the stronger of the two oxidizing agents gains electrons from the stronger reducing agent, with formation of weaker reducing and oxidizing agents.* For example, with the systems $Cl_2/2Cl^-$ and Fe^{+++}/Fe^{++} the stronger oxidizing agent is Cl_2 ($E_0 = +1.36$ V) and the stronger reducing agent is Fe^{++} ($E_0 = +0.77$ V).

Accordingly, the reaction between these two systems proceeds in the direction

$$Cl_2 + 2Fe^{++} \rightarrow 2Cl^- + 2Fe^{+++}$$

i.e., with formation of weaker reducing (Cl^-) and oxidizing (Fe^{+++}) agents than those initially present.

The above rule can also be stated as follows: *an oxidizing agent with a higher potential can oxidize any reducing agent with a lower potential. Similarly, a reducing agent of a lower potential can reduce any oxidizing agent of a higher potential.*

For example, MnO_4^- ions in acid solution ($E_0 = +1.51$ V) can oxidize all the reducing agents above it (in the first column), such as Cl^-, Br^-, Fe^{++}, I^-, SO_3^{--}, $S_2O_3^{--}$, Sn^{++}, S^{--}, etc. Dichromate ions $Cr_2O_7^{--}$ ($E_0 = +1.36$ V) can also oxidize all these reducing agents, with the exception of Cl^-, because the system $Cl_2/2Cl^-$ has the same standard oxidation potential as the system* $Cr_2O_7^{--}/2Cr^{+++}$. Similarly, $Cr_2O_7^{--}$ ions cannot oxidize Mn^{++} ions to MnO_4^-. Conversely, Cr^{+++} ions can reduce MnO_4^-, ions to Mn^{++} ions.

With the aid of this rule and the table of standard oxidation potentials we can predict the direction of any oxidation-reduction reaction, choose suitable oxidizing and reducing agents, and solve a number of other problems important in analytical practice. However, it is necessary to take into account the influence of the concentrations of the individual components of the systems on the oxidation potential, as otherwise erroneous conclusions may be drawn.

79. Influence of Concentrations and the Reaction of the Medium

The relationship between the oxidation potential (E) of any given redox system and the concentrations of the oxidized [Ox.] and reduced [Red.] forms is represented by the Nernst equation, derived from the laws of thermodynamics:

$$E = E_0 + \frac{RT}{nF} \ln \frac{[\text{Ox.}]}{[\text{Red.}]}$$

Here E_0 is the standard oxidation potential** of the given system: R is the gas constant (8.313 joules/mole·deg);

* However, this is valid only when the H^+ and Cl^- ion concentrations in solution correspond to those at which the standard potentials of the corresponding systems were determined. At high enough concentrations Cl^- ions are oxidized.

** The standard potential is the potential of the system when the concentrations of the oxidized and reduced forms are equal. In that case $\ln \frac{[\text{Ox.}]}{[\text{Red.}]} = 0$ and $E = E_0$.

T is the absolute temperature;
F is the Faraday constant (96.500 coulombs/g-eq);
n is the number of electrons (lost or gained).

If we substitute the numerical values of the constants and convert natural to common logarithms, we have for room temperature (20°C):

$$E = E_0 + \frac{0.058}{n} \log \frac{[\text{Ox.}]}{[\text{Red.}]}$$

Thus, for the system Fe^{+++}/Fe^{++}

$$E_{Fe^{+++}/Fe^{++}} = 0.77 + \frac{0.058}{1} \log \frac{[Fe^{+++}]}{[Fe^{++}]}$$

For example, if $[Fe^{+++}] = 1$ g-ion/litre and $[Fe^{++}] = 0.0001$ g-ion/litre, then

$$E_{Fe^{+++}/Fe^{++}} = 0.77 + 0.058 \log \frac{1}{10^{-4}} = 1.002 \text{ V}$$

If the equation for the reaction taking place in the conversion of the oxidized into the reduced form contains stoichiometric coefficients different from unity, they enter the Nernst equation as indices of the respective concentrations. For example, for the system $Br_2/2Br^-$ we can write:

$$E_{Br_2/2Br^-} = 1.07 + \frac{0.058}{2} \log \frac{[Br_2]}{[Br^-]^2}$$

With systems such as Zn^{++}/Zn, where one of the components (Zn) is practically insoluble in water, its concentration is constant and therefore does not enter into the expression for E. Therefore, for this system

$$E_{Zn^{++}/Zn} = E_0 + \frac{0.058}{2} \log [Zn^{++}]$$

Evidently, E_0 (—0.76 V) is the potential of the Zn^{++}/Zn system when $[Zn^{++}] = 1$ g-ion/litre, as it is only then that $\log [Zn^{++}] = 0$ and $E = E_0$.

In the case of oxy-acid anions conversion of the oxidized into the reduced form is very often accompanied by extensive changes in their composition and involves H^+ ions. For example, in oxidation reactions with permanganate and dichromate in acid solutions, MnO_4^- and $Cr_2O_7^{--}$ anions are reduced in accordance with the equations:

$$MnO_4^- + 8H^+ + 5e = Mn^{++} + 4H_2O$$

$$Cr_2O_7^{--} + 14H^+ + 6e = 2Cr^{+++} + 7H_2O$$

etc.

It is evident that E also depends on the H^+ ion concentration in solution. This concentration enters the numerator of the fraction following the logarithm sign, raised to the power equal to the corresponding stoichiometric coefficient, for example*:

$$E_{MnO_4^-/Mn^{++}} = E_0 + \frac{0.058}{5} \log \frac{[MnO_4^-][H^+]^8}{[Mn^{++}]}$$

$$E_{Cr_2O_7^{--}/2Cr^{+++}} = E_0 + \frac{0.058}{6} \log \frac{[Cr_2O_7^{--}][H^+]^{14}}{[Cr^{+++}]^2}$$

etc.

These equations show that in these cases the H^+ ion concentration has a particularly strong influence on the oxidation potential of the solution and therefore on its oxidizing activity.

If the concentrations of individual components of a particular redox system are varied, the oxidation potential is also altered. It may happen that as the result of such a change a system with a higher standard oxidation potential acquires a lower potential than the other system involved.

Therefore, the course of the reaction between such systems becomes the reverse of that indicated by their position in the table of standard oxidation potentials.

This may be illustrated by the following examples. In volumetric analysis copper is determined by an iodometric method based on the reaction:

$$2Cu^{++} + 4I^- = \downarrow 2CuI + I_2$$

This reaction involves the systems: Cu^{++}/Cu^+ ($E = +0.17$ V) and $I_2/2I^-$ ($E_0 = +0.54$ V). The values of the standard potentials suggest that the reaction should proceed in the reverse direction:

$$2CuI + I_2 \rightarrow 2Cu^{++} + 4I^-$$

The reason for this discrepancy between the expectation based on the values of the standard oxidation potentials and the experimental result is the low solubility of CuI, so that the Cu^+ ion concentration is very much lowered and the oxidation potential of the Cu^{++}/Cu^+ system is therefore changed considerably.

If we take the I^- ion concentration in solution to be 10^{-1} g-ion/litre, and take into account that the solubility product of CuI is 10^{-12}, simple calculation gives:

$$[Cu^+] = \frac{10^{-12}}{[I^-]} = \frac{10^{-12}}{10^{-1}} = 10^{-11} \text{ g-ion/litre}$$

* Evidently, the definition of the standard potential in such cases requires not only that the concentrations of the oxidized and reduced forms in solution shall be equal, but also that the H^+ ion concentration must be unity. Only then is the fraction following the logarithm sign equal to unity and $E = E_0$.

Substituting this value of $[Cu^+]$ into the equation for E_{Cu^{++}/Cu^+} we have

$$E_{Cu^{++}/Cu^+} = 0.17 + \frac{0.058}{1} \log \frac{[Cu^{++}]}{10^{-11}} =$$

$$= 0.17 + 0.058 \log [Cu^{++}] - 0.058(-11)$$

and finally

$$E_{Cu^{++}/Cu^+} = 0.808 + 0.058 \log [Cu^{++}]$$

Since 0.808 V is greater than the standard oxidation potential of the system $I_2/2I^-$ (+0.54 V), the direction of the reaction must be

$$2Cu^{++} + 4I^- \longrightarrow \downarrow 2CuI + I_2$$

and not as expected from the standard oxidation potentials of the systems involved.

Such cases are quite common; the direction of a reaction may be changed not only by the decrease in the concentration of a particular ion resulting from the formation of a sparingly soluble compound, but also by the binding of ions in stable complexes.

It is known that the oxidation potential is often influenced very strongly by the H^+ ion concentration in solution; therefore a change of solution pH may sometimes alter the direction of an oxidation-reduction process.

For example, the standard oxidation potentials of the systems AsO_4^{---}/AsO_3^{---} (+0.57 V) and $I_2/2I^-$ (+0.54 V) indicate that the following reaction should take place between them:

$$AsO_4^{---} + 2I^- + 2H^+ \longrightarrow AsO_3^{---} + I_2 + H_2O \quad (1)$$

This is the reaction which occurs in practice if the concentrations of all the ions involved in the reaction are the concentrations used in determination of the standard oxidation potentials of the respective systems. Suppose, however, that the reaction takes place in presence of excess $NaHCO_3$, which maintains the solution pH at about 8. The consequent decrease of the H^+ ion concentration to 10^{-8} g-ion/litre has no effect on the potential of the $I_2/2I^-$ system. However, in the case of the system AsO_4^{---}/AsO_3^{---}, where conversion of the oxidized into the reduced form involves H^+ ions, as is clear from the equation

$$AsO_4^{---} + 2H^+ + 2e \rightleftarrows AsO_3^{---} + H_2O$$

the oxidation potential falls to:

$$E_{AsO_4^{---}/AsO_3^{---}} = 0.57 + \frac{0.058}{2} \log \frac{[AsO_4^{---}](10^{-8})^2}{[AsO_3^{---}]} =$$

$$= 0.57 - \frac{0.058 \times 16}{2} + \frac{0.058}{2} \log \frac{[AsO_4^{---}]}{[AsO_3^{---}]}$$

$$E_{AsO_4^{---}/AsO_3^{---}} = 0.106 + \frac{0.058}{2} \log \frac{[AsO_4^{---}]}{[AsO_3^{---}]}$$

Since 0.106 V is lower than the standard oxidation potential of the $I_2/2I^-$ system, under these conditions AsO_4^{---} ions no longer oxidize I^- ions to I_2, but elemental iodine oxidizes AsO_3^{---} to AsO_4^{---}.

$$AsO_3^{---} + I_2 + H_2O \rightarrow AsO_4^{---} + 2H^+ + 2I^- \qquad (2)$$

Thus, the removal of H^+ ions by addition of $NaHCO_3$

$$H^+ + HCO_3^- = H_2CO_3 = H_2O + CO_2 \uparrow$$

favours reaction (2), which yields these ions. Conversely, increase of H^+ ion concentration, which raises the oxidation potential of the system AsO_4^{---}/AsO_3^{---}, favours reaction (1).

This result can be stated in general form: *if* H^+ *ions are expended in a reaction, it should be conducted in acid solution. Conversely, if they are produced in a reaction, they should be removed by addition of alkali* or of substances such as* $NaHCO_3$. Since the concentrations of H^+ and OH^- ions are interdependent:

$$[H^+][OH^-] = K_{H_2O}$$

removal of OH^- ions is equivalent to formation of H^+ ions, and formation of OH^- ions is equivalent to removal of H^+ ions.

The enormous influence of H^+ ion concentration on the course of oxidation-reduction reactions involving hydrogen ions is demonstrated by the following example. If KI solution is added to a solution of KNO_2, no noticeable changes take place. If a small amount of HCl or H_2SO_4 is then added to the mixture, a violent reaction begins at once, accompanied by evolution of a gas (NO) and formation of a dark grey precipitate (I_2):

$$2NO_2^- + 2I^- + 4H^+ = \downarrow I_2 + 2NO \uparrow + 2H_2O$$

Although H^+ ions were present in the solution even in the absence of added acid, their concentration ($\sim 10^{-7}$ g-ion/litre) was evidently not high enough to raise the oxidation potential of NO_2^-/NO above that of $I_2/2I^-$. Therefore, the reaction could not occur without addition of acid. Calculation with the use of the Nernst equation confirms this explanation. Numerous examples could be given of reactions in which a definite hydrogen ion concentration is required before a redox process can take place.

It is easy to see that the smaller the difference between the standard oxidation potentials of the respective systems the less is the change in the concentration of one of the reacting ions or of the

---

* In the example under consideration addition of alkali is inadmissible, as a side reaction takes place in strongly alkaline solution:

$$I_2 + 2NaOH = NaIO + NaI + H_2O$$

solution pH needed to change the direction of the reaction. For example, in the reaction

$$Pb^{++} + Sn = Pb + Sn^{++}$$

which corresponds to a difference of 0.01 V between the standard potentials, the reaction can be reversed if the Pb^{++} ion concentration is lowered roughly 10-fold relative to the Sn^{++} ion concentration. On the other hand, in the reaction

$$Cu^{++} + Sn = Cu + Sn^{++}$$

where the difference between the potentials is 0.48 V, the Cu^{++} ion concentration would have to be lowered by a factor of 10^{17} or more to reverse the reaction.

In just the same way, the reaction

$$AsO_4^{---} + 2I^- + 2H^+ \rightleftarrows AsO_3^{---} + I_2 + H_2O$$

where the difference between the potentials is 0.03 V, can be easily reversed by an increase of the solution pH. However, no alteration of pH can reverse the reaction

$$Cr_2O_7^{--} + 6Fe^{++} + 14H^+ = 2Cr^{+++} + 6Fe^{+++} + 7H_2O$$

where the difference between the potentials is 0.59 V.*

It follows from the foregoing that *reversal of the course of a reaction is most likely when there is little difference between the standard oxidation potentials of the systems involved.*

80. Equilibrium Constants of Oxidation-Reduction Reactions

The possibility of altering the course of oxidation-reduction reactions in the opposite direction is evidently the consequence of the reversibility of these reactions. We know that chemical equilibrium becomes established in reversible reactions. The equilibrium constant is easy to calculate if the oxidation potentials of both redox systems are known.

Let us perform this calculation for the reaction:

$$Sn^{++} + 2Fe^{+++} \rightleftarrows Sn^{++++} + 2Fe^{++}$$

First we write down equations for the oxidation potentials of the systems Sn^{++++}/Sn^{++} and Fe^{+++}/Fe^{++}:

$$E_{Sn^{++++}/Sn^{++}} = 0.15 + \frac{0.058}{2} \log \frac{[Sn^{++++}]}{[Sn^{++}]} \quad (1)$$

$$E_{Fe^{+++}/Fe^{++}} = 0.77 + 0.058 \log \frac{[Fe^{+++}]}{[Fe^{++}]} \quad (2)$$

* Another reason why this reaction cannot be reversed is that the solution cannot be made alkaline, because Fe^{+++} would be precipitated as $Fe(OH)_3$.

These equations show that as the reaction proceeds and the Sn^{++++} and Fe^{++} ion concentrations increase while the Fe^{+++} and Sn^{++} ion concentrations decrease the potential of the first pair, initially lower, must gradually increase while the potential of the second pair gradually decreases. Eventually the two potentials become equal.

However, we know that transference of electrons is possible only if there is a potential difference, and must cease if the potential difference disappears. Therefore, when

$$E_{Sn^{++++}/Sn^{++}} = E'_{Fe^{+++}/Fe^{++}}$$

equilibrium is established. Substituting the values of $E_{Sn^{++++}/Sn^{++}}$ and $E_{Fe^{+++}/Fe^{++}}$ from Equations (1) and (2) into this equation, we have:

$$0.15 + \frac{0.058}{2} \log \frac{[Sn^{++++}]}{[Sn^{++}]} = 0.77 + 0.058 \log \frac{[Fe^{+++}]}{[Fe^{++}]}$$

and hence

$$\frac{0.058}{2} \log \frac{[Sn^{++++}]}{[Sn^{++}]} - 0.058 \log \frac{[Fe^{+++}]}{[Fe^{++}]} = 0.77 - 0.15$$

The second term in the left-hand side of this last equation can be written as:

$$0.058 \log \frac{[Fe^{+++}]}{[Fe^{++}]} = \frac{0.058}{2}\, 2 \log \frac{[Fe^{+++}]}{[Fe^{++}]} = \frac{0.058}{2} \log \frac{[Fe^{+++}]^2}{[Fe^{++}]^2}$$

The coefficient $\frac{0.058}{2}$ can be taken outside the brackets:

$$\frac{0.058}{2}\left(\log \frac{[Sn^{++++}]}{[Sn^{++}]} - \log \frac{[Fe^{+++}]^2}{[Fe^{++}]^2}\right) = 0.77 - 0.15$$

and hence

$$\log \frac{[Sn^{++++}][Fe^{++}]^2}{[Sn^{++}][Fe^{+++}]^2} = \frac{(0.77 - 0.15) \times 2}{0.058}$$

The expression following the logarithm sign is the equilibrium constant of the reaction; therefore

$$\log K = \frac{(0.77 - 0.15) \times 2}{0.058} \approx 21$$

and hence $K \approx 10^{21}$.

This result shows that at equilibrium the product of the Sn^{++++} and Fe^{++} concentrations is 10^{21} times the product of the concentrations of the unconverted Sn^{++} and Fe^{+++}.

In other words, *the high numerical value of the equilibrium constant indicates that the reaction goes practically to completion.*

This conclusion can be easily confirmed by calculation of the $[Fe^{++}] : [Fe^{+++}]$ and $[Sn^{++++}] : [Sn^{++}]$ concentration ratios at equilibrium at the equivalence point. The reaction equation

$$2Fe^{+++} + Sn^{++} \rightleftarrows 2Fe^{++} + Sn^{++++}$$

shows that at that point the molar $[Fe^{+++}]$ and $[Fe^{++}]$ concentrations at equilibrium should be twice the $[Sn^{++}]$ and $[Sn^{++++}]$ concentrations:

$$[Fe^{+++}] = 2[Sn^{++}]$$

and

$$[Fe^{++}] = 2[Sn^{++++}]$$

Dividing the second equation by the first, we have

$$\frac{[Fe^{++}]}{[Fe^{+++}]} = \frac{[Sn^{++++}]}{[Sn^{++}]} \qquad (3)$$

But earlier we found that

$$K = \frac{[Fe^{++}]^2[Sn^{++++}]}{[Fe^{+++}]^2[Sn^{++}]} = 10^{21}$$

Hence, taking Equation (3) into account, we have at the equivalence point:

$$\frac{[Fe^{++}]^3}{[Fe^{+++}]^3} = \frac{[Sn^{++++}]^3}{[Sn^{++}]^3} = 10^{21}$$

and

$$\frac{[Fe^{++}]}{[Fe^{+++}]} = \frac{[Sn^{++++}]}{[Sn^{++}]} = \sqrt[3]{10^{21}} = 10^7$$

This result shows that at the equivalence point at equilibrium there are 10 million Sn^{++++} (or Fe^{++}) ions to every Sn^{++} (or Fe^{+++}) ion remaining in solution. For example, if 0.1 g-ion of Sn^{++++} was formed at the equivalence point, 10^{-8} g-ion of Sn^{++} remained in solution. Similarly, if 0.2 g-ion of Fe^{++} was formed, 2×10^{-8} g-ion of Fe^{+++} remained unchanged. It follows that in this reaction the conversion of the initial substances is almost complete at the equivalence point.

If the above calculation of the equilibrium constant K is put in general form, we obtain the following equation for any reversible oxidation-reduction process (at 20°C):

$$\log K = \frac{(E_0' - E_0'')\,n}{0.058} \qquad (4)$$

Here E_0' and E_0'' are the standard oxidation potentials of the systems corresponding to the oxidizing agent (E_0') and reducing agent (E_0'') taken;
n is the number of electrons.

Equation (4) shows that *the greater the difference between the standard oxidation potentials of the two systems, the greater must the equilibrium constant be.*

If the difference is large, the reaction goes practically to completion. Conversely, if the difference between the potentials is small the initial substances are not completely converted. To use such a reaction for analytical purposes, we must so choose the concentrations of the substances or ions involved in it that the reaction is as complete as possible.

For example, the reaction which is sometimes used for volumetric determination of quinquivalent arsenic

$$AsO_4^{---} + 2I^- + 2H^+ \rightleftarrows AsO_3^{---} + H_2O + I_2$$

is conducted in strongly acid solution in presence of a large excess of I^- ions, because the potential difference corresponding to the reaction (0.03 V) is small and the equilibrium constant is only about 10.

By the law of mass action, both these factors tend to make the reaction proceed more completely in the desired direction. It was already stated earlier that this reaction can be reversed by addition of excess $NaHCO_3$, which raises the solution pH to about 8.

Since at this pH the value of $E_{AsO_4^{---}/AsO_3^{---}}$ is only $+0.106$ V (p. 320), which is considerably less than the value of $E_{I_2/2I^-}$ ($+0.54$ V), the reaction goes practically to completion under such conditions, so that trivalent arsenic can be determined quantitatively by titration with iodine solution.

The equation

$$\log K = \frac{(E_0' - E_0'')\,n}{0.058}$$

confirms the rule that oxidation-reduction reactions (at the concentrations used for determination of standard potentials) always proceed in the direction of formation of weaker oxidizing and reducing agents than the original substances (p. 315).

If the oxidizing and reducing agents taken are stronger than those formed in the reaction, this means that $E_0' - E_0'' > 0$. In that case $\log K > 0$ and $K > 1$. This shows that the product of the concentrations of the substances formed by the reaction is greater at equilibrium than the product of the concentrations of the original substances, i.e., the reaction proceeds from left to right (→) and if the difference between the standard potentials is large enough the reaction goes almost to completion. Conversely, if $E_0' < E_0''$, i.e., if the original oxidizing and reducing agents are weaker than those which should be formed in the reaction, then $\log E < 0$ and $K < 1$. This means that the reaction tends to go in the opposite direction (←), and the greater the absolute difference between the oxidation potentials the more complete is the reverse reaction.

81. Oxidation-Reduction Titration Curves

In oxidimetric titration the concentrations of the substances or ions involved in the reaction are changing continuously. The oxidation potential of the solution (E) must therefore also change, just as the solution pH changes continuously during titration by the neutralization method. By plotting the oxidation potentials corresponding to different points in the titration we obtain a titration curve similar to the curves for the neutralization method.

As an example, let us calculate and plot the curve for titration of a ferrous iron salt with permanganate in acid solution. The ionic equation for the reaction is:

$$MnO_4^- + 5Fe^{++} + 8H^+ \rightleftarrows Mn^{++} + 5Fe^{+++} + 4H_2O$$

Since the reaction is reversible, the solution always contains both the original ions and the ions formed during the reaction. In other words, at any stage in the titration the solution always contains two redox systems: Fe^{+++}/Fe^{++} and MnO_4^-/Mn^{++}. We therefore have two equations for calculating E:

$$E = 0.77 + \frac{0.058}{1} \log \frac{[Fe^{+++}]}{[Fe^{++}]} \quad (1)$$

$$E = 1.51 + \frac{0.058}{5} \log \frac{[MnO_4^-][H^+]^8}{[Mn^{++}]} \quad (2)$$

Of course, both equations give the same result and either can be used, whichever is the more convenient. So long as not all the ferrous iron has been converted it is very easy to calculate the Fe^{+++} and Fe^{++} concentrations at any point in the titration. The concentrations of the MnO_4^- ions which remain unconverted (owing to the reversibility of the reaction) are much more difficult to calculate. Therefore, Equation (1) is more convenient to use in this case. Conversely, with excess permanganate it is easy to calculate the concentrations of MnO_4^- and Mn^{++} ions in solution and much more difficult to calculate the concentration of the remaining Fe^{++} ions. Therefore, in this case Equation (2) should be used for calculation of E.

Let us calculate the oxidation potential of the solution at the point when 50 ml of $KMnO_4$ solution has been added to 100 ml of $FeSO_4$ solution of the same normality. Evidently, at this point only 50% of the Fe^{++} ions contained in 100 ml of the original solution has been converted into Fe^{+++} ions. We can therefore write*:

$$E = 0.77 + \frac{0.058}{1} \log \frac{50}{50} = 0.77 \text{ V}$$

The points of special interest on the titration curve are those corresponding to 0.1 ml deficiency and 0.1 ml excess of $KMnO_4$, as these points determine the magnitude of the break of potential at the equivalence point. Let us find the first of these points (the start of the abrupt change). At this point 99.9 ml of $KMnO_4$ solution has been added, or 0.1 ml less than is required by the reaction equation; therefore, 0.1 ml of Fe^{++} remains unoxidized in solution and all the rest of the Fe^{++}, which was contained in 99.9 ml of the original solution, has been titrated (i.e., converted into Fe^{+++}). Therefore, at this point

$$E = 0.77 + \frac{0.058}{1} \log \frac{99.9}{0.1} = 0.944 \text{ V}$$

We now find E at the end of the break, i.e., when 100.1 ml of permanganate solution has been added; of this volume, 100 ml was consumed in the reaction with Fe^{++} ions, so that the MnO_4^- in it was reduced to Mn^{++}. The amount of permanganate contained in the added excess (0.1 ml) of solution remains in the form of MnO_4^- ions. Therefore, the ratio $[MnO_4^-] : [Mn^{++}]$ at this point is 0.1 : 100, and

$$E = 1.51 + \frac{0.08}{5} \log \frac{0\ 1 \times [H^+]^8}{100}$$

Assuming that the H^+ ion concentration in the solution is 1 g-ion/litre, we have:

$$E = 1.51 + \frac{0.058}{5} \log 10^{-3} = 1.475 \text{ V}$$

Finally, we calculate E at the equivalence point.

To do this, we multiply Equation (2) by 5 in order to make the coefficients of the logarithmic terms in Equations (1) and (2) equal. The two equations are then added term by term**:

$$E = 0.77 + 0.058 \log \frac{[Fe^{+++}]}{[Fe^{++}]}$$

$$5E = 5 \times 1.51 + 0.058 \log \frac{[MnO_4^-]}{[Mn^{++}]}$$

$$6E = 0.77 + 5 \times 1.51 + 0.058 \log \frac{[Fe^{+++}][MnO_4^-]}{[Fe^{++}][Mn^{++}]} \qquad (3)$$

* Since the Nernst equation contains the *ratio* of the concentrations, $[Fe^{+++}] : [Fe^{++}]$, it can be replaced by the equal ratio of the volumes of the titrated and untitrated parts of the solution (in the present example the original solution volume is 100 ml, and the ratio is 50 : 50).

** The H^+ ion concentration is taken to be 1 M. In both equations E represents the oxidation potential of the given solution and therefore has the same value.

Table XVII

Variations of the Oxidation Potential During Titration of 100 ml of $FeSO_4$ Solution with Permanganate Solution of the Same Normality (at $[H^+]=1$)

$KMnO_4$ added, ml	Excess, ml		$\frac{[Fe^{+++}]}{[Fe^{++}]}$	$\frac{[MnO_4^-]}{[Mn^{++}]}$	Calculations	Oxidation potential E, V
	$FeSO_4$	$KMnO_4$				
50	50	—	$50:50=1$	—	$E=0.77+0.058 \log 1$	0.770
91	9	—	$91:9\approx 10$	—	$E=0.77+0.058 \log 10$	0.828
99	1	—	$99:1\approx 100$	—	$E=0.77+$ $+0.058 \log 100$	0.886
99.9	0.1	—	$99.9:0.1\approx$ $\approx 1,000$	—	$E=0.77+$ $+0.058 \log 1,000$	0.944
100 (equiv. pt.)	—	—	—	—	$E=\frac{0.77+5\times 1.51}{5+1}$	1.387 *
100.1	—	0.1	—	$0.1:100=$ $=0.001$	$E=1.51+$ $+\frac{0.058}{5}\log 0.001$	1.475
101.0	—	1.0	—	$1:100=0.01$	$E=1.51+$ $+\frac{0.058}{5}\log 0.01$	1.487
110.0	—	10	—	$10:100=0.1$	$E=1.51+$ $+\frac{0.058}{5}\log 0.1$	1.498
200.0	—	100	—	$100:100=1$	$E=1.51+$ $+\frac{0.058}{5}\log 1$	1.510

* These figures show that the equivalence point is not in the middle of the break, as was the case in titration curves by the neutralization method.

At the equivalence point the amount of MnO_4^- ions added corresponds to the reaction equation

$$5Fe^{++} + MnO_4^- + 8H^{\cdot} \rightleftarrows 5Fe^{+++} + Mn^{++} + 4H_2O$$

and therefore at equilibrium there must be $5Fe^{++}$ ions for each MnO_4^- ion remaining in solution. Therefore, at the equivalence point the *molar* concentration of Fe^{++} ions is five times the concentration of MnO_4^- ions, i.e.,

$$[Fe^{++}]=5[MnO_4^-]$$

Similarly we find that at the equivalence point

$$[Fe^{+++}] = 5[Mn^{++}]$$

Dividing the second of these equations by the first, we have:

$$\frac{[Fe^{+++}]}{[Fe^{++}]} = \frac{[Mn^{++}]}{[MnO_4^-]} \text{ and } \frac{[Fe^{+++}][MnO_4^-]}{[Fe^{++}][Mn^{++}]} = 1$$

And since $\log 1 = 0$, from Equation (3) we have:

$$6E = 0.77 + 5 \times 1.51$$

and

$$E = \frac{0.77 + 5 \times 1.51}{6} = 1.387 \text{ V}$$

In general, if the standard potentials of the systems corresponding to the oxidizing and reducing agents taken are E'_0 and E''_0, and their stoichiometric coefficients are a and b, the oxidation potential of the solution at the equivalence point is*:

$$E = \frac{bE'_0 + aE''_0}{a+b} \qquad (4)$$

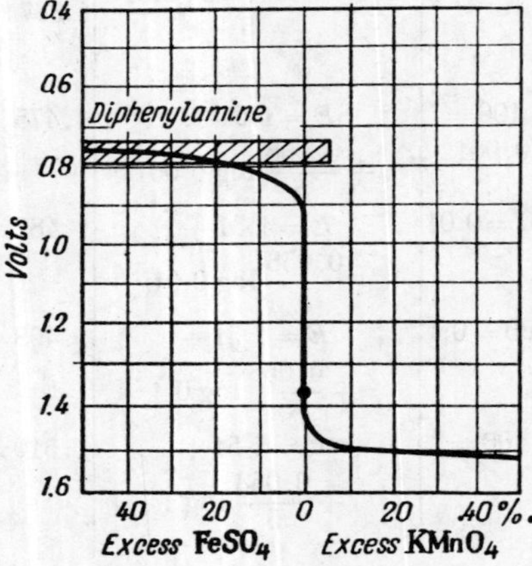

Fig. 57. Curve for titration of $FeSO_4$ solution with permanganate (at $[H^+] = 1$)

The calculation of the titration curve is given in Table XVI, and the curve itself is plotted in Fig. 57.

Figure 57 shows that oxidimetric titration curves are of the same general form as acid-base titration curves. Here again there is an abrupt change of potential near the equivalence point, but the curve is very flat in the remaining regions, which means that E changes very slowly during the titration. The break on the titration curve can be used for precise determination of the equivalence point with the aid of special indicators (fuller details are given in Sec. 82).

---

* If we represent the reaction taking place during the titration by the schematic equation $a\text{Ox.}_1 + b\text{Red.}_2 \rightleftarrows a\text{Red.}_1 + b\text{Ox.}_2$, the concentrations ratio at the equivalence point becomes:

$$\frac{[\text{Red.}_1]}{[\text{Ox.}_1]} = \frac{[\text{Ox.}_2]}{[\text{Red.}_2]} = \sqrt[a+b]{K}$$

where K is the equilibrium constant of the reaction (p. 323).

The magnitude of the potential change evidently depends on the difference between the standard oxidation potentials of the two systems: the greater the difference, the greater the change of potential.

At the same time, oxidimetric titration curves are usually independent of dilution, because the Nernst equation contains the ratio of the concentrations of the oxidized and reduced forms, which does not alter with dilution.*

It must be pointed out, however, that all this is true only if the stoichiometric coefficients of the oxidized and reduced forms in each system are equal. Otherwise the ion concentrations in the numerator and denominator of the logarithmic fraction are raized to different powers. Therefore, both this fraction and the oxidation potential E of the solution would alter with dilution. As the numerator and the denominator of the fraction are raized to different powers, changes of concentration as the solution is diluted influence the value of the potential. For example, in chromatometric determination of ferrous iron the reaction can be represented by the following equation:

$$Cr_2O_7^{--} + 6Fe^{++} + 14H^+ = 2Cr^{+++} + 6Fe^{+++} + 7H_2O$$

The oxidation potential of the $Cr_2O_7^{--}/2Cr^{+++}$ system is given by the expression

$$E = E_0 + \frac{0.058}{6} \log \frac{[Cr_2O_7^{--}][H^+]^{14}}{[Cr^{+++}]^2}$$

If the solution is diluted to double the original volume the ratio $[Cr_2O_7^{--}]$: : $[Cr^{+++}]^2$ is doubled. Moreover, the potential is also strongly influenced by the decrease of H^+ ion concentration. This last factor must be taken into account in all cases where H^+ ions are involved in the titration reaction. In such cases the titration curve is independent of concentration only if $[H^+]$ is maintained practically constant.

The fact that the titration curve is independent of dilution is an advantage of the oxidimetric method over titration by the neutralization method.

Another advantage is that the break on the oxidimetric titration curve can be extended considerably if one of the ions formed in the reaction is combined in the form of a complex; this is sometimes taken advantage of in practice (see Sec. 82).

Suppose, for example, that ions such as PO_4^{---}, F^-, etc., which combine with Fe^{+++} ions to form stable complexes such as $[Fe(PO_4)_2]^{---}$, $[FeF_6]^{---}$, etc., are introduced into the solution. The ordinates of all the points on the titration curve calculated from the formula

$$E = 0.77 + 0.058 \log \frac{[Fe^{+++}]}{[Fe^{++}]}$$

* That is why it is possible to use more dilute solutions in oxidimetry than in neutralization procedures.

are then lowered and the break begins at a lower value of E than in absence of the added ions. For example, if the concentration of Fe^{+++} ions is lowered 10,000-fold owing to their presence, the break on the titration curve begins not at $E = 0.944$ V but at

$$E = 0.77 + 0.058 \log \frac{99.9}{0.1 \times 10^4} = 0.712 \text{ V}$$

It ends, as before, at $E = 1.475$ V. Thus, the extent of the break on the titration curve is increased considerably as the result of complex formation.

82. Indicators Used in Oxidation-Reduction Methods

Turning to indicators used in titrations by the oxidation-reduction method, we must first note that in some cases it is possible to do without them if the colour of the titrating solution undergoes a sharp enough change as the result of the reaction.

Titration *without an indicator* is possible, for example, when various reducing agents are oxidized by permanganate in acid solution. We know that the purple-violet colour of the MnO_4^- ion disappears owing to reduction to the almost colourless Mn^{++} ion. When all the reducing agent has been titrated a single excess drop of permanganate colours the whole solution a distinct pink.

Similarly, reducing agents can be titrated with iodine solution without the use of indicators, because the dark brown colour of iodine disappears as the result of reduction of I_2 to I^- ions. However, since the colour of I_2 solutions is not very deep, it is convenient in such cases to use an indicator—starch solution, which gives an intense blue colour even with very small amounts of free iodine. The use of starch is based on its ability to form a blue adsorption compound with iodine, and is unrelated to the oxidizing properties of I_2.

However, there are indicators which change colour when the oxidation potential of the titrated solution reaches a definite value; such colour changes do not depend on the specific properties of the oxidizing or reducing agents used. Such indicators are known as oxidation-reduction or *redox* indicators.

Such indicators include diphenylamine $NH(C_6H_5)_2$, which is used in qualitative analysis as a reagent for the NO_3^- ion. The latter oxidizes diphenylamine (which is colourless in solution) to another compound (diphenylbenzidine violet),* which has a blue-violet colour.

---

* Its structural formula is:

$C_6H_5{-}N{=}C_6H_4{=}C_6H_4{=}N{-}C_6H_5$

Diphenylamine is also oxidized by many other oxidizing agents with high oxidation potentials, such as $KMnO_4$, $K_2Cr_2O_7$, $KClO_3$, KNO_2, etc. It is therefore essentially a reagent for a definite oxidation potential, just as acid-base indicators are reagents for definite pH values.

It is clear from all this that *redox indicators are substances which can be reversibly oxidized or reduced, with different colours in the oxidized and reduced forms.*

If we denote these forms by the symbols $Ind_{Ox.}$ and $Ind_{Red.}$, their interconversion can be represented by the following equation:

$$Ind_{Ox.} + ne \rightleftarrows Ind_{Red.}$$

Evidently, a system consisting of $Ind_{Ox.}$ and $Ind_{Red.}$ is a redox system. Applying the Nernst equation to it, we have:

$$E = E_0 + \frac{0.058}{n} \log \frac{[Ind_{Ox.}]}{[Ind_{Red.}]} \qquad (1)$$

Here E_0 is the standard oxidation potential of the system, i.e., the potential corresponding to the case when

$$[Ind_{Ox.}] = [Ind_{Red.}]$$

If we add 1-2 drops of a solution of some redox indicator to a solution of a reducing (or oxidizing) agent, the concentrations of the oxidized and reduced forms of the indicator will be in a ratio corresponding to the oxidation potential of the solution. The solution acquires the colour corresponding to that ratio. If this solution is titrated with an oxidizing (or reducing) agent, the oxidation potential E changes. The $\frac{[Ind_{Ox.}]}{[Ind_{Red.}]}$ ratio alters accordingly. However, as with acid-base indicators, not every change of this ratio corresponds to a colour change which can be perceived by the eye. If we assume that the presence of one of the coloured forms can no longer be detected by the eye when its concentration becomes one-tenth of the concentration of the other form, we have the following range of E:

$$E_1 = E_0 + \frac{0.058}{n} \log \frac{1}{10} = E_0 - \frac{0.058}{n} \text{ (colour of } Ind_{Red.})$$

$$E_2 = E_0 + \frac{0.058}{n} \log \frac{10}{1} = E_0 + \frac{0.058}{n} \text{ (colour of } Ind_{Ox.})$$

Consequently*

$$\text{the range} = E_0 \pm \frac{0.058}{n} \qquad (2)$$

---

* Equation (2) is clearly quite analogous to the equation pH range = $= pK \pm 1$ for acid-base indicators (p. 243).

In the case of diphenylamine indicator, for which $E_0 = +0.76$ V and $n = 2$, the range is

$$\text{from } E_1 = 0.76 - \frac{0.058}{2} \approx 0.73 \text{ V}$$

$$\text{to } E_2 = 0.76 + \frac{0.058}{2} \approx 0.79 \text{ V}$$

At potentials below 0.73 V the reduced form of the indicator (diphenylamine) is predominant, and the solution therefore remains colourless. At E = 0.79 V and over the oxidized form (diphenylbenzidine violet) is predominant and the solution has an intense blue-violet colour. Between 0.73 V and 0.79 V the colour of the solution changes gradually from colourless to blue-violet.

The range in which the indicator changes colour must be within the limits of the sharp change of potential on the titration curve in order that the colour change of a redox indicator should be sharp and the indicator error in titration small.

For example, diphenylamine is evidently unsuitable as an indicator in titration of ferrous iron with permanganate (the change of potential extends from E = 0.944 V to E = 1.475 V). In fact, it is evident from Table XVII (p. 327) that its colour would change when only about 50% of the Fe^{++} has been oxidized, and the change would be very slow, as the titration curve is almost horizontal over this region.

However, it was pointed out above (p. 330) that if Fe^{+++} ions are converted into complex form by addition of PO_4^{---} or F^- ions it is possible to lower sharply the potential at which the change begins. In presence of these ions the colour change of diphenylamine is within the range of the potential break and diphenylamine is then quite suitable as an indicator.

Of course, no indicator is necessary in titration with permanganate, but in titration of ferrous salts with dichromate

$$6Fe^{++} + Cr_2O_7^{--} + 14H^+ = 6Fe^{+++} + 2Cr^{+++} + 7H_2O$$

which is a reaction of great practical importance, an indicator is needed. It was for this titration that the first of the redox indicators, diphenylamine, was used for the first time (in 1924).

Since in this case the break on the titration curve extends from E = 0.944 V to E = 1.302 V, all that was said earlier about titration of Fe^{++} with permanganate fully applies here. The titration is performed in presence of H_3PO_4, which converts the Fe^{+++} ion into the stable $[Fe(PO_4)_2]^{---}$ complex, in order that the colour change of the indicator should be sharp and the indicator error negligible.

However, there are redox indicators with higher values of E_0. They include phenylanthranilic acid,* proposed by V. Syrokomsky, V. Stepin, A. Kirsanov, and V. Cherkasov, which has $E_0 = +1.08$ V. In presence of this indicator dichromate can be titrated (in strongly acid solution) with ferrous salts even without addition of H_3PO_4.

The number of redox indicators with various values of E_0 now available is quite large.

The discovery of new indicators is of considerable interest in volumetric analysis, as it extends the application of oxidimetric methods.

Some redox indicators are listed in Table XVIII.

Table XVIII

Redox Indicators

Indicator	Colour		E_0 at $[H^+] = 1$ (V)
	$Ind_{Ox.}$	$Ind_{Red.}$	
Neutral red	Red	Colourless	+0.24
Methylene blue	Greenish blue	Colourless	+0.53
Diphenylamine	Blue-violet	Colourless	+0.76
Diphenylamineazosulphonic acid	Red-violet	Colourless	+0.85
Erioglucin A	Red	Green	+1.00
Phenylanthranilic acid	Red-violet	Colourless	+1.08
Ferroin (complex of *o*-phenanthroline with Fe^{++})	Pale blue	Red	+1.14 *
Diphenylamine-2,2′-dicarboxylic acid	Blue-violet	Colourless	+1.26

* Appreciable colour change at +1.20 V.

In addition to their great advantage, namely, that they can be used in various oxidimetric methods, redox indicators are not without considerable disadvantages. For example, the potential at which one form of an indicator is converted into the other often varies with the solution pH. In some cases the colour change is rather slow or intermediate compounds are formed. Accordingly, titrations with permanganate are still preferably carried out without indicators; iodometric titrations are, as formerly, carried out with the use of starch.

It was shown in Sec. 81 that in an oxidation-reduction titration the oxidation potential of the solution undergoes a more or less abrupt change near the equivalence point. Therefore, if a platinum electrode is immersed in the solution to be titrated and the resultant half-cell is connected to a standard half-cell of accu-

* Also known as diphenylamine-2-carboxylic acid.

rately known potential (for example, a standard hydrogen electrode or, more conveniently, a calomel electrode)* the result is a cell the e.m.f. of which changes sharply near the equivalence point. Therefore, if this e.m.f. is measured periodically by means of a potentiometer during the titration, the sharp change of e.m.f. shows when the equivalence point is reached. This is the principle of *potentiometric titration* of oxidizing and reducing agents.

Potentiometric titration can also be used in the neutralization method. For this the solution being titrated can be converted into a hydrogen half-cell**, which is then connected to a suitable standard half-cell and the e.m.f. of the resultant cell is measured during the titration. Since this e.m.f. depends in this case on the H^+ ion concentration in the solution being titrated, and this concentration changes abruptly at the equivalence point, the latter can be easily detected.

In addition to the conductometric method referred to earlier (p. 191) the potentiometric method greatly extends the applicability of volumetric analysis and is of great practical importance.

83. Rate of Oxidation-Reduction Reactions

Oxidation-reduction reactions have a number of specific features which hinder their use in volumetric analysis.

These features include reversibility which, as was noted earlier, must be prevented in some instances. Another peculiarity is the inadequate rate of many oxidation-reduction reactions. We know that slow reactions are unsuitable for titrations, because not only is the titration very slow, but it cannot be performed accurately enough. Therefore, if it is desired to use such reactions in volumetric analysis, they must be accelerated.

Slow reactions can be accelerated by various methods, foremost of which is increase of the solution temperature. The influence of temperature on the rate of reaction is enormous.

As a rule, *the rate of a reaction is doubled or trebled when the temperature is raised by 10°C*. Therefore, as the temperature is raised in arithmetical progression, the reaction rate increases in geometrical progression.

Therefore, very often a reaction which hardly proceeds at all at room temperature proceeds at an adequate rate on heating. An example important in analysis is the reaction

$$5H_2C_2O_4 + 2KMnO_4 + 3H_2SO_4 = 2MnSO_4 + K_2SO_4 + 8H_2O + 10CO_2\uparrow$$

---

* The calomel electrode consists of metallic mercury in contact with KCl solution saturated with calomel (Hg_2Cl_2). It constitutes the system $Hg_2^{++}/2Hg$, the potential of which is determined by the concentration of Hg_2^{++} ions in solution. This concentration, by the solubility product rule, depends on the Cl^- ion concentration, i.e., on the KCl concentration in solution. If the KCl concentration is 1 *N*, then *E* of the calomel electrode is 0.2816 V (at 25°C).

** This is done in the same way as in construction of a standard hydrogen electrode (p. 313), but the electrolyte is the solution to be titrated instead of H_2SO_4 solution.

which takes place when oxalic acid is titrated with permanganate; this titration should be performed at 70-80°C.

However, it is not always possible to heat the solution, as this may cause either volatilization of one of the reacting substance (for example, of I_2 in iodometric determinations) or oxidation by atmospheric oxygen (oxidation of Fe^{++} during titration of $FeSO_4$ solution with permanganate).

In such cases other methods are used for increasing the rate of reaction; for example, increase of the concentrations of the reacting substances. For instance, the slow reaction

$$6KI + K_2Cr_2O_7 + 7H_2SO_4 = 3I_2 + 4K_2SO_4 + Cr_2(SO_4)_3 + 7H_2O$$

can be accelerated by increase of the H^+ or I^- ion concentrations in solution.

By the law of mass action, the rate of a chemical reaction in a homogeneous medium is directly proportional to the products of the concentrations of the reacting substances if these concentrations are raised to the powers corresponding to the respective stoichiometric coefficients. For example, the rate (v) of the reaction

$$2I^- + H_2O_2 + 2H^+ = I_2 + 2H_2O$$

is, by the law of mass action, given by the equation

$$v = K\,[I^-]^2\,[H_2O_2]\,[H^+]^2$$

where K is the reaction rate constant.

If the concentrations of all three substances are the same and equal to C, we have:

$$v = KC^5$$

However, it is found in practice that the rate of this reaction is proportional to the square and not to the fifth power of the concentration, i.e., $v = KC^2$. Similar deviations from the law of mass action are found with many other oxidation-reduction reactions.

The cause of the deviations lies in the complexity of these reactions. Very often they involve not only transfer of electrons but also a resultant change in the composition of ions taking part in the reaction. Such changes of composition take place, for example, in the reduction of MnO_4^- and $Cr_2O_7^{--}$ ions to Mn^{++} and Cr^{+++} cations.

Complex reactions of this type always pass through a series of intermediate stages, so that the equation for such a reaction does not represent the true course of the process but only the over-all result. The rate of the process as a whole depends on the rates of its individual stages and therefore it cannot be predicted from an over-all equation of this type.

The following considerations show that many oxidation-reduction processes must pass through a series of intermediate stages. Chemical reactions in solutions occur by collisions of the corresponding ions (or molecules). The probability of collision, other things being equal, depends on the number of particles taking part in a given reaction. For example, the probability of collision in a "bimolecular" reaction between two ions, such as

$$Ce^{++++} + Fe^{++} = Ce^{+++} + Fe^{+++}$$

must be far higher than in "trimolecular" reactions such as

$$Sn^{++} + 2Fe^{+++} = Sn^{++++} + 2Fe^{++}$$

or

$$2Fe^{++} + I_2 = 2Fe^{+++} + 2I^-$$

in each of which three particles must collide simultaneously at one point in space in exactly the right proportions. The probability of tetra-, penta-, etc., molecular reactions is so low that such reactions are impossible in practice. All such reactions must inevitably pass through certain intermediate stages each of which is a bi- or trimolecular reaction.

Usually the precise nature of these intermediate stages is unknown. However, in some instances they can be identified and the true course of the process can thus be revealed. For example, the reaction

$$2I^- + H_2O_2 + 2H^+ = I_2 + 2H_2O \qquad \text{(a)}$$

is, according to the above over-all equation, pentamolecular. It has been found experimentally that one of its intermediate stages involves the formation of the hypoiodite ion IO^- by the equation

$$I^- + H_2O_2 = IO^- + H_2O \qquad \text{(b)}$$

The IO^- ions then combine with H^+ ions

$$IO^- + H^+ \rightleftarrows HIO \qquad \text{(c)}$$

and, finally, HIO, being a strong oxidizing agent, oxidizes I^- ions in accordance with the equation

$$HIO + I^- + H^+ \rightleftarrows I_2 + H_2O \qquad \text{(d)}$$

Adding Equations (b), (c) and (d) we have the over-all Equation (a).

It is evident that *the rate of a complex reaction of this type is determined by the rate of its slowest intermediate stage.* The slowest stage of the oxidation-reduction process we are considering here is reaction (b), and since this is a bimolecular reaction the rate of the process as a whole must be proportional to the square of the concentration, as is found to be the case in practice.

Therefore, the deviations of the rates of oxidation-reduction reactions from the law of mass action are merely apparent deviations, which are due to the existence in the oxidation-reduction processes of intermediate stages, generally not known precisely.

In addition to increase of temperature and of concentration, introduction of catalysts may influence the reaction rate.

Catalysts are substances which influence reaction rates but are themselves unchanged by the reactions. In addition to positive catalysts, which accelerate reactions, there are also negative catalysts, which retard them.*

However, the fact that a catalyst is not expended in a reaction does not mean that it takes no part in it.

The action of catalysts in reactions taking place in homogeneous media is associated with intermediate reaction stages in which the catalyst is also involved. However, the catalyst is completely regenerated during the subsequent reaction stages and therefore it is not consumed in the reaction. If these intermediate stages proceed more rapidly in presence of the catalyst than the stages which do not involve the catalyst, the reaction is accelerated.

A well-known example of homogeneous catalysis is the oxidation of thiosulphate by hydrogen peroxide:

$$H_2O_2 + 2S_2O_3^{--} + 2H^+ \rightleftarrows S_4O_6^{--} + 2H_2O$$

This reaction is catalytically accelerated by I^- ions. Their action is clear from the equations for the separate stages of the process:

$$H_2O_2 + I^- \rightarrow IO^- + H_2O \text{ (at a measurable rate)} \qquad \text{(e)}$$

$$IO^- + H^+ \rightleftarrows HIO \text{ (very rapid)} \qquad \text{(f)}$$

$$HIO + I^- + H^+ \rightleftarrows I_2 + H_2O \text{ (very rapid)} \qquad \text{(g)}$$

$$I_2 + I^- \rightleftarrows I_3^- \text{ (very rapid)} \qquad \text{(h)}$$

$$I_3^- + 2S_2O_3^{--} \rightarrow S_4O_6^{--} + 3I^- \text{ (very rapid)} \qquad \text{(i)}$$

Adding the five above equations, we obtain (after cancelling) the over-all reaction equation given above. This equation does not include the catalyst (I^- ions) because all three I^- ions used in stages (e), (g) and (h) are regenerated at stage (i) and are therefore not consumed.

The slowest stage of this reaction is oxidation of I^- ions by hydrogen peroxide (e). However, this is more rapid than the (unknown) stage which determines the reaction rate in absence of I^- ions.

* Such catalysts are usually known as inhibitors.

Another example of homogeneous catalysis important in analysis, which has been studied by N. Shilov, is oxidation of oxalic acid by permanganate

$$5H_2C_2O_4 + 2KMnO_4 + 3H_2SO_4 = K_2SO_4 + 2MnSO_4 + 8H_2O + 10CO_2\uparrow$$

which is catalytically accelerated by addition of $MnSO_4$. The action of $MnSO_4$ can probably be described as follows.

First the added $MnSO_4$ is oxidized by permanganate:

$$3MnSO_4 + 2KMnO_4 + 2H_2O = 5MnO_2 + K_2SO_4 + 2H_2SO_4 \qquad (1)$$

The manganese dioxide so formed at once oxidizes $H_2C_2O_4$ and is itself reduced to a salt of trivalent manganese (III):

$$2MnO_2 + H_2C_2O_4 + 3H_2SO_4 = Mn_2(SO_4)_3 + 4H_2O + 2CO_2 \qquad (2)$$

Finally, $Mn_2(SO_4)_3$ reacts with $H_2C_2O_4$ and is reduced to the original compound $MnSO_4$:

$$H_2C_2O_4 + Mn_2(SO_4)_3 = 2MnSO_4 + 2CO_2 + H_2SO_4 \qquad (3)$$

If we multiply Equation (1) by two and Equations (2) and (3) by five and then add all three equations together, after cancelling we obtain the over-all equation given above. This shows that the $MnSO_4$ added to the solution is completely regenerated and is not consumed in the reaction. However, the reaction is greatly accelerated in its presence, so that the intermediate reactions proceed (on heating) very rapidly.* The catalytic action of Mn^{++} ions may be schematically represented as follows:

$$\begin{array}{ccc} Mn^{++} & \xrightarrow{MnO_4^-} & MnO_2 \\ \uparrow{\scriptstyle H_2C_2O_4} & & \downarrow{\scriptstyle H_2C_2O_4} \\ & Mn^{+++} & \end{array}$$

It should be noted that one of the products in this reaction is a salt of bivalent manganese which catalyses the reaction. Such reactions are known as *autocatalytic.* If $MnSO_4$ is not added previously to the solution then the first few drops of permanganate added during titration of hot acidified $H_2C_2O_4$ solution are decolorized slowly. However, as soon as a small amount of Mn^{++} ions has been formed subsequent decolorization of $KMnO_4$ is virtually instantaneous.

Whereas the direction and the extent of the reaction depend on the sign and magnitude of the potential difference between the two

*** In view of the low probability of reactions involving the simultaneous collision of more than three particles (p. 336) it is likely that the stages detailed above themselves proceed by stages; however, the nature of the latter is unknown.**

systems, the rate of an oxidation-reduction reaction is independent of the potential difference.

For example, the oxidation of gaseous hydrogen by oxygen, which corresponds to a very large difference of standard oxidation potentials (1.23 V), proceeds at an immeasurably low rate at room temperature (to which the corresponding values of E_0 refer). On the other hand, oxidation of Fe^{++} ions by the oxygen of the air is much more rapid, despite the considerably smaller difference of potentials (0.46 V).

This must be taken into account when we use the table of oxidation potentials; not every oxidation-reduction reaction which is possible on the basis of the oxidation potentials of the corresponding systems can be effected in practice, because its rate may be too low.

84. Side Reactions in Oxidation-Reduction Titrations

One complication which hinders the use of redox processes in volumetric analysis is the occurrence (together with the required reaction) of side reactions which consume an unknown amount of the standard solution. As a result the determination itself becomes impossible if steps are not taken to prevent the side reactions.

As one of the most important examples of this, let us consider the permanganate determination of ferrous iron, based on the reaction

$$5Fe^{++} + MnO_4^- + 8H^+ = 5Fe^{+++} + Mn^{++} + 4H_2O$$

It is clear from the above equation that H^+ ions are consumed in the reaction, and so it must be conducted in acid solution. However, the nature of the acid with which H^+ ions are introduced is significant. It is found in practice that in presence of sulphuric acid the amount of permanganate taken corresponds accurately to the Fe^{++} content and a correct result is obtained in the determination. On the other hand, in presence of HCl or chlorides the amount of $KMnO_4$ taken is too high, which shows that permanganate is consumed in a side reaction of some kind. As the solution smells of chlorine during the titration, it is obvious that this side reaction is

$$10Cl^- + 2MnO_4^- + 16H^+ = 2Mn^{++} + 8H_2O + 5Cl_2 \quad (1)$$

Of course, the free chlorine formed in this reaction must itself oxidize Fe^{++} ions:

$$2Fe^{++} + Cl_2 = 2Fe^{+++} + 2Cl^-$$

If all the chlorine remained in solution, the amount of iron oxidized by it would be exactly equivalent to the amount of permanganate used in formation of Cl_2 by reaction (1). In practice, however, some of the chlorine evaporates and this accounts for the excess amount of $KMnO_4$ taken for the titration.

It is interesting to note that although according to the values of the standard oxidation potentials of the systems MnO_4^-/Mn^{++} ($E_0 = +1.51$ V) and $Cl_2/2Cl^-$ ($E_0 = +1.36$ V) oxidation of Cl^- ions by permanganate is possible, in practice this reaction does not occur in absence of Fe^{++} ions at the concentrations used in titration. For example, arsenous and oxalic acids can be titrated with permanganate even in presence of hydrochloric acid.* Therefore, the oxidation of Fe^{++} by permanganate "induces" the side reaction of oxidation of Cl^- ions to Cl_2.

Many such *induced* or *coupled* oxidation-reduction reactions are known. They were studied in detail by N. Shilov (1905).

The occurrence of coupled oxidation-reduction reactions is due to the existence of intermediate stages in the oxidation-reduction process. For example, it was stated earlier that the reaction between I^- ions and hydrogen peroxide proceeds through a number of intermediate stages, where IO^- ions and free hypoiodous acid HIO are first formed; these products contain iodine in a higher state of oxidation (valence + 1) than the final reaction product, I_2 (valence 0).

The intermediate reaction product (HIO) is a very powerful oxidizing agent and as soon as it is formed it oxidizes I^- ions to I_2:

$$HIO + I^- + H^+ = I_2 + H_2O$$

According to the theory put forward by the well-known Russian chemist A. Bakh, analogous formation of more highly oxidized intermediate compounds, having higher oxidizing activity, occurs in many other oxidation-reduction processes. The formation of these compounds, termed "*primary oxides*", is the cause of coupled oxidation-reduction reactions.

For example, there is reason to believe that in the case under consideration Fe^{++} ions are first oxidized by MnO_4^- ions to Fe^{+V} which may be schematically represented as follows:

$$Fe^{++} \xrightarrow{MnO_4^-} Fe^{+V} \text{ (primary oxide)}$$

This primary oxide, being a very powerful oxidizing agent, then oxidizes Fe^{++} to Fe^{+++} as follows:

$$2Fe^{++} + Fe^{+V} = 3Fe^{+++}$$

---

* In the case of $H_2C_2O_4$ the solution must be heated to about 70°C for the titration.

However, if Cl^- ions are present in solution the primary oxide does what permanganate cannot do under the given conditions; it oxidizes part of the Cl^- ions to Cl_2:

$$Fe^{+V} + 2Cl^- = Fe^{+++} + Cl_2 \text{ (coupled reaction)}$$

That is why Cl_2 is formed when Fe^{++} is titrated with permanganate.

It is found in practice that Cl^- ions can be protected against coupled oxidation to Cl_2 if the titration is conducted in the presence of a manganous salt such as $MnSO_4$. Apparently the function of the Mn^{++} ions depends on the fact that they are oxidized more readily than Cl^- ions by the primary oxide. Therefore, in their presence, instead of the above coupled reaction, the following reaction occurs:

$$Fe^{+V} + Mn^{++} = Fe^{+++} + Mn^{+IV}$$

The occurrence of this reaction does not lead to analytical error, because, in contrast to Cl_2, the Mn^{+IV} formed remains in solution and at once oxidizes an equivalent amount of Fe^{++}:

$$2Fe^{++} + Mn^{+IV} = 2Fe^{+++} + Mn^{++}$$

Therefore, in the presence of a bivalent manganese salt ferrous iron can be titrated with permanganate even in the presence of hydrochloric acid. This is of great practical importance in the analysis of iron ores and similar materials which are usually dissolved in hydrochloric acid.

In conclusion, we must draw attention to the following fact. In the neutralization method we deal with whole groups of compounds, such as strong and weak acids, and strong and weak bases. It is then quite immaterial which strong acid (HCl, H_2SO_4 or HNO_3) is used for titrating a given alkali solution. In the same way, solutions of strong alkalies such as NaOH, KOH or $Ba(OH)_2$ are mutually interchangeable.

In oxidation-reduction titrations we cannot replace one oxidizing or reducing agent by another in this way. Each has its specific characteristics, which must be studied. Therefore, the oxidation-reduction method must be subdivided in accordance with the substances used as the principal standard solutions. The four most important subdivisions are permanganometric, chromatometric, iodometric, and bromatometric titrations. These subdivisions are considered in greater detail in the following sections.

QUESTIONS AND PROBLEMS
(on Secs. 78-84)

1. How do oxidation-reduction reactions differ from exchange reactions? What is (a) oxidation, (b) reduction? What are the roles of the oxidizing and reducing agents in the reaction?

2. Explain the difference between weak and strong (a) reducing agents; (b) oxidizing agents. Give examples to illustrate this difference.

3. What are oxidation potentials; how are they determined and what do they characterize?

4. The standard oxidation potential of the Cd^{++}/Cd system is —0.40 V. Name the chemical processes which take place in a cell composed of this system and a standard hydrogen electrode. Write the general equation for the reaction.

5. Do the same for the system Sn^{++++}/Sn^{++} (see Appendix VI).

6. Calculate the oxidation potential of the Mn^{++}/Mn system at Mn^{++} ion concentrations of: (a) 2 g-ions/litre; (b) 0.005 g-ion/litre.

Answer: (a) —1.171 V; (b) —1.124 V.

7. Calculate the oxidation potential of the system Sn^{++++}/Sn^{++} if the Sn^{++++} ion concentration is 0.1 g-ion/litre and the Sn^{++} ion concentration is 0.0001 g-ion/litre.

Answer: 0.237 V.

8. A cell consists of a standard hydrogen electrode and the Ni^{++}/Ni system; with a Ni^{++} concentration of 0.01 g-ion/litre its e.m.f. is 0.192 V, and the nickel electrode is the cathode. Find the standard oxidation potential of the Ni^{++}/Ni system.

Answer: —0.250 V.

9. Calculate the oxidation potential of permanganate if $[MnO_4^-] = [Mn^{++}]$ at hydrogen ion concentrations of: (a) 1 g-ion/litre; (b) 10^{-5} g-ion/litre.

Answer: (a) 1.51 V; (b) 1.046 V.

10. Is it possible: (a) to oxidize $SnCl_2$ to $SnCl_4$ by the action of Cl_2; (b) to oxidize Cl^- to Cl_2 by the action of PbO_2 in acid solution; (c) to oxidize Mn^{++} to MnO_4^-, Br^- ions to Br_2, or Fe^{++} ions to Fe^{+++} ions by the action of HNO_3; (d) to oxidize I^- to I_2 or Cl^- to Cl_2, by the action of $KClO_3$ in acid solution; (e) to oxidize AsO_3^{---} to AsO_4^{---}, Mn^{++} to MnO_4^-, SO_3^{--}, to SO_4^{--}, or SO_4^{--} to $S_2O_8^{--}$ by the action of $K_2Cr_2O_7$ in acid solution?

11. Is it possible to effect the following reductions by the action of Fe^{++}: Cl_2 to Cl^-, I_2 to I^-, Sn^{++++} to Sn^{++}, MnO_4^- in acid solution to Mn^{++}, or $Cr_2O_7^{--}$ in acid solution to Cr^{+++}?

12. Which of the following metals can reduce H^+ ions to H_2 (i.e., displace hydrogen from acid solutions): Cd, Sn, Sb, Al, Ag?

13. The solubility product of AgI is $\sim 1 \times 10^{-16}$. By calculating the required oxidation potential, determine whether metallic silver can displace hydrogen from 1 *N* HI solution.

Answer: Yes ($E \approx -0.128$ V).

14. An equivalent amount of HCl solution is added to an $AgNO_3$ solution which is one of the electrode liquids in a cell consisting of Ag^+/Ag and a standard hydrogen electrode. Use the value of the solubility product of AgCl to determine whether this would reverse the direction of the current in the cell.

Answer: The current would not be reversed.

15. In the cell described in the preceding problem one of the electrode liquids is 0.1 *M* silver nitrate solution. To this solution enough solid KCN is added to make the CN^- ion concentration in solution 1 g-ion/litre. Given that the instability constant of the $[Ag(CN)_2]^-$ complex is 1×10^{-21}, determine whether the direction of the current in the cell is reversed.

Answer: Yes.

16. Use the values of the standard oxidation potentials of the systems MnO_2/Mn^{++} and $Cl_2/2Cl^-$ to determine the course of the reaction between them. Explain how Cl_2 is prepared in the laboratory by the action of concentrated HCl on MnO_2.

17. Derive the formulas for calculating the equilibrium constants of the reactions:

(a) $Sn^{++} + I_2 \rightleftarrows Sn^{++++} + 2I^-$

(b) $MnO_4^- + 8H^+ + 5Fe^{++} \rightleftarrows Mn^{++} + 5Fe^{+++} + 4H_2O$

and find their numerical values. Which of the two reactions goes furthe. to completion?

Answer: (a) $\log K = 13.45$; $K = 2.8 \times 10^{13}$; (b) $\log K = 63.8$; $K = 6.3$ 10^{63}.

18. Calculate the range of break of potential and the position of the equivalence point in titration of a 0.1 *N* solution of a ferrous salt with a 0.1 *N* solution of quadrivalent cerium salt. Take into account that Ce^{++++} ions are reduced to Ce^{+++} and that the standard oxidation potential of the system Ce^{++++}/Ce^{+++} is +1.55 V. Discuss whether the curve for this titration depends on the initial concentrations of the two substances (provided that they are equal to each other) or on the H^+ ion concentration.

Answer: The range is between $E = 0.944$ V and $E = 1.376$ V; the equivalence point is at $E = 1.160$ V; the curve does not depend on the concentrations.

19. Perform the analogous calculations and answer the same questions for titration of a ferrous salt with $KClO_3$ solution if the H^+ ion concentration is 1. Write the equation for the reaction.

Answer: The range is between $E = 0.944$ V and $E = 1.411$ V; the equivalence point at $E = 1.344$ V is independent of the concentrations if the solution pH is kept constant.

20. In the titration of Problem 18, what are the concentrations of unchanged Fe^{++} and Ce^{++++} ions at the equivalence point?

Answer: $[Fe^{++}] = [Ce^{++++}] = 1.9 \times 10^{-8}$ g-ion/litre.

21. What are redox indicators? What chemical process causes them to change colour?

22. (a) Can KI solution be used as a redox indicator? (b) Can starch solution, used in titrations of various reducing agents with I_2 solution, be classed as a redox indicator?

Answer: (a) Yes; (b) no.

23. Calculate the range of the redox indicator ferroin; the conversion of its oxidized form into the reduced form is represented by the equation

$$\underset{\text{Pale blue}}{Fe(C_{12}H_8N_2)_3^{+++}} + e \rightleftarrows \underset{\text{Red}}{Fe(C_{12}H_8N_2)_3^{++}}$$

and its standard oxidation potential is +1.14 V.

Answer: From $E = 1.082$ V to $E = 1.198$ V.

24. What is the colour of ferroin (Problem 23) at oxidation potentials of 0.5 V; 1.0 V; 1.14 V; 1.20 V; 1.50 V? In which cases is the colour the same?

25. What factors determine the rate of an oxidation-reduction reaction? Does the rate depend on the difference between the oxidation potentials of the systems involved in the reaction?
26. Explain why in many cases the influence of concentration on the rate of oxidation-reduction reactions is less than the law of mass action indicates.
27. What evidence is there in favour of the view that oxidation-reduction reactions proceed by way of several intermediate stages?
28. What is the explanation of homogeneous catalysis? Give examples.
29. What is the theory of the formation of primary oxides?
30. How are coupled oxidation effects explained?

PERMANGANATE TITRATIONS

85. General Principles of the Method

The permanganate method is based on reactions of oxidation by the permanganate ion. Oxidation may proceed in acid or in alkaline (or neutral) solution.

When $KMnO_4$ acts as an oxidizing agent in acid solution the septivalent manganese in it is reduced to Mn^{++} cations and a manganous salt of the acid used is formed. For example, if $FeSO_4$ is the reducing agent and if it is oxidized in the presence of sulphuric acid the reaction is represented by the equation

$$10FeSO_4 + 2KMnO_4 + 8H_2SO_4 = 5Fe_2(SO_4)_3 + 2MnSO_4 + K_2SO_4 + 8H_2O$$

or, in ionic form

$$5Fe^{++} + MnO_4^- + 8H^+ = 5Fe^{+++} + Mn^{++} + 4H_2O$$

The decrease of the valence of manganese by 5 shows that the $KMnO_4$ molecule gains 5 electrons. This is also clear from the following equation:

$$MnO_4^- + 8H^+ + 5e = Mn^{++} + 4H_2O$$

It follows that in this case (see p. 209) the gram-equivalent of $KMnO_4$ is

$$\text{g-eq} = \frac{158.03}{5} = 31.61 \text{ g}$$

During oxidation in alkaline or neutral solution septivalent manganese is reduced to quadrivalent manganese with the formation of manganese dioxide,* MnO_2, in the form of a brown precipitate, for example:

$$Cr_2(SO_4)_3 + 2KMnO_4 + 8KOH = 2K_2CrO_4 + \downarrow 2MnO_2 + 2K_2SO_4 + 4H_2O$$

The change taking place in the MnO_4^- ion is represented by the equation

$$MnO_4^- + 4H^+ + 3e = MnO_2 + 2H_2O$$

*** More correctly, the hydrated form $MnO(OH)_2$.**

Therefore, in this case the gram-equivalent of $KMnO_4$ has a different value, namely:

$$\text{g-eq} = \frac{158.03}{3} = 52.68 \text{ g}$$

The different course of the reaction in acid and alkaline solutions can be explained as follows: the Mn^{++} ion and MnO_2 are interconvertible:

$$MnO_2 + 4H^+ + 2e \rightleftarrows Mn^{++} + 2H_2O \qquad (1)$$

The equation shows that with increase of H^+ ion concentration in solution the equilibrium between MnO_2 and Mn^{++} ions shifts towards formation of Mn^{++}. Therefore, even if MnO_2 should be initially formed by oxidation of some substance by permanganate in acid solution, because of the high concentration of H^+ ions it would at once be reduced further to give Mn^{++} ions, in accordance with Equation (1).

Conversely, at low H^+ ion concentrations the equilibrium in reaction (1) is shifted far to the left. Therefore, under such conditions MnO_2 is the more stable, and it is formed if the reaction is conducted in alkaline or neutral solution.

It should be noted that MnO_2 may also be formed if the titration is started in the presence of acid but the amount of acid taken is insufficient for the reaction.

In comparing the two types of titration we must first note that the standard oxidation potential of the MnO_4^-/Mn^{++} sustem (+1.51 V) is considerably higher than that of MnO_4^-/MnO_2 (+0.59 V). Therefore, the oxidizing activity of permanganate is incomparably greater in acid than in alkaline solution, and the reducing agents which can be titrated with it in acid solution are much more numerous.

Further, whereas almost colourless Mn^{++} ions, which remain in solution, are formed by titration in acid solution, titration in alkaline or neutral solution results in the formation of a dark brown precipitate of MnO_2 [or, more correctly, its hydrated form $MnO(OH)_2$], which makes it very difficult to establish the equivalence point accurately during titration. For these reasons oxidation with permanganate in acid solution is generally used in volumetric analysis.

86. Preparation and Storage of Standard $KMnO_4$ Solution

No indicators are used for titrations with permanganate (Sec. 82). Since a single drop of $KMnO_4$ solution, even at a concentration of 0.01 N, confers a distinct pink colour to 50 ml of solution at the end point, there is no need to use 0.1 *N* permanganate solutions. Generally, 0.02 *N* solutions are used.

It should be remembered that permanganate is not pure; it always contains some reduction products such as MnO_2. Moreover, it is easily decomposed by reducing agents—ammonia, organic substances entering the water in the form of dust, etc. Because of this the concentration of a $KMnO_4$ solution falls somewhat after preparation.

From this it follows that *standard permanganate solution cannot be prepared by exact weighing. It has to be standardized, and the solution must be kept for at least 7-10 days after preparation.**

In order that the $KMnO_4$ solution should be stable and its titre should remain unchanged the MnO_2 precipitate present in the $KMnO_4$ solution as an impurity, and any MnO_2 formed by oxidation of organic matter and ammonia dissolved in water by the permanganate, must be removed because it catalytically accelerates farther decomposition of $KMnO_4$. It must also be remembered that permanganate oxidizes rubber, cork, paper, etc. These substances must not be allowed to come in contact with the solution. For example, $KMnO_4$ solution must not be filtered through paper; sintered glass crucibles must be used for this purpose, or the permanganate solution must be decanted from the MnO_2 precipitate by means of a siphon.

Permanganate solution must be kept in a dark place or in dark glass bottles, because light accelerates decomposition of $KMnO_4$ by the reaction:

$$4KMnO_4 + 2H_2O = \downarrow 4MnO_2 + 4KOH + 3O_2 \uparrow$$

In view of all these considerations, $KMnO_4$ solution is prepared as follows. Weigh out on a technical balance the amount of $KMnO_4$ required for 1 litre of 0.02 *N* solution. This amount is 0.02 × 31.61 g, i.e., about 0.63 g. Now measure out 1 litre of distilled water in a large measuring cylinder. As $KMnO_4$ crystals dissolve rather slowly, heat a part of this water almost to boiling and treat the $KMnO_4$ with small portions of it in a beaker or flask, with thorough stirring. From time to time carefully decant the liquid from the crystals into another vessel and add another portion of hot water. When the crystals have been dissolved and the solution has cooled, transfer it into a litre flask. Add the remaining water, mix thoroughly, and leave the solution to stand for 7-10 days. The flask should be

* During this time any reducing agents present in solution would be completely oxidized and the titre of the $KMnO_4$ ceases to change. Oxidation of reducing agents is greatly accelerated if the solution is boiled, so that the whole operation can be completed in 1-2 hours.

stoppered and left in the dark (or covered with opaque paper). At the end of this period carefully siphon the liquid from the precipitated MnO_2 (or filter it through a sintered glass crucible).

87. Standardization of $KMnO_4$ Solution

Many primary standards have been proposed for standardization of $KMnO_4$ solutions; they include $H_2C_2O_4 \cdot 2H_2O$, $Na_2C_2O_4$, As_2O_3, $K_4[Fe(CN)_6] \cdot 3H_2O$, metallic iron, etc.

The most convenient of these are $Na_2C_2O_4$ and $H_2C_2O_4 \cdot 2H_2O$. Both these substances must be chemically pure and must correspond exactly to their formulas.

It is easy to purify $Na_2C_2O_4$ by recrystallization from water and drying at 240-250°C. Sodium oxalate is not hygroscopic, it contains no water of crystallization, and it does not change on keeping. Oxalic acid is rather more difficult to purify than $Na_2C_2O_4$ and is also non-hygroscopic. However, it contains water of crystallization, and, in contrast to $Na_2C_2O_4$, it is efflorescent.

The reactions taking place when these substances are titrated with permanganate are represented by the equations*

$$5Na_2C_2O_4 + 2KMnO_4 + 8H_2SO_4 = 2MnSO_4 + K_2SO_4 + 5Na_2SO_4 + 8H_2O + 10CO_2 \uparrow$$

$$5H_2C_2O_4 + 2KMnO_4 + 3H_2SO_4 = 2MnSO_4 + K_2SO_4 + 8H_2O + 10CO_2 \uparrow$$

In both cases the $C_2O_4^{--}$ ions are oxidized as follows:

$$C_2O_4^{--} - 2e = 2CO_2$$

Therefore, the gram-equivalents of $Na_2C_2O_4$ and $H_2C_2O_4 \cdot 2H_2O$ respectively are:

$$\text{g-eq of } Na_2C_2O_4 = \frac{134.00}{2} = 67.00 \text{ g}$$

$$\text{g-eq of } H_2C_2O_4 \cdot 2H_2O = \frac{126.06}{2} = 63.03 \text{ g}$$

Preparation of the Primary Standard Solution. Weigh out accurately on an analytical balance about $0.02 \times 67.00 \times 0.25 \approx 0.335$ g of $Na_2C_2O_4$ or $0.02 \times 63.03 \times 0.25 \approx 0.315$ g of $H_2C_2O_4 \cdot 2H_2O$, transfer the substance without loss into a 250 ml measuring flask and dissolve it in cold distilled water, make the solution up to the mark with water, and mix thoroughly. Calculate and record the normality of the solution.

---

* See p. 338 for a more detailed account of the mechanism of these reactions.

Titration. Pipette out an aliquot portion (25.00 ml) of the primary standard solution, add 10-15 ml of 2 *N* sulphuric acid solution, and heat the liquid to 75-80°C (do not allow it to boil, because oxalic acid decomposes on boiling). Put the $KMnO_4$ solution in a burette* and adjust the level to the zero mark. If the bottom edge of the meniscus is difficult to see, all the readings may be taken against the top of the meniscus.

Now add the $KMnO_4$ solution drop by drop to the primary standard solution. Each successive drop may be added only after the colour caused by the preceding drop has disappeared. The first drops of $KMnO_4$ fade rather slowly. However, as soon as a small amount of Mn^{++}, which is a catalyst in this reaction (see p. 338 on autocatalysis), has been formed, subsequent fading is almost instantaneous. The end point is reached when one drop of permanganate colours the whole solution a pale pink which persists for 1-2 minutes.**

Perform the accurate titration at least three times and take the average of three concordant results (the difference between them should not exceed 0.1 ml).

Calculation. Find the normality of the permanganate solution in the usual way from the volumes of the $KMnO_4$ and primary standard solutions and the normality of the latter.

88. Determination of Ferrous Iron, Hydrogen Peroxide and Nitrites

Determination of Ferrous Iron. One of the most important determinations by the permanganate method is volumetric determination of ferrous iron. A ferrous salt titrated with $KMnO_4$ is oxidized to a ferric salt:

$$2KMnO_4 + 10FeSO_4 + 8H_2SO_4 = 2MnSO_4 + 5Fe_2(SO_4)_3 + K_2SO_4 + 8H_2O$$

The amount of iron in the unknown solution is easily calculated from the volume of the $KMnO_4$ solution taken for the titration and its normality. As an example, the iron content of a solution of Mohr's salt, which is a double salt of the composition $(NH_4)_2SO_4 \cdot FeSO_4 \cdot 6H_2O$, may be determined as follows.

Weigh out a sample of Mohr's salt, such that an approximately 0.02 *N* solution is obtained when it is dissolved in water in a 250 ml measuring flask.

---

* A burette with a glass tap is preferable. An ordinary burette may also be used, but at the end of the titration the $KMnO_4$ solution must then be poured out immediately and the burette rinsed out with distilled water.

** The colour gradually fades after long standing, because $KMnO_4$ reacts with the manganous salt formed:

$$2KMnO_4 + 3MnSO_4 + 2H_2O = \downarrow 5MnO_2 + K_2SO_4 + 2H_2SO_4$$

When dissolving the salt, pour into the flask (to about a half of its volume) 2 *N* sulphuric acid solution. At the end, add distilled water up to the mark and mix the solution thoroughly. Now proceed with the titration which, in contrast to titration of oxalic acid, is performed with *cold* solution, as ferrous salts are oxidized by atmospheric oxygen on heating.

Pipette out an aliquot portion (25.00 ml) of Mohr's salt solution and titrate it with the $KMnO_4$ solution to a faint pink colour. Repeat the accurate titration once or twice more and take the average of the concordant results.

Calculate the normality of the $FeSO_4$ solution from the volume and normality of the $KMnO_4$ solution used in the titration. From the result calculate, in the usual way, the number of grams of iron in the sample taken (i.e., in 250 ml of solution) and the percentage of iron in Mohr's salt. Since the Fe^{++} loses one electron in the reaction, the gram-equivalent of iron is equal to one gram-atom, or 55.85 g.

Oxalic acid (and its salts), ferrous salts, and many other reducing agents corresponding to oxidation potentials of less than 1.51 V can be determined by permanganate titration. Such substances include nitrites (salts of HNO_2), thiocyanates (salts of HCNS), potassium ferrocyanide $K_4[Fe(CN)_6]$, hydrogen peroxide (H_2O_2), arsenous acid and its salts, etc. Let us consider the determination of H_2O_2 and nitrites in more detail.

Determination of Hydrogen Peroxide, H_2O_2. The determination is based on the reaction:

$$5H_2O_2 + 2MnO_4^- + 6H^+ = \uparrow 5O_2 + 2Mn^{++} + 8H_2O$$

The equation shows that in this reaction H_2O_2 acts as a reducing agent and is oxidized to O_2 as follows:

$$H_2O_2 - 2e = O_2 + 2H^+$$

Therefore:

$$\text{g-eq of } H_2O_2 = \frac{M}{2} = \frac{34 \cdot 02}{2} = 17.01 \text{ g}$$

Since commercial hydrogen peroxide contains about 3% H_2O_2, it must be greatly diluted with water. For the analysis an accurately weighed sample of the hydrogen peroxide solution is diluted with water in a 250 ml measuring flask to give an approximately 0.02 *N* solution. An aliquot portion (25.00 ml) is acidified with 5-10 ml of sulphuric acid solution and titrated with permanganate. The titration is repeated two or three times, the average of the concordant results is taken, and the normality of the H_2O_2 solution is calculated in the usual way. The total amount of H_2O_2 taken (i.e., in 250 ml) is then found and the result is expressed as a percentage.

Determination of Nitrites. This determination is based on the reaction

$$5NO_2^- + 2MnO_4^- + 6H^+ = 5NO_3^- + 2Mn^{++} + 3H_2O$$

Since the oxidation of NO_2^- ions to NO_3^- ions can be written as

$$NO_2^- + H_2O - 2e = NO_3^- + 2H^+$$

the equivalent of a nitrite, such as $NaNO_2$, is

$$\text{g-eq} = \frac{M}{2} = \frac{69.00}{2} = 34.50 \text{ g}$$

A special feature of this determination is that nitrites are readily decomposed by acids to form nitrogen oxides:

$$2NO_2^- + 2H^+ = 2HNO_2 = \uparrow NO + \uparrow NO_2 + H_2O$$

Therefore, the titration procedure must be reversed in order to avoid losses. In this case acidified permanganate solution is titrated with neutral nitrite solution and not vice versa. When the nitrite solution comes into contact with the $KMnO_4$ solution it is oxidized to nitrate almost instantaneously and nitrogen oxides are not formed.

For the determination, an exactly weighed amount of nitrite solution is taken calculated to give an approximately 0.02 *N* solution when dissolved in a 250 ml measuring flask. The burette is filled with this solution. Then 25.00 ml of standard $KMnO_4$ solution is measured out accurately (with a burette or pipette) into a 500 ml conical flask, and roughly the same volume of dilute (1 : 4) H_2SO_4 solution is added. The liquid is diluted with 250 ml of water and warmed *slightly*; it is then titrated with the nitrite solution until one drop decolorizes it. The titration is repeated two or three times, the average of the concordant result is taken, and the normality of the nitrite solution is found from the volumes of nitrite and permanganate solutions and the normality of the permanganate. The amount of nitrite in the sample is found from the normality of the nitrite solution, and the result is expressed as a percentage.

In addition to these "direct" determinations, there are various "indirect" methods, based either on substitution or on back-titration. Some typical examples of such determinations are given below.

89. Determination of Iron in Ferric Chloride Solution

Ferric salts are not oxidized by permanganate. They can be determined in solution only after reduction of Fe^{+++} to Fe^{++}. This reduction can be effected by various reducing agents, such as H_2S, various metals and amalgams, $SnCl_2$ solution, etc.*

* Reduction by the action of metals and amalgams is described in detail in Sec. 93.

In the very useful method described below $FeCl_3$ is reduced by the action of $SnCl_2$ in presence of hydrochloric acid:

$$2FeCl_3 + SnCl = 2FeCl_2 + SnCl_4$$

The excess $SnCl_2$ must be removed completely, as it is also oxidized by $KMnO_4$. This is done by means of mercuric chloride (corrosive sublimate, $HgCl_2$), which reacts with $SnCl_2$ as follows:

$$SnCl_2 + 2HgCl_2 = SnCl_4 + \downarrow Hg_2Cl_2$$

Mercurous chloride (calomel, Hg_2Cl_2) is deposited in the form of a silky white precipitate. This is not filtered off, and the liquid is titrated with $KMnO_4$. The following reaction takes place:

$$5FeCl_2 + KMnO_4 + 8HCl = 5FeCl_3 + MnCl_2 + KCl + 4H_2O$$

The following points must be taken into consideration in this analysis.

1. The precipitated Hg_2Cl_2 can also be oxidized by permanganate. However, if only a small excess of $SnCl_2$ is used in the previous stage the amount of Hg_2Cl_2 precipitate is small, it reacts with the permanganate very slowly, and no appreciable error is introduced into the result. On the other hand, if a large amount of Hg_2Cl_2 is precipitated and, in particular, if it has a grey or dark colour as the result of further reduction to metallic mercury by the reaction

$$Hg_2Cl_2 + SnCl_2 = \downarrow 2Hg + SnCl_4$$

it is oxidized so rapidly during the titration that the result is quite erroneous.

It follows that *a basic condition for accuracy in this method is the use of a very slight excess of* $SnCl_2$. Stannous chloride is added drop by drop until the yellow colour of $FeCl_3$ has disappeared, after which one or two more drops are added.

2. As the result of the reaction between $KMnO_4$ and Hg_2Cl_2, after the end of the titration the pale pink colour of the solution fades fairly rapidly on standing. Therefore, the titration must be ended on the first appearance of a pink colour which persists for 30 seconds. The end point can be seen more easily if the solution is diluted with a large amount of water.

3. Titration of a ferrous salt in presence of hydrochloric acid is accompanied by oxidation of Cl^- ions to Cl_2, so that too much $KMnO_4$ is taken and a wrong result is obtained (see Sec. 84).

To avoid this, the titration should be performed in the presence of a salt of bivalent manganese, which protects Cl^- ions against such oxidation (p. 341). It is also necessary to add phosphoric acid, as the latter converts Fe^{+++} ions into colourless complex $[Fe(PO_4)_2]^{---}$ ions, and thus removes the yellow colour of the solution which is due to hydrolysis of ferric chloride, so that it is easier to detect the end point.

In practice the titration is performed in the presence of a specially prepared preventive solution, containing definite concentrations of $MnSO_4$, H_3PO_4 and H_2SO_4.*

Procedure. The $FeCl_3$ solution to be analysed (containing 0.1-0.3 g of iron) is put in a 250 ml measuring flask, diluted with water to the mark, and stirred thoroughly. Now pipette out an aliquot portion (25.00 ml) of this solution into a large conical flask, add 10 ml of dilute (1 : 1) HCl solution, and heat until boiling begins.** Remove the burner and add very carefully, *drop by drop* with continuous stirring, $SnCl_2$ solution*** to the hot yellow solution. Wait a few seconds after addition of each drop before adding the next. When the yellow colour of the solution has become very faint it is helpful to dilute the $SnCl_2$ solution with an equal volume of water. Add this diluted solution until one drop causes the colour to disappear completely. To make sure that the reduction of Fe^{+++} is complete, add one or two more drops of the $SnCl_2$ solution (but *not more* than that, because an excess of $SnCl_2$ is harmful; see point 1 above).

Cool the solution, dilute it with 100 ml of cold water, add 20 ml of $HgCl_2$ solution**** (*poisonous*), stir thoroughly, and leave to stand for about 2 minutes. A slight silky white precipitate (or turbidity) of Hg_2Cl_2 should be formed. If, as the result of incorrect reduction of Fe^{+++}, an abundant precipitate is formed, and especially if it has a grey colour (liberation of Hg), the determination must be rejected and started again.*****

Without filtering off the precipitate, add 200 ml of cold water and 6-8 ml of preventive solution (see above) to the liquid and then titrate it with permanganate solution until a pink colour, persisting for about 30 seconds, appears (see point 2, above). Add the $KMnO_4$ at such a rate that the drops can be counted. Near the end wait until the colour due to the preceding drop has disappeared before adding the next. Repeat the determination two or three times and take average of the concordant results.

---

* For preparation of the preventive solution 67 g of crystalline $MnSO_4 \cdot 4H_2O$ is dissolved in 500-600 ml of water. To this solution 139 H_3PO_4 (sp. gr. 1.7) and 130 ml of H_2SO_4 (sp. gr. 1.84) is added and the whole is diluted to 1 litre with water.

** The solution becomes bright yellow when heated; this makes it easier to detect the point when reduction of Fe^{+++} by $SnCl_2$ is complete and this colour disappears.

*** Dissolve 150 g of $SnCl_2 \cdot 2H_2O$ in 100 ml of concentrated HCl and dilute with water to 1 litre.

**** Dissolve 60 g of $HgCl_2$ in hot water and dilute to 1 litre.

***** If no precipitate is formed, it means that not enough $SnCl_2$ was used. In this case the determination must also be repeated.

Calculation. Let us perform the calculation expressing the concentration in terms of the titre for the substance being determined. First we find the iron titre of the permanganate, i.e., the number of grams of Fe^{++} which can be oxidized by the permanganate present in 1 ml of the solution. If the normality of the $KMnO_4$ is 0.02025, then 1 ml contains $\frac{0.02025}{1,000}$ gram-equivalents of $KMnO_4$; the same number of gram-equivalents of Fe is oxidized during the reaction. Since the gram-equivalent of iron is 55.85 g, we have

$$T_{KMnO_4/Fe} = \frac{0.02025 \times 55.85}{1,000} = 0.001131 \text{ g Fe in 1 ml}$$

If the average volume of $KMnO_4$ solution taken for titration of 25 ml of the unknown solution was 24.20 ml, then the amount of iron in 250 ml of the solution must be*:

$$Q_{250} = 0.001131 \times 24.20 \times 10 = 0.2737 \text{ g}$$

The determination described above is based on the *substitution method*, because the equivalent quantity of $FeCl_2$, which was titrated, was substituted for the $FeCl_3$ which cannot be titrated with permanganate. The substitution method (preliminary reduction) can also be used for determination of certain other substances, such as salts of molybdic acid, H_2MoO_4, and of vanadic acid, HVO_3; $K_3[Fe(CN)_6]$, and even salts of trivalent chromium, which can be reduced by zinc to salts of bivalent chromium, which are then titrated with $KMnO_4$.

90. Determination of Chromium in Potassium Dichromate Solution

Potassium dichromate, $K_2Cr_2O_7$, is itself an oxidizing agent and therefore, like $FeCl_3$, it cannot be titrated with $KMnO_4$. Neither is it practicable to reduce it to Cr^{+++} ions, which are much weaker reducing agents ($E_0 = +1.36$ V) than Fe^{++} ions ($E_0 = +0.77$ V). However, for permanganate determination of dichromate we can take advantage of the fact that in acid solution dichromate oxidizes ferrous salts, for example:

$$K_2Cr_2O_7 + 6FeSO_4 + 7H_2SO_4 = 3Fe_2(SO_4)_3 + Cr_2(SO_4)_3 + K_2SO_4 + 7H_2O$$

If an accurately measured volume, known to be in excess, of standard $FeSO_4$ solution is added to the unknown $K_2Cr_2O_7$ solution in the presence of H_2SO_4, the residual ferrous sulphate after the

* Of course, it is also possible to carry out the calculation by the usual method, i.e., by first finding the normality of the $FeCl_3$ solution and then calculating the amount of iron in 250 ml.

reaction can be titrated with permanganate and the amount of $FeSO_4$ which reacted with $K_2Cr_2O_7$ can be found by difference. It is then easy to calculate the amount of dichromate in the original solution.

This method, used very frequently in volumetric analysis, is known as the *back-titration method* (or *residual titration*). In this case it is more convenient to use a more stable ferrous compound than $FeSO_4$; namely, Mohr's salt $(NH_4)_2SO_4 \cdot FeSO_4 \cdot 6H_2O$. However, even this salt alters its titre fairly rapidly, so that it must be standardized at the time of the determination.

Procedure. Dilute the $K_2Cr_2O_7$ solution, containing 0.15-0.30 g of the salt, in a 250 ml measuring flask, pipette out 25.00 ml of the diluted solution, and acidify with 10-15 ml of 2 *N* H_2SO_4 solution. From another burette measure out *accurately* into the same flask 40 or 50 ml of approximately 0.02 *N* solution of Mohr's salt. Dilute the resultant green solution (colour of Cr^{+++} ions) with 100 ml of water and titrate the excess Mohr's salt, which did not react with $K_2Cr_2O_7$, with permanganate solution. Aim at obtaining a *greyish* colour (combination of the green colour of Cr^{+++} ions with the pink colour of MnO_4^- ions) by the addition of a single drop of permanganate solution. One or two more drops of permanganate produce a distinct pink colour, but the solution is then overtitrated.

Repeat the titration two or three times and take the average result. At the same time titrate 25.00 ml of the Mohr's salt solution two or three times in the presence of 10-15 ml of sulphuric acid.

Calculation. Suppose that 40.00 ml of Mohr's salt solution was taken with 25.00 ml of $K_2Cr_2O_7$ solution and that titration of the residual Mohr's salt took 14.20 ml of 0.02025 *N* $KMnO_4$ solution. At the same time, 25.00 ml of the Mohr's salt solution takes, say, 24.30 ml of $KMnO_4$ solution in the absence of $K_2Cr_2O_7$. Let us consider the following two methods for calculating the amount of chromium.

1. Let us first find how many millilitres of $KMnO_4$ solution would be needed for titration of the 40.00 ml of Mohr's salt solution in the absence of $K_2Cr_2O_7$. This is done by proportion:

25.00 ml of Mohr's salt takes 24.30 ml of $KMnO_4$

40.00 ml of Mohr's salt takes x ml of $KMnO_4$

$$x = \frac{40.00 \times 24.30}{25.00} = 38.89 \text{ ml}$$

In reality, since part of the Mohr's salt was previously oxidized by $K_2Cr_2O_7$, titration of the solution took less $KMnO_4$ solution, namely, 14.20 ml. Evidently, the amount of $K_2Cr_2O_7$ contained in 25.00 ml of the unknown solution is equivalent to 38.89 — — 14.20 = 24.69 ml of 0.02025 *N* $KMnO_4$ solution. Accordingly, denoting the normality of the $K_2Cr_2O_7$ solution by N, we can write:

$$25.00 \times N = 24.69 \times 0.02025$$

and hence

$$N = \frac{24.69 \times 0.02025}{25.00} = 0.02000$$

It would be quite easy to calculate in the usual way from this result the number of grams of $K_2Cr_2O_7$ in 250 ml of solution and hence to find the amount of Cr. However, it is not necessary to calculate the amount of $K_2Cr_2O_7$. It is more convenient to find the amount of chromium directly, as follows. One gram-equivâlent of $K_2Cr_2O_7$ contains one gram-equivalent of chromium, which is equal to $^1/_3$ of a gram-atom or $\frac{52.00}{3} = 17.33$ g (since one atom of sexivalent chromium gains three electrons in the reaction). Therefore, having found the number of gram-equivalents of $K_2Cr_2O_7$ contained in 250 ml of the solution, we multiply it by the gram-equivalent of chromium. Consequently

$$Q_{250} = \frac{0.02000 \times 250 \times 17.33}{1{,}000} = 0.08665 \text{ g of chromium}$$

2. First we find the normality of the Mohr's salt solution:

$$N \times 25.00 = 0.02025 \times 24.30$$

and hence

$$N = \frac{0.02025 \times 24.30}{25.00} = 0.01969$$

We now calculate how many milligram-equivalents of the respective substances are present in the volumes of the Mohr's salt and permanganate solutions used in the titration. Since 1 ml of Mohr's salt solution contains 0.01969 milligram-equivalent of the salt, 40.00 ml contains

$$0.01969 \times 40.00 = 0.7876 \text{ mg-eq}$$

Similarly we find that the 14.20 ml of 0.02025 N $KMnO_4$ solution used for titration of the residual Mohr's salt contained

$$0.02025 \times 14.20 = 0.2876 \text{ mg-eq}$$

We know (p. 210) that in any reaction equal numbers of milligram-equivalents of both reacting substances are used. Our result therefore shows that of the 0.7876 mg-eq of Mohr's salt taken 0.2876 mg-eq remained after the reaction with $K_2Cr_2O_7$ and was titrated with $KMnO_4$. Therefore, 0.7876 — 0.2876 = 0.5000 mg-eq was consumed in the reaction with $K_2Cr_2O_7$. This is also the number of milligram-equivalents of chromium in 25 ml of the unknown solution. Therefore, 250 ml contained 5.000 mg-eq or

$$5.000 \times 17.33 = 86.65 \text{ mg} = 0.08665 \text{ g of chromium}$$

The above calculation method is convenient if the normalities of both the standard solutions used in the determination are known. If the normality of only one of the solutions is known (as in this case), it is better to use the first calculation method.

This method for determination of chromium is of great practical importance. It is the method used for determining chromium in chromium ores, steels, ferrous alloys, slags, etc.

A weighed sample of ore or slag is usually fused with Na_2O_2 in an iron or nickel crucible, when chromium is oxidized to chromate and Na_2CrO_4 is formed. The solution is acidified with sulphuric acid and chromium is determined as described above. For determination of chromium in an alloy a weighed sample is dissolved in H_2SO_4, ferrous iron and carbides are oxidized by nitric acid, and Cr^{+++} is then oxidized to $Cr_2O_7^{--}$ by the action of ammonium persulphate, $(NH_4)_2S_2O_8$, in the presence of Ag^+ as a catalyst. The MnO_4^- ions (formed in solution by oxidation of the manganese present in the alloy) are reduced by the action of NaCl solution, excess $(NH_4)_2S_2O_8$ is decomposed by boiling, and the determination is completed by the method described above.

Residual titration with permanganate can also be used for determination of certain other oxidizing agents, such as chlorates (salts of $HClO_3$), persulphates (salts of $H_2S_2O_8$), bleaching powder ($CaOCl_2$), etc. Substances such as MnO_2, PbO_2 and Pb_3O_4 can be determined if oxalic acid is used instead of Mohr's salt and the residual oxalic acid is titrated back with permanganate. It will be remembered that back-titration is also used in the neutralization method; for example, in determination of the permanent hardness of water (Sec. 74), of NH_3 in ammonium salts (Sec. 77), etc.

91. Determination of Calcium in Calcium Carbonate

Only indirect methods are used for determination of calcium by permanganate titration; either back-titration or substitution may be used. In the former case an accurately measured excess of oxalic acid solution is added, the precipitated CaC_2O_4 is separated off, and the residual oxalic acid is titrated with permanganate. The amount of $H_2C_2O_4$ required for precipitation of the calcium is found by the difference, and the Ca^{++} content in solution is calculated from the result.

In the substitution method Ca^{++} is precipitated in the form of CaC_2O_4, which is filtered off, washed, and dissolved in H_2SO_4 (or

HCl). The oxalic acid formed is titrated with $KMnO_4$ and Ca^{++} content in solution is calculated from the titration results.

Below we consider only the last method, which is the one most used in practice.

Procedure. Weigh out accurately an amount of $CaCO_3$ sufficient to give an approximately 0.02 *N* solution when dissolved and made up to 250 ml. Since the gram-equivalent of $CaCO_3$ is approximately 50 g, the amount to be weighed out is about

$$\frac{0.02 \times 50 \times 250}{1,000} = 0.25 \text{ g}$$

Transfer the weighed sample through a dry funnel into a 100 ml flask and then rinse the grains remaining on the watch glass and funnel into the same flask. Without taking out the funnel add diluted (1:1) HCl solution into the flask drop by drop, slightly warming and agitating the contents in order to speed up dissolution of the $CaCO_3$. When all the $CaCO_3$ has dissolved in the acid, transfer the solution through the same funnel into a 250 ml measuring flask and rinse the flask and funnel several times with distilled water. At the end wash the outside of the funnel stem (drops of solution may have got on it when the sample was being dissolved), cool the solution, and make up to the mark with water.

Mix the solution thoroughly and pipette out an aliquot portion (25.00 ml) into a conical flask, and add 10 ml of 5% $H_2C_2O_4$ solution, 60-70 ml of water, and one or two drops of methyl orange. Heat the liquid to 70-80°C and add 10% NH_4OH solution diluted with an equal volume of water drop by drop (one or two drops per second) with continuous stirring until the pink colour vanishes.* Then put the flask on a water or sand bath and allow the precipitate to settle out completely.

Cool the liquid, transfer the precipitate to a filter, and wash with cold water. It is best to use a No. 4 sintered glass crucible, but paper (blue band) can also be used. There is no need to try to transfer all the precipitate from the flask onto the filter; it is more convenient to dissolve the precipitate in the flask, so that the less precipitate gets on the filter, the better. If the filtrate is turbid it must be heated for some time and passed again through the same filter when cool.

At the end of the filtration wash the precipitate in the flask and on the filter several times with cold distilled water to remove excess $C_2O_4^{--}$ ions used in the precipitation. If the $C_2O_4^{--}$ ions are not completely removed a certain amount of permanganate would be required to oxidize them and the result of the analysis would be too high. However, too much water must not be used for the washing,

* The conditions for precipitation of CaC_2O_4 are explained in Sec. 43.

because this would lead to appreciable loss by dissolution of the CaC_2O_4 precipitate. A negative reaction for Cl^-, when $AgNO_3$ solution [or $Hg_2(NO_3)_2$] is added to a portion of the washing acidified with HNO_3, shows that the washing is complete.

Dissolve* the washed precipitate in hot 10% (vol.) H_2SO_4 solution. If a paper filter was used for the filtration, first pierce the filter by means of a glass rod and wash the precipitate of the filter into the flask with the minimum quantity of hot water from a wash bottle. Then thoroughly wash the whole filter surface with 80-100 ml of hot 10% H_2SO_4 solution, pouring it in a thin stream down a glass rod. At the end wash the filter two or three times with hot water. Warm the flask slightly until the precipitate dissolves completely.

The CaC_2O_4 precipitate dissolves in H_2SO_4 to form an equivalent amount of $H_2C_2O_4$. Heat the solution to 70-80°C and titrate the oxalic acid with permanganate.

Calculation. Suppose that the titration took 24.60 ml of 0.02025 *N* $KMnO_4$ solution. Therefore the precipitate obtained from 25.00 ml of the unknown solution contained

$$\frac{0.02025 \times 24.60}{1{,}000} \text{ g-eq } CaC_2O_4$$

The gram-equivalent of CaC_2O_4 is $^1/_2$ its gram-molecule, since one $C_2O_4^{--}$ ion loses two electrons when titrated with permanganate:

$$C_2O_4^{--} - 2e = 2CO_2$$

Half a gram-molecule of CaC_2O_4 contains half a gram-atom of Ca, or 20.04 g. Therefore, the amount of Ca^{++} in 25 ml of the solution is

$$\frac{0.02025 \times 24.60 \times 20.04}{1{,}000} = 0.009982 \text{ g}$$

This corresponds to 0.009982 × 10 = 0.09982 g Ca in 250 ml, it only remains to express this amount of calcium as a percentage of the weight taken.

92. Determination of Manganese in Steel (or Cast Iron)

In all the examples of permanganate titrations discussed above a $KMnO_4$ solution was used for titration of various reducing agents. In the method described below for determination of manganese in steel, cast iron, and other substances the sample is dissolved in acid, the Mn^{++} ions present are oxidized to MnO_4^- ions, and the resultant

* It is rather difficult to dissolve CaC_2O_4 in H_2SO_4. Therefore, it is sometimes recommended to put the washed filter into the solution to be titrated. However, when the solution is shaken some types of filter paper disintegrate readily into individual fibres and are oxidized by $KMnO_4$, which leads to errors.

purple solution is titrated with a solution of a reducing agent until colourless.

The oxidizing agent used is ammonium persulphate, the standard oxidation potential of which ($E_0 + 2.01$ V) is higher than that of the system MnO_4^-/Mn^{++} in acid solution (+1.51 V). The reaction proceeds in the presence of a catalyst ($AgNO_3$) on heating:

$$2MnSO_4 + 5(NH_4)_2S_2O_8 + 8H_2O = 2HMnO_4 + 5(NH_4)_2SO_4 + 7H_2SO_4$$

In the absence of a catalyst a brown precipitate of $MnO(OH)_2$ is formed instead of $HMnO_4$.

The permanganic acid formed is usually titrated with a solution of sodium arsenite,* Na_3AsO_3. This is a complex reaction, as in addition to Mn^{++} ions compounds of tri- and quadrivalent manganese are formed in proportions which depend on the experimental conditions. It might seem at first sight that this non-stoichiometric course of the reaction on which calculation of the analytical results is based would make its use impossible. In reality this is not the case. The method is widely used in practice and gives good results. However, the essential condition *is strict adherence to the same experimental conditions in the determinations and in standardization of the sodium arsenite solution.* Under the same conditions the amount of Na_3AsO_3 required for titration of the $HMnO_4$ must be proportional to the manganese content of the steel sample, despite the complex course of the reaction. Of course, the arsenite solution must be standardized against a standard sample (p. 205) of steel of exactly known manganese content, and the titre of the solution must be expressed in terms of manganese.

Suppose, for example, that d grams of steel containing p % of manganese was taken. When it was analysed as described below it was found that titration of the permanganic acid formed by the action of $(NH_4)_2S_2O_8$ took V ml of the standard arsenite solution. Let us find the manganese titre of Na_3AsO_3 ($T_{Na_3AsO_3/Mn}$). To do this, we first calculate the weight of manganese in the sample taken. This weight is $(dp) : 100$ g. To find what weight of manganese corresponds to 1 ml of the standard solution we must divide this weight of manganese by the volume of arsenite solution. This gives:

$$T_{Na_3AsO_3/Mn} = \frac{dp}{100 \times V} \text{ g Mn in 1 ml} \qquad (1)$$

Of course, Equation (1) can also be used for calculating the analytical results in this method, except that in that case the unknown

* To prepare sodium arsenite solution, 5.1-5.2 g of Na_2CO_3 is dissolved in 100 ml of water. To this solution 1.70 g of arsenous anhydride As_2O_3 (*poisonous*) is added and the solution is heated to boiling. After all the As_2O_3 has dissolved the solution is made up to 5 litres and mixed.

quantity is p whereas the manganese titre of the standard solution is known. Therefore

$$p=\frac{T_{Na_3AsO_3/Mn}\times V}{d}\times 100\% \qquad (2)$$

The steel sample is dissolved in a mixture of sulphuric, nitric, and phosphoric acids.* Nitric acid oxidizes Fe^{++} to Fe^{+++} and decomposes carbides (in particular, manganese carbide) while phosphoric acid converts coloured Fe^{+++} ions into the colourless complex form $[Fe(PO_4)_2]^{---}$. Moreover, its presence increases the stability of $HMnO_4$, as it prevents to a considerable extent the decomposition of the latter with the formation of precipitated $MnO(OH)_2$ and liberation of oxygen.

Cobalt, or large amounts (>2%) of chromium, in the steel interfere with the determination. In the presence of cobalt it is impossible to determine the equivalence point owing to the presence of pink Co^{++} ions, while in the presence of chromium determination of the equivalence point is greatly hindered by the formation of $Cr_2O_7^{--}$ ions by the action of $(NH_4)_2S_2O_8$:

$$Cr_2(SO_4)_3+3(NH_4)_2S_2O_8+7H_2O=(NH_4)_2Cr_2O_7+2(NH_4)_2SO_4+7H_2SO_4$$

For these reasons the colour change from pink to yellow at the end of titration is more difficult to detect.

Procedure. Put an accurately weighed sample (about 0.2 to 0.3 g) of steel (or cast iron) into a 250 ml conical flask and dissolve it in the acid mixture by gentle heating in a fume cupboard. When liberation of brown nitrous fumes has ceased (usually after 10-15 minutes of heating), dilute the solution with 50 ml of hot water and add 5 ml of 1% $AgNO_3$ solution and 5-7 ml of 20% $(NH_4)_2S_2O_8$ solution. Now heat the solution to gentle boiling and boil it for 30-40 seconds [*not longer*, otherwise part of the $HMnO_4$ may decompose with precipitation of $MnO(OH)_2$]. Allow the solution to stand for 3-4 minutes to complete the reaction and then cool it at once under the tap as quickly as possible. Titrate the cold solution with standard arsenite solution until it is colourless or (if chromium is present in the steel) until the pink colour changes to yellow. The titration must be *as rapid as possible* because the persulphate present in the solution continues (although slowly, because of the low temperature) to oxidize the manganese reduced during the titration back to $HMnO_4$.

If the titration was carried out with insufficient accuracy or too slowly, it must be repeated. To do this, add 3-5 ml more of $(NH_4)_2S_2O_8$

---

* Add 125 ml of H_2SO_4 (sp. gr. 1.84) *carefully* in a thin stream, with stirring to 500 ml of water. To the cooled solution add 100 ml of H_3PO_4 (sp. gr. 1.70) and 275 ml of HNO_3 (sp. gr. 1.40).

solution to the titrated solution, heat to boiling again, and then proceed as before.

Having found the volume of standard arsenite solution (V) required for the titration, use Equation (2) to find the percentage of manganese in the steel sample.

DICHROMATE TITRATIONS

93. General Principles of the Method

The chromatometric method is based on reactions of oxidation by the dichromate ion. Its oxidizing action is due to conversion of $Cr_2O_7^{--}$ anions containing sexivalent chromium into Cr^{+++} cations:

$$Cr_2O_7^{--} + 14H^+ + 6e = 2Cr^{+++} + 7H_2O$$

This equation shows that if potassium dichromate is used for the oxidation then the gram-equivalent of $K_2Cr_2O_7$ is $^1/_6$ M, or 294.2/6= =49.03 g. Since reduction of $Cr_2O_7^{--}$ to Cr^{+++} requires H^+ ions, dichromate titrations are performed in acid solution.

The oxidation potential of the $Cr_2O_7^{--}/2Cr^{+++}$ system (+1.36 V) is somewhat lower than that of the MnO_4^-/Mn^{++} system (+1.51 V). This is very important, because it is possible to use dichromate for titrations in the presence of hydrochloric acid without risk of oxidation of Cl^- ions, because the oxidation potential of the $Cl_2/2Cl^-$ system (+1.36 V) is equal to that of the $Cr_2O_7^{--}/2Cr^{+++}$ system. However, dichromate oxidizes Cl^- ions to Cl_2 at HCl concentrations above 2 N and also on boiling.

Potassium dichromate also has the following advantages over permanganate:

1. It is easy to prepare the chemically pure substance, strictly corresponding to the formula $K_2Cr_2O_7$, by recrystallization from aqueous solution followed by drying at 200°C. It is therefore possible to prepare standard dichromate solution by exact weighing of the chemically pure salt which is then dissolved in a definite volume.

2. When kept in a closed vessel, $K_2Cr_2O_7$ is exceedingly stable in solution. It does not decompose even when the acidified solution is boiled. Therefore, its titre does not alter on keeping. Dichromate solution may be used even when heating is required for the oxidation.

A disadvantage of $K_2Cr_2O_7$ as an oxidizing agent is that the titration gives rise to Cr^{+++} ions, which confer a green colour to the solution, so that the equivalence point is difficult to detect.

The usual indicator in the dichromate method is diphenylamine, which is a redox indicator (Sec. 82). It has also been proposed to use the sodium or barium salt of diphenylaminesulphonic acid.

This indicator is more soluble than diphenylamine in water, and gives a very sharp colour change from colourless through green to red-violet. It is also possible to use phenylanthranilic acid (p. 333).

Before the introduction of redox indicators into analytical practice, the external indicator $K_3[Fe(CN)_6]$ was used in titrations of ferrous iron with dichromate.

The difference between internal and external indicators is that the latter are not added to the solutions being titrated but are used as spot tests for a particular ion. In the present instance $K_3[Fe(CN)_6]$ is a reagent for the Fe^{++} ion, with which it forms a dark blue precipitate of Turnbull's blue:

$$3Fe^{++} + 2[Fe(CN)_6]^{---} = \downarrow Fe_3[Fe(CN)_6]_2$$

In titrations with $K_3[Fe(CN)_6]$ as indicator, drops of its solution are placed on a porcelain (or glass*) plate. Samples of the titrated solution are withdrawn by means of a glass tube with its end drawn out to a fine capillary, and mixed with drops of the indicator. It is also possible to apply drops of the titrated solution onto filter paper which has been soaked in the indicator solution and dried.

During the first titration spot tests are performed at intervals of 1-2 ml until a blue colour is no longer produced with $K_3[Fe(CN)_6]$. This gives a rough estimate of the volume of $K_2Cr_2O_7$ solution needed; in the next titration similar samples are taken only near the end of the titration at intervals of 0.1-0.2 ml. In the third titration the exact volume of $K_2Cr_2O_7$ solution required for the titration is finally found. In this way the error caused by removal of part of the solution for the spot tests is made negligibly small. However, external indicators are less convenient than internal ones, and they are used only if no suitable internal indicators are available or for titration of turbid or coloured solutions, when internal indicators are useless.

The most important applications of the dichromate method are in determination of iron in ores, slags, alloys, and similar materials. When they are dissolved, the iron is usually (even if only partially) obtained in the form of Fe^{+++} ions, which must be reduced to Fe^{++} before titration. This reduction is performed in the same way as was described for the permanganate method (Sec. 89), by the action of $SnCl_2$ solution with subsequent oxidation of excess stannous chloride by $HgCl_2$ solution. Iron is also often reduced by the action of metals or amalgams. The reducing agent most convenient for this purpose is metallic zinc, which reacts with Fe^{+++} ions as follows:

$$2Fe^{+++} + Zn = 2Fe^{++} + Zn^{++}$$

Excess metal is very easy to remove mechanically, e.g., by filtration through cotton wool.

Reduction of various substances by solid or liquid amalgams of various metals (zinc, cadmium, lead and bismuth) is now extensively used.

---

* A sheet of white paper should be placed under the glass plate to make the colour more distinct.

A very convenient method of reduction is by the use of solid zinc amalgam in a special column known as a *reductor* (Fig. 58).

A perforated porcelain plate is placed at the bottom of the reductor *1*; this is covered with a layer of fibrous asbestos and the column is filled nearly to the top with zinc amalgam containing 20-40% of zinc (grain size 1.5-2 mm) or with zinc shavings treated with 2% $HgCl_2$ solution.

During the determination the flask *2* is connected to a vacuum pump and the reductor is washed through with 150-200 ml of dilute (5%) H_2SO_4. The washings are discarded and the cold acidified* solution to be analysed (total volume 100-150 ml) is run through the reductor at a rate not over 75 ml per minute. Care must be taken not to let the liquid level in the reductor fall below the top of the amalgam, as penetration of air into the reductor leads to error.

When all the iron solution has been passed through the reductor the vessel which had contained this solution is rinsed out with three 25 ml portions of 2.5% H_2SO_4 solution, the washings being added to the solution which had been passed through the reductor; each successive portion is added only after the preceding one has passed completely through the reductor. At the end the reductor is washed through with three portions of pure water, 25-35 ml each.

The flask is separated from the reductor and the end of its tube is rinsed into the flask; the solution is then tested for complete reduction of Fe^{+++} by addition of a drop of the solution to a drop of NH_4CNS on a porcelain tile (no pink colour should appear). The solution is then titrated with dichromate or permanganate.

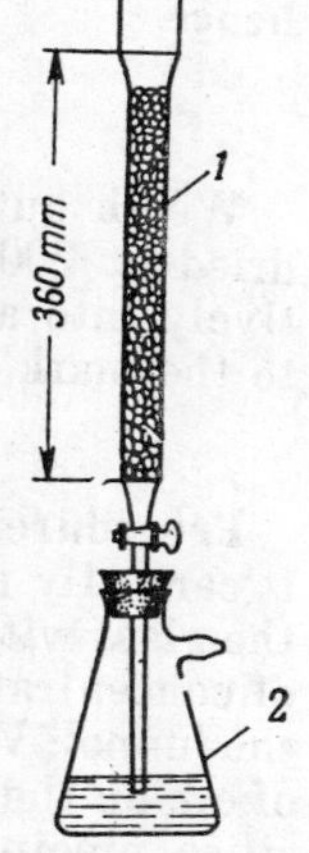

Fig. 58. Reductor
1 — reductor; *2* — flask

Instead of metals or solid amalgams, liquid amalgams may be used; these are considerably more reactive so that less metal is consumed. Moreover, the use of liquid amalgams greatly increases the number of metals which can be used for reduction. It is thus possible to select a metal which reduces only a single strong oxidizing agent in a mixture of oxidizing agents present in solution, without affecting the others (selective titration).

94. Determination of Iron in an Ore

As an example of dichromate determinations, let us consider the determination of iron in an iron ore.

Preparation of Standard $K_2Cr_2O_7$ Solution. In contrast to most of the earlier instances, in which solutions of definite normality were used, we prepare an empirical $K_2Cr_2O_7$ solution (p. 211) of a concentration such that 1 ml corresponds to exactly 0.0025 g Fe. Let us calculate the weight of $K_2Cr_2O_7$ required for preparation of 250 ml of this solution.

The gram-equivalent of $K_2Cr_2O_7$ is $^1/_6$ *M* (Sec. 93), or 49.03 g, and the gram-equivalent of iron is 55.85 g. One litre of the $K_2Cr_2O_7$ solution must correspond to $0.0025 \times 1{,}000 = 2.5$ g Fe, and 250 ml

* Its acidity must be between 0.5 *N* and 5 *N*.

to 0.6250 g Fe. By proportion:

55.85 g Fe is equivalent to 49.03 g $K_2Cr_2O_7$

0.6250 g Fe is equivalent to x g $K_2Cr_2O_7$

hence

$$x = \frac{0.6250 \times 49.03}{55.85} = 0.5488 \text{ g}$$

Weigh out exactly 0.5488 g of the salt, recrystallized twice and dried at 200°C, on an analytical balance and transfer it quantitatively into a 250 ml measuring flask; dissolve it in water, make up to the mark, and mix thoroughly. The iron titre of this solution is*

$$T_{K_2Cr_2O_7/Fe} = 0.002500 \text{ g/ml}$$

Procedure. Weigh out 0.1 g of the ore on a watch glass. Transfer it carefully through a dry funnel into a 100 ml flask, and then weigh the glass with the residual ore again. Treat the sample with 10-15 ml of concentrated HCl, washing the ore grains completely with it from the funnel. Warm the flask gently on a sand bath until the dark grains of ore on the bottom of the flask have disappeared and only a whitish silica precipitate remains. Do not allow the liquid in the flask to boil, as this may lead to partial volatilization of $FeCl_3$.

When the ore has been dissolved reduce the Fe^{+++} ions to Fe^{++}. Tilt the flask, carefully lower into it several pieces of granulated zinc metal,** insert a funnel in the neck of the flask (to retain splashes) and boil the solution until the yellow colour has disappeared entirely; this shows that Fe^{+++} has been completely reduced to Fe^{++}.***

When the solution has become colourless *cool it thoroughly under the tap*, wash the drops of liquid from the funnel into the flask, and take out the funnel. Insert a piece of cotton wool loosely into the funnel and filter the solution through it into a large (500-700 ml) conical flask to remove pieces of unchanged zinc. Wash the small flask, funnel, and cotton wool thoroughly several times with distilled water and dilute the solution to 300-400 ml. This is done so that the chromic salt formed by the reaction

$$K_2Cr_2O_7 + 6FeCl_2 + 14HCl = 2CrCl_3 + 2KCl + 6FeCl_3 + 7H_2O$$

---

* If not exactly 0.5488 g of $K_2Cr_2O_7$ is taken, use the actual weight for calculating to four significant figures the value of $T_{K_2Cr_2O_7/Fe}$ and use this value in the subsequent calculation.

** The zinc must not contain impurities which can be oxidized by $K_2Cr_2O_7$.

*** If the zinc has dissolved completely but the yellow colour persists some more zinc should be added. If a white precipitate (or turbidity) of basic zinc salts is formed, HCl must be added to dissolve them.

interfere as little as possible by its green colour with determination of the equivalence point in the titration.

As was explained in detail in (Sec. 82), titration of iron with diphenylamine indicator must be performed in the presence of H_3PO_4 which converts the Fe^{+++} ions formed by the reaction into the $[Fe(PO_4)_2]^{---}$ complex and thereby lowers the oxidation potential of the solution. Only under this condition does the indicator change colour within the limits of the change of potential on the titration curve. Further, the acidity of the solution must be fairly high. To achieve both these aims, add 25 ml of a special acid mixture* (H_3PO_4 and H_2SO_4) to the solution. Then add one or two drops of diphenylamine indicator solution (not more**) and titrate the solution with the $K_2Cr_2O_7$ solution, adding the latter in small portions, until a persistent blue-violet colour appears.***

Calculation. Multiply the number of millilitres of $K_2Cr_2O_7$ solution taken in the titration by its iron titre, and so find the amount of iron in the sample. Then calculate the percentage of iron in the ore.

IODOMETRY

95. General Principles of the Method

Free iodine, like other halogens, can take electrons from substances which yield them readily (reducing agents), and is therefore an oxidant. Under the influence of substances which are capable of gaining electrons (i.e., oxidants) I^- ions readily give up electrons and therefore act as reducing agents.

The iodometric method of volumetric analysis is based on oxidation-reduction processes involving interconversion of elemental iodine and I^- ions:

$$I_2 + 2e \rightleftarrows 2I^-$$

---

* To prepare the mixture, dissolve 150 ml of H_2SO_4 (sp. gr. 1.84) in 500 ml of distilled water. When the solution is cool, add 150 ml of orthophosphoric acid H_3PO_4 (sp. gr. 1.70) and dilute the mixture with water to 1 litre.

** A 1% solution of diphenylamine in concentrated H_2SO_4 (sp. gr. 1.84). More than the indicated amount of diphenylamine must not be taken because at higher concentrations with insufficient acidity, and also during very slow titration, the indicator undergoes a different type of chemical change which results (in the presence of excess $K_2Cr_2O_7$) in a green colour instead of blue-violet. If this happens, the determination must be rejected and repeated.

*** At first the colour which appears near the end of the titration disappears fairly rapidly owing to interaction of the oxidized form of the indicator, formed in the presence of local excess of $K_2Cr_2O_7$, with the Fe^{++} ions still present in solution. Therefore, a completely stable colouring of the solution must be aimed at.

The standard oxidation potential of the $I_2/2I^-$ system has the relatively low value of $+0.54$ V. It follows that, in contrast to the oxidizing agents already considered ($KMnO_4$ and $K_2Cr_2O_7$), I_2 is a relatively weak oxidant. Conversely, I^- ions are considerably more powerful reducing agents than Cr^{+++} or Mn^{++} ions.

The fact that the system $I_2/2I^-$ is about half-way down the table of oxidation potentials shows that: (a) there are several reducing agents which can be oxidized by free iodine (these include all the reducing agents in the first column of the table above the system $I_2/2I^-$, i.e., those having $E_0 < +0.54$ V); (b) there is also a number of oxidizing agents which can be reduced by I^- ions (all the oxidizing agents in the third column of the table below the system $I_2/2I^-$, having $E_0 > +0.54$ V).

Hence there is thus a dual possibility of using the oxidation-reduction properties of the system $I_2/2I^-$ in volumetric analysis; for determination of reducing agents by oxidation with iodine solution, and for determination of oxidizing agents by reduction with I^- ions.

Let us consider both types of iodometric determinations.

Determination of Reducing Agents. Free iodine reacts with sodium thiosulphate solution as follows:

$$\underset{(+0.08\ V)}{2Na_2S_2O_3} + I_2 = 2NaI + \underset{(+0.54\ V)}{Na_2S_4O_6}$$

The compound $Na_2S_4O_6$ formed in this reaction is sodium tetrathionate, a salt of tetrathionic acid. This most important iodometric reaction may be written in the ionic form as follows:

$$2S_2O_3^{--} + I_2 = 2I^- + S_4O_6^{--}$$

This equation shows that the two $S_2O_3^{--}$ ions, with four excess electrons between them, are converted into a single $S_4O_6^{--}$ ion with only two excess electrons.*

Therefore, two $S_2O_3^{--}$ ions give two electrons to the I_2 molecule as follows:

$$2S_2O_3^{--} - 2e = S_4O_6^{--}$$

The gram-equivalent of sodium thiosulphate is $2M : 2$, or M, which is 248.2 g (corresponding to the formula $Na_2S_2O_3 \cdot 5H_2O$). The gram-equivalent of iodine is equal to the gram-atom of iodine

* In structural form, the reaction may be represented as follows:

```
O   ONa                              O   ONa
 \ /                                  \ /
  S                                    S
 / \  .........                       / \
O   S : Na  :                        O   S
      :     :  + I2   = 2NaI +           |
O   S : Na  :                        O   S
 \ /  :.....:                         \ /
  S                                    S
 / \                                  / \
O   ONa                              O   ONa
2 molecules of Na2S2O3              1 molecule of Na2S4O6
```

(126.9 g) because each atom gains an electron when reduced to an I^- ion.

When a $Na_2S_2O_3$ solution is titrated with iodine solution the characteristic dark brown colour of the iodine vanishes instantly. When all the $Na_2S_2O_3$ has been oxidized one excess drop of iodine solution colours the liquid a pale yellow. Therefore, as in the permanganate method (Sec. 82), it is possible to perform such titrations without an indicator. However, the colour due to iodine at the end point is faint and this makes determination of the equivalence point difficult. It is therefore much more convenient to use a sensitive reagent for iodine as indicator; namely, starch solution, which forms an intense blue adsorption compound with iodine. In titration in the presence of starch solution the end point is determined from the appearance of a permanent blue colour on addition of one excess drop of iodine. It is also possible to titrate iodine solution with thiosulphate until one drop of the latter decolorizes the blue solution. In this case *the starch solution must be added at the very end of the titration*, when very little iodine remains and the solution being titrated has a faint (straw-yellow) colour. If the starch is added earlier, when there is still much iodine in solution, the large amount of the iodine-starch compound formed reacts slowly with the thiosulphate, so that it is easy to add too much thiosulphate.

Knowing the normality of the iodine solution and the volumes of the iodine and thiosulphate solutions used in the titration, we can easily find the normality and titre of the thiosulphate solution. Conversely, the normality and titre of an iodine solution can be calculated from known normality or titre of a $Na_2S_2O_3$ solution.

Various other reducing agents capable of reducing I_2 to I^- ions are determined similarly. They include salts of H_2SO_3, H_3AsO_3 and H_3SbO_3, free H_2S, $SnCl_2$, and other substances. Equations for the reactions taking place when such substances are titrated with iodine are given below ($E_{0 I_2/2I^-} = +0.54$ V)*:

$$\underset{(+0.17\ V)}{SO_3^{--}} + I_2 + H_2O = SO_4^{--} + 2I^- + 2H^+$$

$$\underset{(+0.57\ V)}{AsO_3^{---}} + I_2 + H_2O = AsO_4^{---} + 2I^- + 2H^+$$

$$\underset{(+0.14\ V)}{H_2S} + I_2 = \downarrow S + 2I^- + 2H^+$$

$$\underset{(+0.15\ V)}{Sn^{++}} + I_2 = Sn^{++++} + 2I^-$$

etc.**

---

* The reaction between AsO_3^{---} and I_2 proceeds as indicated only if H^+ ions are removed by addition of $NaHCO_3$ (p. 320).

** The numbers in brackets are the values of E_0 of the respective reducing agents.

Determination of Oxidizing Agents. Since reducing agents are determined by titration with iodine solution, it seems natural to expect that for determination of oxidizing agents, based on reduction by I^- ions, a KI solution should be used for titration. However, in reality this titration cannot be performed because it is impossible to detect the equivalence point. When an oxidant, such as $K_2Cr_2O_7$, is titrated with KI solution the end of the reaction

$$\underset{(+1.36\ V)}{K_2Cr_2O_7} + 6KI + 14HCl = \underset{(+0.54\ V)}{3I_2} + 8KCl + 2CrCl_3 + 7H_2O$$

would be characterized by a cessation of iodine liberation. Obviously this point cannot be detected. As was pointed out earlier, when starch is used as indicator it is easy to detect the instant when I_2 appears in solution (blue colour) or the instant when it disappears (disappearance of blue colour), but not the instant when I_2 formation ceases.

Therefore, an indirect substitution method is used in such cases. To a mixture of potassium iodide and acid solutions (both taken in excess) there is added an exact volume, measured out with a pipette, of the oxidant to be determined,* for example, $K_2Cr_2O_7$ solution.

To complete the reaction (see the above equation) the solution is left to stand for about 5 minutes, and the liberated iodine is then titrated with thiosulphate. It is evident that the number of gram-equivalents of iodine, (the latter being equal to the number of gram-equivalents of thiosulphate taken is equal to the number of gram-equivalents of the oxidizing agent ($K_2Cr_2O_7$). Therefore, although in this determination $K_2Cr_2O_7$ and $Na_2S_2O_3$ do not react directly with each other, nevertheless their respective amounts are equivalent.** Accordingly, the usual formula can be used for the calculation:

$$V_{K_2Cr_2O_7}N_{K_2Cr_2O_7} = V_{Na_2S_2O_3}N_{Na_2S_2O_3}$$

Iodometric determination of oxidizing agents can be schematically represented as follows:

(a) KI + acid (excess in flask) + oxidant to be determined, pipetted out (or weighed) $\rightarrow$ liberation of I_2 (on standing);

(b) $I_2 + 2Na_2S_2O_3 = 2NaI + Na_2S_4O_6$ (titration of iodine with thiosulphate).

---

* Or a weighed sample dissolved in any suitable volume of water (by the method of separate samples).

** Direct titration of thiosulphate with dichromate is not used because the course of the reaction is then complex, with the formation of several products. Moreover, such a sensitive indicator as starch could not be used in this titration.

If H^+ ions are not involved in the reaction between the oxidant and KI, acidification of the solution at stage (a) is superfluous.

Many oxidizing agents capable of oxidizing I^- ions to I_2 can be determined iodometrically by this procedure. They include Cl_2, Br_2, $KMnO_4$, $KClO_3$, bleaching powder $CaOCl_2$, salts of HNO_2, hydrogen peroxide, ferric salts, cupric salts, etc.

Equations for the reactions on which these determinations are based are given below.*

$$\underset{(+1.07\ V)}{Br_2} + 2I^- = 2Br^- + \underset{(+0.54\ V)}{I_2}$$

$$\underset{(+1.51\ V)}{2MnO_4^-} + 10I^- + 16H^+ = 5I_2 + 2Mn^{++} + 8H_2O$$

$$\underset{(+1.45\ V)}{ClO_3^-} + 6I^- + 6H^+ = 3I_2 + Cl^- + 3H_2O$$

$$\underset{(+1.00\ V)}{2NO_2^-} + 2I^- + 4H^+ = I_2 + \uparrow 2NO + 2H_2O$$

$$\underset{(+1.77\ V)}{H_2O_2} + 2I^- + 2H^+ = I_2 + 2H_2O$$

$$\underset{(+0.77\ V)}{2Fe^{+++}} + 2I^- = I_2 + 2Fe^{++}$$

etc.

Determination of Acids. In addition to the above determinations of reducing and oxidizing agents, the iodometric method is also used for determination of acids, based on the reaction

$$KIO_3 + 5KI + 6HCl = 6KCl + 3I_2 + 3H_2O$$

or

$$\underset{(+1.09\ V)}{IO_3^-} + 5I^- + 6H^+ = \underset{(+0.54\ V)}{3I_2} + 3H_2O$$

The equation shows that H^+ ions are consumed in the reaction and an equivalent quantity of free iodine is liberated. The liberated iodine is titrated with thiosulphate, and the normality and titre of the acid solution are calculated from the volume of thiosulphate taken and its normality.

It is evident from all this that the iodometric method of volumetric analysis has very extensive application. Its important advantage is the *high precision* which is due to the great sensitivity of the indicator used (starch solution). The lowest concentration of free

* Values of E_0 of the oxidizing agents and of the system $I_2/2I^-$ are given in brackets.

iodine which can be detected at room temperature by the starch-iodine reaction is between 1×10^{-6} and 2×10^{-5} *N*, provided that the solution contains at least a small amount (0.001 *N* or more) of I^- ions. In the absence of iodide ions the reaction is less sensitive.

Conditions for Iodometric Determinations. 1. It must be remembered that the potential of the $I_2/2I^-$ system is not high, and therefore many iodometric reactions are reversible and do not go to completion; only if suitable conditions are provided do they proceed practically to the end.

2. Since iodine is volatile, *the titration is conducted in the cold.* This is also necessary because the sensitivity of starch as indicator diminishes with rise of temperature. If a starch solution turned blue by a single drop of iodine is heated, the blue colour disappears; when the solution is cooled the colour returns.

3. Iodometric titrations *cannot be performed in strongly alkaline solutions,* because iodine reacts with alkalies in accordance with the equation

$$I_2 + 2NaOH = NaIO + NaI + H_2O$$

or

$$I_2 + 2OH^- = IO^- + I^- + H_2O$$

The presence of hypoiodide (IO^- ions) is inadmissible, because it is a stronger oxidant than I_2 and partially oxidizes thiosulphate to sulphate:

$$S_2O_3^{--} + 4IO^- + 2OH^- = 4I^- + 2SO_4^{--} + H_2O$$

The higher the OH^- ion concentration in solution, the more thiosulphate is converted into sulphate. This side reaction makes exact calculation of the analytical result impossible. Care must therefore be taken that the solution pH does not exceed 9.

If the reaction results in formation of H^+ ions, they must be removed to ensure that the reaction proceeds to practical completion in the required direction; this is done by addition of $NaHCO_3$, which reacts as follows:

$$HCO_3^- + H^+ = H_2CO_3 = H_2O + \uparrow CO_2$$

The solution becomes very slightly alkaline (pH $\approx$ 8), but this does not interfere with the titration.

4. Since the solubility of iodine in water is low, a considerable excess of KI must be used in iodometric determinations of oxidizing agents. The iodine liberated by the reaction then dissolves by forming the unstable complex salt $K[I_3]$ with KI:

$$KI + I_2 \rightleftarrows K[I_3] \text{ or } I^- + I_2 \rightleftarrows [I_3]^-$$

Formation of this compound does not interfere with titration of iodine with thiosulphate, because the solution contains sufficient iodine owing to the reversible character of the above reaction. Subsequently, as free iodine is used up in the reaction with thiosulphate, the equilibrium between I_2 and $[I_3]^-$ ions is disturbed and more I_2 is dissolved.

Moreover, an excess of KI accelerates the reaction between I^- ions and the oxidant and makes it go more completely in the desired direction.

In cases where H^+ ions are consumed in the reaction increase of solution acidity has a similar effect.

5. Despite the use of large amounts of KI and acid, the rate of the reaction between the oxidant and I^- ions is usually too low. Therefore, some time is generally allowed to elapse after addition of the oxidant before the liberated iodine is titrated.

6. When the reaction mixture is left to stand before the start of the titration it is kept in a dark place, because light accelerates the side reaction in which I^- ions are oxidized to I_2 by atmospheric oxygen:

$$4I^- + 4H^+ + O_2 = 2I_2 + 2H_2O$$

96. Preparation of Standard Solutions

Thiosulphate Solution. The high sensitivity of the iodine-starch reaction ensures a quite distinct blue colour in 50 ml of solution with one drop of 0.01 *N* iodine solution. Accordingly, it is possible to use 0.02 *N* rather than 0.1 *N* standard iodine and thiosulphate solutions. It is known (p. 190) that the drop error in titration diminishes with decreasing concentration of the standard solutions. Moreover, in this case the saving of such relatively costly reagents as KI and I_2 is also important.

Sodium thiosulphate, $Na_2S_2O_3 \cdot 5H_2O$, is a crystalline substance. Although it can be obtained chemically pure under the appropriate conditions, standard thiosulphate solutions cannot be prepared by exact weighing, because thiosulphate does not conform to the requirements for primary standards (p. 204). It is a relatively unstable compound; for example, it reacts with carbonic acid dissolved in water as follows:

$$Na_2S_2O_3 + H_2CO_3 = NaHCO_3 + NaHSO_3 + \downarrow S$$

As a result, the normality of the thiosulphate solution increases somewhat. The gram-equivalent of $Na_2S_2O_3$ is 1 *M*, whereas that of $NaHSO_3$ is $^1/_2$ *M*. Therefore, in the above reaction one gram-equivalent of $Na_2S_2O_3$ yields two gram-equivalents of $NaHSO_3$.

The following is evident from this:

(a) It is pointless to weigh $Na_2S_2O_3 \cdot 5H_2O$ out exactly.

(b) The solution must not be standardized at once, but about 10 days after preparation. However, if freshly boiled and cooled distilled water is used and 0.1 g of Na_2CO_3 per litre of solution is added to stabilize the titre,* the solution may be standardized on the day after preparation. The $Na_2S_2O_3$ solution must be kept in bottles protected from CO_2 by a tube containing soda lime or Ascarite, in the same way as NaOH solutions (for example, see Figs. 31*a* and 55).

Subsequently the titre of $Na_2S_2O_3$ gradually decreases, so that it must be checked from time to time.

The decrease of the titre is due to the following causes:

1. Oxidation of $Na_2S_2O_3$ by atmospheric oxygen**:

$$2Na_2S_2O_3 + O_2 = 2Na_2SO_4 + \downarrow 2S$$

2. Decomposition of $Na_2S_2O_3$ by the action of microorganisms (thiobacteria); this is the main cause of the instability of thiosulphate solutions. To prevent this decomposition, 10 mg of mercuric iodide HgI_2 per litre of solution may be added as an antiseptic. The solution should also be effectively protected from light, which favours the growth of these bacteria.

Base your preparation of the thiosulphate solution on the value of its gram-equivalent (248.2 g) and the required normality (about 0.02), and take into account all the points discussed above.

Standardization of thiosulphate solution is described in Sec. 97.

Iodine Solution. Standard iodine solution may be prepared either by exact weighing of chemically pure crystalline iodine, or from commercial iodine. In the latter case the solution is usually standardized against standard thiosulphate solution.

Let us consider both these methods.

Preparation of Iodine Solution by Weighing Chemically Pure Iodine. Commercial iodine contains chlorine, various compounds of iodine with other halogens, such as ICl, IBr and ICl_3, and hygroscopic moisture. The principle on which its purification is based is that the vapour pressure of solid iodine becomes equal to the atmospheric pressure at a temperature below its melting point. Therefore, when solid iodine is heated it passes into the vapour state without melting, and the vapour condenses in the form of crystals on the colder parts of the vessel. This vaporization of a solid without formation of a liquid phase is known as *sublimation*.

---

* CO_3^{--} ions combine with H^+ ions of the carbonic acid:

$$H^+ + CO_3^{--} = HCO_3^-$$

** This reaction is catalytically accelerated by traces of Cu^{++} ions.

Before iodine can be purified by sublimation, the impurities in it must be converted into non-volatile substances. For this, commercial iodine is ground in a jasper or agate mortar* with KI and CaO. Calcium oxide absorbs water and forms $Ca(OH)_2$, while KI reacts with iodine halides to form free iodine and non-volatile salts, e.g.:

$$ICl + KI = KCl + I_2$$
$$IBr + KI = KBr + I_2$$

etc.

A mixture of commercial iodine with KI and CaO is put in a perfectly dry beaker which is covered by a round-bottomed flask filled with cold water, and is warmed cautiously on a hot-plate. From time to time the iodine crystals deposited on the cold flask are transferred by means of a glass rod to a previously weighed watch glass, which is weighed on a technical balance. The sublimation is continued until enough sublimed iodine has been obtained for preparation of the solution. In this case 250 ml of 0.02 *N* iodine solution is sufficient. Since the gram-equivalent of iodine is equal to the gram-atom, 126.9 g, the amount required is

$$\frac{126.9 \times 0.02 \times 250}{1,000} \approx 0.6 \text{ g } I_2$$

When preparing the iodine solution, remember that iodine is volatile and that its vapour poisons the laboratory air and corrodes the metal parts of instruments. Therefore, all operations involving the handling and sublimation of iodine, etc., must be performed in the fume cupboard. The analytical balance, especially, must be protected against the action of iodine vapour. *In no circumstances may iodine be brought into the weighing room in open vessels or weighed in open vessels on analytical balances.*

As already stated, the solubility of iodine in water is very low; it is therefore dissolved in concentrated solutions of KI, with which it forms a soluble red-brown complex compound:

$$I_2 + KI \rightleftarrows K[I_3]$$

At least three times as much KI as iodine by weight should be taken to ensure easy and quick dissolution. Moreover, the volatility of iodine must be taken into account when it is weighed. It is best to weigh iodine in dissolved form, as iodine solutions in KI are less volatile.

---

* Porcelain mortars are unsuitable for this purpose, as their rough walls retain considerable amounts of iodine.

To do this, proceed as follows. First weigh out on the technical balance about 2-3 g of crystalline KI in a weighing bottle and dissolve it in the minimum quantity of water. When the solution has reached the temperature of the surroundings (heat is absorbed when KI dissolves) cover the weighing bottle with its lid and weigh it accurately on the analytical balance. Now transfer the required amount ($\sim$0.6 g) of sublimed iodine from a watch glass into the weighing bottle with the potassium iodide solution (this operation is performed in the fume cupboard), cover at once with the lid, and weigh the bottle accurately again. The difference between the two weighings gives the weight of iodine taken. Cautiously agitate the solution in the stoppered weighing bottle until the iodine crystals dissolve completely* and then pour the solution through a funnel into a 250 ml measuring flask. Rinse the residual iodine from the weighing bottle and funnel carefully into this flask, make the solution up to the mark with water, close the flask with a glass stopper, and mix the solution thoroughly.

Calculate the titre and normality of the solution in the usual way (Sec. 55).

Preparation of the Solution from Commercial (*Unpurified*) *Iodine.* The method for preparing the solution from unpurified iodine is the same, the only difference being that sublimation of the iodine is omitted and about 0.6-0.7 g of commercial iodine is weighed out directly on the technical balance. At the same time about 2-3 g of KI is dissolved in the minimum volume of water. The weighed iodine is put into this solution; when the iodine has dissolved, the solution is diluted with water to 250 ml. It is standardized against thiosulphate as described in Sec. 100.

Starch Solution. For preparation of the starch solution, about 0.5 g of the so-called "soluble starch" is weighed out and mixed thoroughly with 5-7 ml of cold water. The paste is poured into 100 ml of boiling water, which is then boiled for about 2 minutes (until it becomes clear) and filtered while hot. Alternatively, the starch may be allowed to settle to the bottom of the vessel and only the upper layer of quite clear liquid is then used in titrations.

It must be remembered that starch solutions are excellent nutrient media for microorganisms and therefore deteriorate rapidly. A more stable starch solution is obtained if a few milligrams of HgI_2 is added to it (at the time of preparation).

A blue colour should be given by 2-3 ml of starch solution with a drop of 0.02 *N* iodine solution added to 50 ml of water. If the colour is not blue but violet or brownish, the starch has deteriorated and is unsuitable for use as indicator.

---

* If the iodine does not dissolve completely, a little more KI may be added.

97. Standardization of $Na_2S_2O_3$ Solution

Numerous primary standards have been proposed for standardization of $Na_2S_2O_3$; they include solid chemically pure iodine, potassium iodate KIO_3, potassium bromate $KBrO_3$, potassium ferricyanide $K_3[Fe(CN)_6]$, potassium dichromate $K_2Cr_2O_7$, etc. It is possible also to standardize $Na_2S_2O_3$ with the aid of standard $KMnO_4$ solution. This method is interesting because it links the iodometric and the permanganate methods. However, it is less accurate (see p. 345). Potassium dichromate, $K_2Cr_2O_7$, is most often used in practice.

It was stated earlier (p. 361) that chemically pure potassium dichromate, corresponding exactly to its chemical formula, can be obtained by recrystallization from water and drying at 200°C. It is also very stable, both in the solid state and in solution. The only disadvantages of dichromate are the relatively small gram-equivalent and the formation of Cr^{+++} ions, which make determination of the equivalence point difficult because of their green colour, in the reaction. The solution is greatly diluted with water before titration in order to weaken this colour.

Although $K_2Cr_2O_7$, in accordance with its higher oxidation potential ($E_0 = +1.36$ V), can oxidize $Na_2S_2O_3$ ($E_0 = +0.08$ V) directly, the course of the reaction is complex and it cannot be represented by a single equation. Therefore, standardization of $Na_2S_2O_3$ is based on the general principle of iodometric determination of oxidizing agents. First, an exactly measured volume of standard $K_2Cr_2O_7$ solution is added to a mixture of KI and H_2SO_4. The dichromate is then replaced by an equivalent amount of free elemental iodine, which is titrated with the thiosulphate solution to be standardized. The equations for these reactions are given on pp. 366-67.

Preparation of Standard $K_2Cr_2O_7$ Solution. Since the $K_2Cr_2O_7$ molecule gains 6 electrons in the reaction with KI, the gram-equivalent of dichromate is:

$$\text{g-eq of } K_2Cr_2O_7 = M : 6 = 49.03 \text{ g}$$

From the gram-equivalent it is easy to calculate the weight of potassium dichromate which should be taken for 250 ml of an approximately 0.02 N solution.

Weigh the $K_2Cr_2O_7$ accurately on an analytical balance by the usual method, transfer it quantitatively into a 250 ml measuring flask, make it up to the mark with water, and mix thoroughly. Calculate the normality of the solution.

Titration. Fill the burette with the $Na_2S_2O_3$ solution and adjust the liquid level to the zero mark.

Put 5-7 ml of 20% KI solution and 10-15 ml of 2 N H_2SO_4 (from a measuring cylinder) into a large conical flask.* Add an aliquot portion (25.00 ml) of $K_2Cr_2O_7$ solution from a pipette, cover the flask with a watch glass to prevent losses due to volatilization of iodine, and leave the mixture for 5 minutes in a dark place to complete the reaction.

Now remove the watch glass and rinse it with distilled water into the flask. Add about 200 ml of water and titrate the solution with thiosulphate. At first titrate without indicator. When the colour of the solution has changed from dark brown to pale yellowish (straw colour) add about 5 ml of starch solution and continue the titration until a single drop of $Na_2S_2O_3$ solution changes the blue colour to pale green. Add the last drops of thiosulphate slowly, stirring the solution thoroughly each time. Having taken the reading, check the titration by adding one drop (*not more*) of standard $K_2Cr_2O_7$ to the titrated solution. If it has not been overtitrated, a stable blue colour should appear.

Repeat the accurate titration twice more. Take the average of the concordant results (difference not over 0.1 ml).

Calculation. Although $Na_2S_2O_3$ and $K_2Cr_2O_7$ do not interact directly in this determination, nevertheless their quantities are equivalent (p. 368).

Using the formula

$$N_1V_1 = N_2V_2$$

calculate the normality of the thiosulphate solution from the known normality of the dichromate and the volume of the solutions used.

If a standard iodine solution prepared by exact weighing of chemically pure iodine (p. 372) is available in the laboratory, it is useful to check the value found for the titre of the sodium thiosulphate solution. For this, a measured volume of iodine solution is titrated with the thiosulphate solution. Of course, it is possible to standardize the $Na_2S_2O_3$ by the latter method alone, but this is less convenient, because the errors in the two standardizations would be additive.

It is evident that, if a standard thiosulphate solution is available, it is possible to solve the reverse problem, i.e., to determine

* A preliminary experiment must be performed to make sure that elemental iodine is not liberated when the KI and H_2SO_4 solutions are mixed. Iodine is liberated if the KI contains KIO_3 as an impurity, when the solution turns brown (or yellow). If this happens, mix the required amounts of KI and H_2SO_4 in a separate beaker or flask and reduce the liberated iodine by very careful addition of $Na_2S_2O_3$ solution until the colour disappears after the addition of a single drop. *The slightest excess of* $Na_2S_2O_3$ *must be carefully avoided*, because it would give rise to an erroneous (low) result in the subsequent titration. The volume of $Na_2S_2O_3$ used in this operation is, of course, disregarded in the calculation.

the chromium content of a given dichromate solution. Since the CrO_4^{--} ion forms precipitates with Ba^{++} and Pb^{++} ions, this method can also be used for volumetric determination of these ions. The iodometric method is the best for determination of lead. In this determination a measured excess of standard $K_2Cr_2O_7$ solution is added to the unknown solution in the presence of $CH_3COOH +$ $+ CH_3COONa$ buffer, the precipitate is filtered off, and excess $K_2Cr_2O_7$ in the solution is determined by back-titration.

The iodometric method is also used for volumetric determination of sulphates, such as Na_2SO_4. The unknown solution is mixed with excess of a hydrochloric acid solution of $BaCrO_4$, which reacts with Na_2SO_4:

$$Na_2SO_4 + BaCrO_4 = \downarrow BaSO_4 + Na_2CrO_4$$

The solution is neutralized with alkali to remove excess $BaCrO_4$ (which is soluble in strong acids but is insoluble in water); the precipitate ($BaSO_4 + BaCrO_4$) is filtered off and washed. The Na_2CrO_4 in the filtrate and washings is determined iodometrically. Since the amount of Na_2CrO_4 is equivalent to the amount of Na_2SO_4 in the portion of solution taken for analysis, it is easy to calculate the SO_4^{--} ion content of the solution.

98. Determination of Active Chlorine in Bleaching Powder

Bleaching powder is a mixture the most important constituent of which is the double salt $Ca(OCl_2) \cdot CaCl_2$. Its formula is more conveniently written as $CaCl(OCl)$ or $CaOCl_2$. In addition to this salt, bleaching powder contains a considerable amount of lime and small amounts of $Ca(ClO_3)_2$ and $CaCl_2$.

Elemental chlorine is liberated by the action of acids on bleaching powder:

$$CaCl(OCl) + 2HCl = CaCl_2 + H_2O + Cl_2 \uparrow$$

This "active chlorine" content is a measure of the quality of bleaching powder.

The determination of active chlorine is based on the following reaction:

$$CaCl(OCl) + 2KI + 2HCl = I_2 + 2KCl + CaCl_2 + H_2O$$

The iodine liberated (the amount of which is equivalent to the amount of active chlorine in the bleaching powder) is titrated with thiosulphate in the presence of starch. Accurate results cannot be obtained by determination of active chlorine in an aqueous extract of bleaching powder, because lime strongly adsorbs certain chlorine compounds. A suspension must therefore be used.

Procedure. Weigh out 0.4-0.6 g of bleaching powder in a stoppered weighing bottle on an analytical balance. Grind the sample thoroughly with 5 ml of water in a mortar with a pouring lip and transfer the suspension quantitatively through a funnel into a 250 ml measuring flask. Carefully rinse the remaining suspension from the pestle, mortar, and funnel into the same flask. Make up the contents of the flask to the mark with water and shake the flask thoroughly. *Immediately*, before the particles have settled, pipette out 25.00 ml of the suspension into a titration flask and add 5-7 ml of 20% KI solution and 20 ml of 4 *N* HCl solution. Titrate the liberated iodine with thiosulphate solution in the usual way, adding starch solution (5 ml) at the very end of the titration. Repeat the determination two or three times more, remembering to shake the suspension thoroughly before taking each aliquot portion for analysis.

Take the average of the concordant readings.

Calculation. First calculate the chlorine titre of the thiosulphate. For example, if the normality of the $Na_2S_2O_3$ is 0.02106, then 1 ml of this solution contains $\frac{0.02106}{1,000}$ gram-equivalent of sodium thiosulphate, which corresponds to the same number of gram-equivalents of I_2 and Cl_2. Since the gram-equivalent of chlorine is the same as its gram-atom, 35.45 g, we can write:

$$T_{Na_2S_2O_3/Cl} = \frac{0.02106 \times 35.46}{1,000} = 0.0007464 \text{ g of chlorine per 1 ml}$$

Now calculate the number of millilitres of the thiosulphate solution required for titration of the whole sample taken (i.e., 250 ml of the suspension), multiply this volume of $Na_2S_2O_3$ by its chlorine titre, and so find the chlorine content of the sample first in grams and then as a percentage.

99. Determination of Copper in Copper Sulphate

One of the most important applications of iodometry is in volumetric determination of copper, widely used in analysis of alloys, ores, etc. This determination is based on the reaction:

$$2Cu^{++} + 4I^- = \downarrow 2CuI + I_2$$

The equation shows that each Cu^{++} ion gains an electron from the I^- ions and is reduced to a Cu^+ ion which is then precipitated in the form of the sparingly soluble cuprous iodide CuI (solubility product $\approx 10^{-12}$). Therefore, the oxidation gram-equivalents of copper and $CuSO_4 \cdot 5H_2O$ in this case are equal to the gram-atom (63.54 g Cu) and the gram-molecule (249.7 g $CuSO_4 \cdot 5H_2O$) respectively.

The values of the standard oxidation potentials of the systems Cu^{++}/Cu^{+} (+0.17 V) and $I_2/2I^-$ (+0.54 V) might suggest that the reaction should proceed in the reverse direction.

As was explained in detail in Sec. 79 (p. 318) the discrepancy between the course of the reaction indicated by the values of the standard oxidation potentials and the actual course of the reaction is due to the low solubility of CuI. Therefore, the concentration of the reduced form in solution, i.e., Cu^+ ions, is greatly reduced and the potential of the Cu^{++}/Cu^{+} system becomes greater than that of $I_2/2I^-$.

A large excess of KI is needed to make this reversible reaction proceed sufficiently fully in the required direction; the greater the excess of KI, the lower the Cu^{++} concentration and the higher the oxidation potential of the Cu^{++}/Cu^{+} system.

Although H^+ ions do not take part in this reaction, it is helpful to have a faintly acid solution in order to suppress hydrolysis of cupric salts, which lowers the oxidation potential of the Cu^{++}/Cu^{+} system and slows down the reaction.

Procedure. Weigh out enough $CuSO_4 \cdot 5H_2O$ on the analytical balance to give an approximately 0.02 *N* solution when dissolved in a 250 ml measuring flask. After the sample has been dissolved acidify it with 15 ml of 2 *N* CH_3COOH solution, make the solution up to the mark, and mix thoroughly.

Measure out 15 ml of 20% KI solution from a measuring cylinder into a titration flask, add an aliquot portion (25.00 ml) of the $CuSO_4$ solution, cover the flask with a watch glass, and leave it in the dark for about 5 minutes to complete the reaction. Now titrate it with $Na_2S_2O_3$ solution, adding starch (5 ml) as before, at the very end of the reaction, when the solution with its suspended precipitate has a straw colour. Titrate until the blue colour disappears on addition of a single drop of $Na_2S_2O_3$ and does not return after several minutes (the CuI precipitate suspended in the liquid is the colour of ivory at the end point*). Repeat the accurate titration two or three times and take the average of the concordant results.

Calculation. Having found the normality of the $CuSO_4$ solution, calculate the number of gram-equivalents of the salt, and therefore of copper, present in the sample (i.e., in 250 ml of solution). Since the gram-equivalent of copper is 63.54 g, it is easy to find the number of grams of copper and its percentage content in the sample. If the recrystallized salt was taken for analysis, calculate the theoretical percentage of Cu in $CuSO_4 \cdot 5H_2O$ and compare it with your result.

---

* To make sure that the solution is not overtitrated, take the burette reading and then add a drop of the $CuSO_4$ solution. A permanent blue colour should then appear.

100. Determination of Arsenic in Sodium Arsenite Solution

As an example of iodometric determination of reducing agents, let us consider the determination of arsenic in a solution of sodium arsenite, Na_3AsO_3.

This determination is based on the reaction

$$Na_3AsO_3 + I_2 + H_2O \rightleftarrows Na_3AsO_4 + 2HI$$

or

$$AsO_3^{---} + I_2 + H_2O \rightleftarrows AsO_4^{---} + 2I^- + 2H^+$$

It was already pointed out in Sec. 79 that in accordance with the standard oxidation potentials of the systems AsO_4^{---}/AsO_3^{---} (+0.57 V) and $I_2/2I^-$ (+0.54 V) this reaction tends to go in the reverse direction. To make it go fully enough in the desired direction it is necessary to remove the H^+ ions formed. In this case alkali or Na_2CO_3 cannot be added (p. 370), and therefore the reaction is conducted in presence of excess $NaHCO_3$, which gives pH ≈ 8 in the solution.

In addition, it must be remembered that Na_3AsO_3 solution is usually prepared by dissolution of As_2O_3 in NaOH

$$As_2O_3 + 6NaOH = 2Na_3AsO_3 + 3H_2O$$

and therefore it contains free alkali. Obviously, the latter must first be neutralized with acid.

Preparation and Standardization of Iodine Solution. In this determination the solution to be analysed has to be titrated with iodine; therefore prepare 250 ml of approximately 0.02 *N* iodine solution (pp. 373). If the solution is prepared from commercial (unpurified) iodine (p. 374), it must first be standardized. For the standardization, put the prepared iodine solution into a burette with a glass tap.* Measure out 25.00 ml of standard $Na_2S_2O_3$ solution with a pipette (or burette) into a conical flask, add 1-2 ml of starch solution, and titrate with iodine solution until a single drop produces a stable blue colour.

Repeat the titration once or twice more and take the average of the concordant readings. Calculate the normality of the iodine solution from the known normality of the $Na_2S_2O_3$.

Procedure. Put the Na_2AsO_3 solution into a 250 ml measuring flask, dilute it with approximately 70-100 ml of distilled water, and neutralize it with 2 *N* H_2SO_4 solution in the presence of two or three drops of phenolphthalein. Add the acid drop by drop until

* An ordinary burette may also be used, but this is less advisable, because iodine attacks rubber. In any event, the iodine solution must be run out of the burette immediately after use.

the pink colour disappears. Now put 4-5 g of solid $NaHCO_3$ into the flask and dissolve it, stirring but not heating the solution. If the solution turns red again owing to the presence of Na_2CO_3 in the $NaHCO_3$, add H_2SO_4 drop by drop until the colour vanishes. Now dilute the liquid with water up to the mark and mix it thoroughly.

Pipette out an aliquot portion (25.00 ml) of the arsenite solution by means of a special pipette with a protective bulb (Na_3AsO_3 is *poisonous*) into a conical flask, and add 1-2 ml of starch solution. Titrate the solution with iodine until one drop produces a stable blue colour. Repeat the accurate titration once or twice more and take the average of the concordant results.

Note. The titration sequence in this determination may be reversed in other words, the iodine solution may be pipetted out into a flask and the burette filled with Na_3AsO_3 solution prepared as described above. In this case the starch must, of course, be added as usual at the very end of the titration.This procedure is more convenient if pipettes with protective bulbs, which prevent Na_3AsO_3 solution from entering the mouth, or burettes with glass taps are not available in the laboratory. Of course, in this case the iodine solution must be standardized in the same way, by titration with $Na_2S_2O_3$ solution.

Calculation. Find the normality of the Na_3AsO_3 solution and its arsenic content in grams by the usual method. Remember that since trivalent arsenic is oxidized to the quinquivalent state in the reaction, yielding two electrons, the gram-equivalent of arsenic is

$$\text{g-eq As} = \frac{74.92}{2} = 37.46 \text{ g}$$

101. Determination of Sodium Sulphite

As our second example of the iodometric determination of reducing agents, let us determine the Na_2SO_3 content of commercial sodium sulphite, $Na_2SO_3 \cdot 7H_2O$. This determination is based on the reaction

$$Na_2SO_3 + I_2 + H_2O = Na_2SO_4 + 2HI$$

It might seem that in this case too Na_2SO_3 solution should be titrated with iodine solution. However, it is found in practice that, as in a number of similar cases, such direct titration gives very inaccurate results. The reason is that the reaction of iodine with most reducing agents is relatively slow, especially near the end of the titration, when the concentration of the reducing agent is very low. As a result, the iodine which has not yet reacted with the reducing agent colours the starch before the equivalence point has been reached and the result of the determination is therefore too low. Partial oxidation of the reducing agent by atmospheric oxygen during the titration contributes to this effect. These complications are avoided by back-titration. The reducing agent (Na_2SO_3 in this case) is first treated with an exact volume, known to be in excess of standard iodine solution, and excess iodine is then titrated with thiosulphate.

Procedure. Weigh out accurately a sample of $Na_2SO_3 \cdot 7H_2O$ to give an approximately 0.02 *N* solution when dissolved in 250 ml. Remember that during the reaction the SO_3^{--} ion is oxidized as follows:

$$SO_3^{--} + H_2O - 2e = SO_4^{--} + 2H^+$$

Transfer the sample quantitatively into a 250 ml measuring flask, dissolve it, dilute the solution with water to the mark, and mix thoroughly. Pipette out 25.00 ml of the solution and add an exactly measured volume (40-50 ml) of standard iodine solution (see p. 195) by means of a burette (or pipette). Cover the flask with a watch glass and leave it standing in the dark. After a few minutes titrate the excess iodine with thiosulphate solution. Repeat the accurate titration at least twice. Take the average of the concordant readings.

Calculation. Suppose that after addition of 40.00 ml of 0.01986 *N* iodine solution to 25.00 ml of the sulphite solution (from the sample dissolved in 250 ml) an average of 15.80 ml of 0.02115 *N* $Na_2S_2O_3$ solution was required for the back-titration. First we calculate the volume (V) of iodine solution corresponding to the 15.80 ml of $Na_2S_2O_3$ solution taken for the titration:

$$V \times 0.01986 = 15.80 \times 0.02115$$

and hence

$$V = \frac{15.80 \times 0.02115}{0.01986} = 16.83 \text{ ml}$$

Therefore, of the 40.00 ml of iodine solution added, the volume taken in the reaction with Na_2SO_3 was 40.00—16.83 = 23.17 ml. Use this result to calculate the normality of the Na_2SO_3 solution, the weight of sodium sulphite in the sample, and the percentage content of sulphite in it.

Other reducing agents, such as various sulphides, etc., can be determined in exactly the same way. In determinations of sulphides or H_2S, the S^{--} ions are oxidized to free sulphur on addition of iodine solution, and the sulphur appears in the form of a fine suspension. This does not influence the results of the determinations.

BROMATOMETRY

102. General Principles of the Method

Bromatometry is one of the oxidimetric methods, based on oxidation reactions of the bromate ion, BrO_3^-. In these reactions bromate is reduced to bromide:

$$BrO_3^- + 6H^+ + 6e = Br^- + 3H_2O$$

This equation shows that one gram-equivalent of $KBrO_3$ used as the reagent is $^1/_6$ of its gram-molecule, i. e.,

$$\text{g-eq } KBrO_3 = \frac{167.01}{6} = 27.84 \text{ g}$$

An acid solution is required, because H^+ ions are involved in the conversion of BrO_3^- into Br^- ions.

The relatively high value of the standard oxidation potential of the system BrO_3^-/Br^- ($E_0 = +1.44$ V) shows that potassium bromate is a strong oxidizing agent.

Despite this, the reaction rate in oxidation by the action of bromate is not high enough. To accelerate the reaction, titration is performed in heated and strongly acid solutions.

As already stated, BrO_3^- ions are reduced to Br^- ions during the titration. As soon as a slight excess of bromate appears in solution, the Br^- ions react with BrO_3^- ions:

$$BrO_3^- + 5Br^- + 6H^+ = 3Br_2 + 3H_2O$$

The free bromine so formed colours the solution a pale yellow. This colour is very faint and it cannot be used for exact detection of the equivalence point. However, certain organic dyes are decomposed by free bromine and become colourless in solution. The most widely used of such dyes are the well-known indicators of the neutralization method—methyl orange and methyl red—which can also serve as indicators in bromatometric titration.

It must be pointed out that these substances cannot be classified with the redox indicators. Oxidation of redox indicators is a reversible process leading to equilibrium between the two differently coloured forms:

$$Ind_{Ox.} + ne \rightleftarrows Ind_{Red.}$$

On the other hand, oxidation of methyl orange or methyl red is an irreversible process. This irreversibility must be taken into account in work with these indicators, because the colour may disappear (especially if $KBrO_3$ is added rapidly) before the equivalence point has been reached in the titration. Therefore, a few more drops of indicator must be added at the end of the titration. In replicate titrations the indicator is added only after nearly all the required volume of $KBrO_3$ solution has been added.

The bromatometric method is especially convenient for determination of arsenic and antimony in the trivalent forms; the determination may be performed in the presence of quadrivalent tin. The bromate method for determination of antimony is widely used in analysis of babbitt alloys. It is also used for analysis of certain organic compounds.

It is known that many organic compounds may be brominated by the action of free bromine, for example:

$$\underset{\text{Phenol}}{C_6H_5OH} + 3Br_2 = \underset{\text{Tribromophenol}}{C_6H_2Br_3OH} + 3HBr$$

Elemental bromine is formed by the reaction between $KBrO_3$ and KBr in acid solution (see above). Therefore, the amount of organic substance brominated can be found from the volume of potassium bromate solution required for titration in the presence of excess KBr. This type of reaction is widely used for determination of cations which are precipitated by hydroxyquinoline (Sec. 35). The washed precipitate of the hydroxyquinoline complex is dissolved in HCl and the liberated hydroxyquinoline is titrated with bromate solution in the presence of KBr. This method is discussed in detail in Sec. 104 for determination of magnesium.

The standard solution in bromatometry is 0.1 *N* $KBrO_3$ solution, which can be prepared by accurate weighing of the recrystallized salt, dried at 150-180°C. The weight of the salt required for 1 litre of exactly 0.1 *N* solution is 2.7835 g. The salt is recrystallized from water, approximately this amount is weighed out on the analytical balance, transferred quantitatively into a litre measuring flask, dissolved in water and made up to the mark.*

103. Determination of Antimony in Tartar Emetic

Tartar emetic is a basic tartrate of trivalent antimony. Its composition corresponds to the formula $K(SbO)C_4H_4O_6$. When a solution of this salt is titrated with $KBrO_3$ solution in the presence of HCl the following reaction takes place:

$$3K(SbO)C_4H_4O_6 + KBrO_3 + 15HCl =$$
$$= 3SbCl_5 + 3KHC_4H_4O_6 + KBr + 6H_2O$$

Since each atom of trivalent antimony loses two electrons in this reaction and is oxidized to quinquivalent antimony, the gram-equivalent of antimony is

$$\text{g-eq Sb} = \frac{121.75}{2} = 60.88 \text{ g}$$

Procedure. Weigh out accurately about 4 g of tartar emetic on the analytical balance and dissolve it in a 250 ml measuring flask.

* The normality of this solution can be checked against standard (approximately 0.1 *N*) $Na_2S_2O_3$. An exactly measured volume (20 or 25 ml) of $KBrO_3$ solution is added to a mixture of 10-15 ml of 2 *N* HCl and 5-7 ml of 20% KI solution, the liquid is left to stand for 5 minutes, and the liberated iodine is titrated with thiosulphate with starch added near the end of the titration.

Dilute an aliquot portion (25.00 ml) of the solution with water in a conical flask to 100 ml, add 15 ml of concentrated HCl (sp.gr. 1.19), and heat to 70° C. Add two or three drops of methyl orange or methyl red and titrate the solution with the standard $KBrO_3$ solution. At the end of the titration, when the colour of the solution becomes fainter, add a few more drops of indicator and continue the titration until the colour changes sharply.

In the repeated titration first run in from the burette a volume of $KBrO_3$ solution which is less by 0.5-1 ml than the volume taken in the first (rough) titration, warm the solution again to about 70°C, and only then add the indicator. Titrate slowly until the indicator is decolorized.

Repeat the exact titration once or twice more and take the average result.

Calculation. Calculate the antimony titre of the $KBrO_3$ solution from its normality. It is found from the formula:

$$T_{KBrO_3/Sb} = \frac{N_{KBrO_3} \times 60.88}{1,000}$$

Now calculate the total amount of antimony in the sample (i.e., in 250 ml of solution) and its percentage content.

104. Determination of Magnesium in a Solution of Mg Salt

Determination of magnesium as the pyrophosphate, $Mg_2P_2O_7$, was described in Sec. 45. Let us now consider the hydroxyquinoline method for determination of magnesium. This method is based on the reaction*:

$$MgCl_2 + \underset{\text{Hydroxyquinoline}}{2H(C_9H_6NO)} + 2NH_4OH = \downarrow \underset{\text{Mg hydroxyquinolinate}}{Mg(C_9H_6NO)_2} + 2NH_4Cl + 2H_2O$$

The precipitated magnesium hydroxyquinolinate is filtered off, washed, and dissolved in hydrochloric acid:

$$Mg(C_9H_6NO)_2 + 2HCl = 2HC_9H_6NO + MgCl_2$$

The liberated hydroxyquinoline is titrated with $KBrO_3$ solution in the presence of KBr. The following reactions take place:

$$KBrO_3 + 5KBr + 6HCl = 3Br_2 + 6KCl + 3H_2O$$

$$HC_9H_6NO + 2Br_2 = \underset{\text{Dibromohydroxyquinoline}}{HC_9H_4Br_2NO} + 2HBr$$

These equations show that one atom of magnesium is equivalent to two molecules of hydroxyquinoline, each of which is equivalent

* The structural formula of hydroxyquinoline is given on p. 141.

to four bromine atoms. Therefore, each magnesium atom is equivalent to eight bromine atoms. Then the gram-equivalent of magnesium in this reaction is

$$\text{g-eq Mg} = \frac{A_{Mg}}{8} = \frac{24.31}{8} = 3.04 \text{ g}$$

Consequently, 1 ml of 0.1 *N* $KBrO_3$ solution corresponds to 0.1 mg-eq or 0.304 mg of magnesium.

It follows that even if the titration with $KBrO_3$ solution is carried out to a precision of 0.1 ml, this corresponds to determination of magnesium to a precision of 0.03 mg, which is considerably higher than the precision of the gravimetric determination. In addition to its higher precision, the hydroxyquinoline method is more rapid. As was noted earlier (Sec. 35), one very important advantage of hydroxyquinoline as a precipitant for cations is the almost complete absence of coprecipitation of impurities. In most cases it is easy to obtain pure precipitates by this method.

This method can be used for determination of magnesium in the presence of Al^{+++} and Fe^{+++}, which are previously converted into their tartrate complexes.* It is also possible to determine Mg^{++} in the presence of Ca^{++}, as calcium hydroxyquinolinate is fairly readily soluble in hot ammonia solution. However, reprecipitation is required in this case, because a small amount of Ca^{++} is precipitated during the first precipitation.

The above equations show that magnesium is precipitated by hydroxyquinoline in the presence of ammonia, i.e., an alkaline solution is required (pH = 9.5-12.7).

The titration of hydroxyquinoline with potassium bromate is performed in the usual way, in the presence of methyl orange or methyl red until the indicator is decolorized, and the usual precautions must be taken (p. 383). Alternatively, a certain excess of $KBrO_3$ solution may first be added (until the solution becomes yellow by the liberation of bromine), followed by a small amount of KI, and the iodine liberated is then titrated with thiosulphate solution in the presence of starch. This method, which requires less skill, is described below.

Procedure. To 100-150 ml of solution, containing not more than 0.01 g of magnesium, add 1-2 g of NH_4Cl and 5-10 ml of NH_4OH. If an amorphous precipitate of $Mg(OH)_2$ is formed, it must be dissolved by addition of some more NH_4Cl. Heat the absolutely clear solution to 60-70°C and precipitate the magnesium by addition of a small excess of alcoholic hydroxyquinoline solution. Add it by small portions as usual until the supernatant liquid becomes yellow

* In such cases NaOH is added to the solution instead of NH_4OH.

owing to the formation of the intensely coloured ammonium hydroxyquinolinate.

At the end of the precipitation heat the solution with the precipitate cautiously until it *just begins* to boil, allow the precipitate to settle to the bottom of the beaker, and filter the hot solution through a fast paper filter. Wash the precipitate on the filter and in the beaker with hot water until quite free of added excess hydroxyquinoline, i.e., until the washings become quite colourless.

Dissolve the washed precipitate of magnesium hydroxyquinolinate on the filter in 2 *N* hydrochloric acid, collecting the solution in the beaker which was used for the precipitation and where part of the precipitate was left. When all the precipitate has dissolved, wash the filter six or seven times with 2 *N* hydrochloric acid, collecting the washings in the same beaker, and then proceed with the titration.

Add 1 g of KBr to the solution; when the KBr has dissolved, add 2-3 drops of methyl orange (or methyl red). Titrate the solution with the $KBrO_3$ solution, stirring the contents of the beaker thoroughly. When the solution has become colourless, continue to add $KBrO_3$ until a distinct yellow colour appears, indicating the presence of free bromine. Note the burette reading, add 5 ml of 10% KI solution, and after 2-3 minutes titrate the liberated iodine with thiosulphate solution. As usual, add starch solution (5 ml) near the end of the titration (when the colour of the solution has become straw-yellow).

Calculation. Suppose that 27.30 ml of 0.1032 *N* $KBrO_3$ solution was added and 8.18 ml of 0.02117 *N* $Na_2S_2O_3$ solution was taken for titration of the liberated iodine. The amount of magnesium can be calculated in various ways. For example, we can calculate the numbers of milligram-equivalents of $KBrO_3$ and $Na_2S_2O_3$ used in the reactions, and find the number of milligram-equivalents of magnesium by the difference, as follows:

$$\text{Number of mg-eq of } KBrO_3 = 27.30 \times 0.1032 = 2.8174$$

$$\text{Number of mg-eq of } Na_2S_2O_3 = 8.18 \times 0.02117 = 0.1732$$

Since 1 mg-eq of $KBrO_3$ corresponds to 1 mg-eq of $Na_2S_2O_3$, the reaction with hydroxyquinoline took 2.8174 — 0.1732 = 2.6442 mg-eq $KBrO_3$. This is equal to the number of milligram-equivalents of magnesium Therefore, the amount of magnesium in the original solution was:

$$x = 2.6442 \times 3.04 = 8.038 \text{ mg} = 0.008038 \text{ g}$$

QUESTIONS AND PROBLEMS
(on Secs. 85-104)

1. How does oxidation by permanganate in acid solution differ from oxidation in alkaline (or neutral) solution, and what is the explanation of the difference? What is the gram-equivalent of $KMnO_4$ in each of the two cases?

2. Explain why standard $KMnO_4$ solution should not be prepared by exact weighing. Why is $KMnO_4$ standardized several days after preparation?

3. Why must precipitated MnO_2 be separated from permanganate solution, and why must the solution be protected from light?

4. In what respect is sodium oxalate more convenient than oxalic acid as a primary standard for $KMnO_4$?

5. Explain why, during titration of oxalic acid (or oxalate), the first few drops of permanganate solution are decolorized slowly but the subsequent loss of colour is almost instantaneous. What should be done so that the first few drops of $KMnO_4$ should also be decolorized instantaneously?

6. The normality of a permanganate solution is 0.02200. What are its titres for $H_2C_2O_4$, Fe and H_2O_2?

Answer: For $H_2C_2O_4$, 0.0009904 g/ml; for Fe, 0.001228 g/ml; for H_2O_2, 0.0003741 g/ml.

7. What is the percentage of iron in a sample of iron wire, if the titration of $FeSO_4$ solution, formed by dissolving 0.1400 g of the wire in H_2SO_4 without excess of air, took 24.85 ml of 0.1000 *N* $KMnO_4$ solution?

Answer: 99.15%.

8. A solution formed by dissolving 0.2500 g of iron ore in HCl was titrated by the method described in Sec. 88, and took 28.00 ml of 0.09950 *N* $KMnO_4$ solution. Calculate the percentage of iron in the ore.

Answer: 62.24%.

9. 0.2000 g of an ore containing MnO_2 was treated with an excess of a mixture of $H_2C_2O_4$ and H_2SO_4. The volume of oxalic acid taken was 25.00 ml, and titration of excess oxalic acid took 20.00 ml of 0.02000 *N* $KMnO_4$. Find the percentage of manganese in the ore, given that 25.00 ml of the $H_2C_2O_4$ solution is equivalent to 45.00 ml of $KMnO_4$.

Answer: 6.87%.

10. 2.0000 g of an ore was dissolved in acid, and the chromium in it was oxidized to $Cr_2O_7^{--}$ by the action of $(NH_4)_2S_2O_8$ (write down the reaction equation). After decomposition of excess $(NH_4)_2S_2O_8$ by boiling the solution was transferred to a 100 ml measuring flask, cooled, and made up to the mark. For the determination, 20.00 ml of this solution was treated with 25.00 ml of $FeSO_4$ solution. Titration of excess $FeSO_4$ took 15.00 ml of 0.04500 *N* $KMnO_4$. Find the percentage of chromium in the ore, given that 25.00 ml of the $FeSO_4$ solution is equivalent to 35.00 ml of $KMnO_4$.

Answer: 3.90%.

11. Find the weight of calcium in 250.0 ml of $CaCl_2$ solution if, after addition of 40.00 ml of $(NH_4)_2C_2O_4$ solution (0.1000 *N*) to 25.00 ml of this $CaCl_2$ solution and separation of the precipitated CaC_2O_4 titration of the residual $(NH_4)_2C_2O_4$ took 15.00 ml of 0.02000 *N* $KMnO_4$ solution.

Answer: 0.7415 g.

12. Calculate the weight of ore, containing about 70% Fe_2O_3, which should be taken for analysis so that after suitable treatment titration of the ferrous salt formed from it should take 20-30 ml of 0.1 *N* $KMnO_4$ solution.

Answer: Between 0.23 and 0.34 g.

13. For determination of manganese in a solution of $MnSO_4$ the solution was titrated in a neutral medium with permanganate solution (write down the reaction equation) the normality of which (for titration in acid solution) was 0.02500. Find the weight of manganese in the solution if 42.00 ml of $KMnO_4$ solution was taken for the titration.

Answer: 0.01730 g.

14. For determination of manganese, a steel sample weighing 0.3000 g was dissolved in acid mixture and the solution was heated with $(NH_4)_2S_2O_8$ solution in the presence of $AgNO_3$ as catalyst. The $MnSO_4$ formed when the steel was dissolved was thereby oxidized to permanganic acid $HMnO_4$ (write down the reaction equation). What is the percentage of manganese in the steel, given that the titration of the permanganic acid took 12.80 ml of Na_3AsO_3 solution of $T_{Na_3AsO_3/Mn}$ = 0.0001510 g/ml?

Answer: ~0.64%.

15. For standardization of sodium arsenite solution, 0.3182 g of a standard steel sample containing 0.84% of manganese was weighed out. Titration of permanganic acid (obtained as described in Problem 14) took 22.27 ml of the arsenite solution. Calculate the manganese titre of the sodium arsenite.

Answer: 0.000120 g/ml.

16. What is the principle of the permanganate method for determination of ferric iron? If $SnCl_2$ is used as the reducing agent, why must excess stannous chloride be removed? How is this done? Why must not a large excess of $SnCl_2$ be used?

17. Explain the coupled oxidation of Cl^- ions during titration of Fe^{++} ions with permanganate. How can this coupled reaction be prevented?

18. How are oxidants determined by the permanganate method? Describe the determination of $KClO_3$ in illustration.

19. Explain why, in determination of calcium by the permanganate method, the CaC_2O_4 precipitate must be washed thoroughly.

20. What are the relative advantages and disadvantages of dichromate and permanganate as oxidizing agents?

21. How is iron determined by the dichromate method? What is the indicator used in this method? What is the purpose of adding mixed acids before the titration?

22. Calculate the weight of iron ore, containing Fe_2O_3, which should be taken so that, after the ore has been dissolved in HCl and reduced by the action of zinc, the $FeCl_2$ solution should be titrated with the number of millilitres of 0.02 *N* dichromate solution equal to the percentage of Fe_2O_3 in the ore.

Answer: 0.1597 g.

23. What are the advantages of liquid amalgams for reduction?

24. What are external indicators? How is Fe^{++} titrated with dichromate with an external indicator?

25. What is the principle of the iodometric method? Discuss the system $I_2/2I^-$ with regard to its position in the table of oxidation potentials and its possible use in analysis.

26. How are (a) reducing agents; (b) oxidizing agents; (c) acids determined by the iodometric method? Give examples in illustration.

27. Explain why only the oxidized and not the reduced forms of the respective systems are used in the permanganate and dichromate methods. Why, in contrast to this, are both forms used in iodometry?

28. List the conditions which must be observed in iodometric determinations.

29. How do NaOH and Na_2CO_3 react with iodine solution? Write the equations for the reactions.

30. How may the influence of reversibility of oxidation-reduction reactions be prevented? Illustrate the answer by the example of the iodometric determination of arsenic.

31. What is the change in the normality of a thiosulphate solution if 1% of the total amount of thiosulphate is decomposed by CO_2 with formation of $NaHSO_3$?

Answer: Increase of 1%.

32. For standardization of thiosulphate against chemically pure iodine, can acidified thiosulphate solution be titrated with iodine?

33. Explain the direction of the reaction used for iodometric determination of copper.

34. Why is a large excess of KI used in iodometric determinations of oxidizing agents?

35. For standardization of sodium thiosulphate solution, 0.1125 g of chemically pure copper was weighed out, dissolved, and treated with KI as in iodometric determination of copper. The iodine liberated was titrated with the thiosulphate solution; 18.99 ml was required. Calculate: (a) the titre of this solution; (b) its titre for Cu; (c) its titre for iodine.

Answer: (a) 0.01473 g/ml; (b) 0.005923 g/ml; (c) 0.01182 g/ml.

36. Calculate the weight of $K_2Cr_2O_7$ which should be taken for standardization of an approximately 0.1 *N* $Na_2S_2O_3$ solution if a 200 ml measuring flask and a 10 ml pipette are to be used and it is aimed to use about 25 ml of thiosulphate solution for titration of the iodine liberated.

Answer: About 2.5 g.

37. Calculate the weight of chlorine in 1 litre of chlorine if titration of the iodine liberated by 25.00 ml of it from KI took 20.10 ml of 0.1100 *N* thiosulphate solution.

Answer: 3.135 g.

38. 0.2000 g of an ore containing MnO_2 was treated with excess HCl. The chlorine formed by the reaction was distilled off and absorbed in KI solution. Titration of the liberated iodine took 42.50 ml of 0.05200 *N* thiosulphate solution. Calculate the percentage of MnO_2 in the ore.

Answer: 48.03%.

39. For determination of lead, 5.0000 g of an ore was weighed out. The ore was dissolved in acid, Pb^{++} was precipitated as $PbCrO_4$, and the precipitate was filtered off, washed, and dissolved in a mixture of HCl and KI (write down the reaction equations). The iodine liberated in this reaction was titrated with 42.00 ml of 0.05000 *N* $Na_2S_2O_3$ solution. Calculate the percentage of lead in the ore.

Answer: 2.90%.

40. In iodometric determination of sulphates (p. 376) SO_4^{--} ions are replaced by an equivalent amount of CrO_4^{--} ions, which are then determined iodometrically. Calculate the amount of Na_2SO_4 in a given solution if titration of the

iodine liberated from KI by the CrO_4^{--} ions equivalent to the SO_4^{--} ions took 30.40 ml of 0.01980 *N* thiosulphate solution.

Answer: 0.02851 g.

41. After combustion of 2 g of steel in a current of oxygen in an electric furnace and absorption in water of the SO_2 formed, titration of the SO_2 solution took 3.33 ml of 0.01125 *N* iodine solution. Find the percentage of sulphur in the steel.

Answer: 0.03%.

42. For determination of H_2S in a solution, 50.00 ml of 0.01960 *N* iodine solution was added to 25.00 ml of the H_2S solution; the excess iodine took 11.00 ml of 0.02040 *N* thiosluphate solution. Find the H_2S content of the solution in grams per litre.

Answer: 0.5150 g per litre.

43. For determination of sulphur content, a steel sample weighing 7.00 g was treated with HCl and the hydrogen sulphide liberated was absorbed in a solution containing a mixture of cadmium and zinc acetates. The solution together with the precipitate (CdS + ZnS) was then treated with 20.00 ml of iodine solution in the presence of HCl and the excess iodine was titrated with 15.27 ml of a thiosulphate solution. Calculate the percentage of sulphur in the steel, given that 1 ml of the iodine solution is equivalent to 0.0004950 g of sulphur and that titration of 10.00 ml of the iodine solution took 10.20 ml of thiosulphate solution.

Answer: 0.0363%.

44. Calculate the weight of HCl in 250 ml of hydrochloric acid solution, given that 24.00 ml of 0.02100 *N* thiosulphate solution is required for titration of the iodine liberated by 25.00 ml of this solution from a mixture of KIO_3 + KI.

Answer: 0.1838 g.

45. What is the principle of the bromatometric method of volumetric analysis? What is the principle of the action of the indicators used in this method? Why cannot these indicators be regarded as redox indicators?

46. Calculate the weight of arsenic in an arsenite solution if titration of this solution took 18.40 ml of 0.1050 *N* $KBrO_3$ solution.

Answer: 0.07238 g.

47. Calculate the titres of 0.1100*N* $KBrO_3$ solution: (a) for As_2O_3; (b) for Sb.
Answer: (a) 0.005441; (b) 0.006697 g/ml.

48. 1.0000 g of babbitt alloy was dissolved in sulphuric acid; the Sb^{+++} in the solution was titrated with 21.40 ml of 0.1100 *N* potassium bromate solution. Tin in the same solution was then reduced by means of metallic lead; titration of the tin took 17.10 ml of iodine solution. Calculate the percentage contents of (a) antimony; (b) tin in the alloy ($T_{I/Sn}$ = 0.00600 g/ml).

Answer: (a) 14.33%; (b) 10.26%.

49. How is magnesium determined by the bromate method? How is the gram-equivalent of magnesium calculated in this determination?

50. What is the gram-equivalent of aluminium if it is determined by precipitation by hydroxyquinoline, the precipitate being dissolved in HCl and the solution titrated with bromate?

Answer: 2.25 g.

CHAPTER VIII

METHODS OF PRECIPITATION AND COMPLEX FORMATION

105. General Principles

The precipitation method is based on titration with the use of reactions accompanied by formation of sparingly soluble compounds. Although very many such reactions are known, only a few of them can be used in volumetric analysis. They must satisfy a number of conditions, namely:

(a) The precipitate must be practically insoluble.

(b) The precipitation should be rapid (i.e., formation of supersaturated solutions should not have an effect).

(c) The titration results should not be distorted appreciably by adsorption (coprecipitation) effects.

(d) It must be possible to detect the equivalence point during the titration.

These conditions restrict severely the range of reactions which are suitable for volumetric analysis. The most important methods are those based on precipitation of insoluble silver salts in accordance with the equation

$$Ag^+ + X^- = \downarrow AgX$$

where X^- represents Cl^-, Br^-, I^-, CNS^-, etc.

Such methods constitute a special section of volumetric analysis, known as *argentometry*. Halogens are also determined by precipitation as the sparingly soluble mercurous salts Hg_2Cl_2 and Hg_2I_2 (*mercurometry*). Certain other precipitation reactions are also sometimes used; for example, precipitation of Zn^{++} as the complex salt $K_2Zn_3[Fe(CN)_6]_2$, or of PO_4^{---} as the double ammonium uranyl phosphate $(UO_2)NH_4PO_4$, etc.

Precipitation titrations are closely allied to volumetric determinations based on reactions of complex formation, such as

$$2CN^- + Ag^+ = [Ag(CN_2)]^-$$

$$Hg^{++} + 4I^- = [HgI_4]^{--}$$

or reactions giving rise to weakly dissociated salts such as $HgCl_2$, $HgBr_2$, $Hg(CNS)_2$, etc.

In addition to precipitation of chlorides and bromides as AgCl and AgBr, they can be determined by the *mercurimetric method*, by means of the reactions:

$$2NaCl + Hg(NO_3)_2 = HgCl_2 + 2NaNO_3$$
$$2KBr + Hg(NO_3)_2 = HgBr_2 + 2KNO_3$$

A serious obstacle to the use of many reactions of complex formation in volumetric analysis is the fact that the same cation and ligand can form complexes differing in composition, i.e., with different proportions of metal and ligand. This makes the reactions complex, as in such cases they do not conform to the same stoichiometric equation.

In recent years, however, organic reagents of a new type have found wide application. They have the general name of *complexones*, the most important of which is known as Trilon B (the trade name of the disodium salt of ethylenediamine tetraacetic acid). This agent, which can form complexes with a large number of different cations, such as the cations of the alkaline earths, many non-ferrous metals (Cu^{++}, Zn^{++}, Ni^{++}, Co^{++}, etc.), ions of the rare-earth elements, iron, zirconium, etc., is free of the above-mentioned disadvantage. Under specified conditions, different cations (even differing in charge) form complex molecules or ions with Trilon B, with the metal and ligand in 1 : 1 molecular ratio. Therefore, stepwise reactions, leading to non-stoichiometric proportions between the metal and the complex former, are excluded in this case. Recently numerous methods have been developed for volumetric determination of various cations by titration of solutions of their salts with standard Trilon B solution. One of the most important applications of this method, for determination of the total hardness of water, is described in Sec. 116.

106. Titration Curves in the Precipitation Method

Titration curves are very important in the precipitation method. Suppose, for example, that 100 ml of 0.1 N NaCl solution is titrated with 0.1 N $AgNO_3$ solution. To simplify the calculation, we shall use a rounded-off value for the solubility product of AgCl (1×10^{-10}) and shall disregard the change of solution volume in the titration.

At the start (i.e., before addition of $AgNO_3$) the Cl^- ion concentration in the solution is equal to the total NaCl concentration (10^{-1} M). Representing the negative logarithm of the concentration (or, more correctly, of the activity) of the Cl^- ions by pCl, we can write:

$$pCl = -\log [Cl^-] = -\log 10^{-1} = 1$$

After 90 ml of $AgNO_3$ solution has been added to the NaCl solution, 90% of all the Cl^- ions is precipitated in the form of AgCl, and their concentration in solution is reduced tenfold, i.e., it becomes 1×10^{-2} g-ion/litre. Accordingly, pCl becomes 2.*

Since $[Cl^-][Ag^+] = 10^{-10}$, the Ag^+ concentration in solution at this stage must be

$$[Ag^+] = \frac{10^{-10}}{[Cl^-]} = \frac{10^{-10}}{10^{-2}} = 10^{-8} \text{ g-ion/litre}$$

Consequently

$$pAg = -\log [Ag^+] = -\log 10^{-8} = 8$$

In the same way, we have for the point when 99 ml of $AgNO_3$ solution has been added (i.e., 99% of the NaCl has been titrated):

$$[Cl^-] = 10^{-3} \qquad pCl = 3$$

$$[Ag^+] = 10^{-7} \qquad pAg = 7$$

When 99.9 ml of $AgNO_3$ solution has been added, we have:

$$[Cl^-] = 10^{-4} \qquad pCl = 4$$

$$[Ag^+] = 10^{-6} \qquad pAg = 6$$

Finally, when the equivalent amount, i.e., exactly 100 ml of 0.1 *N* $AgNO_3$ solution, has been added to 100 ml of 0.1 *N* NaCl solution, a saturated AgCl solution is formed in which the Cl^- and Ag^+ ion concentrations are equal. Therefore, at the equivalence point

$$[Cl^-] = [Ag^+] = \sqrt{10^{-10}} = 10^{-5} \text{ g-ion/litre}$$

$$pCl = pAg = 5$$

When 100.1 ml of $AgNO_3$ has been put in (i.e., 0.1% in excess), the excess of Ag^+ ions is equal to the amount of Ag^+ ions contained in 0.1 ml of $AgNO_3$ solution. This creates a concen ration of Ag^+ ions equal to the concentration of Cl^- ions with 0.1 ml of excess NaCl solution, i.e., 10^{-4} g-ion/litre. Consequently, at this point

$$[Ag^+] = 10^{-4} \qquad pAg = 4$$

$$[Cl^-] = 10^{-6} \qquad pCl = 6$$

When 101.0 ml of $AgNO_3$ has been added, we have

$$[Ag^+] = 10^{-3} \qquad pAg = 3$$

$$[Cl^-] = 10^{-7} \qquad pCl = 7, \text{ etc.}$$

---

* If the change of solution volume is disregarded in reality the concentration is

$$\frac{10}{190} \times 10^{-1} = 5.3 \times 10^{-3} \text{ g-ion/litre, and } pCl = 2.28.$$

The calculated values of pAg and pCl are given in Table XIX and are also plotted in Fig. 59, where the continuous curve represents variations of pCl and the dotted line, variations of pAg during the titration.

Table XIX

Variations of pCl and pAg during Titration of 100 ml of 0.1 *N* NaCl Solution with 0.1 *N* $AgNO_3$ Solution

$AgNO_3$ solution added, ml	$[Cl^-]$	$[Ag^+]$	pCl	pAg
0	10^{-1}	—	1	—
90	10^{-2}	10^{-8}	2	8
99	10^{-3}	10^{-7}	3	7
99.9	10^{-4}	10^{-6}	4	6
100 (equiv. pt.)	10^{-5}	10^{-5}	5	5
100.1	10^{-6}	10^{-4}	6	4
101.0	10^{-7}	10^{-3}	7	3
110.0	10^{-8}	10^{-2}	8	2
200.0	10^{-9}	10^{-1}	9	1

Figure 59 shows that the course of the curves is similar to that found in other methods of volumetric analysis. Near the equivalence point (pCl = pAg = 5) there are sharp changes of pCl (from 4 to 6) and pAg (from 6 to 4).

It is easy to see that the magnitude of the change depends on the concentrations of the solutions. Thus, if the concentrations were 1 *N* and not 0.1 *N* the break would begin at pCl = 3 and end at pCl = 7, i.e., it would be 4 and not 2 pCl units. Conversely, if the concentrations of the NaCl and $AgNO_3$ solutions are decreased the break on the titration curve narrows or even vanishes.

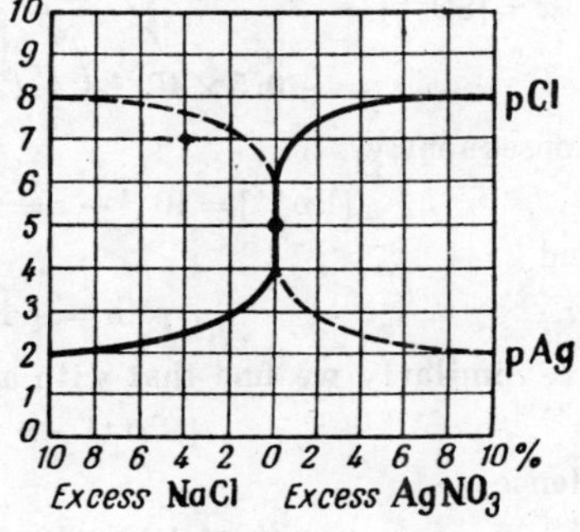

Fig. 59. Titration curve of 0.1 *N* NaCl solution with 0.1 *N* $AgNO_3$ solution (or vice versa)

Apart from the concentrations of the reacting solutions, the break on the titration curve also depends on the solubility product of the precipitate. For example, in the titration of 0.1 *N* KI solution with 0.1 *N* $AgNO_3$ solution the AgI precipitate has SP of app. 1×10^{-16}

which is about one-millionth part of the solubility product of AgCl. Accordingly, the equivalence point in this case is at $[I^-] = [Ag^+] = \sqrt{10^{-16}} = 10^{-8}$ g-ion/litre, i.e., at pI = pAg = 8; the change of pI begins at pI = 4 and ends* at pI = 12, i.e., covers 8 units of pI. Therefore, *the lower the solubility product of the compound formed in the titration, the wider the range of the break on the titration curve.* Conversely, if the SP of the precipitate is large, the range of the break becomes narrower and it may disappear entirely. For example, in titration of 0.1 *N* $Pb(NO_3)_2$ solution with 0.1 *N* Na_2SO_4 solution, $SP_{PbSO_4} = 1 \times 10^{-8}$ and the change of pPb is only about 0.4 of a unit; in the precipitation of $CaSO_4$ (SP = 6×10^{-5}) there is no break at all.

When precipitates such as $PbSO_4$ or $CaSO_4$ are formed, calculation of the titration curves is complicated somewhat, because here we can no longer neglect the amount of ions entering the solution from the precipitate. For example, let us calculate pPb at the start of the break during titration of a lead salt (see above). The Pb^{++} ion concentration at this point is the sum of: (a) 10^{-4} g-ion/litre remaining unchanged by the titration, and (b) x g-ion/litre from the $PbSO_4$ precipitate. As this precipitate gives rise to the same concentration, x g-ion/litre, of SO_4^{--} ions, we can write:

$$x\,(10^{-4}+x)=10^{-8}$$

or

$$x^2+10^{-4}x-10^{-8}=0$$

Solving this quadratic equation, we have:

$$x=[SO_4^{--}]=-\frac{10^{-4}}{2}+\sqrt{\frac{10^{-8}}{4}+10^{-8}}=$$

$$=-0.5\times10^{-4}+1.12\times10^{-4}=0.62\times10^{-4}\ \text{g-ion/litre}$$

Consequently,

$$[Pb^{++}]=10^{-4}+x=10^{-4}+0.62\times10^{-4}=1.62\times10^{-4}$$

and

$$pPb=-\log 1.62\times10^{-4}=3.79$$

Similarly we find that with an excess of 0.1 ml of sulphate solution

$$[Pb^{++}]=x \text{ and } [SO_4^{--}]=10^{-4}+x$$

Hence

$$x\,(10^{-4}+x)=10^{-8};\qquad x=[Pb^{++}]=0.62\times10^{-4}$$

$$pPb=-\log 0.62\times10^{-4}=4.21$$

Therefore, the change in this case is 4.21 — 3.79 = 0.42 pPb unit.

---

* With an excess of 0.1 ml of silver nitrate solution $[Ag^+] = 10^{-4}$ and $[I^-] = \frac{10^{-16}}{10^{-4}} = 10^{-12}$. Therefore, at this point pI = 12.

Since there must be a sufficiently sharp break on the titration curve if the equivalence point is to be determined exactly, this narrowing of the break with increase of the solubility product of the precipitate explains why only precipitation reactions in which the precipitates formed are virtually insoluble (SP of the order of 10^{-10} or less) are used in volumetric analysis.

It should be noted that the above calculations of the titration curves based on the solubility product of the precipitate are approximate only. In reality the situation is complicated by adsorption (coprecipitation) effects, the influence of which is not taken into account in the calculation.

107. Methods of Determining the Equivalence Point

There are several methods for determining the equivalence point in titration by the precipitation method. Here we consider only those which are used in argentometry.

The Gay-Lussac Method (Without Indicator). The following reaction takes place when NaBr solution is titrated with $AgNO_3$ solution (or vice versa):

$$NaBr + AgNO_3 = \downarrow AgBr + NaNO_3$$

It is evident that precipitation of AgBr continues only as long as an excess of Br^- ions is present in solution. Therefore, we can detect accurately the point at which precipitation ceases by taking small portions of the titrated solution at the end of the titration and adding to each a single drop of the $AgNO_3$ solution diluted tenfold. In this instance detection of the end point is made much easier by the fact that near the equivalence point the AgBr precipitate coagulates and collects at the bottom of the vessel in the form of large curdy flakes. The solution clears rapidly; this is facilitated by vigorous stirring or shaking.

In the case of AgCl, the solubility product of which (1.56×10^{-10}) is not as low as that of AgBr (7.7×10^{-13}), the technique is somewhat more complicated. The reason is that the saturated AgCl solution formed at the equivalence point gives a distinct turbidity both with $AgNO_3$ solution and with NaCl solution (decrease of the solubility of AgCl by the introduction of a common ion; see Sec. 19). The turbidity is exactly the same in each case. However, this occurs only at the equivalence point. If the solution is not fully titrated and a small excess of Cl^- ions is present, the turbidity caused by addition of $AgNO_3$ must evidently be greater than that caused by NaCl. Conversely, if the solution is slightly overtitrated, NaCl causes more turbidity than $AgNO_3$.

Therefore, to determine the equivalence point in this case we must take two similar samples of solution before the end of the titration and treat one with a drop of $AgNO_3$ solution and the other with a drop of NaCl solution of the same concentration. The titration is ended when both samples give equal turbidity.

Despite the fact that a certain proportion of the titrated solution must be withdrawn for sampling, this "method of equal turbidity" is one of the most precise methods of volumetric analysis.* However, it requires skill and is rather laborious. Therefore, in practice indicator methods are generally used in argentometric titrations.

Indicator Methods. The most usual indicators in argentometric titrations are potassium chromate solution K_2CrO_4 (the Mohr method) or ferric ammonium alum $NH_4Fe(SO_4)_2$ (the Volhard method).

The use of K_2CrO_4 as indicator is based on the formation of a brickred precipitate of Ag_2CrO_4 by the action of CrO_4^{--} on Ag^+; this precipitate only begins to form after the Cl^- ions have been precipitated almost completely as AgCl.

The cause of this lies in the difference between the solubility products of silver chloride and silver chromate. Suppose that a 0.1 *N* NaCl solution, also containing K_2CrO_4 indicator in 10^{-2} *M* concentration, is titrated with $AgNO_3$ solution. Each of the precipitates (AgCl and Ag_2CrO_4) begins to form only after its solubility product has been exceeded. Since SP_{AgCl} is $\approx 10^{-10}$, the Ag^+ ion concentration in solution needed to reach this value is

$$[Ag^+] = \frac{SP_{AgCl}}{[Cl^-]} = \frac{10^{-10}}{10^{-1}} = 10^{-9} \text{ g-ion/litre}$$

Let us now calculate the concentration of silver ions at which precipitation of Ag_2CrO_4 begins. Its solubility product is

$$[Ag^+]^2[CrO_4^{--}] = SP_{Ag_2CrO_4} = 1.1 \times 10^{-12}$$

Hence:

$$[Ag^+] = \sqrt{\frac{SP_{Ag_2CrO_4}}{[CrO_4^{--}]}} = \sqrt{\frac{1.1 \times 10^{-12}}{10^{-2}}} = 1.05 \times 10^{-5} \text{ g-ion/litre}$$

Therefore, the solubility product of AgCl is reached earlier, i.e., at a lower concentration of Ag^+ ions (10^{-9} g-ion/litre), than that of Ag_2CrO_4 (1.05×10^{-5} g-ion/litre). Consequently, AgCl must be precipitated first. However, since the product $[Ag^+][Cl^-]$ remains (approximately) constant all the time, as the Cl^- ions are precipita-

---

* As was pointed out in the discussion of titrations with external indicators (p. 362), the error due to withdrawal of samples can be made negligibly small. The equal turbidity method, introduced in 1832 by Gay-Lussac, was one of the first methods of volumetric analysis. It was subsequently used for very accurate determinations of the atomic weights of halogens and silver.

ed in the form of AgCl, the Ag^+ ion concentration in the solution must gradually increase.* Eventually the Ag^+ ion concentration corresponding to the solubility product of Ag_2CrO_4:

$$[Ag^+] = \sqrt{\frac{SP_{Ag_2CrO_4}}{[CrO_4^{--}]}} = 1.05 \times 10^{-5} \text{ g-ion/litre}$$

is also reached.

At this point Ag_2CrO_4 begins to be precipitated together with AgCl, and the precipitate suspended in the liquid acquires a red-brown colour; this is taken as the end point. From the equation

$$[Ag^+][Cl^-] = SP_{AgCl}$$

it is easy to calculate the Cl^- ion concentration in the solution at this point:

$$[Cl^-] = \frac{SP_{AgCl}}{[Ag^+]} = \frac{10^{-10}}{1.05 \times 10^{-5}} \approx 9.5 \times 10^{-6} \text{ g-ion/litre}$$

It follows that precipitation of Ag_2CrO_4 begins only after practically all the Cl^- ions have been precipitated as AgCl.

The above concentration of the Cl^- ions remaining in solution corresponds to $pCl = -\log 1.05 \times 10^{-6} \approx 5.03$, which is within the range of the break on the titration curve (4-6). This shows that this indicator at $\sim 10^{-2}$ *M* concentration makes it possible to determine the end point with sufficient accuracy.

It is easy to calculate the concentration of CrO_4^{--} ions at which the start of precipitation exactly coincides with the equivalence point. At that point $[Cl^-] = 10^{-5}$. Therefore, reasoning as before, we can write:

$$\sqrt{\frac{1.1 \times 10^{-12}}{[CrO_4^{--}]}} = \frac{10^{-10}}{10^{-5}}$$

and hence

$$[CrO_4^{--}] = 1.1 \times 10^{-2}\, M$$

The use of the Fe^{+++} as indicator is based on the formation of water-soluble ferric thiocyanate, which has an intense red colour, with CNS^- ions*:

$$Fe^{+++} + 3CNS^- \rightleftarrows Fe(CNS)_3$$

The CNS^- ion also reacts with Ag^+ to form the sparingly soluble salt AgCNS ($SP \approx 1 \times 10^{-12}$). It is therefore possible to titrate solutions of silver salts with NH_4CNS (or KCNS) solutions in the pres-

---

* For example, see Table XIX (p. 395) where this increase of the $[Ag^+]$ ion concentration is seen particularly clearly.

* Researches by A. Babko have shown that in reality various complex ferric thiocyanate ions are formed, such as $[Fe(CNS)]^{++}$, $[Fe(CNS)_2]^+$, etc.

ence of a ferric salt, namely ferric ammonium alum $NH_4Fe(SO_4)_2 \cdot 12H_2O$, as indicator. The reaction is represented by the equation

$$AgNO_3 + NH_4CNS = \downarrow AgCNS + NH_4NO_3$$

Before the equivalence point the concentration of the CNS^- ions remaining in solution is so low that $Fe(CNS)_3$ is not formed. However, the first excess drop of NH_4CNS solution raises this concentration so much that the above reaction occurs and the colour of the solution becomes a more or less intense orange-red.

The thiocyanate method can also be used for determination of bromides and chlorides by back-titration. For example, bromides can be determined as follows:

$$Br^- + Ag^+ \text{ (excess)} \rightarrow \downarrow AgBr + Ag^+ \text{ (residual)}$$

$$Ag^+ \text{ (residual)} + CNS^- \rightarrow \downarrow AgCNS \text{ (titration)}$$

Chlorides are determined similarly. In determination of bromides the end point is very distinct; the first excess drop of the standard NH_4CNS solution produces a stable red colour in the titrated solution. During determination of chlorides, on the other hand, the colour disappears after some time if the liquid is stirred. The explanation is that, in contrast to AgBr ($SP \approx 10^{-13}$), AgCl is more soluble ($SP \approx 10^{-10}$) than AgCNS ($SP \approx 10^{-12}$). Consequently, the Ag^+ ion concentration in saturated AgCl solution is high enough for SP_{AgCNS} to be exceeded, i.e., for the following reaction to occur:

$$Fe(CNS)_3 + 3AgCl \rightleftarrows FeCl_3 + 3AgCNS \tag{1}$$

The disappearance of $Fe(CNS)_3$ from solution causes the colour to disappear. Evidently, the loss of colour ceases only when equilibrium has been established between the two solid phases (AgCl and AgCNS) and the solution. Equilibrium is established when the Ag^+ ion concentration in solution satisfies two equations simultaneously:

$$[Ag^+][Cl^-] = SP_{AgCl} = 1.56 \times 10^{-10}$$

$$[Ag^+][CNS^-] = SP_{AgCNS} = 1.16 \times 10^{-12}$$

Dividing the first equation by the second, we have:

$$\frac{[Cl^{-1}]}{[CNS^-]} = \frac{SP_{AgCl}}{SP_{AgCNS}} = \frac{1.56 \times 10^{-10}}{1.16 \times 10^{-12}} \approx 135$$

Therefore, the concentration of Cl^- ions formed by reaction (1) should be about 135 times as high as the concentration of CNS^- ions before the decolorization can stop. This means that the solution must be considerably overtitrated before a stable colour is produced.

It is not difficult to calculate the extent to which the solution must be overtitrated before the colour caused by formation of $Fe(CNS)_3$ ceases to disappear. It is found in practice that this colour can be detected when the excess of CNS^- ions in solution reaches about 10^{-5} g-ion/litre. Suppose that 0.1 ml of excess 0.1 *N* NH_4CNS solution is added to 100 ml of a suspension of AgCl and AgCNS formed at the equivalence point. This addition introduces $0.1 \times 0.1 = 10^{-2}$ mg-eq of CNS^- ions into the solution, and since these ions are uniformly distributed in a volume of 100 ml each millilitre of solution must contain $10^{-2} \times 100 = 10^{-4}$ mg-eq. This is also the concentration of CNS^- ions in solution (expressed in g-ion/litre) at the first instant after addition of NH_4CNS. Since this concentration is greater than 10^{-5} g-ion/litre, a colour should appear. However, because of the reaction between CNS^- ions and the AgCl precipitate, most of the excess CNS^- ions introduced into the solution (135/136) enter the precipitate, displacing an equivalent quantity of Cl^- ions. After equilibrium has been established, only 1/136 of the total quantity, or $\frac{10^{-4}}{136} \approx 0.007 \times 10^{-4} = 7 \times 10^{-7}$ g-ion/litre remains in solution. Since $7 \times 10^{-7} < 10^{-5}$, the colour disappears.

If the excess of NH_4CNS added to the solution was 1 ml and not 0.1 ml of 0.1 *N* solution the amount of CNS^- ions remaining in solution would be 10 times as much, or 7×10^{-6} g-ion/litre. However, even this is less than 10^{-5}, and therefore the solution becomes decolorized when it is overtitrated by 1 ml. The following condition must be satisfied for the formation of a stable colour:

$$7 \times 10^{-6} \times V \geqslant 10^{-5}$$

and hence

$$V \geqslant 1.4 \text{ ml}$$

where V is the volume of excess titrant.

It is found in practice that the excess must be even greater, about 2.5 ml.

It is clear from all the above that in this titration one should not aim at obtaining a stable colour, but should take advantage of the fact that before the equivalence point is reached the colour disappears very rapidly on stirring. Beyond the equivalence point the disappearance of the colour is relatively slow. The end point can be made more distinct by addition of 1-2 ml of nitrobenzene $C_6H_5NO_2$, carbon tetrachloride CCl_4, or chloroform $CHCl_3$, to the titrated solution. These substances are adsorbed on the AgCl precipitate and greatly retard the reaction between it and $Fe(CNS)_3$.

An even better method is to add a measured excess of $AgNO_3$ solution to the chloride solution in a measuring flask and to make up to the mark with water. Part of the solution is filtered through a dry filter and a definite volume of the filtrate is pipetted out and titrated with thiocyanate solution. In this case the AgCl precipitate is separated from the solution and cannot interfere with the titration.

In addition to the above methods for determining the equivalence point, methods based on adsorption phenomena are also used in argentometry. These are discussed more fully in Sec. 108.

108. Adsorption Effects in Titration. Adsorption Indicators

The precipitates formed during chemical reactions are generally not pure; they contain various impurities as the result of coprecipitation. It is known that one of the commonest causes of coprecipitation is adsorption of various ions on the precipitate particles. In addition to adsorption, coprecipitation may be caused by formation of mixed crystals or chemical compounds of the precipitates with the coprecipitated impurities, etc. (Sec. 27).

Coprecipitation effects must be taken seriously into account in volumetric determinations by the precipitation method, because they introduce a certain error into the results, and may sometimes distort them altogether. The influence of adsorption is especially strong in this respect.

It was noted in Sec. 27 that precipitates with ionic crystal lattices usually adsorb their own ions from solution to a very considerable extent. For example, an AgI precipitate adsorbs Ag^+ or I^- ions most strongly, dependent on which of these ions is present in excess at a given instant in the titrated solution. Therefore, if KI solution is titrated with $AgNO_3$ solution, before the equivalence point is reached the AgI particles adsorb I^- ions from solution, and thereby acquire negative charges. These negatively charged particles attract K^+ "counter-ions" from solution, so that the precipitate contains KI as an impurity.

Conversely, after the equivalence point has been reached or if the order of titration is reversed, the AgI particles adsorb excess Ag^+ ions and NO_3^- counter-ions, so that the precipitate is contaminated with $AgNO_3$ (see Fig. 16).

It is evident from this that *the particle charge becomes reversed during the titration*, passing through the so-called *isoelectric point* at which the particle charge is zero. It is only at this point that the precipitate does not contain either Ag^+ or I^- ions in excess and corresponds exactly to the formula AgI.

Experience shows that the isoelectric point does not necessarily coincide with the equivalence point in titration. For example, near the equivalence point AgI precipitate adsorbs more I^- ions than Ag^+ ions. Therefore, if equivalent amounts of KI and $AgNO_3$ solutions are mixed, the precipitate formed contains I^- ions in certain excess (about 0.1%) over the Ag^+ ions present. Accordingly the concentrations of the Ag^+ and I^- ions in solution are not 10^{-8} g-ion/litre each, as should be at the equivalence point with $SP_{AgI} = 10^{-16}$, but have the following values: $[Ag^+] = 10^{-6}$ g-ion/litre, and $[I^-] = 10^{-10}$ g-ion/litre. It follows that when KI solution is titrated with $AgNO_3$ an excess of Ag^+ ions is obtained in solution somewhat prematurely, i.e., the end point is reached before the equivalence point. Conversely, when $AgNO_3$ solution is titrated with KI an excess of I^- ions appears beyond the equivalence point, because they are adsorbed to the greater extent by the precipitate, and the solution is somewhat overtitrated.

Thus, *the non-correspondence of the isoelectric point and the equivalence point entails a certain error in titration.*

Adsorption may also lead to errors in analysis for another reason. We know that adsorption is a reversible process which leads to equilibrium between adsorbed ions and the same ions in solution. Since the concentration of the ion being determined gradually decreases during titration, the equilibrium is continuously disturbed and the adsorbed ions pass from the precipitate into solution. However, this release of the adsorbed impurities from the precipitate takes time and may therefore be incomplete. The ions which are not removed from the precipitate evidently do not take part in the reaction which occurs during the titration and the result of the analysis is therefore inaccurate.

To avoid this, the titration must be ended very slowly, with vigorous shaking of the flask after addition of each drop of titrant, so that adsorption equilibrium is established more rapidly.

In many cases the error due to adsorption may be greatly reduced (or even eliminated) by decrease of the surface area of the precipitate; this is achieved by allowing the precipitate to stand in contact with the mother liquor, or by heating. For example, the error due to adsorption during precipitation of AgI is prevented if the titration is performed at 95°C (or if the precipitate is left in contact with the mother liquor for some time at the same temperature). Under these conditions the AgI precipitate undergoes rapid "ageing", which is associated with a considerable decrease of its surface area. As a result, adsorption is diminished so much that it no longer affects the analytical result.

However, in many other cases it is impossible to diminish adsorption (or other forms of coprecipitation) to a sufficient extent by any available means. Therefore, the reactions in question cannot be used in volumetric analysis. This applies especially to precipitation of amorphous substances such as $Fe(OH)_3$, as their surface area is enormous and they adsorb very strongly.

For example, it might seem that, because of the very low solubility of $Fe(OH)_3$ and of the ease with which excess OH^- ions can be detected, it should be very easy to determine ferric iron in solution by titration with alkali. In reality, however, such titration is impossible, because adsorption effects greatly distort the results.* The same applies to many other precipitation reactions.

Although adsorption is a serious complication in volumetric analysis by the precipitation method, in some cases it can be used for determination of the equivalence point.

This can be done in the following ways.

Titration to the Clear Point. It was shown earlier that the AgI particles formed during titration of KI solution with $AgNO_3$ adsorb I^- ions and become negatively charged. The charges prevent the particles from forming large aggregates and settling to the bottom of the vessel. Therefore, a colloidal solution of AgI and not a precipitate is first formed during the titration. It has a yellow-green colour and sometimes it is not even opalescent.

However, as more and more I^- ions combine with Ag^+, the AgI particles gradually lose their adsorbed I^- ions (see above) and their charge decreases. Eventually the charge decreases so much that the particles coagulate and are deposited in the form of large curdy flakes. The solution then becomes quite clear. This point, known as the *clear point* depends to a certain extent on the degree of dilution of the iodide solution and on the rate of stirring of the solution during titration.

If the KI solution is very dilute and the stirring is vigorous, the clear point coincides almost exactly with the equivalence point. For quantitative determination of I^- (or Ag^+) ions, the KI solution is diluted to approximately 0.004 *N* concentration (for example, about 500 ml of water is added to 20 ml of approximately 0.1 *N* solution) and titrated with 0.1 *N* $AgNO_3$ solution, the latter being added by small portions with vigorous stirring until the clear point is reached.

It is evident that the titrated solution must not contain bi- or multivalent cations, because these would cause premature coagulation of the AgI sol. In exactly the same way lead salts can be titrated to the clear point with ammonium molybdate, $(NH_4)_2MoO$ ($PbMoO_4$ is precipitated in this reaction).

Titration with Adsorption Indicators. This method is based on adsorption of certain dyes, which then change colour, by precipitates. For example, the dye eosin, which is a relatively weak organic acid, is used as indicator in titration of bromides and iodides with $AgNO_3$ solution. Eosin may be conventionally represented as HEo.

Eosin acts as follows. The Eo^- anions present in the titrated NaBr solution confer a pink colour to it. Before the equivalence point is

---

*** In addition, the use of such reactions is difficult because of the pronounced amphoteric character of many hydroxides.**

reached the particles of AgBr precipitate formed by the reaction adsorb the common Br^- ions which are present in solution in excess. These confer negative charges to the particles and prevent adsorption of the Eo^- anions. However, as the equivalence point* is passed the particle charge is reversed owing to adsorption of Ag^+ ions which are now in excess. As soon as this happens, the positively charged AgBr particles adsorb Eo^- anions. As a result the surface of the precipitate acquires a red-violet colour. This is the end point of the titration.

As the colour changes of dyes such as eosin are associated with adsorption of their ions by the precipitates, such dyes are known as *adsorption indicators*.

Since adsorption occurs on the surface of the precipitate particles, it is advantageous to have this surface as large as possible. The total particle area is especially large in colloidal solutions (with particles from 1 to 100 mμ in size). Therefore, it is very important in titrations with adsorption indicators that the reaction product should be present at least partially in colloidal form. If the colloidal solution coagulates completely the adsorption surface decreases so much that the colour change of the indicator is not sharp. Coagulation of precipitates in titration with adsorption indicators is sometimes prevented by various protective colloids,** such as dextrin, starch, and similar substances.

A given adsorption indicator can be used only if it is not adsorbed too early by the precipitate, as is the case in titration of chlorides in the presence of eosin. In this case the anions (Eo^-) are adsorbed by the AgCl precipitate well before the equivalence point is reached. Therefore, the indicator anions and the Cl^- ions "compete" for the adsorbent surface. This competition must be won by Cl^- ions, even at low concentrations, and not by the indicator ions (which happens if eosin is the indicator). In other words, the precipitate must adsorb the ions to be determined much more strongly than the indicator ions. This condition is satisfied for Cl^- ions by the dye fluorescein, which is used as indicator in titration of chlorides with silver nitrate. Its colour changes from yellow-green to red as the result of adsorption by the AgCl precipitate.

When fluorescein is used, it must be remembered that it is a very weak acid ($K \approx 10^{-8}$). It is therefore evident that H^+ ions must combine with fluorescein anions to give undissociated molecules of the free acid. The concentration of the fluorescein anions is thereby

* More correctly, the isoelectric point.

** Protective colloids are colloidal systems in which the dispersed particles are strongly hydrated and are therefore relatively stable to the action of electrolytes. When AgCl particles adsorb a protective colloid they are stabilized and are not coagulated by electrolytes.

decreased so much that formation of a coloured adsorption layer becomes impossible. Therefore, neutral or weakly alkaline solutions (pH from 7 to 10) must be used in titrations with fluorescein as indicator. Eosin is a much stronger acid than fluorescein, and it can therefore be used in titration of bromides, iodides, and thiocyanates in acid solutions, at pH = 2 or even lower.

Dichlorofluorescein is a stronger acid than fluorescein, and it can be used for titrations in weakly acid solutions (even at pH $\approx$ 4); chlorides can also be titrated in the presence of this indicator.

109. Standardization of Silver Nitrate Solution by the Mohr Method

The Mohr method is based on titration of a halide, such as NaCl, with $AgNO_3$ solution in the presence of K_2CrO_4 as indicator (Sec. 107).

The end point of the titration is the point at which the colour of the suspension changes from pure yellow (due to the presence of CrO_4^{--} ions in solution) to reddish brown. The colour change is caused by the start of precipitation of red insoluble $AgCrO_4$; this occurs, as was shown in Sec. 107, near the equivalence point, i.e., when almost all the Cl^- has been precipitated as AgCl.

The principal standard solution in this method is 0.1 *N* or 0.05 *N* $AgNO_3$. It is prepared by exact weighing of recrystallized chemically pure $AgNO_3$. However, as the titre of $AgNO_3$ solution alters on keeping, it must be checked from time to time. The titre is checked against chemically pure NaCl.

Alternatively, standard $AgNO_3$ solution can be prepared from the commercial salt, which is not quite pure, and standardized against chemically pure NaCl.* Sometimes $AgNO_3$ is standardized gravimetrically, by precipitation of silver chloride from an exactly measured volume of $AgNO_3$ solution by addition of a chloride solution, with subsequent weighing of the precipitated AgCl in accordance with the rules of gravimetric analysis (Sec. 40).

The standardization of $AgNO_3$ solution against NaCl is described below.

Procedure. Weigh out accurately enough chemically pure NaCl to give an approximately 0.1 *N* or 0.05 *N* solution when dissolved

---

* For preparation of chemically pure NaCl for standardization, a concentrated solution of the commercial salt, as pure as possible, is prepared, and concentrated HCl is added (or gaseous hydrogen chloride is passed through the solution). Owing to the common ion effect of Cl^- the solubility of NaCl decreases and it is partially precipitated. The crystals are separated from the solution, washed, and heated over a spirit (not a gas) burner or in an electric furnace at 500-600°C to remove HCl and water.

in water in a 250 ml measuring flask, and calculate the normality of the solution.

Having thus prepared a solution of the primary standard, proceed with standardization of the $AgNO_3$ solution. Pipette out 25.00 ml of the NaCl solution, add 0.5-1 ml of 5% K_2CrO_4 solution, and titrate it with the $AgNO_3$ solution. Shake the flask vigorously during the titration to allow adsorption equilibrium to be established (p. 403). It is necessary to detect the point at which the pure yellow colour of the liquid with the suspended precipitate is changed by a single drop of $AgNO_3$ to a very faint dirty tinge (start of Ag_2CrO_4 precipitation). *On no account pour the contents of the flask down the sink after the titration; they must be collected in a special vessel.* The collected residues of silver chloride are reconverted into $AgNO_3$. This also applies to other argentometric determinations.

Repeat the exact titration two or three times and take the average reading.

Calculation. First find the normality of the $AgNO_3$ solution in the usual way, and then convert it into the chlorine titre of $AgNO_3$ (p. 215).

For example, if the normality of the $AgNO_3$ solution is 0.1012, then

$$T_{AgNO_3/Cl} = \frac{0.1012 \times 35.45}{1,000} = 0.003587 \text{ g/ml of chlorine}$$

By multiplying this value by the number of millilitres of $AgNO_3$ taken in a titration, we find the number of grams of Cl^- in 25.00 ml of a titrated solution. This calculation technique is especially useful in mass determinations of Cl^-. Of course, the ordinary method can also be used.

The Mohr method is used for determination of silver, chlorides, and bromides (it cannot be used for iodides and thiocyanates because the results are greatly distorted by adsorption effects).

Whatever is determined by the Mohr method—halides or silver salts—the titration procedure must always be the same as in standardization of the $AgNO_3$. In other words, *the silver salt solution must always be added from a burette to a measured volume of the halide solution*, because only then is a sharp colour change obtained at the end point.

Further, it must be remembered that *the Mohr method is suitable only for titration in neutral or weakly alkaline solutions* (pH = = 6.5-10), because Ag_2CrO_4 is soluble in acids and cannot be precipitated in their presence.*

* In strongly alkaline solutions (pH $>$ 10) Ag_2O is precipitated. In the presence of ammonium salts the pH range must be narrowed to 6.5-7.2, otherwise the liberated ammonia combines with silver ions to form the complex $[Ag(NH_3)_2]^+$. Obviously, the Mohr method is also unsuitable in the presence of salts which have an acid reaction as the result of hydrolysis.

If the solution for analysis is acid, it is neutralized by a solution of borax $Na_2B_4O_7 \cdot 10H_2O$ or sodium bicarbonate $NaHCO_3$. These substances, of course, must be free from chlorides. This must be checked as follows. A small amount of the salt is dissolved in water, acidified with HNO_3, and $AgNO_3$ solution is added.

Another condition for applicability of the Mohr method is *absence of cations which form precipitates with* CrO_4^{--} *in the solution to be titrated.* Such cations include Ba^{++}, Pb^{++}, Bi^{+++}, and others. Certain anions which form precipitates with Ag^+ ions also interfere (PO_4^{---}, AsO_4^{---}, CO_3^{--}, $C_2O_4^{--}$, etc.). All this greatly restricts the application of the method. The thiocyanate method (the Volhard method) is more widely used.

110. Standardization of Ammonium Thiocyanate Solution

As already stated (Sec. 106), the thiocyanate method for determination of silver and halides is based on the reaction:

$$AgNO_3 + NH_4CNS = \downarrow AgCNS + NH_4NO_3$$

The indicator in this method is Fe^{+++} ion, which makes it possible to detect excess NH_4CNS owing to formation of ferric thiocyanate $Fe(CNS)_3$, which is a soluble red compound. The indicator used in practice is a saturated solution of ferric ammonium alum $NH_4Fe(SO_4)_2 \cdot 12H_2O$, to which a little concentrated HNO_3 is added to suppress hydrolysis and to destroy the consequent brown colour of the solution. In contrast to the Mohr method, in the Volhard method *the presence of acid does not interfere with the titration but, on the contrary, improves the precision of the results.* The presence of Ba^{++}, Pb^{++}, Bi^{+++} ions, etc., does not interfere either. Only mercury salts and oxidizing agents interfere, because the former precipitate the CNS^- ion while the latter oxidize it.

The main standard solutions are $AgNO_3$ and NH_4CNS (or KCNS) solutions. The silver nitrate may be standardized by the Mohr method as described in the preceding section. Standardization of thiocyanate solution is described below.*

Procedure. Put the approximately 0.1 *N* (or 0.05 *N*) NH_4CNS (or KCNS) solution to be standardized in a burette and titrate an $AgNO_3$ solution of known concentration with it, having previously

* By the rule given on p. 205, et seq., it would be more accurate to determine the ratio between the titres of the NH_4CNS and $AgNO_3$ solutions as described in this section and then to standardize the $AgNO_3$ solution (see Sec. 111) against a weighed quantity of a chemically pure halide (for example, NaBr). Instead of this, in order to save time, we describe a less precise method, which connects the thiocyanate method with the Mohr method.

diluted the latter to 100 ml with water and added 2-3 ml of indicator solution. Add the NH_4CNS, briskly stirring the liquid, and continue until a permanent reddish colour appears. Repeat the exact titration two or three times and take the average of the results.

Calculation. Calculate the normality and the titre of NH_4CNS solution for silver by the usual method.

It is convenient to express the concentration of the NH_4CNS solution in the form of its titre for silver because the solution is used for mass determinations of silver in its salts and alloys. Silver alloys are dissolved in HNO_3 and the solutions are titrated with NH_4CNS in the same way as was described for standardization of the latter.

111. Thiocyanate Determination of Halides

As was already stated in Sec. 107, the thiocyanate method can be used for determination of halides as well as of silver.

Procedure. Weigh out accurately on the analytical balance any halide, such as NaBr, to give an approximately 0.1 *N* (or 0.05 *N*) solution when dissolved in water in a measuring flask.

Pipette out an aliquot portion (25.00 ml) of this solution and add from a burette a known excess (say, 40.00 ml) of standard $AgNO_3$ solution. Without filtering off the precipitate titrate the excess $AgNO_3$ with NH_4CNS solution as described in the preceding section. Repeat the determination two or three times and take the average result.

Calculation. The calculation may be performed in various ways. For example, the equation $N_1V_1 = N_2V_2$ can be used for calculating the number of millilitres of $AgNO_3$ solution equivalent to the volume of NH_4CNS solution taken for the back-titration. The volume of $AgNO_3$ solution required for precipitation of Br is found by difference. Then, remembering that a gram-equivalent of bromine is the same as the gram-atom (79.91 g), we find in the usual way the normality of the NaBr solution and the total amount and percentage content of bromine in the sample taken.

Alternatively, we can first find the numbers of milligram-equivalents of $AgNO_3$ and NH_4CNS used in the determination (i.e., the values of the product *NV* for the two solutions). The difference gives the number of milligram-equivalents of $AgNO_3$ used for precipitation of Br^-, and hence the number of milligram-equivalents of bromine in the titrated volume of NaBr solution. It is then easy to calculate the total bromine content and the percentage of bromine in the sample.

If Cl^- is determined instead of Br^-, it is more difficult to detect the equivalence point (Sec. 107) because of the reaction

$$3AgCl + Fe(CNS)_3 = \downarrow 3AgCNS + FeCl_3$$

which causes gradual disappearance of the colour of $Fe(CNS)_3$ when the contents of the flask are stirred.

To make the colour more stable, 1-2 ml of nitrobenzene* ($C_6H_5NO_2$) is added to the solution; adsorption of nitrobenzene by the AgCl precipitate slows down the above reaction. It is even better to remove the AgCl precipitate by filtration from an aliquot portion of the solution (p. 401) and to titrate and filtrate with $AgNO_3$ solution.

The thiocyanate method is not always suitable for determination of chlorides. For example, it cannot be used if the solution itself has an intense colouring (pink in the case of cobalt salts, green in the case of nickel salts, blue in the case of cupric salts, etc.) The presence of peptizing agents (as in analysis of DDT emulsions) also interferes because they increase the total surface area of the precipitate and so accelerate the reaction between iron thiocyanate and AgCl, thereby making the end point very indistinct, despite the addition of nitrobenzene. The solution must also be free of oxidizing agents which can oxidize CNS^- ions.

112. Determination of Halides by Titration with Silver Nitrate in Presence of Adsorption Indicators

The theory of adsorption indicators was discussed in Sec. 108. Therefore, we shall now describe only the procedure for determination of halides by titration with $AgNO_3$ in the presence of adsorption indicators.

Determination of Chlorides. Weigh out enough of the chloride (NaCl or KCl) on an analytical balance to give an approximately 0.1 *N* or (0.05 *N*) solution when dissolved in water in a 250 ml measuring flask. To an aliquot portion (25.00 ml) add an approximately equal volume of water, 3-5 drops of 0.5% fluorescein solution, and 10 ml of 0.5% dextrin (or starch) solution free from Cl^-. Titrate the solution with continuous stirring, *in diffused light*, with $AgNO_3$ solution until the green colour of the liquid in the flask changes sharply to pinkish red. Repeat the exact titration two or three times and take the average reading.

Calculate the chlorine content of the sample in the usual way and express the result as a percentage.

It will be remembered that dextrin is added as a protective colloid to prevent coagulation of AgCl. The titration can be performed without it, but the colour change is then less sharp. In titration with fluorescein as indicator the solution must be neutral or weakly

* Carbon tetrachloride (CCl_4) or chloroform ($CHCl_3$) may be used instead of nitrobenzene.

alkaline (pH = 6.5-10). If dichlorofluorescein is used instead, the titrated solution may be weakly acid. The titrated solution must be protected from direct sunlight, because silver halides containing adsorbed indicator are highly sensitive to the action of light. In bright sunlight the reddened precipitate quickly becomes grey and then black (because of decomposition).

Determination of Bromides or Iodides (and Thiocyanates). This determination is performed with eosin as indicator*; the colour change is from pink to red-violet. Before the end of the titration the solution should be shaken vigorously. The titration may be performed in acid (at pH $\geqslant$ 2) as well as is neutral solution. It is better to acidify neutral solutions slightly with acetic acid.

In this case addition of a protective colloid does not improve the colour change, which is sharp enough even in very dilute solutions.

113. Mercurometric Determination of Chlorides

In the mercurometric method chlorides are determined by titration with mercurous nitrate solution. The reaction is represented by the equation

$$2NaCl + Hg_2(NO_3)_2 = \downarrow Hg_2Cl_2 + 2NaNO_3$$

The indicator may be either $Fe(CNS)_3$ solution or a solution of the organic reagent diphenylcarbazone.

Let us consider both methods more fully.

1. In the first method a solution of $Fe(CNS)_3$ indicator is formed by addition of 1 ml of 0.05 N NH_4CNS solution and 2-3 ml of concentrated $Fe(NO_3)_3$ solution** to the solution for titration. The indicator acts as follows. As soon as an excess of Hg_2^{++} ions appears in solution after precipitation of Cl^- ions is complete, they react with CNS^- ions so that $Fe(CNS)_3$ is decomposed and the red colour of the solution disappears. The volume of $Hg_2(NO_3)_2$ solution required for the reaction with the indicator must be found by a blank experiment. This volume is subtracted from the volume of $Hg_2(NO_3)_2$ taken for titration of the chloride.

When working with mercury salts, remember that all mercury compounds are strong poisons. Therefore, observe all the safety precautions, wash the hands frequently, do not spill the solutions, do not bring food into the laboratory, do not drink out of chemical glassware, etc.

---

* A 0.5% aqueous solution of the sodium salt of eosin is used. Four to six drops of the indicator are taken per 25 ml of 0.1 N solution.

** To prepare $Fe(NO_3)_3$ iron wire is dissolved in 30% nitric acid, the solution is evaporated to dryness, and the required amount of the dry residue is dissolved in water slightly acidified with HNO_3.

As it is impossible to obtain $Hg_2(NO_3)_2 \cdot 2H_2O$ sufficiently pure, the solution (approximately 0.1 *N*) is prepared from the commercial salt and standardized against chemically pure NaCl. For preparation of the solution 30 g of the commercial salt is dissolved in 1 litre of approximately 0.2 *N* HNO_3 solution. The resultant solution usually contains a considerable amount of Hg^{++} ions, which react both with CNS^- ions and with Cl^- ions. For reduction of Hg^{++} to Hg_2^{++} a small amount of metallic mercury is put into the flask containing the solution which is shaken thoroughly and left to stand for at least 24 hours. Only then should the solution be standardized. The titre of $Hg_2(NO_3)_2$ solution remains unchanged for several months.

Procedure. Weigh out the chloride to be analysed (or chemically pure NaCl if the mercurous nitrate solution is to be standardized). The weight taken should be enough to give an approximately 0.1 *N* solution when dissolved in a 250 ml measuring flask. Put an aliquot portion (25.00 ml) of the solution in a 250 ml measuring flask and add 1 ml (20 drops) of 0.05 *N* NH_4CNS solution and 2-3 ml of concentrated $Fe(NO_3)_3$ solution. The liquid then becomes an intense red colour.

Titrate the coloured solution with the standard $Hg_2(NO_3)_2$ solution with continuous and vigorous stirring until the colour disappears entirely after the addition of a single drop. Repeat the exact titration two or three times and take the average of the concordant results.

At the same time determine the volume of $Hg_2(NO_3)_2$ solution required to decolorize the volume of indicator used. To 25 ml of water add the same volumes of NH_4CNS and $Fe(NO_3)_3$ solutions as were used for the titration, and add $Hg_2(NO_3)_2$ solution drop by drop until the colour disappears. Note down the volume required.

Calculation. Subtract the volume of $Hg_2(NO_3)_2$ solution required to decolorize the indicator from the volume taken for the titration; this gives the volume required for precipitation of Cl^- ions. Now calculate the amount of chlorine in the sample in the usual way, and express the result as a percentage.

2. The indicator used in the second method is a 1-2% solution of diphenylcarbazone, which forms with Hg_2^{++} ions a blue precipitate soluble in 6 *N* HNO_3 solution. The acidity in the determination can range from 0.2 *N* to 5 *N* HNO_3. Among the advantages of this method is the possibility of titration in strongly acid solution, of back-titration, and of titration of coloured and turbid solutions (as the colour of the precipitate at the end point is very bright).

In contrast to the thiocyanate method, this titration is also possible in the presence of peptizing agents. Hydrogen peroxide, even at concentrations as high as 5 *M*, does not interfere either. This makes it possible to determine chlorides in the presence of a number of reducing agents and of certain oxidants (such as sulphite, sulphide, nitrite, permanganate and chromate), which are decomposed by the action of excess H_2O_2 in acid solution.

The determination by this method is performed as follows. The solution to be analysed is first acidified with nitric acid (free from chlorides) so that the concentration of the acid is within the range of 0.2-5 *N*. The indicator is added and a first rough titration is carried out to an accuracy of 1 ml. As the $Hg_2(NO_3)_2$ solution is added, the liquid gradually turns blue. At the equivalence point the colour at once changes to blue-violet. In order that the pale blue colour should not interfere with the determination of the equivalence point, in the replicate titrations the indicator is added only when only 1-2 ml of the titrant remains to be added before the end point. In this case no correction for the indicator is necessary.

This titration should not be performed in direct sunlight.

114. Mercurimetric Determination of Chlorides

In distinction from the mercurometric method described above for determination of chlorides, which is based on precipitation of Cl^- ions by Hg_2^{++} ions, in the mercurimetric method* Cl^- ions are combined with Hg^{++} ions to form the weakly dissociated salt $HgCl_2$. A solution of mercuric nitrate is used for the titration. The equation for the reaction is:

$$2NaCl + Hg(NO_3)_2 = HgCl_2 + 2NaNO_3$$

The indicator is a solution of sodium nitroprusside $Na_2[Fe(CN)_5NO]$, which forms a sparingly soluble salt with Hg^{++} ions. However, the degree of dissociation of $HgCl_2$ is so low that the amount of Hg^{++} ions formed is insufficient to reach the solubility product of mercuric nitroprusside. Therefore, the latter compound is not precipitated until all the chloride has been titrated and a certain excess of the highly dissociated mercuric nitrate $Hg(NO_3)_2$ has formed in solution. A correction, equal to 0.17 ml with 0.1 *N* solutions, must be applied to allow for this excess.

An even more convenient indicator for this titration is a solution of diphenylcarbazone, which forms an intense blue precipitate with mercuric ions.

It must be remembered that *all safety precautions must be observed in work with mercury salts* (see p. 411).

---

* The terms "mercurometric" and "mercurimetric" are derived from the terms for mercurous (univalent) and mercuric (bivalent) mercury.

The titrant used in this method is 0.1 *N* $Hg(NO_3)_2$ solution. To prepare this solution, 17 g of $Hg(NO_3)_2 \cdot {}^1/_2H_2O$ is weighed out on a technical balance, transferred to a 1 litre measuring flask, and about 2 ml of concentrated HNO_3 (to prevent hydrolysis of the mercuric salt) and a small amount of water are added. When the salt has completely dissolved the solution is made up to the mark with water and stirred thoroughly. The solution is standardized against standard approximately 0.1 *N* NaCl solution. 20.00-25.00 ml of the NaCl solution is diluted with water to 100 ml and then titrated as described below.

Procedure. 100 ml of neutral chloride solution is acidified with 4 ml of 0.2 *N* HNO_3 and 10 drops of 1% alcoholic diphenylcarbazone solution are added. The solution is titrated with $Hg(NO_3)_2$ solution until a blue-violet colour appears. The calculation is performed in the usual way.

This method can also be used for determination of bromides, but here the acidity of the solution must be 0.15-0.20 *N*.

L. Kulberg and N. Mustafin proposed β-nitroso-α-naphthol as a convenient indicator for mercurimetric titrations. In aqueous solutions at pH $\leqslant$ 6.5 this compound does not react with $HgCl_2$ but forms a red precipitate with $Hg(NO_3)_2$. This indicator is added to the weakly acidic solution to be analysed, in the proportion of not less than 0.15 ml of saturated alcoholic solution to 10 ml of the solution to be titrated, and the liquid is then titrated with $Hg(NO_3)_2$ solution of not less than 0.025 *N* concentration. The titrated solution remains yellow almost up to the equivalence point. Immediately before this point the colour changes to orange, and at the actual equivalence point a pink turbidity or a red precipitate appears. The titration must be ended slowly, because the precipitated mercury compound readily forms supersaturated solutions.

115. Determination of Zinc by Precipitation with Potassium Ferrocyanide

The method is based on precipitation of Zn^{++} in neutral or weakly acid solution by standard $K_4[Fe(CN)_6]$ solution. In the case of $ZnSO_4$ the reaction is:

$$3ZnSO_4 + 2K_4[Fe(CN_6)] = \downarrow K_2Zn_3[Fe(CN)_6]_2 + 3K_2SO_4$$

Until recently the equivalence point in this titration was determined by means of various external indicators, the best of which is uranyl nitrate, which forms a brick-red precipitate of a uranyl salt with $K_4[Fe(CN)_6]$. A more convenient internal indicator is now used; this is diphenylamine (see Sec. 82), which belongs to the class of redox indicators.

Potassium ferrocyanide $K_4[Fe(CN)_6]$ is a complex salt of ferrous iron and, like other ferrous compounds, it has reducing properties.

When $K_4[Fe(CN)_6]$ is oxidized, the corresponding ferric salt is formed; this is potassium ferricyanide $K_3[Fe(CN)_6]$, an oxidizing agent. A mixture of the two salts is a redox system the potential of which is given by the equation:

$$E = 0.36 + \frac{0.058}{1} \log \frac{[Fe(CN)_6]^{---}}{[Fe(CN)_6]^{==}} \qquad (1)$$

If a small amount of $K_3[Fe(CN)_6]$ solution is added to a measured volume of standard $K_4[Fe(CN)_6]$ solution, the oxidation potential of the mixture is considerably below the value required to change the colour of the added diphenylamine indicator (transition range 0.73-0.79 V), and the latter remains colourless. If the solution is titrated with a solution of zinc salt, as the $[Fe(CN)_6]^{==}$ ions are precipitated in the form of $K_2Zn_3[Fe(CN)_6]_2$ the oxidation potential of the solution increases in accordance with Equation (1). When nearly all the $[Fe(CN)_6]^{==}$ ions have been precipitated the potential rises to the value at which the colour of diphenylamine changes to blue-violet.

The titration can also be reversed. Solutions of $K_3[Fe(CN)_6]$ and diphenylamine are added to an acid solution of a zinc salt; the solution then acquires a blue-violet colour. When this solution is titrated with $K_4[Fe(CN)_6]$, the latter is used up for precipitation of Zn^{++} ions and therefore the colour remains blue-violet until Zn^{++} has been precipitated almost completely in the form of $K_2Zn_3[Fe(CN)_6]_2$. After this the first excess drop of $K_4[Fe(CN)_6]$ lowers the oxidation potential of the solution so much that it becomes colourless.

The standard solutions used in this method are approximately 0.05 *M* $K_4[Fe(CN)_6]$ and 0.1 *M* $ZnSO_4$. The former may be prepared by exact weighing of $K_4[Fe(CN)_6]$, which is obtained as the chemically pure anhydrous salt by recrystallization and drying to constant weight at 100°C; its composition corresponds exactly to the above formula. However, it is better to standardize $K_4[Fe(CN)_6]$ by titrating the other solution, $ZnSO_4$, with it. The latter is prepared from an exact weight (about 6.5 g per litre) of chemically pure zinc, which is dissolved in 2 *N* H_2SO_4. The solution is transferred to a 1 litre measuring flask and made up to the mark with water.

The titres of both solutions are best expressed in terms of zinc. For example, to find $T_{ZnSO_4/Zn}$ the weight of metallic zinc taken is divided by the volume of the $ZnSO_4$ solution prepared from it. The titre of the $K_4[Fe(CN)_6]$ is either found from the equation for the reaction taking place in the titration (if an exact weight of $K_4[Fe(CN)_6]$ was taken), or calculated by division of the number of grams of zinc consumed in the titration by the volume of the

$K_4[Fe(CN)_6]$ solution (in standardization by titration of $ZnSO_4$).*

Procedure. Weigh out accurately enough $ZnSO_4 \cdot 7H_2O$ to give an approximately 0.1 *M* solution when dissolved in water in a 250 ml measuring flask. To an aliquot portion (25.00 ml) add about 50 ml of water, 2 g of $(NH_4)_2SO_4$, about 20 ml of 6 *N* H_2SO_4 solution, two or three drops of $K_3[Fe(CN)_6]$ solution,** and three drops of indicator—1% solution of diphenylamine in concentrated sulphuric acid. After some time, when a blue colour has appeared in the solution, titrate it with the approximately 0.05 *M* $K_4[Fe(CN)_6]$ standard solution. Continue the titration until the solution has been overtitrated by 1-2 ml (until the colour has become yellow-green).

Now titrate the added excess of $K_4[Fe(CN)_6]$ slowly with the standard zinc sulphate solution until the colour changes sharply after addition of a single drop. Repeat the exact titration two or three times and take the average reading.

Apply an indicator correction, equal to 0.05 ml (for three drops of indicator), to the volume of $K_4[Fe(CN)_6]$ solution taken in the titration.

Calculation. Suppose that 34.00 ml of $K_4[Fe(CN)_6]$ solution with the titre $T_{K_4[Fe(CN_6)]/Zn} = 0.004912$ g/ml was initially added to 25.00 ml of the zinc salt solution.

Back-titration of the excess $K_4[Fe(CN)_6]$ took 1.25 ml of $ZnSO_4$ solution with the titre $T_{ZnSO_4/Zn} = 0.006480$ g/ml.

After applying the correction to the volume of $K_4[Fe(CN)_6]$ taken we have 34.05 ml, which corresponds to $34.05 \times 0.004912 = 0.1673$ g of zinc. However, $1.25 \times 0.006480 = 0.0081$ g of zinc was added to the solution during the back-titration.

Therefore, 25.00 ml of the zinc salt solution contains $0.1673 - 0.0081 = 0.1592$ g of zinc. This corresponds to 1.592 g of zinc for the whole amount weighed out (250 ml of solution). This amount of zinc must now be expressed as a percentage of the sample taken.

116. Complexometric Determination of the Total Hardness of Water

As was already stated in Sec. 105, in recent years (since 1946) organic reagents of a new type, known generally as the complexones, have been introduced into analytical practice for volumetric determination of various cations. Complexones are certain aminopolycarboxylic acids and their salts. The one most commonly used

---

* For example, if $T_{ZnSO_4/Zn} = 0.006480$ g/ml and the volume of solution taken for the titration is 28.00 ml, then the total weight of zinc in this volume is 0.006480×28.00 g. This is divided by the volume of the $K_4[Fe(CN)_6]$ solution taken for the titration to give its titre for zinc.

** 1% solution of $K_3[Fe(CN)_6]$ solution in water free from CO_2 is used. It should be kept in a dark glass bottle.

is known as Trilon B, the disodium salt of ethylenediamine tetra-acetic acid (EDTA). The structural formula of Trilon B is

$$\begin{matrix} NaOOC-CH_2 \\ HOOC-CH_2 \end{matrix} \!\!>\!\! N-CH_2-CH_2-N \!\!<\!\! \begin{matrix} CH_2-COONa \\ CH_2-COOH \end{matrix} \quad 2H_2O$$

Trilon B, like other complexones, forms very stable soluble internal complex salts with many metals. The metal replaces hydrogen atoms of the —COOH groups and is also linked by coordinate bonds to nitrogen atoms, as the following structural formula shows:

$$\begin{matrix} HOOCH_2C \\ NaOOCH_2C \end{matrix} \!\!>\!\! N-CH_2-CH_2-N \!\!<\!\! \begin{matrix} CH_2COONa \\ CH_2COOH \end{matrix} + Me^{++} =$$

$$= \begin{matrix} -OOCH_2C \\ NaOOCH_2C \end{matrix} \!\!>\!\! N-CH_2-CH_2-N \!\!<\!\! \begin{matrix} CH_2COONa \\ CH_2COO- \end{matrix} + 2H^+$$

(both N atoms coordinated to Me, which is also bonded to the two carboxylate groups)

The very low instability constants of such complexes, ranging from 10^{-9} to 10^{-26}, indicate that these internal complex salts are highly stable. In particular, $K_{inst.}$ of the Ca^{++} complex is 2.7×10^{-11} and that of the Mg^{++} complex is 2×10^{-9}.

The complex-forming ability of Trilon B can be easily demonstrated experimentally by treating precipitates such as CaC_2O_4 or $BaSO_4$ with a concentrated solution of it; the precipitates dissolve. This occurs because the respective cations are combined into complexes so that their concentrations fall so much that the products of the ionic concentrations $[Ca^{++}]\cdot[C_2O_4^{--}]$ and $[Ba^{++}]\cdot[SO_4^{--}]$ become less than the respective solubility products. If we represent the formula of Trilon B schematically as $Na_2[H_2EDTA]$, the reaction with $BaSO_4$ can be represented by the equation

$$BaSO_4 + Na_2[H_2EDTA] \rightleftarrows Na_2[BaEDTA] + H_2SO_4$$

It is important to note that the precipitates are dissolved *only in alkaline solution*; for example, in the presence of NH_4OH. When the solutions are acidified the complexes are decomposed and $BaSO_4$ or CaC_2O_4 are again precipitated. The explanation is that, as the above equation shows, the formation of complexes with Trilon B is accompanied by accumulation of acid in the solutions. Consequently, if H^+ ions combine with OH^- ions from an alkali the equilibrium shifts to the right, favouring complex formation; conversely, if the solution is acidified the reaction equilibrium shifts to the left and the complex decomposes. This applies to the formation of complexes of any metals with Trilon B. A weakly alkaline solution (pH = 8-10), produced by addition of ammoniacal buffer mixture ($NH_4OH + NH_4Cl$ mixture), is the most favourable for these reactions.

Trilon B and other complexones have various uses in analysis. For example, they are used as masking agents in separation of cations with hydroxyquinoline, and in electrochemical methods of analysis. However, their most important use is for volumetric determination of various cations. As an important practical example of such determinations, we describe below the complexometric determination of the total hardness of water, i.e., the total content of calcium and magnesium salts. This method is much more convenient than the acidimetric methods for determination of hardness (see Sec. 74), and is more precise. In this method the water is made alkaline by addition of ammoniacal buffer mixture and titrated with standard Trilon B solution. The usual indicator is Eriochrome Black T, which forms soluble wine-red complexes with Ca^{++} and Mg^{++} ions.* These complexes are less stable, i.e., they have higher $K_{inst.}$** than the complexes of the same metals with Trilon B.

When the indicator is added to the water to be analysed, it forms complexes with Ca^{++} and Mg^{++} ions and the colour of the solution becomes wine-red. When the water is titrated with Trilon B these complexes are decomposed as the result of removal of Ca^{++} and Mg^{++} ions, which form more stable (i.e., less dissociated) complexes with Trilon B, and the indicator anions go into solution. At the equivalence point the wine-red colour of the solution changes to blue owing to accumulation of the indicator anions. If the indicator is represented schematically by H_2R, all the processes taking place during the titration may be represented as follows:

$$\underset{\text{Dark lilac}}{H_2R} \rightleftarrows 2H^+ + \underset{\text{Blue}}{R^{--}}$$

$$Ca^{++} + \underset{\text{Blue}}{R^{--}} \rightleftarrows \underset{\text{Wine-red}}{CaR} \quad (\text{at pH} = 8\text{-}10)$$

$$\underset{\text{Wine-red}}{CaR} + \underset{\text{Colourless}}{Na_2[H_2EDTA]} = \underset{\text{Colourless}}{Na_2[CaEDTA]} + \underset{\text{Blue}}{R^{--}} + 2H^+ \quad (\text{at pH} = 8\text{-}10)$$

---

* This indicator is also known as Chromogen Black Special ET-00. Its structural formula is

OH OH
NaO_3S — — N = N —
O_2N

** The values of $K_{inst.}$ of the complexes formed by the indicator with Ca^{++} and Mg^{++} ions are 3.9×10^{-6} and 1×10^{-7} respectively.

The indicator Eriochrome Black T is used either in solution* or (because the solution is unstable) in solid form. In the latter case the indicator is mixed in the proportions of 1 : 200 with some indifferent "filler" such as NaCl or KCl. The mixture is ground thoroughly in a mortar, and about 20-30 mg is added to the solution before titration.

Standard Trilon B solutions are used in various concentrations: 0.1 *N*, 0.05 *N*, and 0.01 *N*. The molecular weight of Trilon B is 372.3, and its gram-equivalent is 186.1 g. Therefore, 18.6 g of Trilon B must be weighed out for preparation of 1 litre of 0.1 *N* solution, and 9.3 g for 1 litre of 0.05 *N* solution. The solution is standardized against a solution of a calcium or a magnesium salt of accurately known concentration; for example, 0.01 *N* magnesium sulphate solution prepared from Fixanal.

The presence of Cu^{++}, Zn^{++} and Mn^{++} ions interferes with determination of hardness by this method. Copper and zinc ions are removed by addition of 1 ml of 1.5-2% Na_2S solution; the solution is then titrated with Trilon B in the usual way without filtering off the precipitated sulphides. If manganese is present in the water, 5 drops of a 1% solution of hydroxylamine hydrochloride $NH_2OH \cdot HCl$ is added before the reagents. (This is done in order to prevent oxidation of Mn^{++} ions by atmospheric oxygen, as it is the oxidation products which interfere with the subsequent determination of hardness.)

Procedure. Pipette out a volume of water which does not contain more than 0.5 mg-eq of Ca^{++} and Mg^{++}, so that the titration should not take more than 5 ml of 0.1 *N* or 10 ml of 0.05 *N* Trilon B solution. Dilute this sample to about 100 ml with distilled water and add 5 ml of ammoniacal buffer mixture.** Now add 7-8 drops of the indicator (or put in 20-30 mg of its mixture with NaCl or KCl by means of a spatula and stir until dissolved), and titrate the liquid with standard Trilon B solution until the wine-red colour changes to blue (with a greenish tinge). Near the end of the titration add the Trilon B drop by drop and aim at complete disappearance of the reddish tinge. If there is any doubt about the end point, take the reading and add another drop of solution. If the colour changes, the end point has not been reached.

Calculation. We know (Sec. 73) that the hardness of water is expressed in terms of the number of milligram-equivalents of calcium

* 0.5 g of Eriochrome Black T is dissolved in 10 ml of ammoniacal buffer mixture and the volume is made up to 100 ml with ethyl alcohol. This solution does not keep for longer than 10 days.

** This is prepared by mixing 100 ml of 20% NH_4Cl solution with 100 ml of 20% NH_4OH solution and diluting the mixture to 1 litre with distilled water.

and magnesium per litre of water. If the normality of the Trilon B solution is N, then one millilitre of it corresponds to N milligram-equivalents of these metals in the volume of water taken for analysis. By calculating for 1 litre of water, we find the total hardness in milligram-equivalents.

QUESTIONS AND PROBLEMS
(on Secs. 105-116)

1. State the conditions which a given precipitation reaction must satisfy before it can be used in volumetric analysis.

2. Calculate and plot the curve for titration of 0.1 N $AgNO_3$ solution with 0.1 N NH_4CNS solution ($SP_{AgCNS} \approx 10^{-12}$).

3. What factors determine the extent of the break on the titration curve in the precipitation method?

4. A 0.1 N $CaCl_2$ solution is titrated with 0.1 N Na_2SO_4 solution. Find the value of pCa at the beginning of the break, at the equivalence point, and at the end of the break, taking SP_{CaSO_4} as 6×10^{-5}.

Answer: The three values of pCa almost coincide (to within 0.01) at 2.11.

5. What is the principle of titration of bromides and chlorides with $AgNO_3$ solution without indicators?

6. How does K_2CrO_4 act as an indicator in titration of chlorides with $AgNO_3$ solution?

7. Silver nitrate solution is added to a solution containing Cl^- and I^- ions. Which salt, AgCl ($SP \approx 10^{-10}$) or AgI ($SP \approx 10^{-16}$) is the first to be precipitated?

What is the concentration of the first anion to be precipitated at which precipitation of the other anion begins, if the initial concentrations of both anions were 0.01 g-ion/litre?

Answer: 10^{-8} g-ion/litre.

8. A solution of $(NH_4)_2C_2O_4$ is added to a solution containing 1 g-ion/litre of Ba^{++} and 0.01 g-ion/litre of Ca^{++}. Which of these cations is precipitated first, and what percentage of it is precipitated at the point when the precipitation of the other cation begins?

Answer: Ba^{++}; 38%.

9. In what limits may the concentration of CrO_4^{--} ions in a 0.1 N chloride solution be varied so that the start of precipitation of $AgCrO_4$ during titration with 0.1 N $AgNO_3$ should not be outside the break on the titration curve?

Answer: Between 9×10^{-4} and 0.9 g-ion/litre.

10. What should be the titration sequence in determination of silver by the Mohr method?

11. State the conditions for application of the Mohr method.

12. What is the principle of the thiocyanate method for determination of silver? What indicator is used? Why is thiocyanate titration performed in acid solution?

13. What are the complications introduced by adsorption effects into titration by the precipitation method? Explain why Fe^{+++}, Cu^{++}, and other cations cannot be determined quantitatively by titration of their salts with alkali solution.

14. How does the charge of AgCl particles change when a chloride solution is titrated with silver nitrate solution? How does it change when the titration sequence is reversed? What is the isoelectric point?

15. What is the principle of titration to the "clear point"? Which ions are determined by this method in practice?

16. Explain the action of adsorption indicators. Illustrate your answer by examples.

17. Why cannot chlorides be titrated with eosin as indicator? What is the significance of the solution pH in titrations with adsorption indicators?

18. What is the principle of mercurometric determination of chlorides? What indicators are used in this method?

19. What is the principle of mercurimetric determination of chlorides? What indicators are used in this method?

20. Explain the action of diphenylamine in determination of zinc by titration with $K_4[Fe(CN)_6]$ solution. Describe how the titration is performed and the results calculated.

21. What are the titres of 0.05605 *N* $AgNO_3$ solution for: (a) Cl; (b) NaCl?
Answer: (a) 0.001987 g/ml; (b) 0.03276 g/ml.

22. Find the percentage of silver in an alloy, if the solution formed by dissolving 0.3000 g of the alloy in HNO_3 took 23.80 ml of 0.1000 *N* NH_4CNS solution.

Answer: 85.63%.

23. Find the weight of KCl in 250 ml of a solution if 25.00 ml of the solution took 34.00 ml of 0.1050 *N* $AgNO_3$.

Answer: 2.662 g.

24. Find the weight of chlorine in a solution of NH_4Cl if its titration took 30.00 ml of an $AgNO_3$ solution, the chlorine titre of which was 0.003512 g/ml.

Answer: 0.1054 g.

25. Find the weight of $BaCl_2$ in 250 ml of solution, given that after addition of 40.00 ml of 0.1020 *N* $AgNO_3$ solution to 25.00 ml of the $BaCl_2$ solution back-titration of the excess silver nitrate took 15.00 ml of 0.0980 *N* NH_4CNS solution.

Answer: 2.714 g.

26. What are complexones, and for what purposes are they used?

27. How is the total hardness of water determined with the use of Trilon B? What is the significance of the pH in this determination? Explain your answer.

CHAPTER IX

COLORIMETRY

117. The Principle of the Method

In analytical practice it is often necessary to determine very small quantities ("traces") of substances present as impurities in various materials. For example, the impurity contents of technically pure metals may be measured in thousandths of one per cent, the iron or chlorine contents of reagent-grade sulphuric acid should not exceed a few ten-thousandth parts of one per cent, etc.

Such small quantities are virtually impossible to determine by the usual gravimetric or volumetric methods, because very large samples of the materials would have to be taken to ensure adequate concentrations of the impurities in solution. In such cases it becomes necessary to use special methods of analysis; one such method is *colorimetry*.

In colorimetric determinations the quantity of an element (*or ion*) *present is estimated from the intensity of the colour of the solution due to the presence of a coloured compound of that element.* The more intense the colour, the higher the concentration of the element (or ion) in solution. If two solutions under identical conditions and containing the same coloured compound have colour of the same intensity, the concentrations of the given element (or ion) in them are also equal. Therefore, if we make, by dilution, the colour of an unknown solution exactly the same as that of a so-called *standard solution*, containing the element to be determined in a suitable and accurately known concentration, we also make the concentrations of the two solutions equal. If we know how much one of the solutions had to be diluted for this, we can easily calculate its concentration from the known concentration of the standard solution.

Colorimetric determinations usually boil down to such matching of the colours of unknown and standard solutions (which may be effected by methods other than dilution).

A coloured solution may be sometimes formed as soon as the substance is dissolved, if this involves the production of ions (such as MnO_4^-, CrO_4^{--}, etc.) or molecules which have sufficiently intense colour.

However, much more often a colour must be produced by addition of some reagent which reacts chemically with the element or ion to be determined. For example, in colorimetric determination of iron, ammonium thiocyanate NH_4CNS is added to the unknown solution; it reacts with Fe^{+++} to form the compound $Fe(CNS)_3$, which has an intense blood-red colour; titanium is determined by the addition of hydrogen peroxide (H_2O_2), which gives rise to an orange-yellow colour due to the formation of the peroxide titanium compound $[TiO(H_2O_2)]SO_4$*, etc.

It may also be necessary to use reagents which cause coloration of the solution in cases when the ion to be determined is coloured, but the colour is not intense enough. For example, copper salts are coloured blue, but this colour is too weak. Therefore, for colorimetric determination of copper it is usually preferable to convert the Cu^{++} ion by the action of NH_4OH into the much more intensely coloured complex $[Cu(NH_3)_4]^{++}$, which is of an azure-blue colour.

Reactions involving the formation of intensely coloured complex ions by interaction of metal cations with ammonia, CNS^- ions, various organic compounds, etc., are very often used for other colorimetric determinations. It is known that complex ions can dissociate to various extents into their constituent simple ions (or ions and molecules). For example, the $[Cu(NH_3)_4]^{++}$ ion partially dissociates in solution as follows:

$$[Cu(NH_3)_4]^{++} \rightleftarrows Cu^{++} + 4NH_3$$

It is also known that the dissociation of a complex may be characterized by its *instability constant*. In this case the instability constant is:

$$\frac{[Cu^{++}]\,[NH_3]^4}{[Cu\,(NH_3)_4]^{++}} = K_{inst.} = 5 \times 10^{-14}$$

The lower the value of $K_{inst.}$, the less does the complex dissociate and the stabler it is.

Values of $K_{inst.}$ of coloured complexes are very important in colorimetric analysis. Apart from the intensity of its colour, the suitability of a complex also depends on its stability, characterized by its $K_{inst.}$. The lower the value of $K_{inst.}$, the more complete is the reaction of complex formation. Therefore, in the case of complexes with low $K_{inst.}$ even a slight excess of reagent is sufficient to convert the ion almost completely into the complex form, i.e., to produce a colour which does not alter when more reagent is added. Conversely, in the case of complexes of high $K_{inst.}$ the colour of the solution depends very strongly on the amount of excess reagent.

* This compound is often called pertitanic acid in conformity with the previous way of presenting its formula as $H_2[TiO_2(SO_4)_2]$.

It follows that the precision with which the reagent must be measured out depends on $K_{inst.}$ of the complex; the higher the value of $K_{inst.}$ the more precise must this measurement be.

Complexes with high instability constants are also inconvenient for colorimetric analysis for another reason. There is the possibility that they may be converted into other complexes, such as chloride or sulphate complexes, because of the presence of HCl or H_2SO_4 which are commonly used for dissolving the substance to be analysed. Such conversion would, of course, affect the colour of the solution and might lead to errors in the determination. However, it is known that interconversion of complex ions occurs easily only if the complex so formed is more stable, i.e., has a lower $K_{inst.}$, than the original complex. It follows that the possibility of complications caused by the presence of extraneous ions (such as Cl^-, SO_4^{--}, etc.) in solution increases with increasing $K_{inst.}$ of the coloured complex used.

When reactions of complex formation are used in colorimetric analysis, selection of a suitable solvent, which influences $K_{inst.}$ of the complex, and such reaction conditions as concentration of the reagent used, solution pH, etc., are of great importance.

Apart from complex formation, other reactions, such as oxidation-reduction, organic synthesis, etc., are used in colorimetry. For example, manganese and chromium are determined colorimetrically by oxidation to MnO_4^- and CrO_4^{--} ions, which are coloured; determination of nitrites is based on reactions with the organic reagents α-naphthylamine and sulphanilic acid, which form an intense red azo dye with NO_2^- ions, etc. Reactions involving the formation of coloured peroxide compounds, such as $[TiO(H_2O_2)]SO_4$ in determination of titanium, are sometimes used.

Colorimetric methods are highly sensitive, i.e., they are suitable for determining elements at very low concentrations. In addition, they are usually simple and are generally much more rapid than gravimetric and in some cases volumetric determinations. For these reasons colorimetry is ever more widely used in industrial and research laboratories.

The *nephelometric* and *turbidimetric* methods of quantitative analysis are closely allied to colorimetry. In distinction from the latter, these methods are based on reactions involving the formation of sparingly soluble compounds; the amount of an element present is estimated from the turbidity produced in the solution by comparison with the turbidity of an appropriate standard solution.

In turbidimetric determinations the solution is examined in passing light, i.e., the decrease of light intensity caused by the presence of suspended particles of the solid phase is measured. In contrast, in nephelometric determinations the solution is examined in a direction at right angles to the light beam. In this case the intensity of the light scattered by the particles of the solid phase is observed. The difference between the two methods is shown schematically in Fig. 60.

The physical basis of all three methods is measurement of the quantity of light absorbed or scattered by particles of a substance dissolved or suspended in a liquid. These methods are jointly known as *photometric methods* of analysis. Only colorimetric methods are considered in this book. In colorimetric determinations the colours

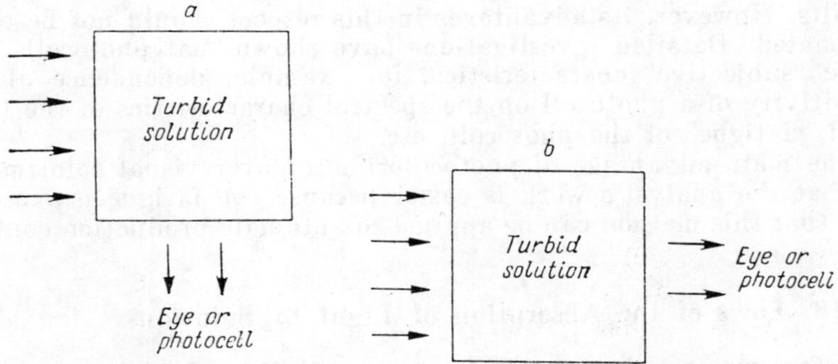

Fig. 60. Schematic representation of nephelometric (*a*) and turbidimetric (*b*) determinations

of an unknown and a standard solution are compared either visually or with the aid of photocells, i.e., instruments which, when exposed to light, yield electric current, the strength of which depends on the intensity of the incident light. The colour measurements in this case are replaced by measurements of the deflection of the needle of a galvanometer in the circuit.

In accordance with the observation method used, a distinction is made between *visual colorimetry* and *photocolorimetry*.

In visual colorimetry the result of a determination depends to a considerable extent on the subjective characteristics of the analyst (the ability to perceive slight colour differences). Eye fatigue, which may lead to considerable errors, also has a strong influence on the precision of the determinations. Because of all this, the relative error in visual colorimetric determinations is comparatively high. At the best it is 2-5% of the quantity measured, but it may be 10% or more. It should be remembered, however, that with very low contents of the element to be determined the degree of precision required is usually different from that needed with high contents. For example, in most cases it is quite immaterial whether the content of some element in a substance is 0.0010% or 0.0011%, although the relative difference is 10%.

On the other hand, it should be taken into account that in such cases the gravimetric or volumetric methods would give even larger errors (if they could be used at all). Because of all this we must attach a different significance to the magnitude of the relative error in determination of traces of impurities than in determinations previously described.

There is no doubt that the photocolorimetric method is more objective than visual colorimetry and can therefore give more precise results. However, its advantages in this respect should not be overestimated. Detailed investigations have shown that photocells also have "subjective" characteristics, for example, dependence of the sensitivity of a photocell on the spectral characteristics of the light used, "fatigue" of the photocell, etc.

The main advantage of photocolorimetry over visual colorimetry is that the analyst's work is easier because eye fatigue is avoided, and that this method can be applied to automate production control.

118. Laws of the Absorption of Light by Solutions

Before we consider methods used for colorimetric determinations, we must examine the laws governing the absorption of light by coloured solutions.

If a beam of monochromatic light of intensity I_0 falls on a homogeneous layer of some substance, part of the light (of intensity I_r) is reflected from the substance, part (I_a) is absorbed, and part (I_t) is transmitted through the layer, so that

$$I_0 = I_r + I_a + I_t \tag{1}$$

In the case of aqueous solutions, which are generally used in colorimetry, I_r is small in comparison with I_a and I_t and may be disregarded without appreciable error. We therefore have

$$I_0 \approx I_a + I_t \tag{2}$$

The value of I_a depends almost entirely on the presence in solution of molecules or ions of a coloured substance which absorbs light much more than the solvent (water, alcohol, ether, etc.).

Thus, in passing through the solution the light beam loses some of its intensity; the loss increases with the number of molecules or ions of the coloured substance which it meets in its path. However, the number of molecules or ions met by the light, and therefore the loss of intensity, depends, in addition to the nature of the substance absorbing the light, on the concentration (C) and the thickness of the layer of solution (h) through which the light passes.

This relationship can be represented by the following formula:

$$\log \frac{I_0}{I_t} = \varepsilon hC \tag{3}$$

Here the quantity $\log \frac{I_0}{I_t}$, which is a measure of the weakening of the light as it passes through the solution, is known as the *extinction* or the *optical density* of the solution.*

The constant ε depends on the nature of the absorbing substance and on the wave length of the light. If the concentration C is expressed in moles per litre this constant is known as the *molar extinction coefficient* of the solution.

Formula (3) is an expression of the law for absorption of light by coloured solutions. This law (the Lambert-Beer law) may be stated as follows: *the optical density of a solution is proportional to the product of the concentration of the absorbing (coloured) substance and the thickness of the layer of solution.*

From Equation (3) we have

$$\frac{I_0}{I_t} = 10^{\varepsilon hC}$$

and hence

$$I_t = I_0 \times 10^{-\varepsilon hC} \tag{4}$$

The theoretical derivation of this law is based on the following reasoning.

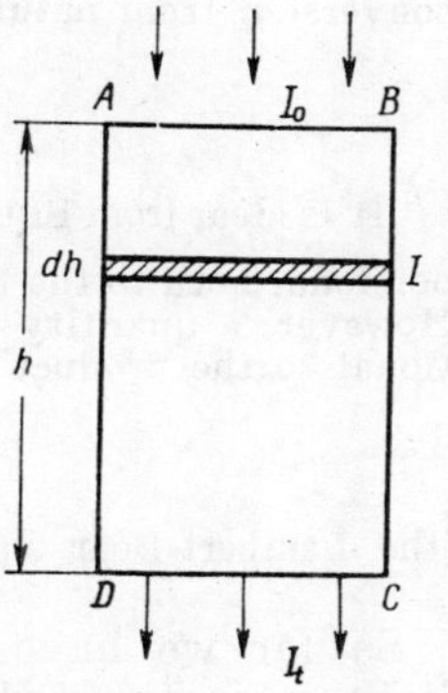

Fig. 61. Absorption of light by a solution

Suppose that a light beam passes through a column of solution $ABCD$ (Fig. 61) in the direction indicated by the arrows. Consider, within this column, an infinitesimally thin layer of thickness dh; in passing through this layer the intensity of the light changes by $-dI$. Since dI is vanishingly small, we may assume that the intensity of the light (I) passing through this layer is constant.

Assuming the decrease of light intensity ($-dI$) proportional to the intensity I in the layer and to the thickness dh of the layer, we can write:

$$-dI = K_1 I\, dh$$

or

$$\frac{dI}{I} = -K_1\, dh \tag{5}$$

where K_1 is a proportionality factor.

Integrating this equation, we have:

$$\int_{I_t}^{I_0} \frac{dI}{I} = -K_1 \int_h^0 dh$$

* The optical density of a solution is sometimes denoted by D.

or

$$\ln \frac{I_0}{I_t} = K_1 h \tag{6}$$

Converting from natural to common logarithms, we have:

$$\log \frac{I_0}{I_t} = 0.4343\, K_1 h = \varepsilon_1 h \tag{7}$$

where $\varepsilon_1 = 0.4343\, K_1$.

In just the same way, assuming the change of light intensity ($-dI$) due to an infinitesimal increase in the concentration of the absorbing substance to be proportional to I and dC, we have

$$-dI = K_2 I\, dC$$

Integration of this equation between I_0 and I_t and between 0 and C and conversion from natural to common logarithms gives the expression

$$\log \frac{I_0}{I_t} = \varepsilon_2 C \tag{8}$$

It is clear from Equations (7) and (8) that the optical density $\left(\log \frac{I_0}{I_t}\right)$ is proportional both to the thickness of the layer of solution and to its concentration. However, a quantity which is proportional to two other quantities is proportional to the product of those quantities. We can therefore write:

$$\log \frac{I_0}{I_t} = \varepsilon h C$$

(the Lambert-Bear equations).

So far we have considered the transmission of monochromatic light, accompanied by a decrease of its intensity from I_0 to I_t. In the case of white light, because of the unequal absorption of light of different wave lengths by the coloured substance, the solution acquires a colour complementary to the colour corresponding to the absorbed light. The colour intensity should vary with the concentration and the thickness of the layer of solution in accordance with the Lambert-Beer law. Therefore, this law can be applied to colorimetric determinations based on comparison of the colours of solutions.

Let us consider a corollary of the Lambert-Beer law as used in comparison of colours in visual colorimetry. Suppose that we have two solutions (unknown and standard) containing the same coloured substance at concentrations of $C_{\text{un.}}$ and $C_{\text{st.}}$ with layer thicknesses of $h_{\text{un.}}$ and $h_{\text{st.}}$ (cm) respectively. Using the Lambert-Beer law, we can write for the two solutions:

$$\log \frac{I_0}{I_t} = \varepsilon C_{\text{un.}} h_{\text{un.}}$$

$$\log \frac{I_0}{I'_t} = \varepsilon C_{\text{st.}} h_{\text{st.}}$$

Since the same coloured substance is present in both solutions, the constant ε has the same value in both equations. The same applies to I_0, since both solutions are illuminated equally. If the thicknesses of the solution layers through which the light passes are so chosen that both solutions appear of the same colour, I_t and I'_t must also be equal. The left-hand sides of the two equations are then equal to each other, and therefore the right-hand sides must also be equal, i.e.,

$$\varepsilon C_{un.}\, h_{un.} = \varepsilon C_{st.}\, h_{st.}$$

and

$$C_{un.}\, h_{un.} = C_{st.}\, h_{st.} \tag{9}$$

Equation (9) shows that *when the colours are of the same intensity the product of the concentration and layer thickness is the same for both solutions.*

Since the concentration of one of the solutions is known, we can find experimentally the ratio of the layer thicknesses $h_{st.}: h_{un.}$ when the colours are equal, and then calculate the unknown concentration $C_{un.}$ from Equation (9). This concentration is

$$C_{un.} = C_{st.} \frac{h_{st.}}{h_{un.}} \tag{10}$$

The above explains the principle of the *balancing method* for equalization of the colours of the unknown and standard solutions, which is the method most commonly used in visual colorimetry.

119. Conditions for Applicability of the Lambert-Beer Law. Influence of the Medium pH

The applicability of the balancing method in colorimetric determinations depends on the conformity of solutions of a given coloured substance to the Lambert-Beer law. However, this law is valid over wide ranges of concentrations only provided that the structure of the coloured ions (or molecules, in the case of non-electrolytes) does not alter with changes of concentration. This is true for solutions of permanganates, chromates, many organic dyes, etc. However, quite often a coloured substance undergoes chemical changes which influence its colour, when the concentration is varied. Solutions of such substances do not obey the Lambert-Beer law. In such cases the molar extinction coefficient ε, which by this law should be a constant for the given substance, varies with the concentration. Evidently, Equation (9) is then inapplicable and the balancing method cannot be used.

In illustration, let us consider the example of picric acid. This is a weak organic acid*, which, for the sake of simplicity, we represent by the formula HA. When this acid is dissolved, the following equilibria are established**:

$$HA_0 \rightleftarrows HA \rightleftarrows H^+ + A^- \quad (1)$$

Colourless Yellow Yellow

The (apparent) dissociation constant of picric acid is calculated from the equation***:

$$\frac{[H^+][A^-]}{[HA_0]} = K$$

This equation shows that when a solution of picric acid is diluted the colourless HA_0 molecules should disappear from solution while the content of the yellow A^- anions should increase.

If the thickness of the liquid layer is halved, the light passing through the solution meets exactly one half as many light-absorbing molecules (or ions). The same is true if the solution concentration is halved, provided that the substance obeys the Lambert-Beer law. However, when a solution of picric acid is diluted, equilibrium (1) is disturbed and the concentration of A^- anions is decreased by less than one half. Therefore, we cannot assume that the one is equivalent to the other, as is done in the matching method. The same applies to most other cases when equilibrium between differently coloured forms of a particular substance is disturbed by a change of concentration. For example, in the most usual case of formation of a coloured complex (XR) by the reaction between an ion to be determined (X) and a reagent (R), the reaction equilibrium

$$X + R \rightleftarrows XR$$

is determined by the equation for the instability constant of the complex:

$$\frac{[X][R]}{[XR]} = K_{inst}.$$

This equation shows that the coloured complex should dissociate when the solution is diluted. Therefore, the decrease of the colour intensity when the solution is diluted is more rapid than the decrease of the total concentration of the complex. It follows that the Lambert-Beer law is inapplicable in this case too. However, if an excess of the reagent (R) is used, dissociation of the complex XR can be

* Its formula is $C_6H_2(NO_2)_3OH$.

** Here HA_0 and HA represent two tautomeric forms of picric acid, which have different colours.

*** The derivation of this equation is given on p. 240.

suppressed so much that deviations from the Lambert-Beer law become negligible. In order to achieve this, the solution is usually diluted not with water but with a solution of the reagent, the concentration of which is thereby kept constant.

The magnitude of the observed deviations from the Lambert-Beer law also depends on the value of $K_{inst.}$ of the complex. The lower this value, the less are the deviations and the less is the excess of reagent needed to suppress the dissociation of the complex.

Hydrolysis of a coloured substance, increasing with dilution, may be another cause of deviations from the Lambert-Beer law. It is known that hydrolysis is prevented by adjustment of the solution pH. The influence of pH must also be taken into account in other cases. For example, the colour of a picric acid solution must evidently be very much influenced by the pH of the solution. The concentration of the coloured anions must increase with increase of pH (i.e., with decrease of $[H^+]$), and vice versa.

Similarly, the pH of the medium influences the colour if the substance is a weak acid with coloured anions or a weak base with coloured cations. It was noted in Sec. 23 that solution pH must also be taken into account during formation of complexes if the ligands are NH_3 molecules or anions of weak acids, which can combine with hydrogen ions to form the more stable complex NH_4^+ or undissociated molecules of the respective weak acids.

For example, the complex $[Cu(NH_3)_4]^{++}$ decomposes as follows when its solutions are acidified:

$$[Cu(NH_3)_4]^{++} + 4H^+ = Cu^{++} + 4NH_4^+$$

and the intense blue colour changes to pale blue. It is known (Sec. 78) that the H^+ ion concentration also has a very strong influence on the course of many oxidation-reduction processes.

120. Influence of Extraneous Ions on the Colour of Solutions

In colorimetric analysis the ion which is to be determined is usually present in solution together with various extraneous ions which may also influence the colour of the solution. This may occur in the following cases:

(1) the extraneous ions form coloured complexes with the reagent used, or combine with it without forming a coloured product;

(2) the extraneous ions are themselves coloured;

(3) the extraneous ions, being anions, combine with the cations to be determined to form a compound or complex of a low degree of dissociation.

Of course, in colorimetric determinations the influence of extraneous ions on the colour of the solution must be eliminated. This may be done either by chemical or by physical methods.* Let us consider the most important chemical methods.

The most important and commonly used method for eliminating the influence of extraneous ions is masking. This method, widely used in qualitative analysis, was considered in detail in Sec. 23. The interfering extraneous ion (M) is combined in the form of a colourless complex (MQ) by addition of a suitable "masking agent" (Q). For this masking to occur, the complex (MQ) should be more stable than the complex (MR) formed by the interfering ion (M) with the reagent (R).

An example of the use of masking in colorimetry is provided by the colorimetric determination of the Co^{++} ion in the form of the thiocyanate complex $[Co(CNS)_4]^{--}$; here the interfering effect of Fe^{+++} ions is eliminated by addition of NaF or NH_4F to the solution, so that the ferric ions form the very stable colourless complex $[FeF_6]^{---}$. The influence of Fe^{+++} ions can also be eliminated by means of tartaric or citric acid, pyrophosphate, and certain other substances.

An interfering ion can also be eliminated by a change of its valence. For example, formation of $Fe(CNS)_3$ can also be prevented by reduction of Fe^{+++} to Fe^{++}, which does not form coloured compounds with NH_4CNS.

Sometimes the desired effect is achieved by a decrease of the concentration of the reagent (R) to a level at which it does not form a complex with the extraneous cation (MR), whereas the more stable complex with the cation to be determined (XR) is formed.

Extraneous ions may interfere not only when they form coloured complexes (MR) with the reagent (R), but also when such a complex is colourless but the concentration of the reagent in solution is greatly lowered by its formation.

To prevent this, an excess of reagent is added so that enough is present to combine both with the cation to be determined (X) and with the extraneous cation (M).

In colorimetric determination of cations it may be necessary to take into account the presence of anions which can form compounds or complexes of a low degree of dissociation with the cation to be determined. It is usually much simpler to eliminate such anions than to eliminate interfering cations, especially since the anions are generally introduced with the solvent, the choice of which depends to some extent on the analyst.

In practice it is necessary to reckon with the effects of Cl^-, SO_4^{--} and PO_4^{---} anions which, by forming chloride, sulphate or phosphate complexes with the X cation, make formation of the coloured

* See p. 439 with reference to the use of the comparator.

XR complex incomplete and thereby weaken the colour. This effect of the anions (p. 423) becomes appreciable only if the XR complex is insufficiently stable. In order to diminish the influence of these anions on the result they are often added in roughly the same concentrations to the corresponding standard solutions.

If for any reason it is impossible to eliminate the interfering influence of extraneous ions by masking or other means, separation reactions have to be used. In colorimetric analysis it is usual to determine extremely small amounts of a particular element in the presence of large amounts of a principal component; *therefore, the element or ion which is to be determined, and not the principal component, should be separated by precipitation* (p. 112).* Otherwise, the result will be much too low because of coprecipitation effects. Sometimes the element to be determined may even be coprecipitated completely.

It was pointed out in Sec. 27 that coprecipitation effects do not always interfere with analysis, but may also be utilized for separation of traces of various impurities from solution by precipitation with a "collector". This technique (p. 103) is of great practical importance and is often used in colorimetric determinations.

For example, in analysis of metallic copper it is necessary to determine very small amounts of arsenic, phosphorus, bismuth, antimony, and other elements. They are first concentrated and separated from the main bulk of the principal component (copper) by precipitation with a collector. A weighed sample of the copper is dissolved in nitric acid, the solution is neutralized, $FeCl_3$ solution is added, and Fe^{+++} ions are precipitated by addition of Na_2CO_3 solution. This gives a very bulky amorphous precipitate, consisting of ferric hydroxide and basic salts, which acts as a collector. All the trace components are precipitated with it almost completely. The "concentrate" is separated from the solution (which contains most of the principal component, copper) and dissolved in a suitable acid. This gives a solution containing the trace components in high enough concentrations for quantitative determination.

Another method is extraction of the ions to be determined; the solution is shaken with an organic solvent which is immiscible with water. The coloured compound of the element to be determined, formed by the action of a suitable reagent, is extracted from the aqueous solution and passes into the layer of organic solvent, so that the ion in question is separated from interfering ions and is concentrated. An example of this method is the extraction of thiocyanate complexes of iron, cobalt, molybdenum, and certain other metals by means of ethyl ether $(C_2H_5)_2O$, amyl alcohol $C_5H_{11}OH$,

* The precipitate is subsequently filtered off, washed, and dissolved, and the solution is analysed.

and similar solvents. It is known (Sec. 35) that the advantage of extraction over precipitation is that the interfacial area in the former method is not large and adsorption effects, which interfere in very many separations, are eliminated almost entirely. In addition, the separation is usually effected much more rapidly than by precipitation with subsequent filtration and washing of the precipitate.

In extraction, *a given substance is distributed between the organic solvent and water so that the ratio of its concentrations in the solvent and water* ($C_0 : C_W$)* *at equilibrium is constant; this ratio is known as the distribution constant.* This *distribution law* can be represented mathematically by the equation

$$\frac{C_0}{C_W} = K \qquad (1)$$

Equation (1) shows that the distribution is independent of the solution concentration. If the concentration of the substance in the aqueous phase (C_W) is decreased, its concentration in the organic layer (C_0) diminishes in the same ratio. Therefore, by successive treatment of a solution with fresh portions of organic solvent we can achieve almost complete extraction of the required substance from aqueous solution if the value of K is sufficiently high. However, in a number of cases complete extraction is not necessary for colorimetric determination. What matters is that the degree of extraction should be the same for both the unknown and the standard solution, and this is in agreement with Equation (1).

We must point out, however, that the above is valid only if the molecular weight of the substance is the same in both phases. If the substance is polymerized in one of the phases, the equilibrium becomes more complicated. If the substance is polymerized by combination of its molecules into pairs when it enters the organic layer

$$\underset{\text{In water}}{2A} \rightleftarrows \underset{\substack{\text{In organic}\\ \text{solvent}}}{A_2}$$

then at equilibrium

$$\frac{C_0}{C_W^2} = K \qquad (2)$$

In this case, if the concentration of the substance in the aqueous phase is halved its concentration in the layer of organic solvent is reduced to one-quarter of the previous value, so that the effectiveness of repeated extractions is greatly diminished and virtually complete extraction is much more difficult to achieve.

---

* Here C_0 and C_W are the concentrations of the substance in the organic solvent and water respectively.

At the same time, complete extraction is necessary in such cases, because here the degree of extraction depends on the concentration and is the same for the unknown and standard solutions only if their concentrations are equal.

121. Methods of Colour Comparison

For determination of the concentration of an unknown solution by comparison of its colour with a standard solution, the two solutions must be compared under identical conditions. Accordingly, the following procedures are adopted in colorimetric determinations.

1. The same reagents are added, in the same sequence and in the same quantities,* to both the standard solution and the unknown solution.
2. The reactions with both solutions are performed simultaneously as very often the colour changes with time.
3. If the unknown solution contains extraneous ions which influence the colour, and their influence cannot be eliminated by any means, approximately the same amounts of these ions are introduced into the standard solution. It is obvious that if the colour due to extraneous ions is too intense colorimetric determination may be impossible.
4. The colours of the unknown and standard solutions are compared in exactly similar vessels, made from the same kind of glass, and the two solutions must be illuminated equally.

The eye is incapable of estimating quantitatively differences of colour intensities; therefore, in visual colorimetry the aim is to equalize the colours of the solutions compared.

If we know how the colours have been equalized, we can easily calculate the concentration of the unknown solution. The following four methods of visual colorimetry are distinguished, in accordance with the method used for equalizing the colours. Of these the *dilution* method and the *balancing* method require that the system obey the Lambert-Beer law (p. 427). The advantage of the *colorimetric titration* and the *standard series methods* is that they may be applied even if the system does not obey this law.

Dilution Method. In this method only one standard solution is prepared, and its concentration is made equal to that of the unknown solution by gradual dilution of the solution with the more intense colour. This dilution is usually performed in glass cylinders

* It has already been stated (p. 423) that equal amounts of reagent must be added when $K_{inst.}$ of the coloured complex is relatively large. In the case of complexes with very low values K_{inst} excess of reagent has virtually no effect on the colour.

(Fig. 62) graduated in millilitres and tenths. The cylinders are placed in a wooden stand with a milk-white glass screen. One of the solutions is diluted until the colours appear exactly similar (when viewed from the side). The volumes of the solutions are measured before and after dilution, and the titre of the unknown solution ($T_{un.}$) is easily calculated from the titre of the standard solution ($T_{st.}$).

Suppose, for example, that one of the cylinders contains a certain volume $V_{st.}$ of the standard solution and after addition of the reagent the solution is diluted with water to volume $V_{st.d.}$.* The other cylinder contains a definite volume $V_{un.}$ of the unknown solution which, after addition of the reagent, is diluted with water to volume $V_{un.d.}$ so that its colour is the same as that of the diluted standard solution. Let us now calculate the titres ($T_{st.d.}$ and $T_{un.d.}$) of the two diluted solutions. One ml of the original standard solution contains $T_{st.}$ grams of the element to be determined. The total weight of the element taken is therefore $T_{st.} V_{st.}$ grams. After dilution this weight of the element is contained in $V_{st.d.}$ ml; therefore

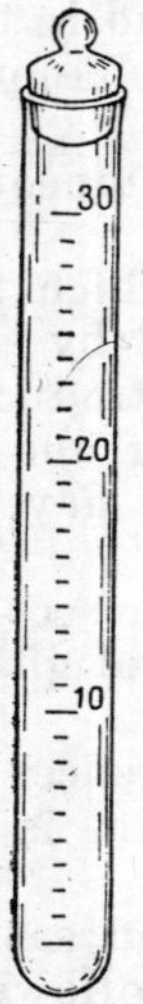

$$T_{st.d.} = \frac{T_{st.} V_{st.}}{V_{st.d.}} \tag{1}$$

Similarly, for the unknown solution we can write

$$T_{un.d.} = \frac{T_{un.} V_{un.}}{V_{un.d.}} \tag{2}$$

Since the colours of the two diluted solutions are the same, we have $T_{un.d.} = T_{st.d.}$. Therefore, from Equations (1) and (2) we have:

$$\frac{T_{un.} V_{un.}}{V_{un.d.}} = \frac{T_{st.} V_{st.}}{V_{st.d.}}$$

and

$$T_{un.} = T_{st.} \frac{V_{st.} V_{un.d.}}{V_{un.} V_{st.d.}} \tag{3}$$

Fig. 62. Graduated cylinder for colorimetric determinations by the dilution method

This formula is used for calculation of the results by the dilution method. This method is suitable if the solutions compared are fairly similar in colour. If the colour difference is considerable, the results are not accurate enough.

Balancing Method. The principle of this, the most useful colorimetric method, based on the Lambert-Beer law, has already been

---

* A diluted stock standard solution is usually called a "working standard" or simply "standard" solution.

discussed. The difference between the colour intensities of the unknown and standard solutions is eliminated and the solutions are "balanced" by suitable alteration of the thickness of one of the layers.

With solutions of coloured substances (p. 429) which obey the Lambert-Beer law, when the colour intensities are equal, the product of the depth (thickness) of the solution layer and its concentration is the same for the standard and the unknown solution, i.e.,

$$C_{un.} h_{un.} = C_{st.} h_{st.}$$

Hence

$$C_{un.} = C_{st.} \frac{h_{st.}}{h_{un.}} \tag{4}$$

This is the formula used for calculations of the results obtained by the balancing method.

Special instruments, known as *colorimeters*, are used for comparison of colours by variation of the depth of one of the solutions. The more widely used types of colorimeters are described below (p. 440 et seq).

Colorimetric Titration. In this method too only one standard solution is prepared, but its colour is adjusted to match the colour of the unknown solution by a gradual increase of its concentration on addition of a standard solution of the component to be determined from a burette.

Exactly similar cylinders (or test tubes) 2-2.5 cm in diameter and 25-30 cm high are used for the determinations. One of the cylinders contains the unknown solution with the required amount of the reagent to produce the colour. The other cylinder, used for preparation of the standard solution, contains the same amount of the reagent and, as far as possible, all the impurities (salts, acids, etc.) present in the unknown solution. Both solutions are then made up to the same volume with water and the colorimetric titration is started. A standard solution of the component to be determined is added gradually from a burette, with thorough stirring, into the second cylinder (containing only the reagent and impurities) until the colour exactly matches that of the unknown solution. If the volume of standard solution required for this is considerable, so that the volume of the liquid in that cylinder is increased appreciably, the unknown solution is also gradually diluted with the same amount of water.

The volume of standard solution added is found from the burette reading and is multiplied by its titre; this gives the amount of the element in the standard solution prepared as described above. Since its colour matches that of the unknown solution and the volumes of the two solutions are equal, the amounts of the given element contained in them must also be equal. In colorimetric titration the coloured substance need not conform to the Lambert-Beer law. This method gives fairly accurate results (relative error about 2-5%), and is therefore often used in practice.

Standard Series Method. In this method not one standard solution is prepared but a series, with gradually increasing concentrations of the element to be determined. For example, in the determination of copper by this method, progressively increasing amounts of a standard $CuSO_4$ solution are measured out into a series of similar test tubes, equal volumes of NH_4OH are added to each to convert the Cu^{++} ions into the more intensely coloured $[Cu(NH_3)_4]^{++}$ ions, and each is made up to the same volume (say, 20 ml) with water. This gives a *colorimetric scale*, which indicates the colours corresponding to different concentrations of copper in solution.

The unknown solution is similarly treated with NH_4OH solution and then diluted with water under exactly the same conditions. The colour is compared with the colours of the standard series.

If the solutions compared are placed under the same conditions, equal colours correspond to equal copper contents. For example, if it is found that the colour of the unknown solution is the same as that of a standard solution containing 4.0 mg of Cu^{++} in 20 ml, then this is also the copper content of 20 ml of the unknown solution. If the colour of the latter is more intense than with 4 mg of copper but weaker than with 4.5 mg, its Cu^{++} content may be taken as intermediate between the two, or approximately 4.25 mg per 20 ml.*

Since in the method of standard series the concentrations of the unknown and standard solutions are equal to each other, this method can be used with substances which do not obey the Lambert-Beer law. Its advantages are simplicity and speed. However, it is obvious that this is true only if numerous determinations have to be carried out. With single determinations the time required for preparation of the scale is not justified and this method is not convenient, especially if the colour is unstable and varies with time because of chemical changes in the coloured substance. Such instability makes it necessary to verify and renew the scale frequently. Sometimes this disadvantage can be avoided by preparing the scale not from the coloured compound formed but from other substances, similar to it in colour but more stable chemically.

For example, the colours given by the indicator methyl orange at different pH values can be very successfully imitated by mixture of $FeCl_3$ and $Co(NO_3)_2$ solutions in various proportions, so that a

---

* In this case the Cu^{++} content can be determined more precisely by a combination of this method with the dilution method.

very stable colorimetric scale can be obtained. Sometimes suitably chosen coloured glasses (light filters) or even coloured scales printed on paper are used instead of a series of standard solutions. Such standards may be used if a relatively low accuracy is acceptable.

In the preparation of a colorimetric scale the lowest concentration of the element to be determined is usually taken close to the sensitivity threshold of the reaction used. The highest concentration should not be more than 20 times the lowest, because visual comparison of very intense colours is extremely unreliable.

Selection of the background against which the colours are compared visually is of great importance. Coloured solutions must not be examined against a brightly lit window; too much light enters the eye, which soon becomes tired. It is best to compare colours against a background of milk-white glass or white paper, in a well-lit room under diffused light.

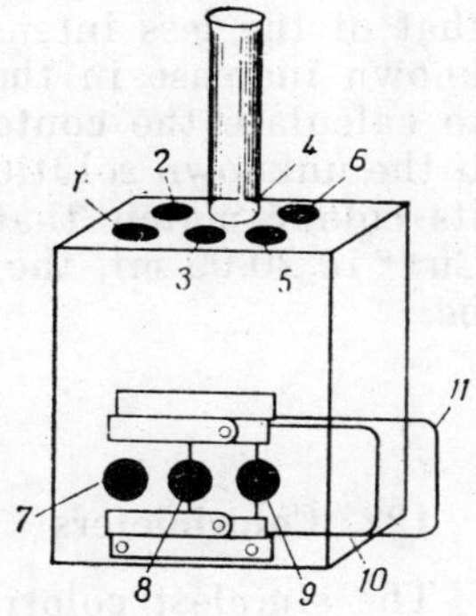

Fig. 63. Comparator: *1, 2, 3, 4, 5, 6*—sockets for test tubes; *7, 8, 9*—horizontal openings; *10, 11*—light filters

The work is made much easier by the use of a *comparator* (Fig. 63). The comparator is also convenient because with its use it is possible to eliminate the influence of the intrinsic colour of the unknown solution (if it is not too intense) on the result. To do this, a test tube with the unknown solution and added reagent is put into socket *4* of the comparator, and a similar test tube containing water is put into socket *3* opposite to it. Sockets *2* and *6* contain tubes with the corresponding standard solutions from the scale, and sockets *1* and *5* contain tubes with the unknown solution without reagent. The colours are examined through the horizontal openings *7*, *8* and *9* which run through the comparator.

The visual impression produced by the unknown solution coloured by the reagent in tube *4* is made up of: (a) the colour of the compound formed by the element to be determined and the reagent; (b) the intrinsic colour of the solution under test, which depends on the presence of coloured extraneous substances or ions. Exactly similar optical addition of colours occurs in the comparator with the standard solutions, as the light passes not only through these solutions but also through the unknown solution not coloured by the reagent (in tubes *1* and *5*). The influence of the intrinsic colour of the solution on the result of the determination is thereby eliminated.

Light filters (*10, 11*) placed behind the horizontal openings (*7, 8, 9*) of the comparator are sometimes used. In their presence the differences between colour intensities are replaced by shade differences, which are easier to detect. For example, if yellow solutions are compared with the use of a blue light filter, they appear more green with increasing intensity of the yellow colour.

If the colour of an unknown solution is intermediate between two solutions in the standard series, a more precise result can be obtained by a combination of the standard series and dilution methods. The unknown solution is diluted with water until its colour matches that of the less intensely coloured solution in the scale. From the known increase in the volume of the unknown solution it is easy to calculate the content of the given element in it. For example, if the unknown solution was diluted from 20.00 to 22.00 ml to make its colour match that of a standard solution containing 4 mg of Cu^{++} in 20.00 ml, the weight of Cu^{++} in the unknown solution must be

$$\frac{4\times 22.00}{20.00}=4.4 \text{ mg}$$

122. Colorimeters

The simplest colorimeter, of the "draining" type (Fig. 64), consists of two exactly similar graduated cylinders contained in a special stand over a milk-white glass screen. These cylinders are provided with taps through which the liquid in them may be drained off. The standard solution is put in one of the cylinders, and the unknown in the other. The cylinders are then viewed from above and the solution of the more intense colour is slowly drained off into a dry beaker placed underneath. When the colours of the solutions are exactly the same the draining is stopped. The depths of the standard and unknown solutions are then read off from the graduations on the cylinders and formula (4) is used to calculate the concentration of the unknown solution. For greater precision the experiment is repeated several times and the average reading is taken for each of the solutions. These average values of $h_{st.}$ and $h_{un.}$ are used in the calculations.

The immersion colorimeter shown in Fig. 65 is the most widely used.

Light falling on the mirror *1* is reflected upwards and passes through the standard and unknown solutions contained in the cups *2* and *2a*. It then passes through the solid (or hollow but sealed at both ends) glass cylinders *3* and *3a*, is internally reflected twice in the prisms *4* and *4a*, and reaches the eye through the lenses *5*. When the observer looks through the eye-piece *6*, he sees the field as a circle split along its diameter into two halves. One half is illuminated by the light which passed through the standard solution, while the other by light from the unknown solution. With this device it is much easier to compare colours and to detect more accurately when matching is obtained by variation of the depth of one of the

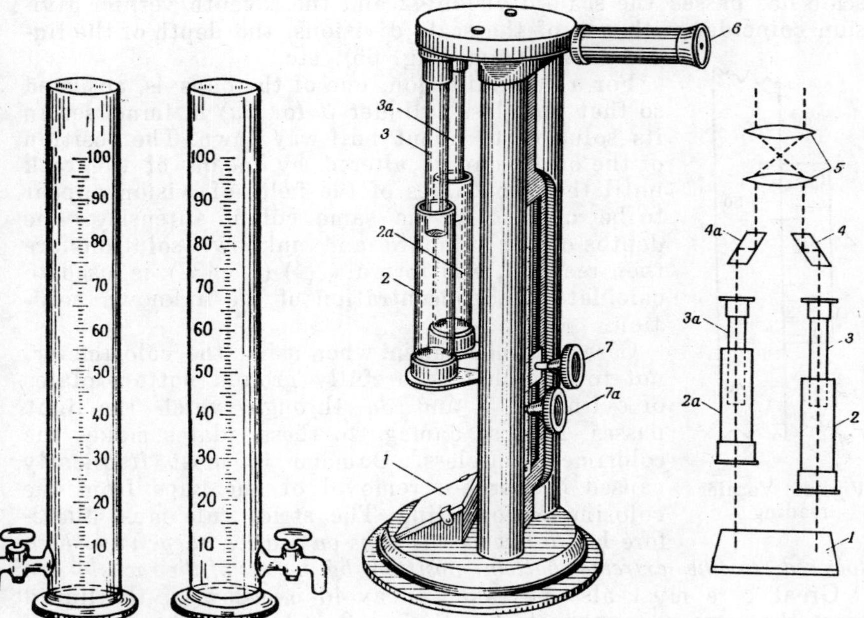

Fig. 64. Simple colorimeter of the draining type

Fig. 65. Immersion colorimeter and the simplified optical path through it:
1—mirror; *2*, *2a*—cups; *3*, *3a*—glass cylinders; *4*, *4a*—prisms; *5*—lenses; *6*—eye-piece; *7*, *7a*—racks

solutions. This variation is effected by raising or lowering one of the cups by means of the racks *7* or *7a* at the back of the instrument. This varies the immersion depth of cylinder *3* (or *3a*) in its solution and therefore the depth of the solution layer through which the light beam passes.

These depths ($h_{st.}$ and $h_{un.}$) of the two solutions are measured by means of scales (with millimetre divisions) placed along the slits at the back of the instrument. In these slits two small vernier scales can be moved by means of racks, so that tenths of a millimetre can be read off. The verniers are connected to the supports of the cups *2* and *2a* and when the knobs are turned they move together with the cups.

When taking a reading, note the division on the scale *1* immediately below the zero division of the vernier *2* (Fig. 66). This gives the number of whole millimetres in the measured depth. To find tenths of a millimetre, note which vernier division coincides with one of the scale divisions. For example, if the zero on the vernier scale has passed the scale division 42 and the seventh vernier division coincides with one of the scale divisions, the depth of the liquid is 42.7 mm (Fig. 66), etc.

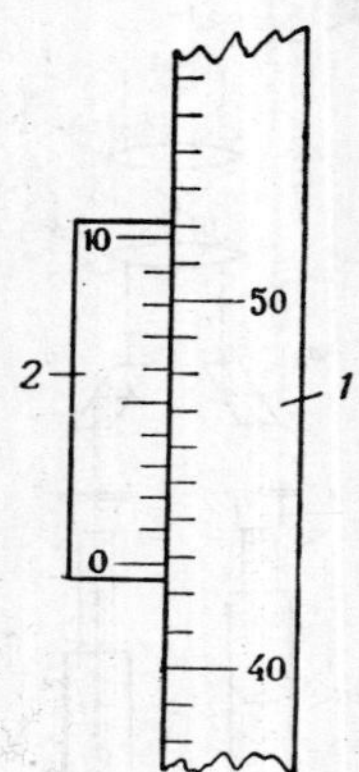

Fig. 66. Vernier reading

For a determination, one of the cups is adjusted so that the glass cylinder *3* (or *3a*) is immersed in its solution to about half-way down. The position of the other cup is altered by means of the rack until the two halves of the field of vision appear to be of exactly the same colour intensity. The depths of the standard and unknown solutions are then read off, and formula (4) (p. 437) is used to calculate the concentration of the unknown solution.

Care must be taken, when using the colorimeter, not to scratch the carefully ground bottom plates of cylinders *3* and *3a* through which the light passes, because damage to these plates makes the colorimeter useless. Damage is most frequently caused by careless removal of the cups from the colorimeter for filling. The strict rule must therefore be *to remove the cups only after they have been lowered to the extreme bottom position by means of the racks.*

Great care must also be taken to avoid overflow of the liquid from the cups when the glass cylinders *3* and *3a* are lowered into them. This can be done as follows. Raise the cups to the extreme top position and fill them almost to the top with distilled water from a wash bottle. Now lower the cups to the extreme bottom position and mark the liquid levels in them with a pencil.

Subsequently the cups are filled with the standard and unknown solutions almost up to these marks.

In using the colorimeter, avoid eye fatigue and strain, as after several observations the eye becomes less sensitive to small variations of colour intensity. Therefore, the observations should be made in a comparatively dark room, and the eyes should be rested for 30-40 seconds at intervals of 20 seconds. It is also possible to make the observations alternately first with one eye and then with the other.

One of the greatest advantages of the colorimeter is that it is easy to carry out replicate observations, which greatly reduce the random error of a single observation (p. 49). Therefore, the matching of the colours of the standard and unknown solution in the colorimeter *must always be repeated several times*. In order to eliminate defects in the optical system of the colorimeter and effects of unequal illumination of the two solutions, after several observations the cups are changed over and the observations are repeated.

Since determinations by the balancing method are based on Equation (4), which is derived from the Lambert-Beer law, the method can be used only if the coloured substance obeys this law fairly accurately (see Sec. 119).

123. Photocolorimetry

Apart from the visual methods described above for comparison of colours, other methods are available. For example, it follows from the equation

$$I_t = I_0 \times 10^{-\varepsilon hC}$$

(p. 427) that the intensity of light passing through a solution changes not only with the concentration (C) or depth of the solution (h), but also with the intensity I_0 of the incident light beam. It is possible to vary I_0 by means of diaphragms through which the light beam passes before entering the solution.

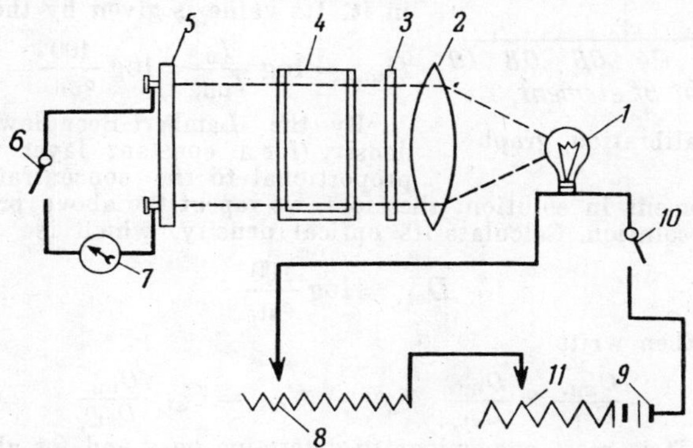

Fig. 67. Schematic diagram of a single-beam photocolorimeter:
1—incandescent lamp; *2*—lens; *3*—light filter; *4*—cuvette; *5*—photocell; *6*—switch; *7*—galvanometer; *8*—rheostat for fine adjustment; *9*—battery; *10*—switch; *11*—rheostat for coarse adjustment

This principle is the basis of the *diaphragm method* which is not considered in detail here.

Similarly, we can give only a very general idea of *photocolorimetry*.

In photocolorimetric determinations (p. 425) the intensity of the light emerging from the solution is estimated by the strength of the photoelectric current produced by illumination of the sensitive surface of a photocell and recorded by a galvanometer in the circuit. Special instruments known as *photocolorimeters* are used for the purpose. They are of two types, known as the "single-beam" and the "double-beam".

A diagram of A. Davydov's single-beam photocolorimeter is given in Fig. 67. Light from the incandescent lamp *1* is converted into a parallel beam by the lens *2*, passes through a suitably chosen light filter *3* and the solution in the cuvette *4* to the photocell *5* connected to the galvanometer *7* through the switch *6*. The light source is a 6-12 V lamp, similar to those used in car headlights, fed from a battery *9*.

Constant light intensity is decisive for accurate operation of the instrument. Heating of the lamp filament is regulated by means of two rheostats in the circuit: *11* (for coarse adjustment) and *8* (for fine regulation).

For the determination, the cuvette *4* is filled with water (or with "blank" solution*), the lamp *1* is switched in by the switch *10*, and heating of the lamp filament is adjusted by the rheostats *11* and *8* so that the galvanometer needle is on the 100 division of the scale. Water (or "blank" solution) is then emptied out of the cuvette, which is filled with the unknown solution (coloured by addition of reagents) and the galvanometer reading is noted (a_{un}). As the deflection of the needle is proportional to the intensity of the light reaching the photocell, these data can be used for calculating the optical density (D_{un}) of the solution due to the presence of the coloured substance in it. Its value is given by the formula:

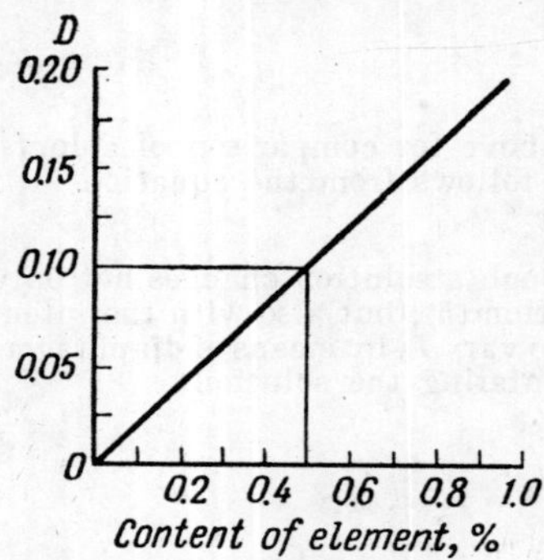

Fig. 68. Calibration graph

$$D_{un.} = \log \frac{I_0}{I_{un.}} = \log \frac{100}{a_{un.}} = 2 - \log a_{un.}$$

By the Lambert-Beer law the optical density (for a constant layer thickness) is proportional to the concentration (C_{un}) of the given element in solution; therefore, we repeat the above procedure with the standard solution. Calculate its optical density, which is

$$D_{st.} = \log \frac{100}{a_{st.}}$$

and we can then write

$$\frac{C_{un.}}{C_{st.}} = \frac{D_{un.}}{D_{st.}} \quad \text{or} \quad C_{un.} = C_{st.} \cdot \frac{D_{un.}}{D_{st.}}$$

However, it is more convenient to determine once and for all the optical densities corresponding to different concentrations of the element with the aid of a series of standard solutions with progressively increasing concentrations. The data so obtained are used for plotting a "calibration graph" (Fig. 68), which is then used in analysis for finding the concentration of the given element graphically.

Double-beam photocolorimeters, also known as differential photocolorimeters, differ from the single-beam type described above in that they have, with a common light source, two similar and symmetrical optical systems (Fig. 69), each provided with a diaphragm. The two photocells are so connected in the common circuit that their respective photoelectric currents are opposite in direction.

Accordingly, if the colours of the standard and the unknown solutions are equal in intensity, the light transmitted through them produces currents of equal strength in the photocells, so that the two currents balance each other. The galvanometer needle is then at zero, which is a sign that the light beams

* A solution containing the same amounts of substances (including the reagents added) as the sample for analysis, but without the element to be determined.

passing through the two solutions are of equal intensity. Conversely, a small difference of intensity causes an easily detected difference between the photoelectric currents, which can be either measured from the deflection of the galvanometer needle or balanced by means of a special recording drum connected to one of the diaphragms. The advantage of this instrument is that the results are entirely independent of any voltage fluctuations in the lamp filament circuit.

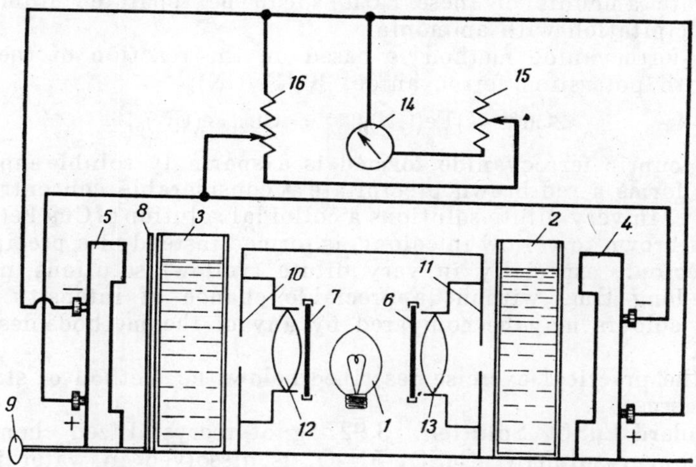

Fig. 69. Diagram of a differential photocolorimeter:
1—incandescent lamp; *2*, *3*—cuvettes; *4*, *5*—selenium photocells; *6*, *7*—light filters; *8*—metal screen; *9*—handle for rotating the screen; *10*, *11*—iris diaphragms (one connected to the recording drum); *12*, *13*—condensing lenses; *14*—galvanometer with 100 scale divisions; *15*, *16*—rheostats

In conclusion, it may be noted that the photocolorimetric method is used in volumetric analysis for determination of the equivalence point in titration.

The theory and methods of colorimetry and photocolorimetry are discussed in detail in special manuals and articles.

124. Determination of Copper in Copper Sulphate Solution

Various methods are available for colorimetric determination of copper. The ammonia and the ferrocyanide methods are the most useful.

The reagent used in the ammonia method for producing the colour is NH_4OH solution, which gives a series of blue ammonia complexes of different coordination numbers with the Cu^{++} ion. Usually in colorimetric determinations the complexes $[Cu(NH_3)_4]^{++}$ and $[Cu(NH_3)_6]^{++}$ are formed; for example:

$$Cu^{++} + 4NH_4OH \rightleftarrows [Cu(NH_3)_4]^{++} + 4H_2O$$

The instability constant of the $[Cu(NH_3)_4]^{++}$ ion is 5×10^{-14}. Nickel and cobalt, which form coloured complexes with ammonia, interfere with determination of copper by the ammonia method. Cations which form insoluble hydroxides with ammonia, such as Fe^{+++}, Al^{+++}, Mn^{++}, Pb^{++}, Sn^{++}, Bi^{+++}, Hg^{++}, etc., also interfere. Moderate amounts of these cations can be separated from Cu^{++} by precipitation with ammonia.

The ferrocyanide method is based on the reaction of the Cu^{++} ion with potassium ferrocyanide, $K_4[Fe(CN)_6]$:

$$2Cu^{++} + [Fe(CN)_6]^{==} = Cu_2[Fe(CN)_6]$$

The cupric ferrocyanide formed is a sparingly soluble substance which forms a red-brown precipitate at considerable concentrations of Cu^{++}. In very dilute solutions a colloidal solution of $Cu_2[Fe(CN)_6]$, yellow-brown to yellow in colour, is formed instead of a precipitate. This colour, especially in very dilute (yellow) solutions, persists for a long time without appreciable change of intensity.

The colours may be compared by any of the methods described above.

In the practical exercise described below the method of standard series is used.

Standard $CuSO_4$ Solution. 3.927 g of recrystallized chemically pure copper sulphate, $CuSO_4 \cdot 5H_2O$, is dissolved in water in a 1 litre measuring flask. The solution is acidified with 5 ml of sulphuric acid (sp. gr. 1.84) to suppress hydrolysis, diluted with water up to the mark, and mixed. One ml of this solution contains 1.0 mg of copper.

Preparation of the Colorimetric Scale. Take 11 exactly similar test tubes 25-30 ml in capacity and make a pencil mark corresponding to a volume of 20 ml on each.* Rinse the test tubes out with distilled water, and measure out into them, with a 5 ml measuring pipette (Fig. 37) or a burette, the following volumes of the standard $CuSO_4$ solution:

Tube	1	2	3	4	5	6	7	8	9	10
Volume of standard solution, ml	0.5	1.0	1.5	2.0	2.5	3.0	3.5	4.0	4.5	5.0

Dilute the solutions in the tubes to about 8-10 ml with water and neutralize the H_2SO_4 by adding 2 N NH_4OH solution drop by drop until the last drop produces a turbidity which does not disappear on stirring. Then add 5.0 ml of 2 N NH_4OH solution to each tube, make the liquid up to the mark with water, and mix.

* These marks should all be at the same height; this indicates that the diameters of the tubes are equal. The marks can be made on strips of paper glued to the tubes.

The tubes should be firmly stoppered so that the colorimetric scale does not alter owing to volatilization of ammonia.

Procedure. Put the unknown solution containing copper in a 100 ml measuring flask, make it up to the mark with water, and mix thoroughly. Measure out exactly 5.0 ml of this solution with a measuring pipette (or burette) into the last (11th) test tube, neutralize it with 2 *N* NH_4OH solution until a permanent turbidity appears, add a further 5.0 ml of the ammonia solution, dilute with water up to the mark, and mix.

Compare the colour of this solution with the colours of the standard solutions in the scale. This is most conveniently done in a comparator (see Fig. 63). Having matched the colour on the scale, calculate the copper content in the total volume of the unknown solution (100 ml) from the copper content of the standard. For example, if the colour of the unknown solution matched that of the standard in tube No. 7, then the copper content of the unknown solution is

$$Q = \frac{3.5 \times 100}{5} = 70 \text{ mg} = 0.070 \text{ g}$$

If the colour of the unknown solution is intermediate between two adjacent colours of the scale, its copper content can be assumed to be the average of the copper contents of the two standard solutions. Should it be found that the colour of the unknown solution is deeper than that of the most concentrated of the standards (in tube No. 10), the experiment must be repeated with a smaller amount of the unknown solution in the test tube.

It is evident that other methods for comparing colours, discussed more fully in Secs. 125 and 126, can be used for this determination.

125. Determination of Titanium in Titanium Sulphate Solution

This determination is based on the formation of yellow pertitanic acid

$$Ti(SO_4)_2 + H_2O = TiOSO_4 + H_2SO_4$$

$$TiOSO_4 + H_2O_2 = [TiO(H_2O_2)]SO_4$$

The reaction is conducted in strongly acid solution with a fairly large excess of H_2O_2. Vanadium, cerium, and molybdenum, which form coloured compounds with hydrogen peroxide, interfere with the determination, as do fluorides and large amounts of phosphates, which combine with Ti^{++++} ions. The Fe^{+++} ion interferes very little in sulphuric or nitric acid solutions. On the other hand, in the presence of Cl^- ions the yellow complex $[FeCl_6]^{---}$ is formed, which interferes with the determination. Small amounts of Fe^{+++} ions may be masked by the addition of phosphoric acid, which forms the more stable colourless complex $[Fe(PO_4)_2]^{---}$ with Fe^{+++}.

The colours may be compared by any of the available methods. The dilution method is described in detail below.

Standard Titanium Solution. About 0.2-0.3 g of TiO_2 is fused in a porcelain (or platinum) crucible with 2-3 g of $KHSO_4$. The melt is cooled and leached with 10% H_2SO_4. The undissolved TiO_2 residue is filtered off and the filtrate is diluted up to 0.5 litre with sulphuric acid so that after dilution the solution contains 5% H_2SO_4. 50-ml samples are taken and the titre of the solution is determined volumetrically (by reduction of Ti^{++++} to Ti^{+++} with zinc followed by titration with $FeCl_3$ solution).*

Procedure. Put the unknown $Ti(SO_4)_2$ solution in a 100 ml measuring flask, dilute to the mark with water, and mix. Take a dry colorimetric cylinder (see Fig. 62), or rinse it out with the standard titanium solution, put in the standard solution *exactly* up to the 10th the division, add 8-10 ml of 3% H_2O_2, dilute to 30 ml with water, and mix thoroughly.

Take another similar cylinder, rinse it out with the unknown solution, and put in 10.00 ml of the unknown solution followed by the same volume as before (8-10 ml) of H_2O_2 solution, mix, and gradually dilute the solution with water until its colour is the same as that of the standard solution.** As a check, change the cylinders over and repeat the colour comparison.

When the colours have been matched, read off the volume of the unknown solution after dilution.

If it is found that even after dilution to 30 ml the colour of the unknown solution is deeper than that of the standard, the determination should be repeated with a smaller initial volume (say, 5.00 ml) of the unknown solution. The titanium content is calculated as described on p. 436.

126. Determination of Iron in a Solution of an Iron Salt

The reaction between Fe^{+++} and CNS^- ions is used for colorimetric determination of iron. In the preceding account it was assumed for simplicity that the reaction is represented by the equation

$$Fe^{+++} + 3CNS^- \rightleftarrows Fe(CNS)_3$$

Research has shown, however, that in reality the reaction is much more complicated, and proceeds with the formation of iron thiocy-

* If a platinum crucible is used for the fusion, the titre of the solution can be determined gravimetrically.

** The cylinders should be turned so that the scale divisions are at the side lest they interfere with observation of the colour.

anate complexes in which the coordination number of iron ranges from one to six. The reactions may be represented by the equations

$$Fe^{+++} + CNS^- \rightleftarrows [Fe(CNS)]^{++}$$

$$[Fe(CNS)]^{++} + CNS^- \rightleftarrows [Fe(CNS)_2]^+$$

etc., up to

$$[Fe(CNS)_5]^{--} + CNS^- \rightleftarrows [Fe(CNS)_6]^{---}$$

At low thiocyanate concentrations (of the order of 5×10^{-3} *M*) most of the iron forms the complex $[Fe(CNS)]^{++}$. With increase of CNS^- ion concentration in the solution this complex is gradually converted into $[Fe(CNS)_2]^+$, $[Fe(CNS)_3]$, $[Fe(CNS)_4]^-$, etc. The colour intensity of the solution also increases. Therefore, in this determination large and *exactly equal* excesses of reagent must be added to both the solutions being compared.

A number of substances interfere with the determination of iron by this method. Primarily, these are all the substances (or ions) which can give more stable complexes with Fe^{+++} or CNS^- ions. These include fluorides, phosphates, arsenates, tartrates*, mercury salts, etc. Acetates and sulphates may interfere if the acidity is low, and chlorides interfere if the reagent is in sufficient excess. Other substances which interfere are reducing agents (such as S^{--}, SO_3^{--}, I^-, Sn^{++}, etc.) which reduce Fe^{+++} to Fe^{++} and oxidants which oxidize the CNS^- ion (such as MnO_4^- or NO_2^- ions, hydrogen peroxide, concentrated HNO_3, etc.).

Ferric salts, especially in dilute solutions, undergo considerable hydrolysis which leads to formation of basic ferric salts or ferric hydroxide:

$$Fe^{+++} + H_2O \rightleftarrows [Fe(OH)]^{++} + H^+$$

$$[Fe(OH)]^{++} + H_2O \rightleftarrows [Fe(OH)_2]^+ + H^+$$

and finally

$$[Fe(OH)_2]^+ + H_2O \rightleftarrows Fe(OH)_3 + H^+$$

In consequence the concentration of Fe^{+++} ions in solution decreases and the colour becomes weaker. This is avoided by suppressing hydrolysis by the addition of acid, preferably nitric.**

The sensitivity of this method (the least amount of Fe^{+++} which can be determined by it) is 0.0025 mg of iron in 50 ml of final volume. If the reaction product is extracted in isoamyl alcohol, the sen-

* Salts of tartaric acid, $H_2C_4H_4O_6$.

** However, its concentration should not be too high, otherwise HNO_3 may oxidize CNS^- ions.

sitivity of the method is raised to 0.0005 mg of iron in 10 ml of extract.

The colour caused by the reaction between Fe^{+++} and CNS^- is unstable. It becomes weaker with time because of reduction of Fe^{+++} ions by CNS^- ions. Therefore, the method of standard series is less convenient in this case. Below we consider the determination of Fe^{+++} by colorimetric titration and by the balancing method.

Standard Solution of Ferric Salt. 0.8640 g of chemically pure ferric ammonium alum $NH_4Fe(SO_4)_2 \cdot 12H_2O$, free from efflorescence, is dissolved in water acidified with 5 ml of H_2SO_4 (sp. gr. 1.84) 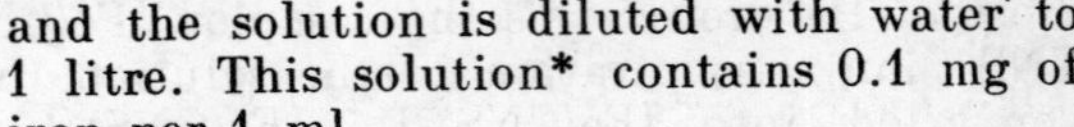 and the solution is diluted with water to 1 litre. This solution* contains 0.1 mg of iron per 1 ml.

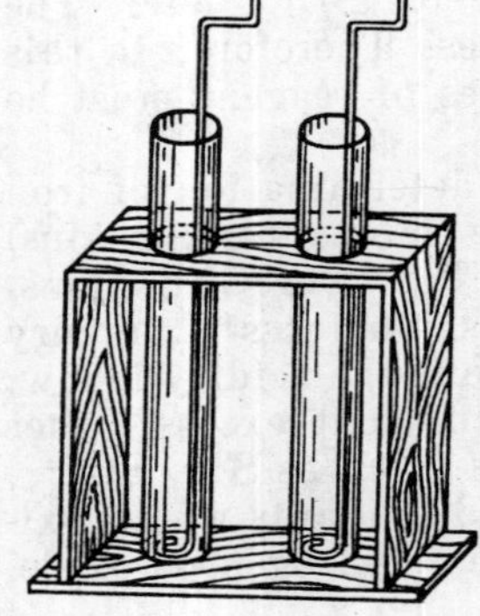

Fig. 70. Stand and cylinders with stirrers for colorimetric titration

Determination of Fe^{+++} by Colorimetric Titration. Put the unknown solution of ferric salt, containing 0.04-0.20 mg of Fe^{+++}, in a 100 ml measuring flask, dilute it with water up to the mark, and mix thoroughly. 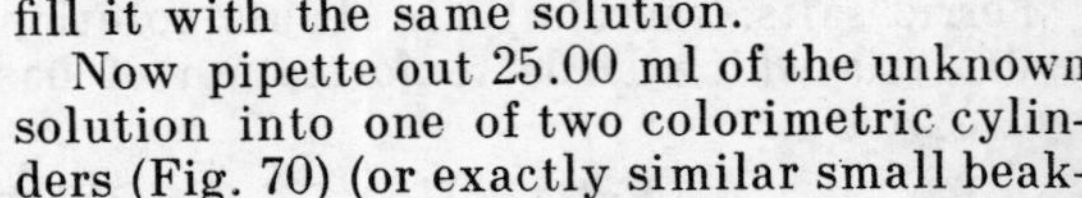 Prepare the solution to be used for the titration in another 100 ml flask. For this, measure out accurately 10.00 ml of the standard ferric ammonium alum solution with a pipette or burette, make up to the mark, and mix thoroughly. The titre of this solution is 0.01 mg of iron per 1 ml; rinse the burette out twice with it, and then fill it with the same solution.

Now pipette out 25.00 ml of the unknown solution into one of two colorimetric cylinders (Fig. 70) (or exactly similar small beakers), and 25.00 ml of water into the other. Add into each cylinder (or beaker) 10 drops of HNO_3 solution (sp. gr. 1.2) and 5 ml of 10% NH_4CNS solution, measuring the latter with a small (10 ml) measuring cylinder or pipette.

Put both cylinders (or beakers) into a special stand or on a sheet of white paper and titrate the colourless solution, containing water and the reagents only, with the standard solution of ferric salt until the colours in the cylinders match exactly. To ensure that the increased volume of the titrated solution does not influence the result, take a burette reading before the end of the titration and add the same volume of water to the unknown solution.

Having obtained a colour match and recorded the burette readings, repeat the experiment once or twice more, taking fresh por-

* The titre of the solution can be checked gravimetrically (Sec. 41) or volumetrically (Sec. 94).

tions of the unknown solution and water each time. Take the average of all the readings. Multiply the result by the titre of the ferric salt solution (0.01 mg/ml) to find the total amount of Fe^{+++} in 25 ml of the unknown solution taken for analysis. Calculate the content in 100 ml of solution and express the result in grams.

Determination of Fe^{+++} by the Balancing Method. Put the unknown solution into a 100 ml measuring flask, make it up to the mark with water, and mix thoroughly. In a similar measuring flask dilute 10.00 ml of the standard ferric ammonium alum solution to 100 ml.

Before starting the determination, adjust the colorimeter (see Fig. 65) so that both halves of the field of vision appear exactly alike when viewed through the eye-piece *6*. Then lower the cups *2* and *2a* to the extreme bottom position by means of the racks and take them carefully out of the colorimeter.

Into one of the cups* measure out 10.00 ml of the unknown solution, and into the other 10.00 ml of the standard solution, and add to each 4 drops of HNO_3 solution (sp. gr. 1.2) and 5.0 ml of 1% NH_4CNS solution. Mix each liquid thoroughly and put the cup with the standard solution in the right-hand socket of the colorimeter, and the cup with the unknown solution in the left-hand socket. Now raise the cups so that the cylinders (*3* and *3a*) are immersed in the liquids to a depth of at least 0.5-1 cm. Now look through the eye-piece *6* and gradually raise, by means of the rack, the solution of deeper colour until both halves of the field appear exactly alike. The eye must be rested frequently, because it tires quickly and becomes unable to perceive slight colour differences.

Having balanced the colours and having checked the balance after resting the eye for 1-2 minutes, read off the scales (p. 442) and calculate the ratio of the heights $h_{st.} : h_{un.}$ If this ratio is close to unity (i.e., if the concentrations of the two solutions do not differ greatly), repeat the experiment at least three times. Then, without changing the position of the colorimeter, change the cups over and again take at least three readings. Write down all the readings.

Colour comparisons in a colorimeter give the best results when the colours are not very different in intensity. Therefore, if the ratio $h_{st.} : h_{un.}$ is very different from unity the solution of the higher concentration must first be diluted with water in a definite proportion. Of course, since this dilution must be taken into account when the result is calculated, it should be performed as accurately as possible, i.e., with a pipette (or burette) and a measuring flask. For example, if the $h_{st.} : h_{un.}$ ratio was found in the first determination to be

* The cups must be clean and absolutely dry; otherwise they must be washed and dried inside and out with a soft cloth. They should on no account be dried in the drying oven.

about 3.6, i.e., if the concentration of the unknown solution is 3.6 times that of the standard, the former must be diluted to exactly $^1/_4$ of its initial concentration.

This can be done as follows. Pipette out a fresh portion (25.00 ml) of the unknown solution and dilute it to 100 ml in a measuring flask. Then use this diluted solution to prepare the coloured solutions in the cups* as described above; compare the colours in the colorimeter, taking at least six readings.

At the end of the experiment empty the colorimeter cups immediately and wash them thoroughly with distilled water.**

Calculation. Suppose that the following readings were obtained in the determination:

Expt. No.	$h_{st.}$	$h_{un.}$	Expt. No.	$h_{st.}$	$h_{un.}$
1	32.0	28.1	4	30.0	27.0
2	32.0	28.5	5	30.0	26.8
3	32.0	27.8	6	30.0	26.1
Average	32.0	28.1	Average	30.0	26.6

First we find the average of the $h_{st.} : h_{un.}$ ratios. The average value is 1.14 with the cups containing the solutions in one position (experiments Nos. 1, 2, and 3) and 1.12 with the cups reversed (experiments Nos. 4, 5, and 6). This gives an average value of 1.13 for $h_{st.} : h_{un.}$.

Hence we find the titre of the unknown solution used in the determination:

$$T_{un.} = T_{st.} \frac{h_{st.}}{h_{un.}} = 0.01 \times 1.13 = 0.0113 \text{ mg/ml}$$

Therefore, 100 ml of this solution contained:

$$Q_{un.} = 0.0113 \times 100 = 1.13 \text{ mg} = 0.00113 \text{ g of iron}$$

If the unknown solution was diluted fourfold with water before the determination then the result must be multiplied by 4. In this case the total amount of iron is

$$Q_{un.} = 0.0113 \times 100 \times 4 = 4.52 \text{ mg} = 0.00452 \text{ g}$$

Besides this thiocyanate method, iron is also determined colorimetrically by Sagaidachny's method, in which the reagent is a solution of salicylic acid, which gives a violet colour with ferric salts (ferrous salts do not give a colour).

* They should first be washed and wiped dry.

** The solutions must not be left in the cups, as this causes damage to the metallic parts of the instrument.

This reaction is highly sensitive: solutions containing 1 part of Fe^{+++} in 10 million parts of water give an appreciable colour. This method gives the best results in acid solutions (pH $\geqslant$ 2) with contents of 0.2-0.3 mg Fe^{+++} per 100 ml of solution. The reagent is a saturated solution of salicylic acid, $C_6H_4(OH)COOH$; 2-4 ml of this solution is taken per 100 ml.

In recent years 1,2,5-sulphosalicylic acid, which has a number of advantages over salicylic acid, has come into extensive use.

127. Determination of Hydrogen Ion Concentration (pH)

The hydrogen ion exponent (pH) can be determined experimentally by a variety of methods, which can be subdivided into potentiometric and colorimetric methods. The potentiometric methods are based on measurement of the e.m.f. of a cell in which the unknown solution is one of the electrode liquids. The electromotive force of such a cell is functionally connected with the H^+ ion concentration in the solution by the Nernst equation (Sec. 79), which is used for calculating the solution pH.

As an example, let us consider a cell composed of the standard hydrogen electrode described on p. 314 (containing H^+ ions at a concentration of 1 g-ion/litre) and another hydrogen electrode which differs from the first only in that the electrolyte in it is the solution of unknown H^+ ion concentration. The potential of the first electrode is taken to be zero. The potential of the second electrode (E_x) as a function of the H^+ ion concentration in the unknown solution is represented by the Nernst equation:

$$E_x = 0 + \frac{0.058}{1} \log [H^+] = 0.058 \log [H^+]$$

But the e.m.f. of the cell (E) is equal to the difference between the potentials of the two electrodes, i.e.,

$$E = 0 - E_x = -E_x = -0.058 \log [H^+]$$

But, since

$$-\log [H^+] = \text{pH, therefore } E = 0.058 \text{ pH}$$

and

$$\text{pH} = \frac{E}{0.058} \qquad (1)$$

This equation is used for finding the pH of the unknown solution from the experimental value of E. In practice, instead of the standard hydrogen electrode the more convenient calomel electrode is commonly used (see footnote to p. 334); its potential (E_{cal}) is accurately known. In this case

$$E = E_{\text{cal.}} - E_x = E_{\text{cal.}} + 0.058 \text{ pH}$$

and

$$\text{pH} = \frac{E - E_{\text{cal.}}}{0.058} \qquad (2)$$

The potentiometric method is the more precise (the precision is of the order of 0.01 pH unit) but it is somewhat laborious and requires the appropriate apparatus. Therefore, in practice pH is more often determined by the simpler colorimetric methods, the precision of which is about 0.1-0.2 pH unit.*

Colorimetric methods are based on the use of pH indicators; the colours of these indicators in the presence of unknown solutions are used for estimating the H^+ ion concentrations of the latter. As was stated earlier (Sec. 60), pH indicators change colour only over a definite pH range, known as the indicator range. It is only within that range that each given colour corresponds to one quite definite solution pH. Outside that range solutions differing greatly in pH may have the same colour. It is clear from this that *a given indicator can be used for* pH *determination only if the* pH *value to be measured lies within the indicator range.* In other words, when the indicator is added to an unknown solution it should assume an intermediate colour and not one of the extreme colours.

Therefore, before pH can be determined colorimetrically, a suitable indicator must be chosen by preliminary tests. The determination itself can be performed in various ways, *with* or *without buffer solutions.*

In the methods with buffer solutions, a suitable indicator is chosen and the table of compositions of buffer solutions (see Appendix VII) is used for preparing a series of buffer solutions with pH values within the range of the chosen indicator and rising progressively by steps of 0.2 pH unit. Equal volumes, say, 10 ml, of the buffer solutions are measured out into a series of similar test tubes, an equal amount (say, 10 drops) of the indicator is added to each, and each liquid is mixed. This gives a colorimetric scale showing the colours of the given indicator at different pH values.

When the scale has been prepared, the same amounts of unknown solution (10 ml) and indicator (10 drops) are put in an exactly similar test tube, the liquid is mixed thoroughly, and the colour is compared with the standard scale of colours. Since the solutions were prepared under the same conditions, equal colours correspond to equal pH values.

This method of pH determination involves the use of standard series. The determinations are very rapid, apart from the time needed for preparation of the scale. Unfortunately, such scales are unstable and must be frequently renewed. This disadvantage has to be accepted if the colours given by the given indicator cannot be imitated by mixing solutions of more stable chemical compounds (for example, see p. 438 with reference to the methyl orange scale).

Methods for pH determination without buffer solutions are also available. There are two variations of such methods. One is based

* For more detailed descriptions of the potentiometric method for pH determination see textbooks on physical chemistry.

on the use of one-colour indicators such as paranitrophenol (p. 236), phenolphthalein, etc. The other method (described in detail below) is based on the use of two-colour indicators. It is very interesting in the theoretical sense as an illustration of the theory of pH indicators, and is also the more precise.

Determinations by this method generally involve the use of six indicators the ranges of which cover the pH range from 3.0 to 9.6, which is of the most practical interest (Table XX).

Table XX

Two-Colour Indicators Used for pH Determination

Indicator	pK	Colour		Method of preparing indicator solution
		Acid form	Alkaline form	
Bromphenol blue	4.1	Yellow	Blue	0.1 g ground with 1.5 ml of 0.1 *N* NaOH and diluted with water to 100 ml
Methyl red	5.0	Red	Yellow	0.1 g dissolved in 300 ml of alcohol and diluted to 500 ml
Bromcresol purple	6.3	Yellow	Purple	0.1 g ground with 1.45 ml of 0.1 *N* NaOH and diluted with water to 100 ml
Phenol red	7.7	Yellow	Red	0.1 g ground with 2.85 ml of 0.1 *N* NaOH and diluted with water to 100 ml
Cresol red	8.1	Yellow	Red	0.1 g ground with 2.65 ml of 0.1 *N* NaOH and diluted with water to 100 ml
Thymol blue	8.8	Yellow	Blue	0.1 g ground with 2.15 ml of 0.1 *N* NaOH and diluted with water to 100 ml

The method is based on the fundamental equation of the theory of pH indicators*:

$$\mathrm{pH} = \mathrm{p}K - \log \frac{C_{\text{acid. f.}}}{C_{\text{alk. f.}}} \tag{3}$$

It follows from the equation that if any pH indicator is added to a particular solution, a definite ratio is established between the concentrations of its acid ($C_{\text{acid. f.}}$) and alkaline ($C_{\text{alk. f.}}$) forms, in accordance with the solution pH.

* The derivation of the equation is given on p. 240.

Since these forms have different colours, the value of the ratio $C_{acid.\,f.} : C_{alk.\,f.}$ determines the colour shade of the indicator at the given pH. For example, with the indicator phenol red at pH equal to its pK (7.7), we have from Equation (1):

$$7.7 = 7.7 - \log \frac{C_{acid.\,f.}}{C_{alk.\,f.}}$$

and hence

$$\log \frac{C_{acid.\,f.}}{C_{alk.\,f.}} = 0 \quad \text{and} \quad \frac{C_{acid.\,f.}}{C_{alk.\,f.}} = 1.$$

From this it follows that when 10 drops of phenol red solution are added to 10 ml of a buffer solution of pH = 7.7 an equilibrium is established between the two differently coloured forms so that exactly one half or 5 drops of the indicator is present in solution as the red alkaline form,* while the other half is present as the yellow acid form.

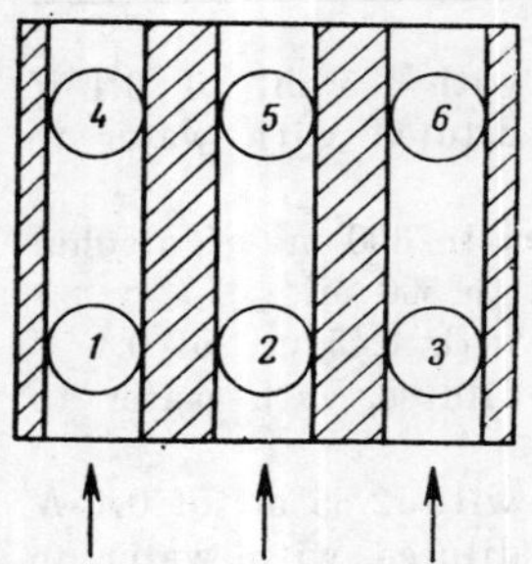

Fig. 71. Arrangement of tubes in the comparator

Optical addition of these colours at the given pH creates the impression of an intermediate orange colour.

Exactly similar optical addition of colours occurs if two similar test tubes are taken, one with acid (HCl) and the other with alkali (NaOH), five drops of phenol red is put in each, the tubes are placed in sockets *2* and *5* of the comparator (Fig. 71), and the two solutions are examined in the direction indicated by the arrows. In the HCl solution practically all the indicator (5 drops) is converted into the acid form ($HInd^0$), while in the NaOH solution it is in the alkaline form (Ind^-). Therefore, if we look through both solutions together we can see an orange colour; although this may differ somewhat from the colour given by a buffer solution of pH = 7.7 (with 10 drops of indicator), this is merely because the thickness of the liquid layer through which the light has to pass is twice as much in the former case (two tubes) as in the latter (one tube). If a tube

* Phenol red is a weak acid which exists in two tautomeric forms $HInd^0$ and HInd. Equilibria in its solutions are represented as follows:

$$\underset{\text{Yellow}}{HInd^0} \rightleftarrows \underset{\text{Red}}{HInd} \rightleftarrows H^+ + \underset{\text{Red}}{Ind^-}$$

Consequently, the acid form here are undissociated $HInd^0$ molecules which accumulate in the solution when it is acidified, and the alkaline form, Ind^- anions towards the formation of which the equilibrium is shifted when H^+ ions are joined by OH^- ions of the alkali.

with water is also put into the comparator behind the buffer solution with 10 drops of indicator, the two colours would be identical.

Therefore, a buffer solution of pH = 7.7 with regard to the colour given by it with 10 drops of phenol red can be satisfactorily replaced by two solutions, acid and alkali, with 5 drops of the given indicator added to each.

Now suppose that two drops of phenol red indicator are put into the tube with acid, and eight drops into the tube with alkali; this means that the total number of drops of indicator in the acid and alkali is 10 as before. To what pH does the colour given by this pair of tubes correspond? To solve this problem, we replace the ratio of the concentrations in Equation (1) by the ratio of the number of drops of indicator in the acid and alkali solutions:

$$\text{pH} = \text{p}K - \log\frac{C_{\text{acid. f.}}}{C_{\text{alk. f.}}} = 7.7 - \log\frac{2}{8} = 8.3$$

Therefore, this pair of solutions gives the same total colour as a buffer solution of pH = 8.3 (with 10 drops of indicator and in the presence of a second tube containing water).

The principle of this method of pH determination is clear from the above examples.

Choice of Indicator. As already stated, the first step in colorimetric determination of pH is the choice of a suitable indicator. This choice is made most conveniently by approximate determination of pH with the aid of the so-called *universal indicators.* These are mixtures of two or more indicators chosen so that their colours alter over a wide pH range.

One of the simplest universal indicators with regard to composition, and at the same time one of the most convenient, is a mixture of methyl red and thymol blue indicators, made up in a particular way.* This indicator undergoes the following colour changes with pH:

pH	Colour	pH	Colour
4	Red	8	Pale green
5	Orange	9	Green
6	Rose-yellow	10	Blue-green
7	Yellow		

An alternative indicator to the above is Kolthoff's universal indicator (EIV-1), which is a mixture of several indicators. Its

* 0.375 g of thymol blue and 0.125 g of methyl red are dissolved in 100 ml of 70% ethyl alcohol.

colour changes with pH are:

pH	Colour	pH	Colour
2 or less	Red-rose	6	Lemon-yellow
3	Red-orange	7	Yellow-green
4	Orange	8	Green
5	Yellow-orange	9	Blue-green
		10 or more	Violet

To use a universal indicator, put 0.5-1 ml (10-20 drops) of the unknown solution in the depression of a tile for spot tests (or in a porcelain crucible) and add a drop of the indicator solution.

It is even more convenient to determine pH approximately by means of universal indicator paper, which is manufactured by the laboratory of the Latvian Division of the D. Mendeleyev Chemical Society of the USSR. A colour scale showing the colours corresponding to different pH values between 1 and 10 is provided with the paper. This scale makes the determination much easier.

Having determined the approximate pH of the unknown solution as described above, use the result for choosing the most suitable of the indicators listed in Table XX. Suppose, for example, that a test with the universal indicator showed that the pH is approximately 6. Therefore, an indicator with pK close to this value should be suitable. In this instance, such an indicator is bromocresol purple (pK = 6.3).

This choice must be confirmed experimentally. Take 10 ml of water and 10 drops of the selected indicator in each of two similar test tubes. Put a drop of 0.05 N HCl in one of these tubes and a drop of 0.05 N NaOH in the other, and mix the contents of each tube. This gives the two extreme colours of the indicator. Measure out 10 ml of the unknown solution and 10 drops of indicator into another similar tube. Compare the colour obtained with the colours of the solutions containing acid and alkali respectively. If it is intermediate between the two, the indicator is suitable. On the other hand, if the colour is the same as either of the other two solutions (with HCl and NaOH), this means that the colour of the universal indicator was assessed wrongly and the wrong indicator was chosen. In that case take another indicator, with pK nearest to the one just tested, and repeat the experiment with it.*

Procedure. Having chosen a suitable indicator, prepare the corresponding colorimetric scale. Take 18 exactly similar test tubes,**

* For example, if the colour of the unknown solution was found to be the same as that of the solution with HCl, methyl red (pK = 5.0) should be taken instead of bromocresol purple.

** It is most convenient to use test tubes with marks (for example, made with a pencil for writing on glass) corresponding to 10 ml volumes.

put 10 ml of water in each, stand them in a wooden rack in two rows, and put one drop of 0.05 *N* HCl solution in each tube of the first row, and one drop of 0.05 *N* NaOH solution in each tube of the second row. To these acid and alkali solutions add the following amounts of the chosen indicator:

	Number of drops of indicator								
Tubes with acid	1	2	3	4	5	6	7	8	9
Tubes with alkali	9	8	7	6	5	4	3	2	1

Label the tubes, indicating the number of drops of indicator in each. Mix the contents of each tube thoroughly.

Having prepared the scale, measure out 10 ml of the unknown solution into a similar tube, add 10 drops of indicator, and mix. Put this coloured solution into socket *2* of the comparator (see Fig. 71), put a test tube with water into socket *5*, and into sockets *1* and *4* (or *3* and *6*) put the pair of tubes from the scale giving the best colour match. Now calculate the pH of the unknown solution as described on p. 457 from the ratio of the numbers of drops of indicator in the acid and alkali in the chosen pair and from the p*K* value of the indicator.

If the colour of the unknown solution is intermediate between the colours of two adjacent pairs of standard solutions in the scale, find the pH values corresponding to the latter and take the average.

The determination can only be accepted as reliable if one of the intermediate pairs and not an end pair of the scale gave a colour match with the unknown solution. Otherwise, the determination should be repeated with another indicator.

QUESTIONS AND PROBLEMS
(on Secs. 117-127)

1. What is the principle of colorimetry? What is its most important field of application?
2. What characteristic of the colorimetric method determined its use if the determinations in question could be performed by the gravimetric or volumetric methods?
3. What are standard solutions in colorimetry?
4. What types of reactions are used in colorimetry for production of coloured solutions?
5. What is the instability constant of a complex? What is the significance in colorimetric analysis of the values of K_{inst} of complexes used in the determinations?
6. What is the principle of the nephelometric method of analysis?
7. State the Lambert-Beer law and the conditions for its applicability. Explain your answer by examples.
8. In what cases does a change of pH influence the colour of a solution? Give examples.
9. In what cases does the presence of extraneous ions in a solution influence its colour?

10. What is masking? Give examples.

11. Name other chemical methods for eliminating the influence of extraneous ions on the colour of solutions.

12. What methods are used for separating interfering ions from those to be determined? Explain why, in determination of traces of impurities, the principal component should not be precipitated.

13. What is precipitation with a collector?

14. Why is separating ions by extraction more advantageous than by precipitation?

15. State the distribution law for the following cases: (a) the molecular weight of the given substance is the same in both solvents; (b) the molecular weight of the substance is three times as much in one solvent as in the other.

16. State in which of the cases named in the preceding question complete extraction (a) is, (b) is not, essential for colorimetric determination.

17. State the conditions which must be observed when colours are compared by means of visual colorimetry.

18. What is the principle of the method of standard series?

19. Explain how the influence of the intrinsic colour of a solution on the result of the determination can be eliminated by means of the comparator. What is the advantage of using light filters with the comparator?

20. What is the principle of the dilution method? Derive the formula for calculating the results of determinations by this method.

21. Describe how colorimetric determinations are performed by the method of colorimetric titration.

22. What is the principle of the balancing method? In what cases is this method unsuitable?

23. Describe the design and operation of draining and immersion colorimeters.

24. What is the principle of photocolorimetry? Describe the use of (a) single-beam, (b) double-beam photocolorimeters.

25. What is the concentration of a certain element in an unknown solution given that it had to be diluted from 20 to 24 ml to give a match with a standard dilute solution containing 0.005 g of the same element per litre?

Answer: About 0.006 g/litre.

26. Two solutions are compared in a colorimeter; the concentration of one is 0.02 mg/ml and the depth of the layer is 10 mm. Find the depth of another solution containing 0.015 mg/ml of the same coloured substance, which would appear to be of the same colour as the first.

Answer: 13.3 mm.

27. Find the percentage of iron in a sample from the following data: 5.00 g of the sample was dissolved and made up to 250 ml, and then 50.00 ml of this solution was diluted further to 1 litre. The Fe^{+++} content of this solution was determined colorimetrically by the balancing method. The standard solution contained 0.01 mg Fe^{+++} per ml, and when the colours were matched in a colorimeter a depth of 30 mm of the standard solution corresponded to a depth of 40 mm of the unknown solution.

Answer: 0.75%.

28. Find the percentage of manganese in a steel sample from the following data: 0.2000 g of the steel was dissolved, the solution was made up to 100 ml and 25.00 ml of this solution was diluted further to 250 ml. A 25.00 ml portion of this diluted solution was then treated with $(NH_4)_2S_2O_8$ on heating with $AgNO_3$ as catalyst, and after dilution to 50.00 ml it was subjected to colorim-

etric investigation. The standard solution contained $KMnO_4$ in a quantity corresponding to 0.001 mg of manganese per ml. The depths of the matching layers in the colorimeter were 25 mm of the standard solution, and 20 mm of the unknown solution.

Answer: 1.25%.

29. For determination of molybdenum in steel, a 2.00 g steel sample was dissolved and after suitable treatment the volume was made up to 500 ml. An aliquot portion (25.00 ml) of this solution was transferred to a colorimetric cylinder and solutions of H_2SO_4, NH_4CNS, and $SnCl_2$ were added. The solution, which became red owing to the formation of quinquivalent molybdenum thiocyanate $Mo[(CNS)_5]$, was diluted to 50 ml. In a second cylinder, to which the same reagents had been added, the volume was made up to 45.00 ml and 1.50 ml of a standard solution containing 0.1 mg of molybdenum per ml was added; the solutions were then of the same colour intensity (if viewed horizontally). Find the percentage of molybdenum in the steel.

Answer: 0.16%.

30. What is the principle of the potentiometric method for pH determination? What is the precision of this method?

31. What is the basis of the colorimetric method of pH determination? What is its precision?

32. Describe how pH is determined colorimetrically (a) with buffer solutions; (b) without buffer solutions.

33. In a pH determination without buffer solutions an unknown solution on addition of 10 drops of cresol red indicator acquired the same colour as a pair of standard solutions, one of which contained three drops of the same indicator in acid, and the other contained seven drops of the indicator in alkali. Find the pH of the solution.

Answer: About 8.5.

CHAPTER X

ELECTROCHEMICAL METHODS OF ANALYSIS

128. General Principles of Electrogravimetric Analysis

Of the numerous methods of electrochemical analysis, the electrogravimetric method is considered in detail in this book.

Electrogravimetric analysis is a physico-chemical method of analysis. At the same time it is a form of gravimetric analysis. Its characteristic feature is deposition of the element to be determined on a weighed electrode by electrolysis.

Electrogravimetric analysis is used for determination of metals almost exclusively. Metals are usually present in solutions as cations, which migrate to the cathode during electrolysis, are discharged, and deposited as the free metals. The amount of metal deposited is found from the increase in the weight of the cathode.

Very few metals are deposited on the anode during electrolysis. They include manganese and lead, which are oxidized to MnO_2 and PbO_2 during electrolysis.

Since cathodic metal deposits in most cases conform very satisfactorily to the requirements for precipitated and weighed forms, it is possible by electrolysis to determine the contents of certain metals in solutions of their salts with a high degree of precision. With the aid of suitable instruments and verified techniques the determinations can be performed relatively rapidly. Therefore, electrogravimetric analysis is used very extensively in practice, especially in investigations of non-ferrous metals and alloys. However, several metals do not give sufficiently dense deposits on the electrode during electrolysis.* On the other hand, if the solution contains not one cation but several, they may be discharged and deposited together on the cathode, or some extraneous ions (such as H^+ ions) may be discharged instead.

All these factors, and the high cost of platinum electrodes, greatly restrict the use of electrolysis in analytical practice. Platinum

* If the metal deposit is loose, losses occur during the various analytical operations (washing, drying, and weighing of the electrode), and therefore such deposits are unsuitable.

electrodes are used because platinum conforms best to the requirements for electrode materials in electrogravimetric analysis.

These requirements are:

(1) the electrodes must not dissolve, either by the action of current or as the result of chemical interaction with substances present in solution, including acids;

(2) the electrolytic deposit must adhere firmly to the electrode;

(3) the electrode must remain unchanged when kept in air; otherwise it would be impossible to determine accurately the weight of metal deposited by electrolysis.

Because of the high cost of platinum, it is necessary to look for cheaper metals or alloys to substitute platinum as an electrode material. Nevertheless, the anodes are made of platinum because, firstly, anodes made from other metals may dissolve during electrolysis and, secondly, the size (and therefore the weight) of the anode need not be large. Cathodes are sometimes made of cheaper materials, such as copper, etc. However, it must be pointed out that so far no electrode material equivalent to platinum in its properties has been found. For example, copper electrodes are oxidized relatively easily by atmospheric oxygen, which leads to changes in weight and a lower accuracy in the determinations.

It must be borne in mind, however, that certain metals (such as zinc) should not be deposited on platinum, as they form compounds with it. As a result the electrode is severely damaged when the deposit is removed. To avoid this, the platinum electrode should first be coated with a metal which has no action on platinum, such as copper, and the element to be determined (Zn) is then deposited on the copper-plated electrode.

The electrode used for deposition of metals to be determined should have the largest possible area and the lowest possible weight, and must not interfere with mixing of the liquid. Grid electrodes conform best to all these requirements, and they are the most commonly used electrodes in practice. In most cases the anode is a platinum wire in spiral form. The usual apparatus for electrolysis is shown in Fig. 73.

129. Chemical Processes During Electrolysis

It is known that electrolyte ions undergo reduction or oxidation at the electrodes. For example, in the electrolysis of $CuCl_2$ solution the cathode, which receives electrons from the source of current, transfers them to the Cu^{++} ions, which are thereby reduced to metallic copper which is deposited on the cathode surface. At the same time the Cl^- ions reach the anode, give up their excess electrons, and are oxidized to elemental chlorine, which is liberated as a gas after saturation of the solution.

The processes taking place during electrolysis of $CuCl_2$ solution may be schematically represented as follows:

at the cathode (—)	at the anode (+)
$Cu^{++} + 2e = \downarrow Cu$	$2Cl^- - 2e = \uparrow Cl_2$

Thus, *cations are reduced at the cathode, and anions are oxidized at the anode.*

This simple scheme of electrolysis may become more complicated if the H^+ and OH^- ions which are always present in aqueous solutions are discharged (i.e., reduced or oxidized) more easily than the ions of the salt undergoing electrolysis.

For example, in the electrolysis of $CuSO_4$ solution metallic copper is liberated at the cathode as before. However, at the anode the OH^- ions of water, which give up electrons more readily than SO_4^{--} ions, are discharged instead of the latter.

In this case the electrolysis may be schematically represented as follows:

at the cathode (—)

$$2Cu^{++} + 4e = \downarrow 2Cu$$

at the anode (+)

$$\begin{aligned} 4H_2O &\rightleftarrows 4H^+ + 4OH^- \\ 4OH^- - 4e &= 2H_2O + O_2 \\ \hline 2H_2O - 4e &= 4H^+ + \uparrow O_2 \end{aligned}$$

Oxygen is liberated at the anode and escapes in the form of gas, while H^+ ions accumulate in the solution near the anode. However, hydrogen ions can be present only together with an equivalent amount of anions. These are SO_4^{--} anions, which migrate towards the anode during electrolysis and accumulate there together with H^+ ions. Therefore, sulphuric acid (in the form of its ions) is formed at the anode in addition to oxygen.

In just the same way, during electrolysis of $Cu(NO_3)_2$ solution oxygen and nitric acid are formed at the anode because OH^- ions are oxidized more readily than NO_3^- ions. When solutions of Na_2SO_4, KNO_3, etc., are electrolyzed, H^+ ions of water are reduced at the cathode rather than Na^+, K^+ cations, etc., because hydrogen ions have a greater tendency to attach electrons than K^+ or Na^+ ions, in accordance with the higher oxidation potential. Therefore, the processes taking place during electrolysis can be represented as follows:

at the cathode (—)

$$\begin{aligned} 4H_2O &= 4H^+ + 4OH^- \\ 4H^+ + 4e &= 2H_2 \\ \hline 4H_2O + 4e &= \uparrow 2H_2 + 4OH^- \end{aligned}$$

at the anode (+)

$$\begin{aligned} 4H_2O &= 4H^+ + 4OH^- \\ 4OH^- - 4e &= 2H_2O + O_2 \\ \hline 2H_2O - 4e &= \uparrow O_2 + 4H^+ \end{aligned}$$

In this case electrolysis results in decomposition of water with liberation of H_2 and O_2, while OH^- and H^+ ions accumulate near the electrodes (i.e., the corresponding free alkalies and acids are formed).*

Other oxidation-reduction processes may also occur during electrolysis. For example, Fe^{++} ions are oxidized at the anode to Fe^{+++} ions, Pb^{++} and Mn^{++} ions to Pb^{++++} and Mn^{++++} ions. Since the latter form oxides in the presence of water

$$Pb^{++++} + 2H_2O = \downarrow PbO_2 + 4H^+$$
$$Mn^{++++} + 2H_2O = \downarrow MnO_2 + 4H^+$$

manganese and lead are deposited at the anode as PbO_2 and MnO_2.

If the anode is made not of platinum but of some other metal, it may also take part in the oxidation-reduction processes taking place during electrolysis. For example, it was stated earlier that during electrolysis of $CuSO_4$ solution with platinum anode the OH^- ions of water are oxidized to O_2 at the anode. If copper is used instead of platinum as the anode material, then the electrode itself, i.e., metallic copper, which gives up electrons even more readily than OH^- ions, is oxidized instead of OH^- ions. The anode therefore dissolves with the formation of Cu^{++} ions; the reaction proceeds as follows:

$$Cu - 2e = Cu^{++}$$

At the same time an equivalent amount of copper is deposited on the cathode from the solution. In other words, the effect is to transfer copper from the anode to the cathode. This process is used for purification (refining) of copper, and also in electroforming.

If a halide, such as NaCl, is electrolyzed with a silver anode, metallic silver and not Cl^- ions would be oxidized at the anode, in accordance with the lower oxidation potential of Ag^+/Ag (+0.80 V) as compared with $Cl_2/2Cl^-$ (+1.36 V). The Ag^+ ions so formed would be deposited on the anode in the form of AgCl. These processes are used for electrogravimetric determination of Cl^-, Br^- and I^-.

* It should be pointed out that formerly the formation of H_2 and O_2 during electrolysis was regarded as the result of "secondary reactions" between the products of electrolysis and water. It was considered that in the case of Na_2SO_4 these products were metallic sodium and uncharged SO_4 groups, which cannot exist in the presence of water and enter into the following secondary reactions with it as soon as they are formed:

$$4Na + 4H_2O = 4NaOH + 2H_2\uparrow$$
$$2SO_4 + 2H_2O = 2H_2SO_4 + O_2\uparrow$$

This viewpoint has now been abandoned, as it is not justified experimentally and is not consistent with modern views on the direction of oxidation-reduction processes (Secs. 78-80).

130. The Laws of Electrolysis

The relationships between the amounts of substances liberated at the electrodes and the quantity of electricity passed through the circuit are represented by Faraday's two laws of electrolysis.

1. *The amounts of substances liberated at the electrodes are directly proportional to the quantity of electricity passed through the solution.* With 10, 100, etc., coulombs of electricity passed through copper sulphate solution the amounts of copper liberated at the cathode and of oxygen liberated at the anode are respectively 10, 100, etc., times the amounts liberated by the passage of 1 coulomb.

2. *The amounts of different substances liberated at the electrodes by the same quantity of electricity are proportional to their chemical equivalents.*

For example, it has been established experimentally that when 96,500 coulombs of electricity is passed through silver nitrate solution 1 gram-equivalent (107.88 g) of silver is deposited at the cathode. By Faraday's second law, in the electrolysis of other electrolyte solutions the same quantity of electricity liberates an equivalent amount (i.e., 1 gram-equivalent) of any other element; for example, 1.008 g of H_2, $\frac{63.54}{2}$ g of Cu, $\frac{65.37}{2}$ g of Zn, $\frac{208.98}{3}$ g of Bi, 35.453 g of Cl, etc. *The quantity of electricity which must be passed in order to liberate 1 gram-equivalent of any substance at the electrode is called the faraday* (*or Faraday's number*), *denoted by the symbol F** One faraday is

$$1F = 96{,}500 \text{ coulombs}$$

Faraday's laws are easily explained in terms of the modern theory of the nature of electrolysis. It is known that electricity is carried through solutions only by ions, which move towards the oppositely charged electrodes during electrolysis and are discharged there. It follows that the more electricity is passed through a solution the greater are the amounts of the substances liberated at the electrodes (Faraday's first law).

One gram-atom of every element contains the same number (6.02×10^{23}) of atoms. At the same time every Ag^+ ion discharged at the cathode gains one electron. Therefore, 6.02×10^{23} electrons are needed for liberation of one gram-atom or 107.87 g of silver at the cathode. Their total charge is 1 F = 96,500 coulombs.

When the same quantity of electricity is passed through $CuSO_4$ solution, since each Cu^{++} ion gains two electrons at the cathode the number of copper atoms liberated at the cathode is halved in

* The faraday must not be confused with the *farad*, the unit of electrical capacity.

comparison with the number of Ag atoms; it is $\left(\frac{6.02\times10^{23}}{2}\right)$ atoms of copper, or half a gram-atom $\left(\frac{63.54}{2}\text{ g}\right)$. However, half a gram-atom of copper and one gram-atom of silver correspond to the gram-equivalents of these elements. Therefore, the same quantity of electricity is needed to liberate equal numbers of gram-equivalents of different substances (Faraday's second law).

Faraday's two laws may be summarized mathematically as follows:

$$q=\frac{e}{F}\cdot i\cdot t \qquad (1)$$

where q is the amount of substance liberated at the electrode; $\frac{e}{F}$ (the quotient obtained by dividing the gram-equivalent e by 96,500) is known as the *electrochemical equivalent* of the substance, or the number of grams liberated at the electrode by 1 coulomb of electricity; i is the current strength in amperes, and t is the time in seconds.

When the current strength is 1 ampere, 1 coulomb of electricity passes through the solution per second; therefore, the product $i\cdot t$ is the total number of coulombs passed through the solution. Since 1 coulomb liberates $\frac{e}{F}$ g of substance, we can derive Equation (1) above.

Equation (1) can be used for solving various problems associated with electrolysis; for example, calculating the quantity of electricity needed for liberation of a given amount of substance, duration of electrolysis at a given current intensity, etc. It must be borne in mind, however, that usually such calculations give only approximate results.

In practice the time required for electrolysis is greater than that given by Equation (1). This is because the principal electrode reaction is usually accompanied by various side processes. For example, during electrolysis of $CuSO_4$ solution part of the copper deposited on the cathode may be oxidized by the oxygen dissolved in the solution and return to the electrolyte in the form of Cu^{++} ions. Sometimes (especially near the end of electrolysis) H^+ ions are partially discharged together with Cu^{++} ions, etc. All these side processes consume additional electricity. Therefore, the current efficiency is nearly always less than 100% which accounts for the discrepancies between experimental results and data calculated from Equation (1).

131. Decomposition Voltage

When a current of electricity is passed through a solution, products of electrolysis are liberated at the electrodes. These products, present together with the ions from which they were formed, constitute oxidation-reduction systems (Sec. 78). For example, in electrolysis of $CuCl_2$ solution the system Cu^{++}/Cu is formed at the cathode, and $Cl_2/2Cl^-$ at the anode. In the same way, in electrolysis of $CuSO_4$ the system Cu^{++}/Cu is formed at the cathode and $O_2 + 4H^+/2H_2O$ at the anode; electrolysis of H_2SO_4 gives rise to $2H^+/H_2$ (at the cathode) and $O_2 + 4H^+/2H_2O$ (at the anode), etc.

Each of these systems has a definite oxidation potential and constitutes a half-cell. Since the two systems are electrically connected they constitute a galvanic cell with its own electromotive force (e.m.f.). The direction of this e.m.f. is opposite to the external e.m.f. applied during electrolysis. For example, in electrolysis of 1 *M* $CuCl_2$ solution the potential of the Cu^{++}/Cu system at the cathode is equal to its standard potential or +0.34 V (since the Cu^{++} ion concentration is 1 g-ion/litre), while the potential of the $Cl_2/2Cl^-$ system is +1.36 V. We know that the system with the lower potential (Cu^{++}/Cu) must act as the negative pole in the cell, i.e., it yields electrons into the circuit. Therefore, the following process takes place at the cathode in the operation of the galvanic cell which arises as the result of electrolysis:

$$Cu - 2e = Cu^{++}$$

This process, and the direction of the current in the circuit, are opposite to those resulting from the application of the external e.m.f. during electrolysis; in the latter case Cu^{++} ions are reduced to metallic copper which is deposited on the cathode, but here the copper is oxidized to Cu^{++} ions and redissolves. In electrolysis electrons move from the battery to the cathode, but here they move away from the cathode in the direction of the battery and towards the anode. In just the same way processes the reverse of those taking place during electrolysis (gain of electrons and reduction of free chlorine to Cl^- ions) also occur at the anode.

Thus, *an e.m.f. opposite to the external e.m.f. of the current source arises in the system as the result of liberation of electrolysis products at the electrodes.* This effect is known as *electrochemical polarization*, and the resultant back e.m.f. is called the *electromotive force of polarization.*

Its existence is easy to demonstrate as follows. If the current source is disconnected during electrolysis and the electrodes are connected to the terminals of a galvanometer, the galvanometer needle is deflected in the opposite direction to its deflection under the influence of the external e.m.f. during electrolysis.

Electrochemical polarization is independent of current density* and it arises when electrolysis products different from the electrode

* Current density is the current intensity per unit electrode area (number of amperes per square centimetre, A/cm^2).

materials are liberated at the electrodes. It can be eliminated by addition of substances known as *depolarizers*, which combine with or remove the electrolysis products. For example, if oxygen or chlorine is liberated at the electrode, the depolarizer used is hydroxylamine hydrochloride ($NH_2OH \cdot HCl$), which reduces them to the corresponding anions.

In the same way, if hydrogen is liberated at the electrode, oxidizing agents such as HNO_3, $(NH_4)_2S_2O_8$, etc., are used as depolarizers.

Polarization may be caused not only by the formation of new oxidation-reduction systems at the electrodes, as in the case discussed above, but also by changes of ion concentrations during electrolysis. For example, in electrolysis of $CuSO_4$ solution with copper electrodes copper is dissolved at the anode and deposited on the cathode. Therefore, the same system Cu^{++}/Cu is present at both electrodes.

However, since its potential depends on the concentration of Cu^{++} ions in accordance with the Nernst equation

$$E = 0.34 + \frac{0.058}{2} \log [Cu^{++}]$$

and the concentration increases near the anode and decreases near the cathode during electrolysis, polarization e.m.f. arises in this case too (concentration polarization).

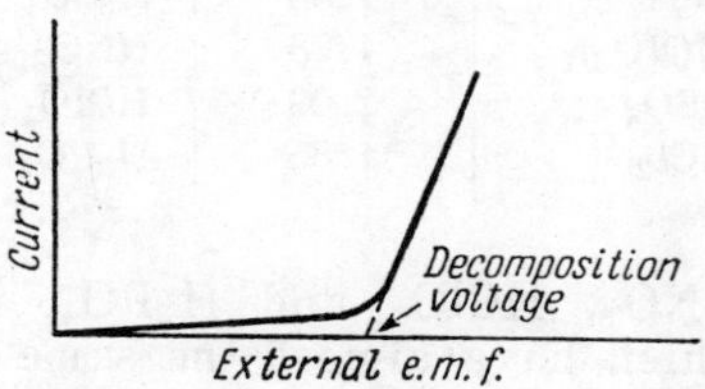

Fig. 72. Variation of current strength with increased voltage during electrolysis

It is therefore clear that a voltage in excess of the polarization e.m.f. must be applied to the electrodes for electrolysis to occur. This is fully confirmed by experiment. For example, in electrolysis of $CdSO_4$ solution acidified with sulphuric acid, if an e.m.f. of less than 2.03 V is applied, electrolysis begins for an instant but the current strength in the circuit drops at once almost to zero and further liberation of electrolysis products ceases. Conversely, at voltages above 2.03 V electrolysis proceeds continuously, and the current strength increases rapidly as the voltage is raised above this value: this is illustrated by the curve in Fig. 72.

The minimum potential difference which must be applied to the electrodes in order to bring about continuous electrolysis of a given electrolyte is known as its decomposition voltage (E_d).

The decomposition voltages of various electrolytes are given in Table XXI.

The decomposition voltage depends both on the cation and on the anion of the electrolyte. For example, sulphates of different metals have different decomposition voltages (here the nature of the cation has an influence). In the same way, the decomposition voltages of the chloride and sulphate of the same metal are different, owing to the nature of the anion. The exceptions are oxy-acids such as H_2SO_4,

Table XXI

Decomposition Voltages of 1 N Solutions of Some Electrolytes

Electrolyte	Decomposition voltage, V	Electrolyte	Decomposition voltage, V	Electrolyte	Decomposition voltage, V
$ZnSO_4$	2.35	$Pb(NO_3)_2$	1.52	HCl	1.31
$ZnBr_2$	1.80	$AgNO_3$	0.70	HBr	0.94
$CdSO_4$	2.03	$CuSO_4$	1.36	HI	0.52
$CdCl_2$	1.88	H_2SO_4	1.67	NaOH	1.69
$Cd(NO_3)_2$	1.98	HNO_3	1.69	KOH	1.67
$NiSO_4$	2.09	$HClO_4$	1.65	NH_4OH	1.74
$NiCl_2$	1.85	H_3PO_4	1.70		

HNO_3, $HClO_4$ and H_3PO_4, and caustic alkalies (KOH, NaOH), which have almost the same decomposition voltage (about 1.7 V) irrespective of the differences in composition. This is because in electrolysis of solutions of all these compounds the same ions are discharged at the electrodes: H^+ ions at the cathode and OH^- ions at the anode.*

It has already been mentioned that the decomposition voltage must be equal to the polarization e.m.f. The latter represents the difference between the oxidation potentials of the two oxidation-reduction systems arising at the electrodes (Sec. 78). These potentials are calculated from the Nernst equation. For example, in electrolysis of 1 *M* $CdSO_4$ solution acidified to pH = 0 (i.e., to $[H^+] = 1$) the potential of the Cd^{++}/Cd system is equal to its standard potential $E_c = -0.40$ V. Similarly, the potential of the system $O_2 + 4H^+/2H_2O$ at $[H^+] = 1$ is equal to its standard potential $E_a = +1.23$ V. It is therefore to be expected that the decomposition voltage of 1 *M* $CdSO_4$ solution should be equal to the e.m.f. of the cell formed from these systems, i.e.,

$$E_d = E_a - E_c = 1.23 - (-0.40) = 1.63 \text{ V}$$

However, this value for E_d is less than the experimental value (2.03 V). The reason is that the so-called *overvoltage* at the electrodes

---

* The equal decomposition voltages provide experimental proof of the view that the ions discharged are in fact hydrogen and hydroxyl, and not SO_4^{--}, NO_3^-, ClO_4^-, or Na^+ and K^+; otherwise the decomposition voltages of all these acids and alkalies would be different.

was not taken into account in the calculation of E_d. The gaseous half-cells such as $2H^+/H_2$, $O_2 + 4H^+/2H_2O$, $Cl_2/2Cl^-$, etc., formed during electrolysis are not under the conditions for which their standard oxidation potentials are determined. In the latter case the electrode is always a platinized platinum plate (coated with a layer of platinum black), whereas during electrolysis the gas is liberated on the surface of a smooth (bright) platinum plate (or wire).

It is found experimentally that this difference in the conditions for conversion of H^+ into elemental hydrogen or of water into elemental oxygen and H^+ ions leads to a change in the potentials of the respective systems. For example, whereas the standard potential of the $2H^+/H_2$ system is zero (on the hydrogen scale), it is —0.07 V at the same hydrogen ion concentration and gaseous hydrogen pressure at a smooth platinum electrode. The potential of this system also changes in the same way if electrodes of other metals, such as copper, lead, mercury, etc., are used.

This change of the potential of a given system when a platinized electrode is replaced by some other material is known as the overvoltage of the particular element (hydrogen, oxygen, chlorine, etc.) at the given electrode.

Hydrogen overvoltages at electrodes made from different metals, at room temperature and current density 0.01 A/cm^2, are given below.

Cathode metal	Pt (bright)	Au	Fe	Cu	Zn	Hg	Sn	Pb
Overvoltage, V	—0.07	—0.39	—0.56	—0.58	—0.75	—1.04	—1.08	—1.09

The above results show that the hydrogen overvoltage can be very high at certain electrodes (especially electrodes made of mercury, lead or tin). For example, the standard potential of $2H^+/H_2$ at a mercury electrode is 1.04 V on the negative side of the potential at an electrode made of platinized platinum. The magnitude of the hydrogen overvoltage is of great importance in electroanalysis, as it makes possible the cathodic liberation of metals which should not be liberated according to their oxidation potentials.

In addition to the nature and the surface state of the metal, the overvoltage depends on the current density and temperature.

Overvoltage decreases with rise of temperature. On the other hand, it increases with increase of current density. For example, at a current density of 0.1 A/cm^2 the hydrogen overvoltage on copper is 0.85 V, whereas at 0.01 A/cm^2 it is 0.58 V.

Overvoltage is also observed with other gaseous half-cells. For example, the oxygen overvoltage at a smooth platinum anode in acid solution is about +0.4 V. In other words, the standard potential of $O_2 + 4H^+/2H_2O$ system when determined at such an electrode is 0.40 V on the positive side of the value determined at a platinized platinum electrode, i.e., its value is 1.23 + 0.40 = 1.63 V. In alkaline solution the oxygen overvoltage is about +1.4 V.

Overvoltage occurs also in the liberation of metals. However, at moderate current densities it is usually so small that it may be disregarded.

Several theories have been put forward to explain the overvoltage effect. For example, hydrogen overvoltage may be attributed to retarded combination of the electrically neutral hydrogen atoms, formed by discharge of H^+ ions, to form H_2 molecules, and retarded removal of the gas bubbles from the electrode surface. By a more recent theory, advanced by Academician A. Frumkin, who has made a detailed study of the overvoltage effect, it is due to retarded discharge of hydrogen ions.*

Because of the existence of overvoltage, in calculations of decomposition voltages we must take into account not only the oxidation potentials of the systems at the anode (E_a) and cathode (E_c) but also the overvoltages at these electrodes (P_a and P_c). The formula for calculating the decomposition potential becomes:

$$E_d = (E_a + P_a) - (E_c + P_c) \qquad (1)$$

As an example, let us use this formula for calculating the decomposition voltage of 1 *M* H_2SO_4 solution. During electrolysis the system $2H^+/H_2$ is formed at the cathode and the system $O_2 + + 4H^+/2H_2O$ at the anode. Therefore, $E_a = 1.23$ V, and $E_c = 0$. If smooth platinum electrodes are used, then $P_a = 0.40$ V and $P_c = = -0.07$ V; hence

$$E_d = (1.23 + 0.40) - (0 - 0.07) = 1.70 \text{ V}$$

This result is in quite good agreement with the experimental value (1.67 V). For the electrolysis of 1 *M* acid solution of $CdSO_4$, considered earlier, we have, in complete agreement with the experimental result:

$$E_d = (1.23 + 0.40) - (-0.40 + 0) = 2.03 \text{ V}$$

If the electrolyte concentration is not 1 *M*, the values of E_a and E_c in formula (1) are found from the Nernst equation. A matter of special interest is calculation of the decomposition voltage corresponding to practically complete liberation of a given metal at the

---

* Theories of overvoltage are put forward in greater detail in textbooks on physical chemistry.

cathode. Liberation can be assumed complete when the concentration of the corresponding ion in solution has fallen to 10^{-6} g-ion/litre. For electrolysis of $CdSO_4$ this Cd^{++} ion concentration corresponds to the value $E_c = -0.40 + \frac{0.058}{2} \log 10^{-6} \approx -0.57$ V. On the other hand, the potential of the system $O_2 + 4H^+/2H_2O$ changes so little during electrolysis that the change may be disregarded.

This is confirmed by the following calculation. Since the solubility of oxygen is low, the solution near the anode is saturated with it. Therefore, the O_2 concentration is constant, and as such does not enter into the Nernst equation, like the virtually constant concentration of H_2O. Therefore, the Nernst equation for the given system becomes:

$$E = 1.23 + \frac{0.058}{4} \log [H^+]^4 \text{ or}$$

$$E = 1.23 + 0.058 \log [H^+]$$

If the initial acidity of the solution was $[H^+] = 1$, and the concentration of the $CdSO_4$ taken for electrolysis was 0.1 *M*, then liberation of 0.1 g-ion of Cd^{++} at the cathode is accompanied by formation of an equivalent quantity (0.2 g-ion) of H^+ at the anode. Therefore, the H^+ ion concentration increases from 1 to 1.2 g-ion/litre. We then have:

$$E_a = 1.23 + 0.058 \log 1.2 = 1.23 + 0.005 \approx 1.23 \text{ V}$$

Therefore

$$E_d = (1.23 + 0.40) - (-0.57 + 0) = 2.20 \text{ V}$$

This result shows that complete deposition of Cd^{++} at the cathode can be achieved only if a potential difference of not less than 2.20 V is applied to the electrodes. The required voltage in other cases can be calculated similarly.

132. Electrolytic Separation of Metals

Liberation of any metal at the cathode requires the application of an e.m.f. greater than the decomposition voltage of the salt subjected to electrolysis. Therefore, if a solution to be analysed contains salts of different metals and their decomposition voltages differ sufficiently (by 0.2-0.4 V or more), the respective metals can be isolated from the solution and determined quantitatively one after the other. This can be explained by the following example. Suppose that a mixture of Ag_2SO_4 and $CdSO_4$ solutions, each of 0.1 *M* concentration, is electrolyzed. We find the voltage needed for complete liberation of the silver ($E_0 = 0.80$ V):

$$E_c = 0.80 + 0.058 \log 10^{-6} = 0.45 \text{ V}$$

$$E_d = (1.23 + 0.40) - (0.45 + 0) = 1.18 \text{ V}$$

We now compare this voltage with the voltage required for deposition of cadmium to begin ($E_0 = -0.40$ V):

$$E_c = -0.40 + \frac{0.058}{2} \log 0.1 \approx -0.43 \text{ V}$$

$$E_d = (1.23 + 0.40) - (-0.43 + 0) = 2.06 \text{ V}$$

The values found for E_d show that if the voltage is suitably chosen we can first liberate silver at the cathode and determine it, and then repeat the process for cadmium. For liberation of silver the e.m.f. must be between 1.18 and 2.06 V, and for liberation of cadmium it must exceed 2.2 V. In practice silver is usually deposited at voltages not higher than 1.35-1.38 V, and cadmium at 2.6-2.7 V. If the unknown solution contains, in addition to the above-named salts, also copper sulphate ($E_d \approx 1.36$ V), it is possible to deposit first silver, then copper, and finally cadmium.

It follows from these examples that *metals are liberated during electrolysis in the order of decreasing oxidation potentials.* The reason is not difficult to see. Metals with high potentials are more "noble", i.e., more difficult to oxidize, than metals with lower potentials. On the other hand, the cations formed by the noble metals are stronger oxidizing agents and therefore they are easier to reduce during electrolysis, requiring lower voltages and therefore less energy consumption.

However, it is known that the oxidation potential of a given system depends not only on the nature of the metal but on the concentration of its ions in solution. Therefore, by varying the concentrations of ions by binding them in complexes we can sometimes alter the sequence in which they are liberated during electrolysis. For example, it was stated above that copper is deposited first from a mixture of $CuSO_4$ and $CdSO_4$ solutions. However, if a sufficient amount of KCN is added to the solution, it is possible to deposit cadmium quantitatively on the cathode at ~2.5 V while all the copper remains in solution. The reason is that cations of both metals form the complex ions $[Cd(CN)_4]^{--}$ ($K_{inst.} = 7.7 \times 10^{-18}$) and $[Cu(CN)]_4^{---}$ ($K_{inst.} = 5.1 \times 10^{-31}$). Because of the lower value of $K_{inst.}$ of the copper complex the Cu^+ ion* concentration in solution falls much more than the Cd^{++} ion concentration. Accordingly the oxidation potential of the Cu^+/Cu system becomes less than that of the Cd^{++}/Cd system. Therefore, under these conditions copper

* The action of KCN first reduces Cu^{++} ions to Cu^+, and the latter then form the complex $[Cu(CN)_4]^{---}$.

behaves as the less noble metal and is liberated at a higher voltage than cadmium.

This example clearly demonstrates the significance of complex formation in electrolytic separation of metals.

133. Effect of Solution pH

In discussing the role of solution pH in electrolysis we must be guided by considerations analogous to those put forward above. It should not be forgotten that aqueous electrolyte solutions always contain H^+ ions, which may be discharged at the cathode instead of the cations of the metal being determined. However, this happens only if the voltage required for liberation of a given metal is higher than the voltage of hydrogen liberation. Therefore, knowing the oxidation potentials of the metal and hydrogen at the given concentrations of their ions in solution, and taking into account the hydrogen overvoltage on the metal, we can easily predict theoretically what should be liberated at the cathode.

In illustration, let us consider the following problem: is it possible to electrolyze 0.1 *M* $CuSO_4$ solution at pH = 0, i.e., at $[H^+] =$ $= 1$ g-ion/litre? First we find the oxidation potential of the Cu^{++}/Cu system when $[Cu^{++}] = 0.1$ g-ion/litre. Its value is

$$E = 0.34 + \frac{0.058}{2} \log 0.1 \approx 0.31 \text{ V}$$

The oxidation potential of the system $2H^+/H_2$ at $[H^+] = 1$ is zero. However, since the cathode becomes coated with copper during electrolysis, we must take into account the hydrogen overvoltage on copper. This overvoltage is —0.58 V (at current density 0.01 A/cm^2). Therefore, a cathode potential of —0.58 V corresponds to liberation of hydrogen, and +0.31 V to liberation of copper. Therefore, the acid solution would not interfere with deposition of copper on the cathode. Liberation of hydrogen can begin only when the Cu^{++} ion concentration has fallen to a value corresponding to a potential of —0.58 V. This concentration can be easily found from the equation

$$-0.58 = 0.34 + \frac{0.058}{2} \log [Cu^{++}]$$

hence

$$\log [Cu^{++}[= -\frac{(0.34 + 0.58)\,2}{0.058} = -31.7$$

and

$$[Cu^{++}] = 10^{-31.7} = 2 \times 10^{-32} \text{ g-ion/litre}$$

Therefore, hydrogen is not liberated until the deposition of Cu^{++} ions has been practically completed.

If we take $CdSO_4$ solution instead of $CuSO_4$, since the standard oxidation potential of the Cd^{++}/Cd system is negative ($E_0 = -0.40$ V) it might seem at first sight that hydrogen would be liberated during electrolysis. However, we must take into account the hydrogen overvoltage on cadmium, which is about -0.7 V Therefore, although the potential of cadmium is negative, it can be deposited from acid solutions; this is confirmed by experiment.

It is even possible to deposit zinc ($E_0 = -0.76$ V) from acid solutions, because of the high hydrogen overvoltage on zinc (-0.75 V). However, the deposition of zinc is not complete at a considerable H^+ ion concentration. Deposition becomes more complete if the acid concentration is decreased or, even better, if a strong acid is replaced by a weak one. For example, good results are obtained in determination of zinc in the presence of $CH_3COOH + CH_3COONa$ buffer mixture, which gives a pH of about 6 in solution, i.e., an H^+ ion concentration of the order of 10^{-6} g-ion/litre. Under these conditions the oxidation potential of the $2H^+/H_2$ system falls to

$$E = 0 + 0.058 \log 10^{-6} \approx -0.35 \text{ V}$$

Zinc is also often determined in alkaline or ammoniacal solution. The decrease of H^+ ion concentration which results from the presence of alkali greatly lowers the oxidation potential of $2H^+/H_2$. Thus, at pH = 14, its value is

$$E = 0 + \frac{0.058}{1} \log 10^{-14} = -0.81 \text{ V}$$

Moreover, the hydrogen overvoltage is also higher in alkaline solution. However, this is accompanied by lowering the oxidation potential of the Zn^{++}/Zn system, because under the specified conditions most of the Zn^{++} ions are converted into ZnO_2^{--} anions (with excess of strong alkali) or into $[Zn(NH_3)_4]^{++}$ cations (in ammoniacal solution).

Quantitative consideration of all the opposing effects here is rather complicated, and requires a knowledge of the decomposition constants of the complexes and of the hydrogen overvoltage at various pH values. However, it has been found in practice that electrolytic determination of many metals (zinc, nickel, etc.) in solutions containing ammoniacal, cyanide, oxalate, and other complexes is quite practicable and usually gives good results. This procedure always has to be used if it is required to deposit electrolytically from alkaline solution a metal the hydroxide of which is sparingly soluble. Another method for preventing the liberation of hydrogen during electrolysis, in addition to lowering the H^+ ion concentration and thus reducing the potential of the $2H^+/H_2$ system, is by the use of a mercury cathode for electrolysis. The hydrogen overvoltage on mercury is particularly high (about —1 V). Therefore, if a mercury cathode is used it is possible to deposit quantitatively many metals which cannot be deposited on platinum because hydrogen is liberated there instead. Another advantage of the mercury cathode is that liberated metals form amalgams with mercury. Since amalgams are dilute solutions of these metals in mercury, they are dissolved (i.e., oxidized) much less than the corresponding metals in the pure state, i.e., they behave like nobler metals. Because of this, even alkali metals can be liberated at a mercury cathode (at low H^+ ion concentrations). The use of mercury cathodes for separation of Fe^{+++} and a number of other cations from Al^{+++}, Ti^{++++}, etc., is very important.

134. Significance of Current Density in Electrolysis. Accelerated Electrolysis

The current strength in the circuit as well as the voltage must be taken into account in electrolysis. By Ohm's law, the current strength (I) is directly proportional to the applied voltage (E) and inversely proportional to the resistance (R). However, in the case of electrolyte solutions we must take into account the polarization e.m.f., which opposes the current, and therefore must be subtracted from the applied voltage in calculations of current strength. Since the polarization e.m.f. is numerically equal to the decomposition voltage (E_d) of a given electrolyte, Ohm's law in this case is represented by the formula

$$I = \frac{E - E_d}{R} \cdot (1)$$

It should be noted that the *current density* rather than the absolute value of the current strength is significant in electrolysis. The current density is the ratio of the current strength (in amperes) to the area of the electrode (in cm^2) at which a given element is liberated. For example, if the current strength is 1.0 A and the cathode area is 100 cm^2, the cathodic current density is $\frac{1.0}{100} = 0.01$ A/cm^2.

From this it is clear that in order to determine the current density we must know the electrode area. If the electrode is in the form of a rectangular plate or a hollow cylinder, its surface area is evidently double the area of the rectangle or double the area of the curved face of the cylinder. The area of a wire mesh electrode can be calculated with sufficient accuracy for practical purposes assuming that the electrode is solid.

The wire gauze or mesh electrodes generally used are made from pieces of gauze 10 cm long and 5 cm wide. The area of such an electrode may be assumed equal to 100 cm^2.

The area of a gauze electrode can be calculated more exactly from the formula

$$S = 2\pi dlb\sqrt{n}$$

where d is the thickness of the wire;
l is the length of the gauze;
b is the width of the gauze;
n is the number of wire intersections per cm^2.

The higher the current density, the more metal is deposited on the electrode surface per unit time and the sooner is the electrolysis completed.

It must be borne in mind, however, that if the current density is too high the deposit formed is loose (spongy) and adheres badly to the electrode, so that it is easy to lose some of it. In addition, such deposits have enormous surface area and are therefore oxidized more easily by atmospheric oxygen; this is another source of error in analysis.

The explanation of the spongy structure of metal deposits is that at a high current density more metal ions are discharged at the cathode per unit time than can reach the cathode from the solution. Therefore, the solution near the cathode becomes so impoverished in respect of these ions that H^+ ions begin to discharge instead.* The gaseous hydrogen covers the cathode surface with bubbles, which make the metal looser during subsequent deposition. The metal is thus permeated by an enormous number of small pores and adheres badly to the electrode.

At lower current densities the loss of the ions near the cathode is counterbalanced by diffusion of these ions from other parts of the solution. In consequence, the potential of the oxidation-reduction system formed at the cathode, for example Cu^{++}/Cu, is continuously maintained at the required level until deposition of Cu^{++} is practically complete. Hydrogen liberation is thereby prevented and a compact and bright copper deposit is formed on the cathode; this deposit adheres very firmly and has a small area. Therefore, the errors due to loss or oxidation of the deposit are eliminated and an accurate result is obtained in the determination.

Thus, because the diffusion of ions is a slow process, in order to obtain good deposits the electrolysis must be conducted at low current density, which slows it down considerably. Therefore, stirring of the electrolyte, used by N. Klobukov as long ago as 1886, is a very successful solution of this difficulty. Considerably higher cur-

* For example, it was shown earlier (p. 475) that if the Cu^{++} ion concentration at the cathode falls to 2×10^{-32} g-ion/litre the potential of the Cu^{++}/Cu system becomes equal to the potential (-0.58 V) at which H^+ ions are dis charged at a copper-coated electrode and gaseous hydrogen is formed.

rent densities can be used if the electrolyte is stirred, so that the process is greatly accelerated.

Stirring can be effected by a variety of methods. For example, a stream of some indifferent gas can be passed through the solution by means of a glass tube. A certain degree of mixing is also achieved if the solution is heated non-uniformly; this is done by moving the burner flame from the centre of the bottom of the vessel to the side, so that convection currents arise in the liquid.

Increase of the solution temperature also greatly increases the rate of diffusion and, in addition, because the viscosity of the liquid decreases on heating, the resistance of the liquid to migration of ions through the solution diminishes, improving the electrolysis conditions. More effective stirring is achieved by the use of various automatic stirrers driven by electric motors. Often one of the electrodes acts as a stirrer. For example, N. Klobukov used a rotating anode in the form of a corrugated disc.

Alternatively, a rotating cathode is often used. This is usually in the form of a platinum gauze cylinder on a frame of thick platinum wire. The electrolysis is conducted in a beaker, and the anode is a similar platinum cylinder, but of larger diameter, concentric with the cathode.

Sometimes stirring is effected electromagnetically. The beaker with the electrolyte is surrounded by a coil through which a direct current is passed. A strong magnetic field is created in the coil, and this causes fairly rapid rotation of the electrolyte. Electromagnetic stirrers which are immersed directly into the solution are also used.

The data in Table XXII show how electrolysis is accelerated by automatic stirring of the solution.

With reference to the formation of metal deposits which satisfy the requirements of electrogravimetric analysis, we may note the

Table XXII

Acceleration of Electrogravimetric Determinations by Stirring

Metal determined	Solution	Stationary electrode		Rapidly moving electrode	
		Amount of metal deposited, g	Minimum deposition time, hours	Amount of metal deposited, g	Minimum deposition time, minutes
Cu	Acid	0.25	$1\frac{1}{3}$	0.3	10
Ni	Ammoniacal	0.25	$\frac{3}{4}$	0.2	20
Zn	Alkaline (NaOH)	0.25	3	0.4	15

significance of using complex compounds of metals for electrolysis. It is found in practice that electrolysis of such compounds gives more uniform and compact cathodic metal deposits than electrolysis of simple salts.

This is explained as follows. Current always travels by the shortest path, i.e., by the path which offers least resistance. The following effect often occurs in the electrolysis of a simple salt, in which the concentration of metal ions is high and is effectively maintained by diffusion and by transfer of ions under the influence of the applied voltage (if the current density is not too high). The first metal crystals to be deposited on the cathode surface form projections on it; further amounts of metal are deposited predominantly on these projections, because there the distance to the anode (and therefore the resistance) is least. This results in the formation of long growths of crystals stretching towards the anode. Such growths do not adhere firmly to the cathode and readily crumble away.

In contrast, in electrolysis of a complex salt the concentration of the metal ions is very much lower. The loss is usually made up only by diffusion, and not by transfer under the influence of current, because most of the metal to be determined is in the majority of cases present in complex anions, which migrate towards the anode during electrolysis. In consequence the solution becomes very impoverished with respect to cations at the points of the cathode surface where the metal crystals are deposited. Therefore, discharge of cations begins at other points of the cathode surface, where their concentration is higher. Deposition is therefore more uniform over the entire cathode, and the deposit is more even and compact. Because of this, and also for the reasons stated earlier (p. 474) complex compounds of metals are very often used in electrogravimetric analysis.

135. Determination of Copper in Copper Sulphate Solution

Copper can be determined electrolytically either in acid or in ammoniacal solution. Especially accurate results are obtained when copper is deposited from solution containing nitric acid, because HNO_3 acts as a depolarizer and prevents liberation of hydrogen at the cathode (p. 469). In its presence NO_3^- ions are reduced at the cathode to NH_4^+. The reaction, represented by the equation

$$NO_3^- + 10H^+ + 8e = NH_4^+ + 3H_2O$$

requires a lower voltage than the reduction of H^+ ions to H_2.

However, in this case the electrolysis is very lengthy (6-8 hours). Therefore, if very high precision is not required, it is preferable to use sulphuric acid solution with an addition of a certain amount of HNO_3 as depolarizer. The nitric acid should be free from nitrous acid, which retards deposition of copper and which may cause deposition of CuO. It is possible to remove HNO_2 by previous boiling of the nitric acid, or by addition of a small amount of urea $CO(NH_2)_2$, which reduces nitrous acid to nitrogen.

The acidity of the solution is very important to deposition of copper. The best results are obtained with H_2SO_4 solution of about 0.2 *N* concentration. At lower acidities the deposit is dark owing to partial oxidation of copper by the oxygen formed at the anode, so that the results are too high. Conversely, at excessively high acidities the deposition of copper slows down. The solution is heated to 50-70°C to accelerate the electrolysis.

Before the determination the electrolysis apparatus must be assembled.

Preparation of the Apparatus. The apparatus for electrolysis is shown in Fig. 73. The cathode is a platinum gauze *1* supported on a

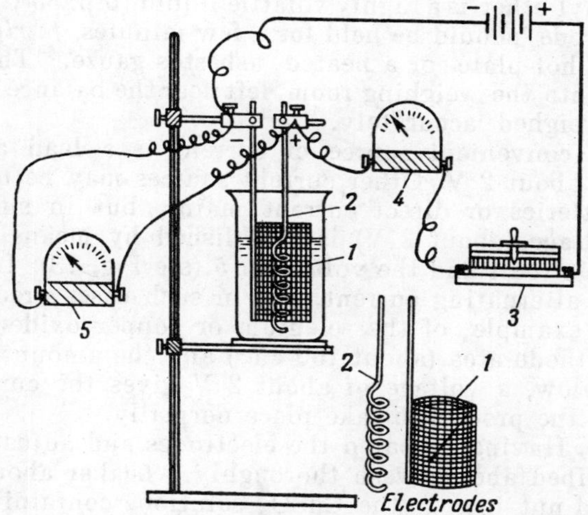

Fig. 73. Apparatus for electrogravimetric analysis, and its individual components:

1—platinum gauze (cathode); *2*—platinum spiral (anode); *3*—rheostat; *4*—ammeter; *5*— voltmeter

frame of thick platinum wire, and the anode is a platinum spiral *2*. When assembling the apparatus, remember that *the electrodes must be handled with great care.* Never touch the working parts of the electrodes with the hands, as this inevitably contaminates the electrodes with grease, and copper is not deposited on greasy cathode surfaces.

In consequence, the current density at other regions of the surface may rise above the permissible level. The electrodes must be picked up only by the very tops of the rods. When the rods are fixed in the terminals, they must not be screwed in too tight.

Before the apparatus is assembled, the electrodes must be thoroughly cleaned. For this, they are immersed for some time into hot dilute (1 : 1) nitric acid to dissolve any metal which may remain from previous determinations and to remove other contaminations. The electrodes are then taken out of the HNO_3 solution, allowed to drain completely, and washed thoroughly first with tap and then with distilled water. The HNO_3 solution should not be poured away, as it can be used repeatedly.

This completes the preparation of the anode. The cathode must be dried thoroughly before it is weighed. To speed up the drying, the cathode is dipped into ethyl alcohol and then into ethyl ether (*highly inflammable*; *keep away from lighted burners*!) to remove the alcohol. Ethyl ether is a highly volatile liquid (b.p. 35°C); to remove it, the electrode should be held for a few minutes *fairly high* above an electric hot-plate or a heated asbestos gauze.* The cathode is then taken into the weighing room, left near the balance for 2-3 minutes, and weighed accurately.

The most convenient source of current is a lead accumulator, which gives about 2 V. Other current sources may be used, such as alkaline batteries or direct current mains, but in such cases the required voltage (about 2 V) is established by means of the rheostat *3* in the circuit and the voltmeter *5* (see Fig. 73). It is also possible to use alternating current, but in such cases a rectifier is necessary (for example, of the selenium or copper oxide type). With the usual cathode area (about 100 cm^2) and the amounts of reagents indicated below, a voltage of about 2 V gives the current density required for the process to take place normally.

Procedure. Having prepared the electrodes and adjusted the voltage as described above, wash thoroughly a beaker about 150 ml in capacity and put into it the $CuSO_4$ solution, containing not more than 0.1 g of copper. Add 7-8 ml of 2 *N* HNO_3 and 3 ml of dilute (1 : 4) H_2SO_4 solution. Put the beaker with the solution in the ring of a stand.

Lower the weighed gauze cathode into the beaker and fix it in a clamp so that it does not touch the bottom or sides of the beaker and is everywhere equidistant from them. Fix the platinum spiral (anode) in another clamp so that the anode is at the centre of the

* After the cathode has been washed in distilled water, it is permissible to wash it with alcohol only; in this case longer heating is needed for drying, and this is best done in a drying oven. The alcohol and ether should be stored in well-stoppered bottles after use; they can be used repeatedly.

gauze cathode. This is important; otherwise copper would be deposited predominantly on the regions of the cathode surface closest to the anode. The current density at such regions would be much higher than elsewhere, and a spongy and easily crumbled copper deposit may be formed. The end of the spiral should project a little beyond the gauze, a few millimetres short of the bottom of the beaker.

Having fixed the electrodes, dilute the solution with distilled water until the liquid level in the beaker is about 1 cm below the top edge of the gauze.

Cover the beaker with two halves of a cut watch glass, and then join the gauze cathode to the negative pole and the spiral (anode) to the positive pole of the current source by means of wires, check the voltage again and adjust it by means of the rheostat. The ends of the leads joining the electrodes to the current source must be well cleaned and fixed so as to ensure good contact.

To speed up the electrolysis, heat the solution gently (to 50-70°C) over a small flame of a special gas microburner or spirit lamp. It is better to have the flame nearer to one side of the beaker rather than in the centre, because this favours better mixing of the liquid as the result of convection (p. 479).

Continue the electrolysis until the solution is completely colourless (this usually takes about an hour), and then test for complete deposition of copper. To do this, add distilled water into the beaker (having rinsed the watch glasses with it) until the liquid level has risen by 2-3 mm, and then continue the electrolysis for about 10 minutes. If a coating of copper, of a golden tinge, does not appear on the newly immersed part of the electrode, take a drop of the solution on a dropping plate (or a watch glass) and add 2-3 drops of sodium acetate solution followed by a drop of $K_4[Fe(CN)_6]$ solution. If a reddish brown turbidity due to $Cu_2[Fe(CN)_6]$ does not appear, the deposition may be regarded as a complete. Conversely, if a copper deposit appears on the newly immersed part of the cathode, more water must be added and the electrolysis continued until the test for complete deposition of copper gives a negative result; the above test for Cu^{++} by the action of $K_4[Fe(CN)_6]$ in the presence of CH_3COONa* must then be repeated.

When the deposition of copper is complete, turn out the burner and wash the electrodes. *The current must not be disconnected*, otherwise the copper deposited on the cathode begins to dissolve immediately in the hot acid mixture containing HNO_3.

Several different methods may be used for washing the electrodes.

---

* CH_3COONa is used for replacement of the strong acids present in solution by the weak acetic acid.

1. Raise the horizontal rod of the stand carrying the clamps with the electrodes fixed in them,* remove the beaker with the solution, and quickly replace it by another, filled with distilled water. Raise this second beaker so that the gauze is completely immersed in the water. After one minute replace this beaker by another, with a fresh portion of distilled water. Change the water in this way about four times until liberation of oxygen bubbles at the anode ceases. When changing the beakers, take care that the electrodes are not exposed to the air for more than a few seconds.

2. Having removed the electrodes as described above, put an empty beaker quickly under them and wash them immediately with a jet of water from a wash bottle.

3. Carefully introduce a siphon tube filled with water into the beaker almost to the bottom, trying not to touch the cathode, and siphon off the solution into a beaker or jar below. At the same time, add distilled water into the beaker so that the electrodes are always submerged to the top of the gauze. Add water until liberation of oxygen at the anode ceases.

When the washing is completed, and only then, disconnect the current and take the electrodes out of the clamps. Put the cathode on a piece of filter paper, allow the water to drain, wash the cathode with alcohol and ether, and then dry and weigh it. All these operations are performed as in the preparation of the cathode for the determination (see above). The difference between the weights of the cathode before and after electrolysis is the weight of copper deposited. With proper working, the copper deposit on the cathode should be compact, of a golden colour, without dark spots indicating partial oxidation of copper with the formation of CuO. If the deposit is spongy or dark, the determination must be rejected and repeated.

At the end of the determination clean the electrodes, keeping them in hot dilute (1 : 1) HNO_3 solution until the copper has dissolved completely. Then wash them thoroughly first with tap and then with distilled water.

136. Separation and Determination of Copper and Nickel in Solution

The separation and consecutive determination of copper and nickel in solution is based on the difference between the decomposition voltages of their salts and on appropriate regulation of the solution pH. For example, copper, the oxidation potential of which is +0.34 V is reduced at the cathode much more easily than nickel,

* If the construction of the stand permits, lower the beaker with the solution enough to allow another beaker to be put in its place.

the standard potential of which is negative ($E_0 = -0.25$ V). At a potential of about 2 V copper is deposited completely on the cathode even from strongly acid solutions, whereas nickel is not deposited under these conditions. For complete deposition of nickel from the solution after deposition of copper it is necessary not only to raise the voltage to 3-4 V but also to lower the H^+ ion concentration considerably by making the solution alkaline with ammonia. This converts the Ni^{++} ions into complex $[Ni(NH_3)_4]^{++}$ cations which remain in the solution while Fe^{+++} ions and certain other cations which do not form complexes with ammonia (if such are present in solution) are precipitated as the hydroxides and can be separated by filtration.

If, instead of this, a nickel salt is electrolyzed in even a very weakly acidic solution, then nickel is not deposited completely because of the negative value of the standard oxidation potential of the Ni^{++}/Ni system and the low hydrogen overvoltage on nickel, as H^+ ions begin to discharge at the cathode instead of Ni^{++} ions long before the deposition is complete. In ammoniacal solution the oxidation potential of the $2H^+/H_2$ system falls to about -0.7 V and becomes less than the potential of the Ni^{++}/Ni system, despite the fact that the concentration of Ni^{++} ions in solution decreases as the result of formation of the $[Ni(NH_3)_4]^{++}$ complex.

Deposition in ammoniacal solution is advantageous also because most of the nickel is then present in solution in the form of complex ions and it therefore forms a more compact and even layer on the cathode (p. 480).

Procedure. Put the solution, containing not more than 0.1 g each of copper and nickel, into a 150 ml beaker and determine its copper (Sec. 135). The solution remaining after separation of the copper, together with the first portion of the washings (the first beaker with water in the method 1 described on p. 484), must then be evaporated to remove HNO_3 (which prevents complete deposition of nickel) on a sand bath in a fume cupboard until dense white "smoke" of SO_3 appears.* Transfer the solution for evaporation to a porcelain basin and heat it so that it evaporates but does not boil, because splashing is inevitable during boiling.

At the end of the evaporation allow the contents of the basin to cool completely; then dilute the contents cautiously with 25 ml of distilled water and warm until all the salts have dissolved. If necessary, add a little dilute (1 : 4) H_2SO_4 solution.

* The SO_3 "smoke" (more correctly described as mist) consists of minute droplets of H_2SO_4 formed by the reaction of SO_3 with atmospheric moisture. Its appearance indicates complete removal of water and nitric acid from solution and conversion of all nitrates into sulphates, i.e., removal of the NO_3^- ions which interfere with the determination.

Now neutralize the sulphuric acid present in the solution with pure 25% ammonia solution,* adding the latter until the colour of the solution changes from green to bluish (colour of $[Ni(NH_3)_4]^{++}$ ions) or until a weak odour of NH_3 can be detected. Then add 20 ml more of ammonia solution to the nearly neutral solution, and dilute it to 100 ml with distilled water.

Before starting the electrolysis remove the deposited copper from the cathode by means of hot dilute (1 : 1) HNO_3 solution and prepare the electrodes (as for determination of copper). Having assembled the apparatus and adjusted the voltage to 3.5-4 V (if lead accumulators are used, two must be connected in series), perform the electrolysis in the usual way. In this case part of the cathode should not be left outside the liquid, because the deposited nickel differs little from platinum in appearance and completeness of deposition cannot be checked, as in the case of copper, by addition of water and consequent increase of the immersion depth of the cathode.

The electrolysis should be conducted at a temperature of about 60°C, because in the cold nickel can absorb considerable amounts of hydrogen and the deposit may flake off easily in places.

When the solution is quite colourless continue the electrolysis for 5 more minutes; then take a drop of the solution onto a tile or watch glass and act on it with a drop of $(NH_4)_2S$ solution. If there is no brown colour as the result of NiS formation, continue the electrolysis for 5 more minutes and then wash the electrodes and dry and weigh the cathode.

The electrolysis should not be continued too long, because the platinum anode then begins to dissolve and the platinum is deposited on the cathode, giving too high a result.

When the determination is ended, dissolve the deposited nickel by boiling the cathode for 15 minutes in dilute (1 : 1) nitric acid. The dissolution is accelerated if Cu^{++} ions are present in the HNO_3. It is even better to dissolve the nickel by electrolysis. For this, the gauze electrode with the deposited nickel is made the anode (i.e., connected to the positive pole of the current source), with copper wire as the cathode. The electrolyte is dilute nitric acid.

At the end of the process the electrode must be carefully examined; its surface must be free from traces of undissolved nickel.

If black flakes appear when the metal deposited on the cathode is dissolved in HNO_3, this means that platinum is being deposited together with nickel owing to partial dissolution of the platinum anode (see above). In such cases the determination must be rejected and repeated, care being taken not to continue the electrolysis longer than is necessary.

---

* The ammonia solution must not contain any admixture of organic compounds.

137. Separation of Ions at a Mercury Cathode. Determination of Titanium in Steel

Because of the high hydrogen overvoltage on mercury (about 1 V) and the ability of mercury to form amalgams with lower oxidation potentials than those of the metals liberated during electrolysis, various separations of great practical importance can be performed by electrolysis with a mercury cathode. An example of such separation is the determination of titanium in steel (or cast iron).

A weighed sample of steel (or cast iron) is dissolved in acid, and the solution is electrolyzed with a mercury cathode in weakly acid solution. Iron, chromium, manganese and other metals are deposited on the mercury cathode and form amalgams, while titanium, aluminium, and vanadium remain in solution as the respective ions.

For determination of titanium in this solution, it is precipitated in weakly acid solution by the organic reagent cupferron.* The reaction is represented by the equation:

$$4\,C_6H_5{-}N\left\langle{N{=}O \atop ONH_4}\right. + Ti(SO_4)_2 = \downarrow \left[C_6H_5{-}N\left\langle{N{=}O \atop O}\right\rangle\right]_4 Ti + 2(NH_4)_2SO_4$$

Cupferron — Yellow precipitate

When the precipitate is ignited it is converted into TiO_2, which is weighed.

Procedure. Weigh out 1-2 g of steel (or cast iron) and dissolve it on heating (in a fume cupboard) on an electric heater or sand bath in dilute (1 : 5) H_2SO_4. When hydrogen evolution has ceased, oxidize the solution by adding concentrated HNO_3 drop by drop until frothing stops. Remove excess HNO_3 by careful evaporation of the soluton until white SO_3 "smoke" appears. Cool the liquid, add carefully 70-80 ml of cold water, and warm the mixture until the salts have dissolved completely.

Filter off the undissolved silicic acid and graphite and wash the residue two or three times with acidified hot water and two or three times with hot water without acid.** Neutralize the solution together with the washings by adding Na_2CO_3 or ammonia solution until a turbidity (precipitate) appears and does not vanish on stirring; add a slight excess (not more than 1-2 ml) of H_2SO_4 to dissolve this

---

* As stated on p. 142 cupferron is the ammonium salt of nitrosophenylhydroxylamine. Three grams of the substance is dissolved in 100 ml of cold water. The solution is unstable and must not be kept longer than two days.

** For particularly accurate determinations, the filtered and washed residue must be fused with 2-3 g of $K_2S_2O_7$; the melt is leached with 2% sulphuric acid, the residue is filtered off and the filtrates are combined.

precipitate. The total volume of the final solution should not exceed 100 ml.

Having prepared the solution as described above, proceed with the electrolysis. Transfer the solution quantitatively into the electrolysis vessel shown in Fig. 74, containing 150-200 g of mercury. *In work with mercury great care must be taken not to spill a single drop, because mercury vapour is poisonous and spilt mercury slowly evaporates and contaminates the air in the room for a long time.*

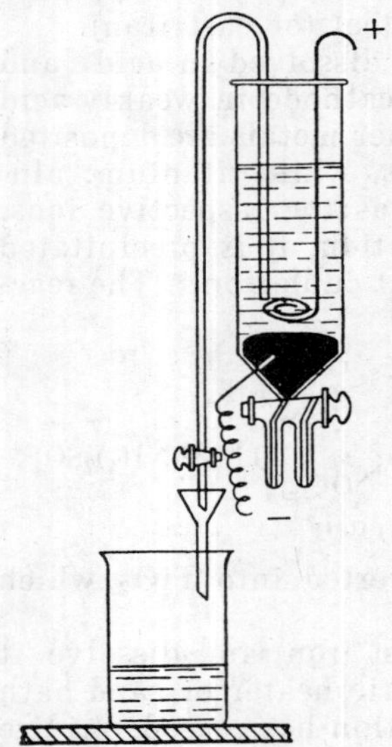

Fig. 74. Apparatus for electrolysis with a mercury cathode

Connect the mercury to the negative pole and the platinum spiral to the positive pole of the current source. Pass a current of 3-4 A at 5-7 V to effect electrolysis.

Continue the electrolysis until the solution becomes colourless; after 15-30 minutes of further electrolysis test a drop of the solution for Fe^{++} by means of $K_3[Fe(CN)_6]$ solution. If the colour produced is pale yellow, and not blue (or green), stop the electrolysis. Without interrupting the current even for a minute, run all the mercury out through the tap into a vessel for the purpose, and then siphon the solution into a large beaker, previously filtering it in order to retain any drops of amalgam which might be carried over. In the same way, taking care not to interrupt the current, wash the electrolysis vessel two or three times with water. The total volume of the solution with the washings should be about 300 ml.

When the washing is complete, switch off the current and add to the solution 15 ml of H_2SO_4 (sp. gr. 1.84) and then cool it to 5-10°C. Now add 3% cupferron solution drop by drop with continuous stirring to precipitate titanium. Continue the addition until a white turbidity (which vanishes easily) appears; this indicates an excess of the reagent.

Leave the yellow precipitate to settle for 40-50 minutes, filter the solution through a filter containing a small amount of paper pulp (see p. 114), and wash the precipitate thoroughly first with 5% (vol.) H_2SO_4 and then two or three times with pure water.

After the washing allow the liquid to drain as fully as possible from the precipitate and then transfer the precipitate on the filter into a weighed crucible which has been taken to constant weight. Dry the filter carefully, then ash it slowly without letting it catch fire, and finally ignite the precipitate in an electric muffle furnace (or over the full burner flame) at 1100°C to constant weight.

From the weight of the TiO_2 precipitate calculate the amount of titanium in the sample and the percentage of titanium in the steel.

The filtrate on separation of titanium contains all the aluminium; this can be precipitated by hydroxyquinoline and determined as described in Sec. 42.

138. Internal Electrolysis

The electrolysis processes discussed above are effected by application of an external e.m.f. from a source of current. However, the latter is not essential. It is possible to carry out electrolysis so that the solution with electrodes immersed in it constitutes a galvanic cell which produces its own current; this current causes electrolytic deposition of the metal to be determined on a weighed cathode.

This method, known as *internal electrolysis*, may be illustrated by the following example. Electrodes, one of which is made of platinum gauze and the other is a zinc plate, are immersed in a beaker with $CuSO_4$ solution. The electrodes are then joined by means of a copper wire or clamp (Fig. 75). The resultant system is evidently a galvanic cell in which the less noble metal (Zn) yields electrons and goes into solution in the form of Zn^{++} ions:

$$Zn - 2e = Zn^{++}$$

The released electrons travel along the wire to the platinum electrode and are transferred there to Cu^{++} ions, which are thus reduced to metallic copper which is deposited on the electrode:

$$Cu^{++} + 2e = \downarrow Cu$$

Adding the two equations, we have:

$$Cu^{++} + Zn = \downarrow Cu + Zn^{++}$$

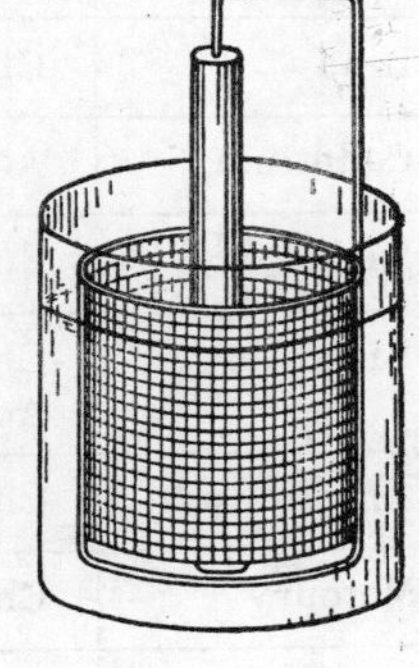

Fig. 75. Apparatus for internal electrolysis without a diaphragm

Thus, Cu^{++} ions are reduced by metallic zinc during the action of the cell. Other metals, such as Al, Fe, Pb, etc., can be used as the anode instead of zinc. However, these metals must be less noble than the metal to be deposited (Cu), i.e., they must have lower (more negative) oxidation potentials.

In other words, *only metals with higher oxidation potentials than the anode are deposited on the cathode. Metals with lower oxidation potentials remain in solution.*

It is therefore possible, by choosing the anodes suitably and by using different salts (simple and complex) and regulating the medium, to achieve very sharp separation of metals even if their oxidation potentials are close to each other.

Table XXIII indicates the anodes and solutions with which various cations are determined by the method of internal electrolysis.

The current in internal electrolysis is weak and very uniform, so that even extremely small amounts of metal can be obtained in the form of a very even and compact deposit on the cathode.

Table XXIII

Solutions and Anodes for Internal Electrolysis

Cation determined	Solution	Anode
Copper	Chloride Acetate Sulphate	Lead Iron Zinc Aluminium
Lead	Chloride	Cadmium
Cadmium	Acetate	Zinc
Nickel	Sulphate	Zinc
Bismuth	Chloride Acetate	Lead Aluminium
Antimony	Chloride	Iron
Mercury	Chloride	Copper
Silver	Nitrate	Copper
Tin	Chloride Oxalate	Zinc Aluminium

It should also be pointed out that in internal electrolysis the only oxidation process at the anode is dissolution of the latter, i.e., its conversion into the corresponding ions, while in ordinary electrolysis various oxidation processes take place at the anode, and these sometimes interfere with deposition of the required element and, in general, introduce complications into the process.

The main danger in internal electrolysis is what is known as "contact precipitation", or discharge of some of the ions of the metal to be determined at the anode itself. To prevent contact precipitation, the cathode and anode are usually separated by a partition (diaphragm), usually of collodion. Some investigations have involved the use of rather complicated apparatus, containing two electrolytes: the catholyte, which was the solution to be analysed, and the anolyte, a solution of a salt in which the anode was immersed. One or even both solutions had to be stirred by means of special electric stirrers.

Soviet chemists have simplified this rather complex technique. For example, Y. Chernikhov and his associates found that it is not necessary to use two solutions. It is quite sufficient to cover the anode with a semipermeable collodion membrane in order to prevent contact precipitation. Similarly, instead of mechanical stirring, agitation of the solution could be effected by a current of inert gas passed through it. This much simpler apparatus gives very good results in determinations of even relatively large amounts (of the order of 0.2 g) of various metals, such as Cu, Bi, etc.

The technique of internal electrolysis has been simplified still further by Y. Lurye, who found that the use of diaphragms is not necessary if the amount of metal to be determined is small (not more than 20 mg) and if certain conditions are observed. His method of internal electrolysis is especially simple and convenient in practice.

In this method the connected electrodes (see Fig. 75) are immersed in the solution to be analysed, contained in a beaker. The apparatus is left until the end of electrolysis, without stirring, after which the electrodes are taken out, the platinum gauze is washed, separated from the anode plate, dried and weighed. The metal deposited on the cathode can also be dissolved in acid, and the determination is then completed by the colorimetric or some other method.

To avoid contact precipitation it is essential that the flow of current is not interrupted, because of bad contacts during the electrolysis. Therefore, all metal contacts are thoroughly cleaned with emery paper before each experiment. The anode metal should also be of the highest possible chemical purity. Its surface must be small, and it must be thoroughly polished with fine emery paper. The solution must not contain substances which cause appreciable destruction of the anode, such as strong acids at high concentrations, certain complex formers, etc.

If these conditions are complied with, the method gives good results.

As an example of internal electrolysis, let us consider the determination of copper in a magnesium alloy.

Procedure. Dissolve a weighed sample of the alloy (1 g) in a mixture of 100 ml of dilute (1 : 4) H_2SO_4 and 1 ml of dilute (1 : 1) HNO_3. When the metal has dissolved, add several ml of 10% hydrazine sulphate solution ($N_2H_4 \cdot H_2SO_4$) to reduce nitrous acid and oxides of nitrogen, which interfere with deposition of copper on the cathode. Dilute the solution to 150 ml, warm it to 60-65°C, and subject it to internal electrolysis. For this, immerse into the solution an electrode system consisting of a zinc anode and a platinum gauze cathode, assembled as shown in Fig. 75.* Previously, thoroughly

* The cathode must be washed, dried and weighed as described on p. 482.

clean the anode and cathode contacts and the surface of the zinc anode and fix them firmly in the appropriate terminals.

Keeping the solution hot, leave the electrodes in it for about 1-$1^1/_2$ hours. Then test for completeness of deposition of copper by adding enough water to the solution to raise the liquid level by about 1 cm; if no deposition of copper can be seen after 10-15 minutes on the freshly immersed part of the cathode, test a drop of the solution with $K_4[Fe(CN)_6]$ solution (p. 483).

When deposition of copper is complete, take the electrodes out of the solution without disconnecting them, and wash them thoroughly. Finally wash the cathode with alcohol and ether (or with alcohol only) in the usual way, and dry and weigh it. Calculate the percentage of copper in the alloy from the increase in the weight of the cathode.

Alternatively, Y. Chernikhov's method of internal electrolysis with a diaphragm can be used. The anode is first immersed two or three times into collodion solution and left in the air to allow the collodion film to dry. The electrolysis is conducted in the cold for 50-70 minutes.

139. The Principle of the Polarographic Method of Analysis

In the polarographic method, introduced in 1922 by the Czech scientist J. Heyrovsky, the solution under investigation is electrolyzed with a dropping-mercury cathode under a steadily increasing potential.

The electrolysis is conducted in a special instrument known as a polarograph, which automatically records a *current-voltage curve* or *polarogram*, which shows the variation of the current passing through the solution with change of voltage. By means of this curve the cations present in solution can be determined quantitatively as well as qualitatively.

If the solution contains a salt of one cation only, the polarogram is in the form of an S-shaped curve (Fig. 76).

This curve shows that until the applied voltage has reached a certain value (p. 469) the current remains constant and very close to zero (residual current). However, as soon as this value of the voltage is exceeded the current increases rapidly with the voltage and the curve rises steeply. However, very soon the current again ceases to increase and the curve becomes a straight line parallel to the abscissa axis (limiting or diffusion current). The current-voltage curve is therefore of a stepwise character, and is known as a "polarographic wave".

The potential at which the curve begins to rise steeply depends on the concentration of the ion being reduced and on the method of measurement. Therefore, it cannot be used for characterization of an unknown substance. However, if we take the middle point of the steep portion of the curve instead of its initial point, and drop a perpendicular from this middle point onto the abscissa axis, and measure the corresponding potential (intercept AC on Fig. 76), we find what is known as the *half-wave potential* which is independent of the concentration and the method of measurement, and which is specific for a particular ion. Therefore, *the cation present in the solution can be qualitatively identified by its half-wave potential.*

Quantitative determination is based on measurement of the height of the polarographic wave, i.e., of the limiting current. To understand this, we should note that as the voltage rises the rate of reduction of the metal ions at the cathode increases continuously and the layer of solution in immediate contact with the cathode becomes progressively poorer in these ions. Eventually, the system reaches a state in which the amount of ions discharged per unit time at the cathode is exactly equal to the amount reaching it by diffusion from more distant parts of the solution. From this point the current cannot increase further with increase of voltage. This gives rise to the limiting current, which is also known as the diffusion current because of its connection with the rate of diffusion.

However, the rate of diffusion is proportional to the difference between the concentrations of the ion in solution and in the layer adjacent to the cathode, where the concentration is virtually zero under limiting current conditions.

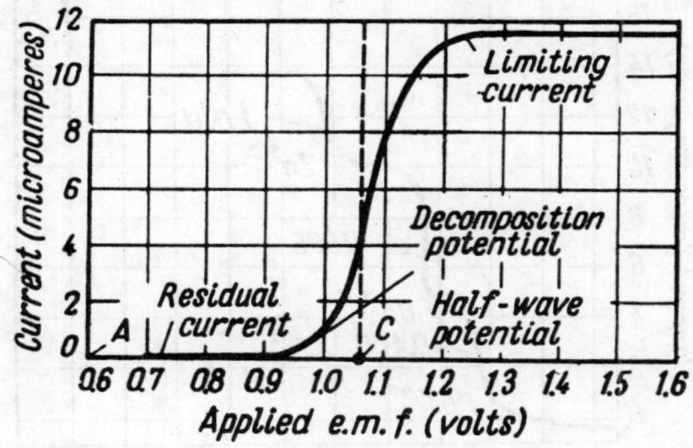

Fig. 76. Polarogram of a solution containing one type of cation only

It follows that *the height of the polarographic wave is directly proportional to the concentration of the ion being reduced at the cathode* (*i.e., the ion being determined*).

Therefore, if we obtain, under identical conditions, the polarograms of an unknown solution and of a standard solution containing the given ion in precisely known concentration ($C_{st.}$), denoting the heights of the polarographic waves by H_x and $H_{st.}$ we can write the proportion:

$$\frac{C_x}{C_{st.}} = \frac{H_x}{H_{st.}}$$

from which we can easily find the unknown concentration in the solution for analysis (C_x):

$$C_x = C_{st.} \cdot \frac{H_x}{H_{st.}}$$

For mass determinations it is more convenient to use a series of standard solutions and to plot a calibration curve showing the heights of the polarographic wave corresponding to different concentrations of a given ion, and to use this curve for finding the required concentrations during analysis.

It was stated earlier that when a definite voltage is reached the current ceases to change whatever the increase in voltage. However, this is only true if the solution does not contain any other ions which can be reduced at the mercury cathode. If such ions are present, as the voltage is raised after the limiting current for one ion has been reached, eventually the potential rises to a value at which cations of another metal are reduced. Consequently, the current voltage curve begins to rise again after the horizontal stretch. In other words, one polarographic wave is followed by another, and this by a third (if a third cation is present), etc. If the reduction potentials of these ions differ sufficiently (by more than 0.2 V), the ions can be detected qualitatively and determined quantitatively from the polarogram. Fig. 77 shows the polarogram of a solution containing Pb^{++}, Cd^{++}, Zn^{++} and K^{+} cations.

A schematic diagram of a polarograph is shown in Fig. 78. The cathode is a drop of mercury flowing out of a glass capillary tube with a drawn-out

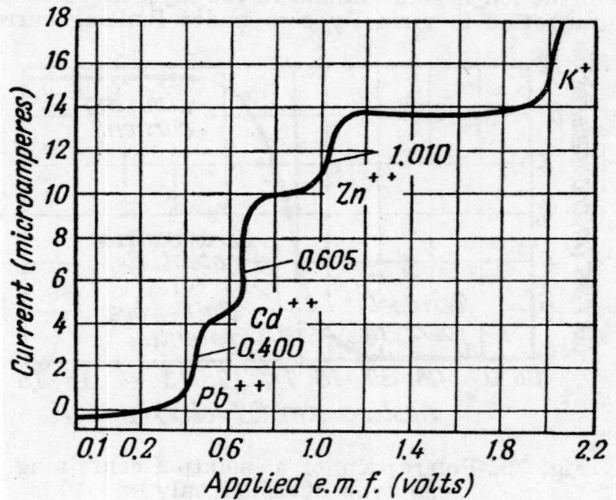

Fig. 77. Polarogram of a solution containing a mixture of cations

end, inserted through a bung into the electrolysis vessel *1* and connected by a rubber tube to a mercury reservoir *2*. The anode is a layer of mercury on the bottom of the vessel *1*, containing the unknown solution on top of the mercury. The cathode area (the area of a drop of mercury) is very small in comparison with the anode area. Accordingly the anode potential remains almost constant during electrolysis and changes of applied voltage influence the cathode potential only.

The characteristic feature of the dropping cathode is that its surface is continuously renewed. Therefore, it always has the same properties, because the same effects are reproduced at each successive drop. The properties of the anode change gradually (although very slowly) as drops of mercury carrying the metal deposited from solution accumulate in it.

The current source is a 2 V (or 4 V) storage battery *5*. As the circuit includes a potentiometer wire of high resistance, at the start of the experiment the voltage across the solution is close to zero. However, by rotation (by means of the electric motor *4*) of the drum *3* on which this wire is wound an increasing length of the wire is cut out of the circuit with the aid of the sliding contact *9*. The resistance in the circuit therefore diminishes and the applied voltage rises continuously from 0 to 2 (or 4) V.

Each complete revolution of the drum *3* corresponds to an increase of 1/20 of the total e.m.f. of the storage battery, i.e., 0.1 V (or 0.2 V).

The rotating drum *3* is geared to a cylinder *6* covered with photosensitive (photographic) paper which is firmly attached to it and enclosed in a case with a narrow longitudinal slit. The sensitive paper is displaced by 1 cm in one complete revolution of the drum *3*. The mirror of the sensitive galvanometer *7*, illuminated by the light source *8* reflects the light beam which reaches the sensitive paper through the longitudinal slit in the case.

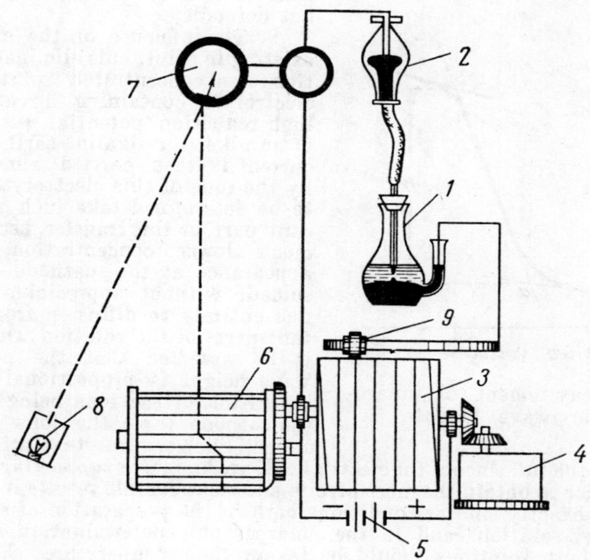

Fig. 78. Diagram of a polarograph with photographic recording:
1—vessel for electrolysis; *2*—mercury reservoir; *3*—rotating drum; *4*—electric motor; *5*—battery; *6*—cylinder with sensitive paper; *7*—galvanometer; *8*—light source; *9*—sliding contact

The higher the current intensity, the greater the deflection of the galvanometer mirror *7*. The light beam reflected from the mirror leaves a thin line on the paper, visible after development. Thus the instrument automatically records a current-voltage curve together with a series of parallel lines 1 cm apart, which corresponds to an increase of 0.1 (or 0.2) V. Fig. 79 shows a polarogram obtained experimentally, and indicates the method used for measuring the polarographic wave height (intercept h), from which the concentration of the given ion in solution is determined. The following conditions must be observed in polarographic analysis:

1. The solution for analysis must not react with mercury.
2. The electrolysis must be conducted without stirring of the solution, in order to avoid breakdown of the diffusion layers surrounding the electrode.
3. The capillary must be immersed in the solution; the rate of flow of the mercury drops from it is regulated by variation of the height of the reservoir *2* (see Fig. 78) so that 20-30 drops flow out per minute. The dropping rate

must, of course, be the same in analysis of the unknown and the standard solution.

4. Oxygen contained in the solution for analysis is removed by a current of nitrogen or hydrogen, passed through it for 10-20 minutes (or by addition of sulphite if the solution is neutral or acid)*.

5. The solution pH must be appropriately adjusted or substances forming complexes with particular ions must be added in order that the reduction potentials of two (or more) cations should not coincide.

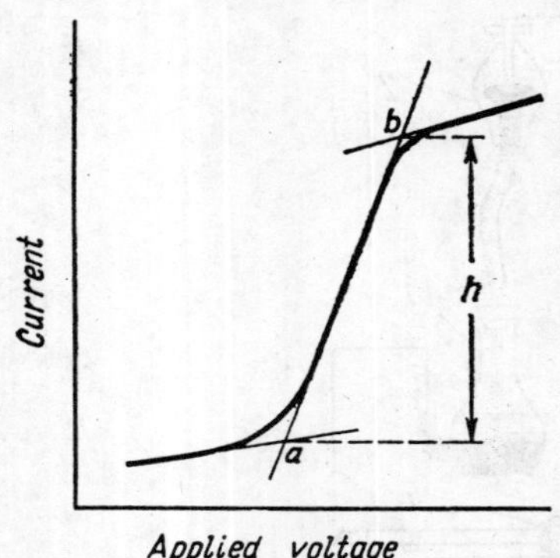

Fig. 79. Measurement of polarographic wave height

6. The influence of the electric field existing in solution is eliminated by addition of a concentrated solution of some electrolyte containing a cation with a high reduction potential (usually a salt of an alkali or alkaline-earth metal). The current is then carried almost entirely by the ions of this electrolyte. The ions to be determined take such an insignificant part in this transfer, because of their much lower concentration, that their appearance at the cathode may be assumed, without appreciable error, to be due entirely to diffusion from more distant parts of the solution. Only then can it be assumed that the polarographic wave height is proportional to the concentration of the ions being reduced at the cathode (i.e., the ions being determined). Such electrolyte solutions, used for eliminating the influence of the electric field, are known as *supporting electrolytes*.

7. In order to obtain the most precise and reproducible results it is necessary to maintain exactly similar conditions both in the preparation of the unknown and standard solutions and in the polarographic determination itself (equal volumes of both solutions should be taken, their temperatures should be the same, the mercury dropping rate should be equal, etc.).

The polarographic method is coming to be more and more widely used in research and industrial laboratories. Its principal advantages are:

1. The high sensitivity of the method, which makes it suitable for determination of very small amounts of impurities, that cannot be determined by the usual chemical methods.

2. Several different elements can be determined in the same solution, both qualitatively and quantitatively without the need for chemical separation.

3. The same solution can be used for a series of repeated determinations, because the solution concentration remains almost unchanged after each electrolysis, since the polarographic current is very weak.

4. Determinations can be performed with small volumes of solutions (about 1 ml or even less) or with small weights of substances (0.1-0.05 g). Therefore, polarographic determinations can be performed by semimicro- and micromethods.

---

* Oxygen present in solution interferes strongly with polarographic determination of the elements indicated above, as it gives 2 polarographic waves when reduced at the cathode. The first corresponds to reduction of O_2 to H_2O_2, and the second, to reduction to H_2O or OH^- ions. Dependent on the solution pH, the first wave is obtained at potentials from +0.15 to —0.15 V, and the second, from —0.5 to +1.2 V.

5. Automatic (photographic) recording of polarograms eliminates subjective errors. Moreover, the determination is *very rapid* (two or three determinations can be performed in 10-15 minutes).

The precision of polarographic analysis is about 5-10% (relative). As already stated (p. 425) such precision is usually sufficient for practical purposes in determinations of small amounts of impurities which cannot be determined by the usual chemical methods.

QUESTIONS AND PROBLEMS
(on Secs. 128-139)

1. What is the principle of electrogravimetric analysis? What are the advantages and disadvantages?

2. State the properties which electrodes used for electrogravimetric analysis should have.

3. What chemical processes take place at the anode and cathode in electrolysis of the following solutions: HCl, $Ni(NO_3)_2$, K_2SO_4 and NaOH?

4. Which metals are liberated at the anode in electrolysis, and why?

5. State Faraday's laws and calculate the electrochemical equivalents of: (a) silver; (b) copper.

Answer: (a) 0.001119 g/coulomb; (b) 0.0003293 g/coulomb.

6. What weight of nickel is liberated at the cathode by a current of 3.85 A in 15 minutes?

Answer: 1.054 g.

7. Calculate the weight of cadmium sulphate which can be decomposed by a current of 2.5 A in 12 minutes.

Answer: 1.944 g.

8. What volume (ml) of hydrogen is liberated during electrolysis of Na_2SO_4 solution by a current of 2.3 A in 6 minutes?

Answer: Approximately 96 ml.

9. Calculate the time during which a current of 5 A should be passed through zinc chloride solution in order to decompose 2.456 g of $ZnCl_2$.

Answer: Approximately 11.5 min.

10. What is (a) electrochemical polarization? (b) concentration polarization? Explain the existence of a definite decomposition voltage.

11. How can the decomposition voltage be calculated theoretically? What is overvoltage?

12. What is the decomposition voltage of $CuSO_4$ in 1 *M* solution at pH = 0? How does this value change at the point of practically complete deposition of copper (i.e., with decrease of the copper ion concentration in solution to 10^{-6} g-ion/litre)?

Answer: 1.29 V; rises to 1.46 V.

13. In what sequence are metals liberated as the voltage increases?

14. The standard oxidation potential of the system Co^{++}/Co is —0.28 V, and that of Cd^{++}/Cd, —0.40 V. Use those values to find by calculation whether cobalt and cadmium can be quantitatively separated by electrolysis of a mixture containing 0.1 *M* each $CoSO_4$ and $CdSO_4$ per litre (at pH = 0).

Answer: Liberation of Co begins at 1.929 V and is practically complete at 2.074 V; liberation of Cd begins at 2.059 V, i.e., before liberation of Co is complete. Therefore, these metals cannot be separated electrolytically under the specific conditions.

15. To 1 *M* solution of a zinc salt solid KCN was added to give a CN^- ion concentration of 1 g-ion/litre. What is the potential of a zinc electrode immersed in this solution if K_{inst} of the $[Zn(CN)_4]^{--}$ complex is approximately 1×10^{-16}?

Answer: —1.224 V.

16. In electrolytic separations of metals, what are the advantages of binding their ions in the form of complexes?

17. What is the role of H^+ ion concentration in solution during electrolysis?

18. Explain why despite the negative value of the standard oxidation potential of the system Cd^{++}/Cd, it is nevertheless possible to deposit cadmium by electrolysis from acid solutions.

19. Calculate the oxidation potential of the system $2H^+/H_2$: (a) at pH = 4; (b) at pH = 7; (c) at pH = 14.

Answer: (a) —0.232 V; (b) —0.406 V; (c) —0.812 V.

20. What conditions should be satisfied by metal deposits formed by electrolysis? What are the disadvantages of coarsely crystalline and spongy deposits?

21. What is current density? What is its role in electrolysis? What are the advantages and disadvantages of electrolysis at relatively high current densities?

22. What advantages are gained by stirring the solution during electrolysis? What is accelerated electrolysis? How is acceleration achieved?

23. Why are oxidizing or reducing agents sometimes added to solutions for electrolysis?

24. Explain why, at the end of electrolysis of $CuSO_4$ solution, the current is not switched off until the electrodes have been washed.

25. What is the purpose of washing electrodes with alcohol and ether?

26. Why is nickel deposited electrolytically from ammoniacal solution? What is the principle of separation of copper from nickel?

27. What are the advantages of electrolysis with a mercury cathode. Why is it possible to liberate even alkali and alkaline-earth metals at a mercury cathode? Under what conditions is such liberation possible?

28. How is titanium separated from iron, manganese, chromium, and other elements in the analysis of steel? What ions remain with Ti^{++++} in such separation? How is the titanium content subsequently determined?

29. What is the principle of internal electrolysis, and what are its advantages over external electrolysis?

30. What anode may be selected for separation of zinc and nickel by internal electrolysis?

31. What is contact precipitation in internal electrolysis? How may it be prevented?

32. What are the advantages and disadvantages of internal electrolysis with a diaphragm, and without a diaphragm?

33. What is the principle of the polarographic method of analysis? Explain how cations present in solution are detected qualitatively and determined quantitatively by this method.

34. Why is the height of the polarographic wave proportional to the concentration of the cation which is being reduced at the cathode?

35. What is the function of the supporting electrolyte in polarographic determinations?

36. State the conditions for conducting polarographic determinations.

37. What are the advantages of the polarographic method? What is its precision? How rapid are the determinations?

APPENDICES

I. ATOMIC WEIGHTS

Element	Symbol	Atomic number	Atomic weight	Element	Symbol	Atomic number	Atomic weight
Actinium	Ac	89	[227]	Mendelevium	Md	101	[256]
Aluminium	Al	13	26.9815	Mercury	Hg	80	200.59
Americium	Am	95	[243]	Molybdenum	Mo	42	95.94
Antimony	Sb	51	121.75	Neodymium	Nd	60	144.24
Argon	Ar	18	39.948	Neon	Ne	10	20.183
Arsenic	As	33	74.9216	Neptunium	Np	93	[237]
Astatine	At	85	[210]	Nickel	Ni	28	58.71
Barium	Ba	56	137.34	Niobium	Nb	41	92.906
Berkelium	Bk	97	[247]	Nitrogen	N	7	14.0067
Beryllium	Be	4	9.0122	Osmium	Os	76	190.2
Bismuth	Bi	83	208.980	Oxygen	O	8	15.9994
Boron	B	5	10.811	Palladium	Pd	46	106.4
Bromine	Br	35	79.909	Phosphorus	P	15	30.9738
Cadmium	Cd	48	112.40	Platinum	Pt	78	195.09
Calcium	Ca	20	40.08	Plutonium	Pu	94	[244]
Californium	Cf	98	[251]	Polonium	Po	84	[209]
Carbon	C	6	12.01115	Potassium	K	19	39.102
Caesium	Cs	55	132.905	Praseodymium	Pr	59	140.907
Cerium	Ce	58	140.12	Promethium	Pm	61	[145]
Chlorine	Cl	17	35.453	Protactinium	Pa	91	[231]
Chromium	Cr	24	51.996	Radium	Ra	88	[226]

Cobalt	Co	27	58.9332	Radon	Rn	86	[222]
Copper	Cu	29	63.546	Rhenium	Re	75	186.2
Curium	Cm	96	[247]	Rhodium	Rh	45	102.905
Dysprosium	Dy	66	162.50	Rubidium	Rb	37	85.47
Einsteinium	Es	99	[254]	Ruthenium	Ru	44	101.07
Erbium	Er	68	167.26	Samarium	Sm	62	150.35
Europium	Eu	63	151.96	Scandium	Sc	21	44.956
Fermium	Fm	100	[253]	Selenium	Se	34	78.96
Fluorine	F	9	18.9984	Silicon	Si	14	28.086
Francium	Fr	87	[223]	Silver	Ag	47	107.870
Gadolinium	Gd	64	157.25	Sodium	Na	11	22.9898
Gallium	Ga	31	69.72	Strontium	Sr	38	87.62
Germanium	Ge	32	72.59	Sulphur	S	16	32.064
Gold	Au	79	196.967	Tantalum	Ta	73	180.948
Hafnium	Hf	72	178.49	Technetium	Tc	43	[99]
Helium	He	2	4.0026	Tellurium	Te	52	127.60
Holmium	Ho	67	164.930	Terbium	Tb	65	158.924
Hydrogen	H	1	1.00797	Thallium	Tl	81	204.37
Indium	In	49	114.82	Thorium	Th	90	232.038
Iodine	I	53	126.9044	Thulium	Tu	69	168.934
Iridium	Ir	77	192.2	Tin	Sn	50	118.69
Iron	Fe	26	55.847	Titanium	Ti	22	47.90
Krypton	Kr	36	83.80	Tungsten	W	74	183.85
Lanthanum	La	57	138.91	Uranium	U	92	238.03
Lowrencium	Lr	103	[257]	Vanadium	V	23	50.942
Lead	Pb	82	207.19	Xenon	Xe	54	131.30
Lithium	Li	3	6.939	Ytterbium	Yb	70	173.04
Lutetium	Lu	71	174.97	Yttrium	Y	39	88.905
Magnesium	Mg	12	24.312	Zinc	Zn	30	65.37
Manganese	Mn	25	54.9381	Zirconium	Zr	40	91.22

II. DISSOCIATION CONSTANTS AND STRENGTH EXPONENTS (p*K*) OF SOME WEAK ELECTROLYTES

Electrolyte	Dissociation constant	$pK = -\log K$	Electrolyte	Dissociation constant	$pK = -\log K$
			Acids		
			Inorganic		
Nitrous acid, HNO_2	4×10^{-4}	3.40	Hydrogen peroxide, H_2O_2	2.4×10^{-12}	11.62
Boric acid, H_3BO_3			Hydrofluoric acid, H_2F_2	7.4×10^{-4}	3.13
1st stage	5.70×10^{-10}	9.24	Sulphurous acid, H_2SO_3		
Water, H_2O	1.8×10^{-16}	15.74	1st stage	1.30×10^{-2}	1.89
			2nd stage	6.3×10^{-8}	7.20
Iodic acid, HIO_3	1.67×10^{-1}	0.78			
			Hydrogen sulphide, H_2S		
Arsenic acid, H_3AsO_4			1st stage	5.7×10^{-8}	7.24
1st stage	5.62×10^{-3}	2.25	2nd stage	1.2×10^{-15}	14.92
2nd stage	1.10×10^{-7}	6.77			
3rd stage	2.95×10^{-12}	11.53	Hydrocyanic acid, HCN	7.2×10^{-10}	9.14
Arsenous acid, H_3AsO_3			Carbonic acid, H_2CO_3		
1st stage	5.8×10^{-10}	9.24	1st stage	4.31×10^{-7}	6.37
2nd stage	3×10^{-14}	13.52	2nd stage	5.61×10^{-11}	10.25
Orthophosphoric acid, H_3PO_4					
1st stage	7.51×10^{-3}	2.12	Chromic acid, H_2CrO_4		
2nd stage	6.23×10^{-8}	7.21	1st stage	1.8×10^{-1}	0.75
3rd stage	2.2×10^{-13}	12.67	2nd stage	3.2×10^{-7}	6.50

Continued

Electrolyte	Dissociation constant	$pK = -\log K$
Acids		
Organic		
Tartaric acid, $H_2C_4H_4O_6$		
1st stage	1.04×10^{-3}	2.98
2nd stage	6.9×10^{-5}	4.16
Citric acid, $H_3C_6H_5O_7$		
1st stage	1.2×10^{-3}	2.92
2nd stage	7.3×10^{-5}	4.14
3rd stage	1.5×10^{-6}	5.82
Formic acid, HCOOH	1.77×10^{-4}	3.75
Acetic acid, CH_3COOH	1.86×10^{-5}	4.73
Oxalic acid, $H_2C_2O_4$		
1st stage	5.9×10^{-2}	1.23
2nd stage	6.4×10^{-5}	4.19
Succinic acid, $H_2C_4H_4O_4$		
1st stage	6.9×10^{-5}	4.16
2nd stage	2.5×10^{-6}	5.61

Electrolyte	Dissociation constant	$pK = -\log K$
Bases		
Inorganic		
Ammonium hydroxide, NH_4OH	1.79×10^{-5}	4.75
Barium hydroxide, $Ba(OH)_2$ 2nd stage	2.3×10^{-1}	0.64
Calcium hydroxide, $Ca(OH)_2$		
2nd stage	3×10^{-2}	1.50
Lead hydroxide, $Pb(OH)_2$		
1st stage	9.6×10^{-4}	3.02
2nd stage	3×10^{-8}	7.52
Organic		
Aniline, $C_6H_5NH_2$	4.0×10^{-10}	9.40
Benzidine, $(NH_2C_6H_4)_2$		
1st stage	9.3×10^{-10}	9.03
2nd stage	5.6×10^{-11}	10.25
Pyridine, C_5H_5N	2.04×10^{-9}	8.69
Quinoline, C_6H_7N	6.3×10^{-10}	9.20
Ethylamine, $C_2H_5NH_2$	5.6×10^{-4}	3.25

III. SOLUBILITIES AND SOLUBILITY PRODUCTS OF SOME SPARINGLY SOLUBLE ELECTROLYTES AT ROOM TEMPERATURE

Formula of electrolyte	Product of ionic concentrations	Numerical values	
		Solubility product SP	Solubility (mole/litre)
		Hydroxides	
$Ag(OH)$	$[Ag^+]\cdot[OH^-]$	2×10^{-8}	1.4×10^{-4}
$Al(OH)_3$	$[Al^{+++}]\cdot[OH^-]^3$	1.0×10^{-32}	4.4×10^{-9}
$Cd(OH)_2$	$[Cd^{++}]\cdot[OH^-]^2$	1.2×10^{-14}	1.4×10^{-5}
$Cr(OH)_3$	$[Cr^{+++}]\cdot[OH^-]^3$	5.4×10^{-31}	1.2×10^{-7}
$Cu(OH)_2$	$[Cu^{++}]\cdot[OH^-]^2$	5.6×10^{-20}	2.4×10^{-7}
$Fe(OH)_2$	$[Fe^{++}]\cdot[OH^-]^2$	1.0×10^{-15}	6.3×10^{-6}
$Fe(OH)_3$	$[Fe^{+++}]\cdot[OH^-]^3$	3.8×10^{-38}	1.9×10^{-10}
$Mg(OH)_2$	$[Mg^{++}]\cdot[OH^-]^2$	5×10^{-12}	1.1×10^{-4}
$Mn(OH)_2$	$[Mn^{++}]\cdot[OH^-]^2$	4×10^{-14}	2.1×10^{-5}
$Ni(OH)_2$	$[Ni^{++}]\cdot[OH^-]^2$	6.3×10^{-16}	5.4×10^{-6}
$Co(OH)_2$	$[Co^{++}]\cdot[OH^-]^2$	2.0×10^{-16}	3.7×10^{-6}
$Sb(OH)_3$	$[Sb^{+++}]\cdot[OH^-]^3$	4×10^{-42}	2×10^{-11}
$Sn(OH)_2$	$[Sn^{++}]\cdot[OH^-]^2$	5×10^{-26}	2.3×10^{-9}
$Zn(OH)_2$	$[Zn^{++}]\cdot[OH^-]^2$	1×10^{-17}	1.3×10^{-6}
		Sulphides	
Ag_2S	$[Ag^+]^2\cdot[S^{--}]$	6.3×10^{-50}	2.5×10^{-17}
Bi_2S_3	$[Bi^{+++}]^2\cdot[S^{--}]^3$	1.0×10^{-97}	1.6×10^{-20}
CdS	$[Cd^{++}]\cdot[S^{--}]$	7.9×10^{-27}	8.8×10^{-14}
CoS_α	$[Co^{++}]\cdot[S^{--}]$	4×10^{-21}	6.3×10^{-11}
CoS_β	$[Co^{++}]\cdot[S^{--}]$	2×10^{-25}	4.5×10^{-13}
CuS	$[Cu^{++}]\cdot[S^{--}]$	6.3×10^{-36}	2.5×10^{-18}
Cu_2S	$[Cu^+]^2\cdot[S^{--}]$	2.5×10^{-48}	1.8×10^{-27}
FeS	$[Fe^{++}]\cdot[S^{--}]$	3.2×10^{-18}	6.8×10^{-9}
HgS	$[Hg^{++}]\cdot[S^{--}]$	4×10^{-53}	6.3×10^{-27}
MnS	$[Mn^{++}]\cdot[S^{--}]$	1.4×10^{-15}	3.7×10^{-8}
NiS_α	$[Ni^{++}]\cdot[S^{--}]$	3.2×10^{-19}	5.7×10^{-10}
NiS_γ	$[Ni^{++}]\cdot[S^{--}]$	2×10^{-26}	1.4×10^{-13}
PbS	$[Pb^{++}]\cdot[S^{--}]$	2.5×10^{-27}	5.0×10^{-14}
SnS	$[Sn^{++}]\cdot[S^{--}]$	1.0×10^{-25}	3.2×10^{-13}
ZnS	$[Zn^{++}]\cdot[S^{--}]$	1.2×10^{-23}	3.5×10^{-12}
		Chlorides	
$AgCl$	$[Ag^+]\cdot[Cl^-]$	1.6×10^{-10}	1.2×10^{-5}
Hg_2Cl_2	$[Hg_2^{++}]\cdot[Cl^-]^2$	1.1×10^{-18}	6.5×10^{-7}
$PbCl_2$	$[Pb^{++}]\cdot[Cl^-]^2$	1.6×10^{-5}	1.6×10^{-2}

Continued

Formula of electrolyte	Product of ionic concentrations	Numerical values	
		Solubility product SP	Solubility (mole/litre)
	Bromides		
AgBr	$[Ag^+] \cdot [Br^-]$	7.7×10^{-13}	8.8×10^{-7}
Hg_2Br_2	$[Hg_2^{++}] \cdot [Br^-]^2$	5.2×10^{-23}	2.8×10^{-8}
$PbBr_2$	$[Pb^{++}] \cdot [Br^-]^2$	9.1×10^{-6}	1.3×10^{-2}
	Iodides		
AgI	$[Ag^+] \cdot [I^-]$	1.5×10^{-16}	1.2×10^{-8}
Hg_2I_2	$[Hg_2^{++}] \cdot [I^-]^2$	4.5×10^{-29}	2.2×10^{-10}
PbI_2	$[Pb^{++}] \cdot [I^-]^2$	1.1×10^{-9}	6.5×10^{-4}
CuI	$[Cu^+] \cdot [I^-]$	1.1×10^{-12}	1.05×10^{-6}
	Sulphates		
Ag_2SO_4	$[Ag^+]^2 \cdot [SO_4^{--}]$	7.7×10^{-5}	2.6×10^{-2}
$BaSO_4$	$[Ba^{++}] \cdot [SO_4^{--}]$	1.1×10^{-10}	1.05×10^{-5}
$CaSO_4 \cdot 2H_2O$	$[Ca^{++}] \cdot [SO_4^{--}]$	6.1×10^{-5}	7.8×10^{-3}
$PbSO_4$	$[Pb^{++}] \cdot [SO_4^{--}]$	2.2×10^{-8}	1.5×10^{-4}
$SrSO_4$	$[Sr^{++}] \cdot [SO_4^{--}]$	2.8×10^{-7}	5.3×10^{-4}
Hg_2SO_4	$[Hg_2^{++}] \cdot [SO_4^{--}]$	6.3×10^{-7}	7.9×10^{-4}
	Carbonates		
Ag_2CO_3	$[Ag^+]^2 \cdot [CO_3^{--}]$	6.1×10^{-12}	1.15×10^{-4}
$BaCO_3$	$[Ba^{++}] \cdot [CO_3^{--}]$	8×10^{-9}	8.9×10^{-5}
$CaCO_3$	$[Ca^{++}] \cdot [CO_3^{--}]$	4.8×10^{-9}	1.9×10^{-5}
$MgCO_3$	$[Mg^{++}] \cdot [CO_3^{--}]$	1.0×10^{-5}	3.2×10^{-3}
$SrCO_3$	$[Sr^{++}] \cdot [CO_3^{--}]$	1.1×10^{-10}	1.05×10^{-5}
$CdCO_3$	$[Cd^{++}] \cdot [CO_3^{--}]$	5.2×10^{-12}	2.3×10^{-6}
$PbCO_3$	$[Pb^{++}] \cdot [CO_3^{--}]$	1.5×10^{-13}	3.9×10^{-7}
	Oxalates		
$BaC_2O_4 \cdot 2H_2O$	$[Ba^{++}] \cdot [C_2O_4^{--}]$	1.6×10^{-7}	4×10^{-4}
$CaC_2O_4 \cdot 2H_2O$	$[Ca^{++}] \cdot [C_2O_4^{--}]$	2.6×10^{-9}	5.1×10^{-5}
MgC_2O_4	$[Mg^{++}] \cdot [C_2O_4^{--}]$	8.6×10^{-5}	9.1×10^{-3}
PbC_2O_4	$[Pb^{++}] \cdot [C_2O_4^{--}]$	3.2×10^{-11}	5.6×10^{-6}
$SrC_2O_4 \cdot H_2O$	$[Sr^{++}] \cdot [C_2O_4^{--}]$	5.6×10^{-8}	2.4×10^{-4}
ZnC_2O_4	$[Zn^{++}] \cdot [C_2O_4^{--}]$	7.5×10^{-9}	8.7×10^{-5}
	Chromates		
Ag_2CrO_4	$[Ag^+]^2 \cdot [CrO_4^{--}]$	1.1×10^{-12}	6.5×10^{-5}
$BaCrO_4$	$[Ba^{++}] \cdot [CrO_4^{--}]$	2.4×10^{-10}	1.5×10^{-5}
$PbCrO_4$	$[Pb^{++}] \cdot [CrO_4^{--}]$	1.8×10^{-14}	1.3×10^{-7}
$SrCrO_4$	$[Sr^{++}] \cdot [CrO_4^{--}]$	3.5×10^{-5}	5.4×10^{-3}

Continued

Formula of electrolyte	Product of ionic concentrations	Numerical values: Solubility product SP	Numerical values: Solubility (mole/litre)
	Phosphates		
Ag_3PO_4	$[Ag^+]^3 \cdot [PO_4^{---}]$	1.3×10^{-20}	4.6×10^{-6}
$MgNH_4PO_4$	$[Mg^{++}] \cdot [NH_4^+] \cdot [PO_4^{---}]$	2.5×10^{-13}	6.3×10^{-5}
$Pb_3(PO_4)_2$	$[Pb^{++}]^3 \cdot [PO_4^{---}]^2$	7.9×10^{-43}	1.5×10^{-5}
	Salts of Various Acids		
$AgBrO_3$	$[Ag^+] \cdot [BrO_3^-]$	5.8×10^{-5}	7.6×10^{-3}
$AgCNS$	$[Ag^+] \cdot [CNS^-]$	1.16×10^{-12}	1.1×10^{-6}
$Ag_4[Fe(CN)_6]$	$[Ag^+]^4 \cdot [Fe(CN)_6]^{==}$	1.5×10^{-41}	2.2×10^{-9}
$Ag_3[Fe(CN)_6]$	$[Ag^+]^3 \cdot [Fe(CN)_6]^{---}$	9.8×10^{-25}	4.3×10^{-7}
Ag_3AsO_3	$[Ag^+]^3 \cdot [AsO_3^{---}]$	4.5×10^{-19}	1.1×10^{-6}
Ag_3AsO_4	$[Ag^+]^3 \cdot [AsO_4^{---}]$	1.0×10^{-19}	7.8×10^{-6}
CaF_2	$[Ca^{++}] \cdot [F^-]^2$	4×10^{-11}	2.1×10^{-4}
$KHC_4H_4O_6$	$[K^+] \cdot [HC_4H_4O_6^-]$	3×10^{-4}	1.7×10^{-2}

IV. INSTABILITY CONSTANTS OF CERTAIN COMPLEXES

Complex former	Equation for dissociation of complex	Instability constant $K_{inst.}$	$pK_{inst.} = -\log K_{inst.}$
Ag^+	$[Ag(NH_3)_2]^+ \rightleftarrows Ag^+ + 2NH_3$	6.8×10^{-8}	7.2
	$[Ag(S_2O_3)]^- \rightleftarrows Ag^+ + S_2O_3^{--}$	1×10^{-13}	13.0
	$[Ag(CN)_2]^- \rightleftarrows Ag^+ + 2CN^-$	1×10^{-21}	21.0
Al^{+++}	$[AlF_6]^{---} \rightleftarrows Al^{+++} + 6F^-$	1.45×10^{-20}	19.84
Cd^{++}	$[Cd(NH_3)_4]^{++} \rightleftarrows Cd^{++} + 4NH_3$	1×10^{-7}	7.0
	$[CdCl_4]^{--} \rightleftarrows Cd^{++} + 4Cl^-$	9×10^{-3}	2.05
	$[Cd(CN)_4]^{--} \rightleftarrows Cd^{++} + 4CN^-$	7.7×10^{-18}	17.11
Co^{++}	$[Co(NH_3)_6]^{++} \rightleftarrows Co^{++} + 6NH_3$	1.25×10^{-5}	4.91
	$[Co(CNS)_4]^{--} \rightleftarrows Co^{++} + 4CNS^-$	5.5×10^{-3}	2.26
Co^{+++}	$[Co(NH_3)_6]^{+++} \rightleftarrows Co^{+++} + 6NH_3$	6×10^{-36}	35.22
Cu^{++}	$[Cu(NH_3)_4]^{++} \rightleftarrows Cu^{++} + 4NH_3$	4.6×10^{-14}	13.34
Cu^+	$[Cu(CN)_4]^{---} \rightleftarrows Cu^+ + 4CN^-$	5.1×10^{-31}	30.29
Fe^{++}	$[Fe(CN_6)]^{==} \rightleftarrows Fe^{++} + 6CN^-$	1×10^{-24}	24.31
Fe^{+++}	$[Fe(CN)_6]^{---} \rightleftarrows Fe^{+++} + 6CN^-$	1×10^{-31}	31.0
Hg^{++}	$[Hg(CNS)_4]^{--} \rightleftarrows Hg^{++} + 4CNS^-$	1×10^{-22}	22.0
	$[HgCl_4]^{--} \rightleftarrows Hg^{++} + 4Cl^-$	6×10^{-16}	15.22
	$[HgI_4]^{--} \rightleftarrows Hg^{++} + 4I^-$	5×10^{-31}	30.30

Continued

Complex former	Equation for dissociation of complex	Instability constant $K_{inst.}$	$pK_{inst.} = -\log K_{inst.}$
Ni^{++}	$[Ni(NH_3)_6]^{++} \rightleftarrows Ni^{++} + 6NH_3$	6×10^{-9}	8.22
	$[Ni(CN)_4]^{--} \rightleftarrows Ni^{++} + 4CN^-$	1×10^{-22}	22.0
Sn^{++++}	$[SnCl_6]^{--} \rightleftarrows Sn^{++++} + 6Cl^-$	1.5×10^{-1}	0.82
Zn^{++}	$[Zn(NH_3)_4]^{++} \rightleftarrows Zn^{++} + 4NH_3$	2.0×10^{-9}	8.70
	$[Zn(CN)_4]^{--} \rightleftarrows Zn^{++} + 4CN^-$	2×10^{-16}	16.0
	$[Zn(C_2O_4)_3]^{----} \rightleftarrows Zn^{++} + 3C_2O_4^{--}$	1×10^{-9}	9.0

V. DENSITY OF SOLUTIONS

Ammonia solutions

Density g/cm³	g NH_3 per 100 g solution (% by wt)	Density g/cm³	g NH_3 per 100 g solution (% by wt)	Density g/cm³	g NH_3 per 100 g solution (% by wt)
0.880	34.35	0.920	20.88	0.960	9.34
0.884	32.84	0.924	19.67	0.964	8.29
0.888	31.37	0.928	18.45	0.968	7.26
0.892	30.00	0.932	17.24	0.972	6.25
0.896	28.67	0.936	16.06	0.976	5.25
0.900	27.33	0.940	14.88	0.980	4.27
0.904	26.00	0.944	13.71	0.984	3.30
0.908	24.68	0.948	11.58	0.988	2.35
0.912	23.39	0.952	11.49	0.992	1.43
0.916	22.12	0.956	10.40	0.996	0.512

Solutions of strong acids and alkalis

Density g/cm³	Grams per 100 g of solution (% by wt)				
	H_2SO_4	HNO_3	HCl	KOH	NaOH
1.000	0.2609	1.333	0.360	0.197	0.159
1.020	3.242	3.982	4.388	2.38	1.94
1.040	6.237	7.530	8.490	4.58	3.74
1.060	9.129	10.97	12.51	6.74	5.56
1.080	11.96	14.31	16.47	8.89	7.38
1.100	14.73	17.58	20.39	11.03	9.12
1.120	17.43	20.97	24.25	13.14	11.01
1.140	20.08	23.94	28.18	15.22	12.83

Continued

Density g/cm³	Grams per 100 g of solution (% by wt)				
	H_2SO_4	HNO_3	HCl	KOH	NaOH
1.160	22.67	27.00	32.14	17.29	14.64
1.180	25.21	30.00	36.23	19.35	16.44
1.200	27.72	32.94	—	21,38	18.25
1.220	30.18	35.93	—	23.38	20.07
1.240	32.61	39.02	—	25.36	21.90
1.260	35.01	42.14	—	27.32	23.73
1.280	37.36	45.27	—	29.25	25.56
1.300	39.68	48.42	—	31.15	27.41
1.320	41.95	51.71	—	33.03	29.26
1.340	44.17	55.13	—	34.90	31.14
1.360	46.33	58.78	—	36.73	33.06
1.380	48.45	62.70	—	38.56	35.01
1.400	50.50	66.97	—	40.37	36.99
1.420	52.51	71.63	—	42.15	38.99
1.440	54.49	76.71	—	43.92	41.03
1.460	56.41	82.39	—	45,66	43.12
1.480	58.31	89.07	—	47.39	45.22
1.500	60.17	96.73	—	49.10	47.33
1.520	62.00	—	—	50.80	49.44
1.540	63.81	—	—	—	—
1.560	65.59	—	—	—	—
1.580	67.35	—	—	—	—
1.600	69.09	—	—	—	—
1.620	70.82	—	—	—	—
1.640	72.52	—	—	—	—
1.660	74.22	—	—	—	—
1.680	75.92	—	—	—	—
1.700	77.63	—	—	—	—
1.720	79.37	—	—	—	—
1.740	81.16	—	—	—	—
1.760	83.06	—	—	—	—
1.780	85.16	—	—	—	—
1.800	87.69	—	—	—	—
1.820	91.11	—	—	—	—

VI. NORMAL OXIDATION-REDUCTION POTENTIALS

Highest degree of oxidation (oxidants)	Number of electrons	Lowest degree of oxidation (reductants)	Potential E_0 (V)
F_2 (*g*)	+2	$2F^-$	+2.87
$S_2O_8^{--}$	+2	$2SO_4^{--}$	+2.01
$NaBiO_3 + 4H^+$	+2	$BiO^+ + Na^+ + 2H_2O$	(+1.08)
$H_2O_2 + 2H^+$	+2	$2H_2O$	+1.77
PbO_2 (*s*) $+ 4H^+$	+2	$Pb^{++} + 2H_2O$	+1.68
Ce^{++++}	+1	Ce^{+++}	+1.55
$MnO_4^- + 8H^+$	+5	$Mn^{++} + 4H_2O$	+1.51
$ClO_3^- + 6H^+$	+6	$Cl^- + 3H_2O$	+1.45
$BrO_3^- + 6H^+$	+6	$Br^- + 3H_2O$	+1.44
Cl_2 (*g*)	+2	$2Cl^-$	+1.36
$Cr_2O_7^{--} + 14H^+$	+6	$2Cr^{+++} + 7H_2O$	+1.36
MnO_2 (*s*) $+ 4H^+$	+2	$Mn^{++} + 2H_2O$	+1.23
$O_2 + 4H^+$	+4	$2H_2O$	+1.23
$IO_3^- + 6H^+$	+6	$I^- + 3H_2O$	+1.09
Br_2 (*l*)	+2	$2Br^-$	+1.07
$HNO_2 + H^+$	+1	NO (*g*) $+ H_2O$	+1.00
$NO_3^- + 4H^+$	+3	NO (*g*) $+ 2H_2O$	+0.96
$NO_3^- + 3H^+$	+2	$HNO_2 + H_2O$	+0.94
Ag^+	+1	Ag (*s*)	+0.80
$NO_3 + 2H^+$	+1	NO_2 (*g*) $+ H_2O$	+0.79
Fe^{+++}	+1	Fe^{++}	+0.77
$BrO_3^- + 3H_2O$	+6	$Br^- + 6OH^-$	+0.60
$MnO_4^{---} + 2H_2O$	+2	MnO_2 (*s*) $+ 4OH^-$	+0.60
$AsO_4^{---} + 2H^+$	+2	$AsO_3^{---} + H_2O$	+0.57
I_2 (*s*)	+2	$2I^-$	+0.54
Cu^+	+1	Cu (*s*)	+0.52
$[Fe(CN)_6]^{---}$	+1	$[Fe(CN)_6]^{=}$	+0.36
$VO^{++} + 2H^+$	+1	$V^{+++} + H_2O$	+0.36
Cu^{++}	+2	Cu (*s*)	+0.34
$SO_4^{--} + 2H^+$	+2	$SO_3^{--} + H_2O$	+0.17
Cu^{++}	+1	Cu^+	+0.17
Sn^{++++}	+2	Sn^{++}	+0.15
S (*s*) $+ 2H^+$	+2	H_2S	+0.14
$TiO^{++} + 2H^+$	+1	$Ti^{+++} + H_2O$	+0.10
$S_4O_6^{--}$	+2	$2S_2O_3^{--}$	+0.08
$2H^+$	+2	H_2 (*g*)	±0.00
Pb^{++}	+2	Pb (*s*)	−0.13
$CrO_4^{--} + H_2O$	+3	$CrO_3^{---} + 2OH^-$	−0.13

Continued

Highest degree of oxidation (oxidants)	Number of electrons	Lowest degree of oxidation (reductants)	Potential E_0 (V)
Sn^{++}	+2	Sn (*s*)	−0.14
$2CO_2$	+2	$C_2O_4^{--}$	(−0.2)
V^{+++}	+1	V^{++}	−0.25
Ni^{++}	+2	Ni (*s*)	−0.25
Cd^{++}	+2	Cd (*s*)	−0.40
Cr^{+++}	+1	Cr^{++}	−0.41
Fe^{++}	+2	Fe (*s*)	−0.44
$As + 3H^+$	+3	AsH_3	−0.60
Zn^{++}	+2	Zn (*s*)	−0.76
Mn^{++}	+2	Mn (*s*)	−1.18
$ZnO_2^{--} + 2H_2O$	+2	Zn (*s*) + $4OH^-$	−1.22
Al^{+++}	+3	Al (*s*)	−1.70
Mg^{++}	+2	Mg (*s*)	−2.37
Na^+	+1	Na (*s*)	−2.71
Li^+	+1	Li (*s*)	−3.04

VII. BUFFER MIXTURES FOR pH DETERMINATIONS

Phosphate Mixtures for the pH Range 2.2-8.0

pH	0.2 *M* Na_2HPO_4, ml	0.1 *M* citric acid, ml	pH	0.2 *M* Na_2HPO_4, ml	0.1 *M* citric acid, ml
2.2	0.40	19.60	5.2	10.72	9.28
2.4	1.24	18.76	5.4	11.15	8.85
2.6	2.18	17.82	5.6	11.60	8.40
2.8	3.17	16.83	5.8	12.09	7.91
3.0	4.11	15.89	6.0	12.63	7.37
3.2	4.94	15.06	6.2	13.22	6.78
3.4	5.70	14.30	6.4	13.85	6.15
3.6	6.44	13.56	6.6	14.55	5.45
3.8	7.10	12.90	6.8	15.45	4.55
4.0	7.71	12.29	7.0	16.47	3.53
4.2	8.28	11.72	7.2	17.39	2.61
4.4	8.82	11.18	7.4	18.17	1.83
4.6	9.35	10.65	7.6	18.73	1.27
4.8	9.86	10.14	7.8	19.15	0.85
5.0	10.30	9.70	8.0	19.45	0.55

Universal Mixtures for the pH Range 1.81-11.93 (at 18°C)

V ml of 0.2 *N* NaOH solution is added to 100 ml of a mixture of equal volumes of 0.04 *M* H_3PO_4, 0.04*N* CH_3COOH, and 0.04 *M* H_3BO_3

V	pH	V	pH	V	pH	V	pH
0	1.81	27.5	4.35	52.5	7.00	77.5	9.91
2.5	1.89	30.0	4.56	55.0	7.24	80.0	10.38
5.0	1.98	32.5	4.78	57.5	7.54	82.5	10.88
7.5	2.09	35.0	5.02	60.0	7.96	85.0	11.20
10.0	2.21	37.5	5.33	62.5	8.36	87.5	11.40
12.5	2.36	40.0	5.72	65.0	8.69	90.0	11.58
15.0	2.56	42.5	6.09	67.5	8.95	92.5	11.70
17.5	2.87	45.0	6.37	70.0	9.15	95.0	11.82
20.0	3.29	47.5	6.59	72.5	9.37	97.5	11.92
22.5	3.78	50.0	6.80	75.0	9.62	100.0	11.98
25.0	4.10						

VIII. VALUES OF t_α FOR DIFFERENT VALUES OF CONFIDENCE (α) AND DIFFERENT NUMBERS OF DETERMINATIONS (n)

α / $K=n-1$	0.5	0.7	0.9	0.95	0.99	0.999
1	1.00	1.96	6.31	12.71	63.66	636.62
2	0.82	1.34	2.92	4.30	9.92	31.60
3	0.76	1.25	2.35	3.18	5.84	12.94
4	0.74	1.19	2.13	2.78	4.60	8.61
5	0.73	1.16	2.01	2.57	4.03	6.86
6	0.72	1.13	1.94	2.45	3.71	5.60
7	0.71	1.12	1.89	2.36	3.50	5.40
8	0.71	1.11	1.86	2.31	3.35	5.04
9	0.70	1.10	1.83	2.26	3.25	4.78
10	0.70	1.09	1.81	2.23	3.17	4.59
20	0.69	1.06	1.72	2.09	2.84	3.85
30	0.68	0.05	1.70	2.04	2.75	3.65
60	0.68	1.05	1.67	2.00	2.66	3.46
120	0.68	1.04	1.66	1.98	2.62	3.37
∞	0.67	1.04	1.64	1.96	2.58	3.29

INDEX

TO THE READER

Mir Publishers welcome your comments on the content, translation and design of this book.

We would also be pleased to receive any proposals you care to make about our future publications.

Our address is:

Mir Publishers 2, Pervy Rizhsky Pereulok, Moscow, USSR.